Thieme

Self-Ligating Brackets in Orthodontics

Current Concepts and Techniques

Bjoern Ludwig, MD
University of Homburg/Saar
Private Practice, Traben-Trarbach
Germany

Dirk Bister, MD, DD
Consultant Orthodontist
Guy's and St. Thomas' Dental Hospital
London
Addenbrooke's Hospital
Cambridge
UK

Sebastian Baumgaertel, DMD, MSD, FRCD(C)
Clinical Associate Professor
Department of Orthodontics
School of Dental Medicine
Case Western Reserve University
Cleveland, Ohio
USA

With contributions by
Franziska Bock, Jens Bock, Bettina Glasl, Heiko Goldbecher, Thomas Lietz, Joerg A. Lisson

1470 illustrations

Thieme
Stuttgart · New York

Library of Congress Cataloging-in-Publication Data is available from the publisher.

This book is an authorized translation of the German edition published and copyrighted 2010 by Georg Thieme Verlag, Stuttgart. Title of the German edition: Selbstligierende Brackets: Konzepte und Behandlung.

Translator: Dirk Bister

Reviewer: Sebastian Baumgaertel

Important note: Medicine is an ever-changing science undergoing continual development. Research and clinical experience are continually expanding our knowledge, in particular our knowledge of proper treatment and drug therapy. Insofar as this book mentions any dosage or application, readers may rest assured that the authors, editors, and publishers have made every effort to ensure that such references are in accordance with **the state of knowledge at the time of production of the book.**

Nevertheless, this does not involve, imply, or express any guarantee or responsibility on the part of the publishers in respect to any dosage instructions and forms of applications stated in the book. **Every user is requested to examine carefully** the manufacturers' leaflets accompanying each drug and to check, if necessary in consultation with a physician or specialist, whether the dosage schedules mentioned therein or the contraindications stated by the manufacturers differ from the statements made in the present book. Such examination is particularly important with drugs that are either rarely used or have been newly released on the market. Every dosage schedule or every form of application used is entirely at the user's own risk and responsibility. The authors and publishers request every user to report to the publishers any discrepancies or inaccuracies noticed. If errors in this work are found after publication, errata will be posted at www.thieme.com on the product description page.

Rüdigerstrasse 14, 70469 Stuttgart, Germany
http://www.thieme.de
Thieme New York, 333 Seventh Avenue,
New York, NY 10001, USA
http://www.thieme.com

Cover design: Thieme Publishing Group
Typesetting by: Primustype Robert Hurler GmbH, Notzingen, Germany
Printed in Italy by L.E.G.O. S.p.A., Vicenza
ISBN 978-3-13-154701-9 1 2 3 4 5 6

List of Contributors

Franziska Bock, MD
Private Practice
Fulda
Germany

Jens Bock, MD
Private Practice
Fulda
Germany

Bettina Glasl, MD
University of Homburg/Saar
Private Practice
Traben-Trarbach
Germany

Heiko Goldbecher, MD
Private Practice
Halle
Germany

Thomas Lietz
Private Practice
Neulingen
Germany

Joerg A. Lisson, MD
Professor
Department of Orthodontics
University of Homburg/Saar
Germany

Bjoern Ludwig, MD
University of Homburg/Saar
Private Practice, Traben-Trarbach
Germany

Foreword

Since the early beginning of orthodontics, clinicians have progressively produced modifications and enhancements to improve force delivery of the appliances and clinician's efficiency. Major advances since the last century included the development by Dr. Angle of the Edgewise appliance, the introduction of enamel direct and indirect bonding techniques, the advent of the Preadjusted Straight Wire appliances and the development of fully customized Lingual Appliances (IBraces or Incognito). In the last 10 years, self-ligating appliances have captured the imagination of many clinicians and are increasing in popularity. Those brackets have been developed to overcome the limitations of stainless steel and elastomeric ligatures in terms of ergonomics, efficiency, plastic deformation, discoloration, plaque accumulation, and friction.

A self-ligating bracket is a ligature-less system with a mechanical device built in to close off the edgewise slot. Secure engagement may be produced by a built-in clip mechanism replacing the stainless steel or elastomeric ligature. Both active and passive self-ligating brackets have been manufactured, referring to the bracket/archwire interaction. The active type has a spring clip that presses against the archwire. In the passive type, the clip or rigid door does not actively press against the archwire. Active self-ligating appliances may allow better torque control with undersize archwires than can be achieved with passive appliances; a spring clip might also enhance the potential for bucco-lingual alignment. The resistance to sliding is thought to be lower for passive appliances, however, which may improve the aligning capability of these systems. Self-ligating systems outperform conventional brackets in the in-vitro situation, producing considerably less friction within the appliance systems, but this effect is less marked in-vivo. Clinical data documenting the efficiency of rotational correction and space closure with self-ligating systems remain limited. Use of self-ligating brackets results in a marginal reduction in chairtime required for appliance manipulation. Also, there is limited, retrospective evidence pointing to reduced overall treatment time with fewer scheduled appointments with the use of self-ligating systems.

While many clinicians recommend selected self-ligating appliances to facilitate expansion in non-extraction treatment, there are no published long-term follow-up studies on the stability of this approach.

Vittorio Cacciafesta, DDS, MSc, PhD
Milan, Italy

Foreword

Teeth don't know what is pushing them—they are made that way: aloof. For a tooth to move, significant biologic responses must take place within the periodontal tissues. As we know today, teeth cannot run faster than the remodeling rate of periodontal tissues.

It is empirically noted time and again that a single tooth can be moved with minimal ingenuity. The lightest, or the heaviest, of forces can elicit tooth movement in any imaginable direction. When a group of teeth are connected, however, the clinician's trouble starts. United teeth stand, whereas divided they fall. Despite this common knowledge, common observation, and common sense, it is common to place brackets on all teeth and stretch a piece of wire from one ear to the other. The wisdom of such mechanotherapy, obviously, is against the clinician's polemic to move teeth efficiently.

One must assume efficient tooth movement happens when teeth move fast and without much provocation. This line of logic leads to the argument that teeth must move independently without any influence from the adjacent teeth, yet stay within a group. But is it doable?

Teeth don't know what is pushing them, but they do know the laws of the universe such as gravity, electromagnetism, Newton's laws of motion, and the like. Because of such an upbringing, with these universal truths, teeth have good manners: they obey. They cannot accept any force unless the force is pitted against something else, any more than Abraham Lincoln could accept bribery. It stands to reason therefore, that friction must be created somewhere along or near the dental arch for a tooth to move freely. Interestingly, this phenomenon is termed anchorage in orthodontics.

If there must be anchorage, the slithering of brackets along an archwire is not possible without friction created at the adjacent bracket. It is stated above that a singular tooth moves effortlessly, but not a cluster of teeth attached to each other. So what does a tooth know that a bracket doesn't? Teeth know the periodontal apparatus is the decision maker, whether it is to slide or be stubbornly stationary. Inadvertently, the self-ligating bracket seems to take advantage of the biological determinants of periodontal response to force more than a stainless-steel ligature tightened around a bracket with the aid of Coon tying pliers. Ligatures *force* the movement, whereas movement is *allowed* with the self-ligating bracket.

The discussion is just as profound as the debate between the Platonic and Hippocratic schools of thought. Should the orthodontist induce tooth movement by using the biological response of the periodontal tissues or by forcing a full-size wire into the bracket slot, letting the bends in the wire in combination with the bracket slot express the kinetic potential, as both will work?

This book is dedicated to answering such queries.

Orhan C. Tuncay, DMD, FCPP
Professor and Chairman
Department of Orthodontics
Temple University Kornberg School of Dentistry
Philadelphia, USA

Preface

Self-ligating brackets—in recent years these words have taken on almost unbelievable magic powers. It is now almost impossible to envisage orthodontic treatment without such brackets. Keywords supporting this idea are: greater user comfort; better differentiation from competitors; more marketing possibilities, economical, shorter chair times, easy-to-use, patient comfort, perfect for your patients, and so on. The conclusion is: everything works easier and quicker. Sometimes the phrase "intelligent system" is used. Somewhat exaggerated, it seems as if the bracket at last can inform the tooth who is now in charge of moving from the false to the correct position. And the tooth? It follows the new brackets obediently, friction-free, and at a breathtaking pace.

By putting this rather ironic text at the front of a specialist book, the authors attempt to make it clear that they are attempting to replace suggestive remarks with facts and to be critical about advertising slogans. All the authors have been working with self-ligating brackets for a long time and will be presenting their investigations and experiences accordingly in this book.

Sometimes it may seem that self-ligating (SL) brackets are a recent invention. This is not the case. The first experiments with brackets that fixed the wire into the slot date back to the 1930s. The era of modern SL brackets began with Speed Brackets around 1980. For almost two further decades the SL brackets existed in the background. The growing number of systems and concepts from recent years is difficult to explain. The explosive growth in popularity became quite uncontrolled, and this book will try to clear the undergrowth as it were.

There have been many publications on this topic during recent years. A lot of experience has been gained regarding friction and treatment times as well as the requirements for clinical use and treatment possibilities. The aim of the authors is to summarize existing knowledge and to complement it with their own experiences and study results, in order to provide readers with an overview of SL brackets that is as comprehensive as can be. Following a chapter on the history of SL brackets, the first part of the book presents aspects dealing with material and techniques, including the evaluation of selected systems. The second part of the book is dedicated to clinical practice. Here also the authors have tried to demonstrate the complexity of the topic from the first to the final treatment steps. Statements are illustrated using numerous case studies. The conclusion drawn from this section could be: SL brackets are and will remain interesting tools, if they are properly used. They are just one of the many therapeutic choices in the hands of a doctor, and not a "magic pill."

This book is intended to be both a guide and a compendium, teaching beginners how to use this method, helping advanced users to detect sources of errors, and encouraging readers to go in a new, creative direction.

The authors thank everyone who played a part in completing the manuscript by giving advice and help, whether directly or indirectly, and those who motivated us to invest a great amount of work to reach our goal. Without this help the project would not have been realized so quickly. Our special thanks go to the Editorial Department of Thieme Publishers in Stuttgart for their excellent cooperation and the way in which they were able to turn our not always simple ideas into reality.

Bjoern Ludwig, MD
Dirk Bister, MD, DD
Sebastian Baumgaertel, DMD, MSD, FRCD(C)

Contents

I Basics

1 The Development and History of Fixed Appliances

Franziska Bock

2 Materials

Bjoern Ludwig and Bettina Glasl

3 Bracket Systems

Heiko Goldbecher

II Treatment

4 Diagnosis

Bjoern Ludwig and Bettina Glasl

5 Oral Hygiene

Heiko Goldbecher and Jens Bock

6 Bonding Techniques

Heiko Goldbecher and Jens Bock

7 Treatment

Bjoern Ludwig and Bettina Glasl

8 Auxiliary Equipment and Techniques

Bjoern Ludwig, Bettina Glasl, and Thomas Lietz

9 Retention and Stability

Bettina Glasl and Bjoern Ludwig

I Basics

The Development and History of Fixed Appliances

Franziska Bock

1

For many centuries, in many regions and cultures of the world, attempts have been made to correct malocclusions caused by malaligned teeth, skeletal discrepancies of the jaws, or a combination of the two. The Habsburg dynasty, for example—one of Europe's most powerful reigning families—shaped Europe politically, but there was one thing that, despite all their wealth and influence, they were powerless against: the male Habsburgs, regardless of whether they had been crowned or not, were unable to overcome their class III malocclusion. Throughout the history of dentistry, the profession was well aware of malocclusions and sought ways to treat them. Pierre Fauchard, for example, dedicated an entire chapter of his 1728 textbook—the first dental textbook ever written—to the correction of malocclusions.

Fauchard's text is the first description in the literature of the use of fixed appliances. The fixed appliance he described was quite simple by today's standards and consisted of gold bands and either silk ties or metal wires that were attached to a misaligned tooth and the neighboring teeth.[29] Many other authors have since described a large number of fixed appliances that used bands. Other appliances featuring very varied designs and adjuncts, such as wooden wedges, special ligatures, as well as "caps" or crowns, were also used to treat poorly aligned teeth.[22] Further refining treatment mechanics, some orthodontists also used developments that were originally described by engineers; Carabelli (1842) developed a number of appliances in this way. He is also known as the first orthodontist who fitted appliances not directly on the patient but used plaster models of fixed appliances, which allowed him to manufacture the fixed appliances in the laboratory.[22] Whilst most of the above-mentioned appliances were only suitable for treating specific malocclusions, Edward H. Angle was the first orthodontist to develop a 'standardized' fixed appliance. Angle not only established orthodontics as the first dental specialty, but also developed and categorized malocclusions, and his classification is still in use today. The appliances he developed were intended to be suitable for treating the types of malocclusion he identified. The expansion arch (E-arch, 1887) consisted of a band that was activated with a screw and an arch with a threaded end, which was fitted into a tube and tightened using a screw nut. The arch itself was then connected by ligatures to the individual teeth in order to align them.

NOTE

The ribbon arch developed by Angle in 1916 was the starting point for the development of bracket systems whicht are still in use today.

In 1910, Angle developed the 'pin-and-tube' appliance in which small pins were soldered to the arch and then inserted into vertical tubes. Further development of the appliance utilising bands with vertical slots, also known as the ribbon arch appliance (Angle 1916), allowed three-dimensional control of tooth movement. This was the first fixed appliance that used a rectangular slot in a bracket, which was then soldered to a band. The ribbon arch appliance marked the birth of modern orthodontics; all of today's fixed appliances are derived from it.[23] Subsequent improvements on the concept by Angle led to the invention of the 'Edgewise' appliance in 1928. This was another milestone, as a change in the archwire dimensions (turning the wire on its 'edge') allowed controlled expression of torque, tip, and rotation.[23,24] All later developments of fixed appliances copied these early developments in bracket design, eventually leading to contemporary fixed appliance designs in terms of slot shape, size, and position, the number of slots, the contour of the bracket and its base, as well as the mechanism for ligating the archwire to the bracket.[18] Advances in the manufacture of brackets were another (often underestimated) factor involved in further developments. With the invention of metal injection molding, it became possible to produce very complex bracket shapes of an extremely high level of precision and in large quantities, making it easy to incorporate precise values for torque, tip, and angulation in the bracket.[16] In addition, the manufacturing technique allows smaller and flatter bracket designs.

Development of Self-Ligating Bracket Systems

The technique today uses metal or elastomeric ligatures to attach an archwire to a bracket. Ligating the archwire to the bracket slot in this way can be quite time-consuming, particularly when metal ligatures are used, and this is why self-ligating brackets were first developed. The earliest examples (all developed in the United States) date back to the 1930s.

NOTE

The term "self-ligating bracket" (SL bracket) is used for brackets that incorporate a locking mechanism (such as a ring, spring, or door mechanism) that holds the archwire in the bracket slot.

There are essentially two main types of self-ligating bracket, depending on the design of the locking mechanism, the dimensions of the slot, and the dimensions of the archwires: active brackets and passive brackets. In passive systems (such as the Damon System, Ormco Corporation, Orange, California; and Discovery SL, Dentaurum Ltd., Ispringen, Germany), the slot is locked or shut with a rigid locking mechanism. Once it is engaged, the bracket is effectively turned into a tube, ideally allowing archwires to slide freely within the tube. In active systems (such as Quick, Forestadent Ltd., Pforzheim, Germany; and

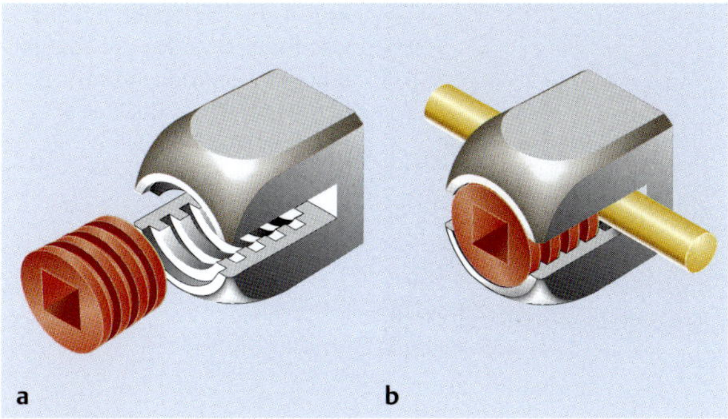

Fig. 1.1 a, b Russell attachment (1935)
a Open.
b Closed.

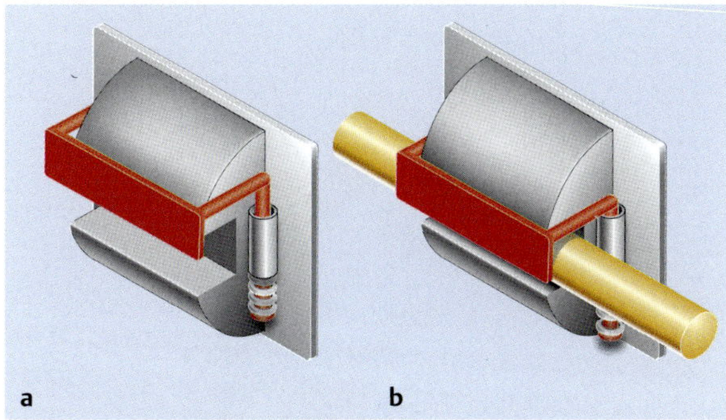

Fig. 1.2 a, b Boyd bracket (1933)
a Archwire slot open.
b Archwire slot closed.

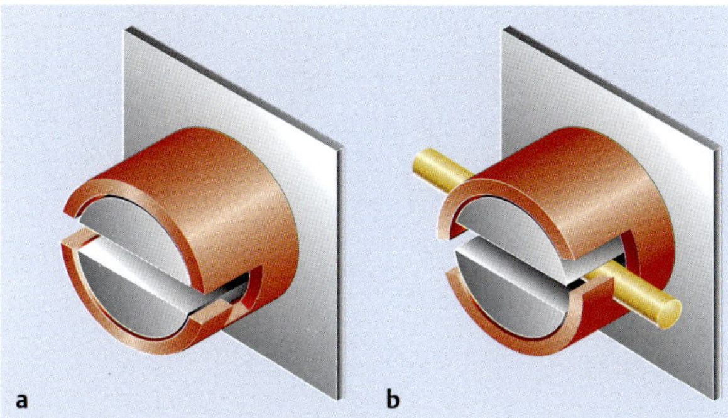

Fig. 1.3 a, b Ford bracket (1933)
a Slot open.
b Slot closed.

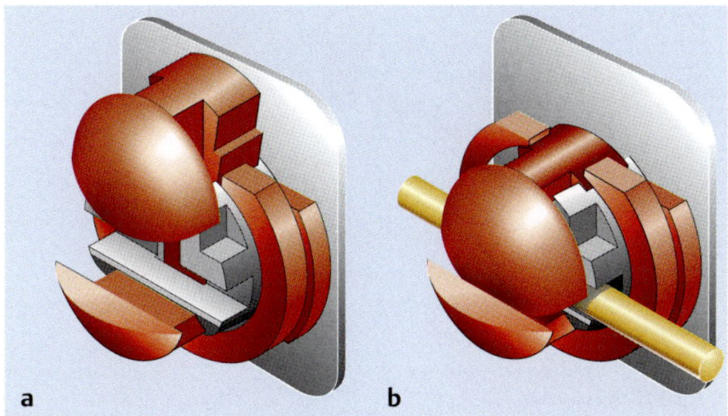

Fig. 1.4 a, b EdgeLok bracket (**a**). The bracket slot is closed with a sliding mechanism (**b**)

SPEED, Strite Industries, Cambridge, Ontario, Canada), the locking mechanism generally consists of a flexible but resilient clip that can actively engage wire into the bracket slot once the archwire reaches a certain size or deflection.[26]

Stolzenberg invented the Russell attachment in 1935 and is one of the pioneers of self-ligating brackets (**Fig. 1.1**).[5,12,25] Although Boyd (1933) (**Fig. 1.2**) and Ford (1933) (**Fig. 1.3**) developed passive, ligature-free systems earlier, these were never widely used.[10] Other designs were patented, but only very few of them eventually became commercially available.

It was not until the 1970s that interest in the development of self-ligating brackets resurfaced. In 1972, Wildman introduced the passive EdgeLok bracket,[10,12,30] which in its earlier incarnations had a round bracket body as well as a labial sliding door (**Figs. 1.4** and **1.5**). This was the first self-ligating bracket to become widely available commercially, but it was eventually taken out of production as more advanced systems appeared. At about the same time (1973), the Mobil-Lock bracket (**Fig. 1.6**) was introduced by Sander.[27] This was the first self-ligating twin bracket that had a variable slot. Due to the eccentric movement of the locking system, the wire could either be locked tightly into the bracket or, with proper adjustment, achieve partial ligation, which was designed to allow the wire to glide freely through the slot.[20] These were all passive systems, and none of them are still in use today, as they have been superseded by newer and improved designs.

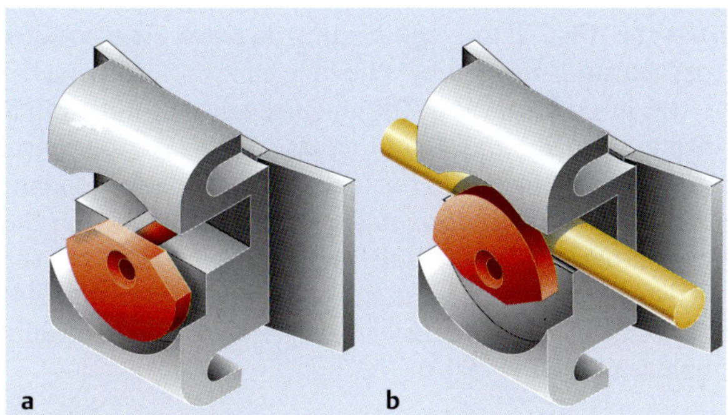

Fig. 1.5 a, b EdgeLok bracket
a Slot open.
b Slot closed.

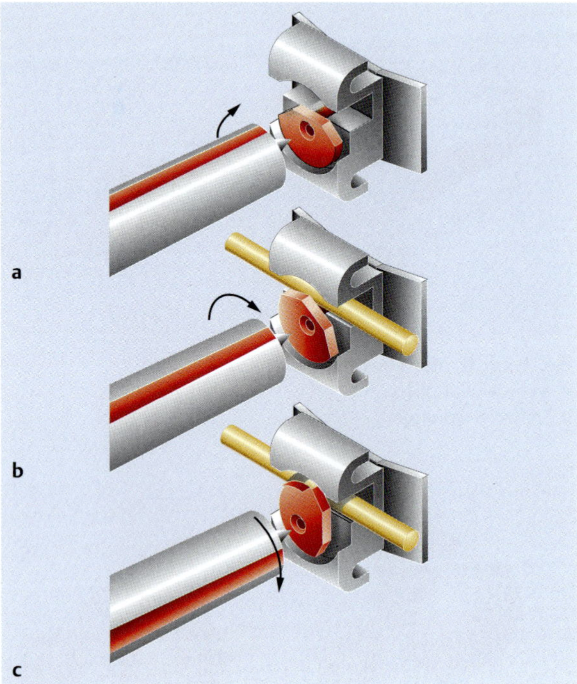

Fig. 1.6 a–c Mobil-Lock bracket
a Open.
b Closed—sliding.
c Closed—locked.

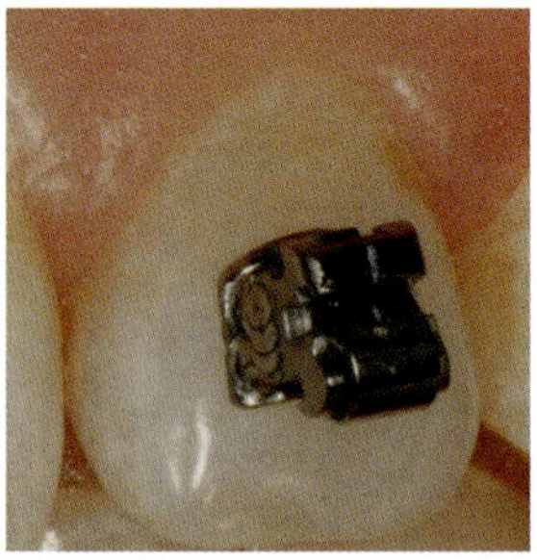

Fig. 1.7 The Speed bracket was the first active self-ligating bracket. (Reproduced with permission from Bock et al.[2])

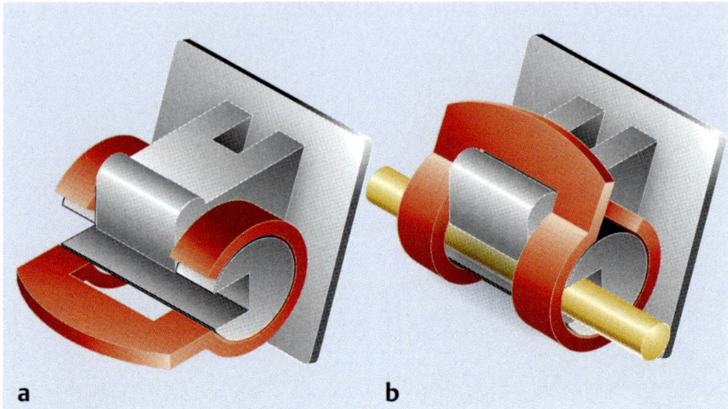

Fig. 1.8 a, b Activa bracket
a Slot open.
b Slot closed.

The 1980s

In the 1980s, Hanson developed a completely new approach to self-ligation: the SPEED bracket (**Fig. 1.7**). This was the first active self-ligating bracket. The locking mechanism is formed by a flexible clip.[5,9,12] This bracket is still in use today, but has undergone significant modifications during the past 20 years of clinical experience. As mentioned earlier in the text, changes in bracket manufacture techniques have had a significant impact on the bracket design. For example, the locking mechanism, the resilient spring had originally been made from stainless steel, but this has recently been replaced with nickel–titanium (NiTi).

NOTE

The SPEED bracket was quickly accepted in clinical practice and is still in use today.

Following the clinical acceptance and commercial success of the SPEED bracket, further self-ligating systems were developed in quick succession. Since the 1980s, a number of very different designs for self-ligating brackets have entered the market and Plechtner introduced the Activa bracket in 1986 (**Fig. 1.8**).[5,12] This passive system consisted of a mechanism that rotated around the body of the bracket and locked in an occlusogingival direction; this rotating "door" closes and opens the slot.[10]

The 1990s

In the 1990s, Heiser developed the Time bracket (**Fig. 1.9**), which is also an active system.[12] A hinging movement opens the locking mechanism in the direction of the gingiva. The Flair bracket (**Fig. 1.10**), which has been commercially available since 2005, is a further development of the Time bracket. It is significantly smaller than the Time bracket and has different in-out values and an improved locking mechanism.

Wildman also carried out further development of the EdgeLok bracket. Maintaining the concept of the vertical sliding door on the labial side, he introduced the TwinLock bracket in 1998 (**Fig. 1.11**). In this twin bracket, the flat, rectangular door sits between the two tie-wings.[12]

Another self-ligating bracket with a vertical mechanism was developed by Dwight Damon and first introduced in 1999 (**Fig. 1.12**). The Damon 2 bracket was developed later using a different locking mechanism.[5,12] Like the TwinLock bracket, it uses a rectangular sliding door mechanism between the wings of the bracket (**Fig. 1.13**). The Damon system was marketed very successfully in combination with a treatment philosophy that is mainly based on a nonextraction approach. Particular archwire sizes, shapes, dimensions, and materials are all part of the concept. To further develop and satisfy the demand for an esthetic self-ligating bracket, the Damon 3 bracket was introduced in 2004. The bracket consists of a tooth-colored acrylic base material (**Fig. 1.14**) but the locking mechanism remained.

A hybrid between a conventional twin bracket and a SPEED bracket, known as the In-Ovation bracket, was developed by Voudouris in 1997.[5,12,19] An improved design has been available since 2002, marketed as In-Ovation R (**Fig. 1.15**). An esthetic version of this system (In-Ovation C) was introduced in 2007 in the form of a ceramic bracket, in which the metal clip has been produced in such a way that it is matt in appearance and thus does not reflect light as much as a polished surface would (**Fig. 1.16**).

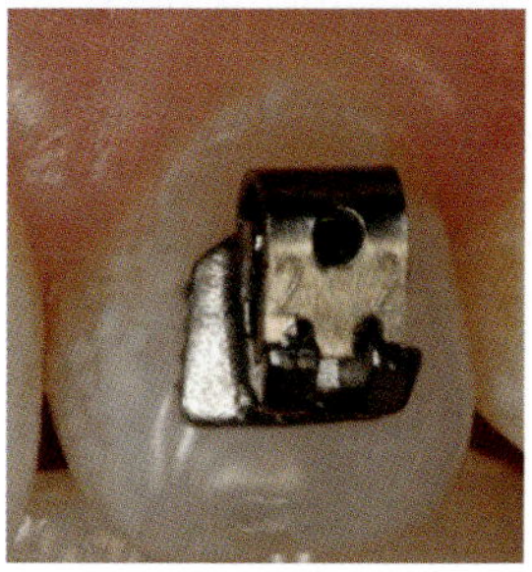

Fig. 1.9 The Time bracket. (Reproduced with permission from Bock et al.[2])

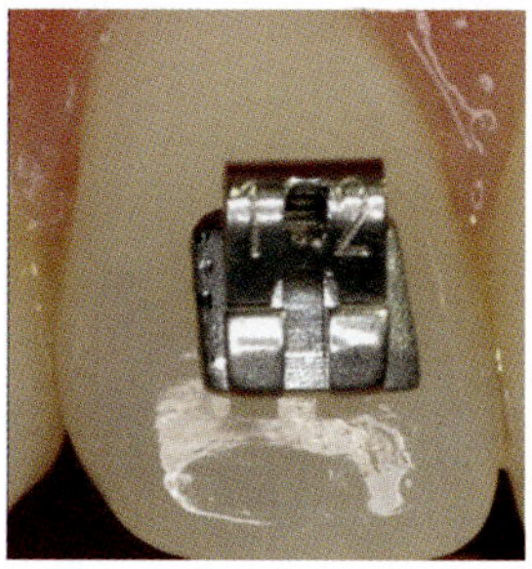

Fig. 1.10 The Flair bracket was a further development of the Time bracket.

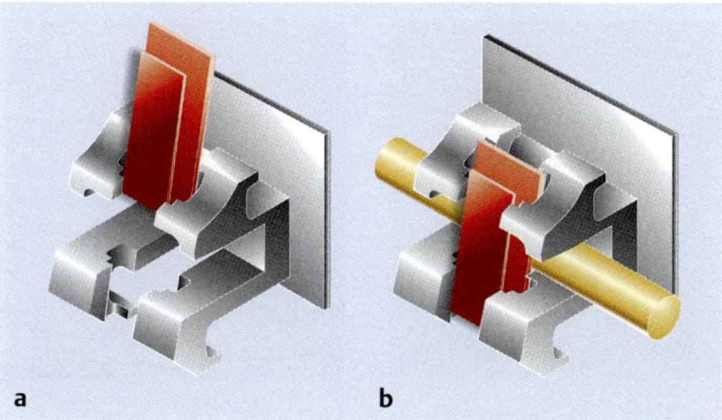

Fig. 1.11 a, b The TwinLock bracket is based on the same locking concept used in the EdgeLok bracket.
a Open.
b Closed.

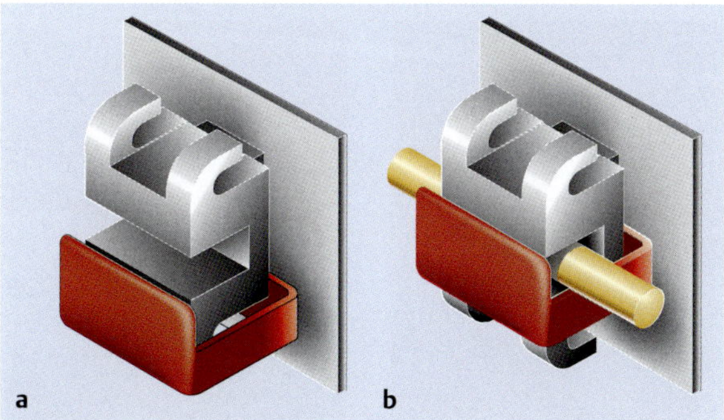

Fig. 1.12 a, b The first-generation Damon self-ligating bracket.
a Open.
b Closed.

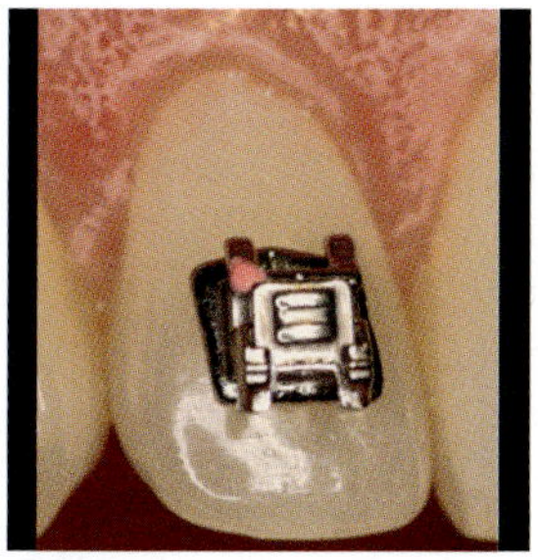

Fig. 1.13 The second-generation Damon bracket.

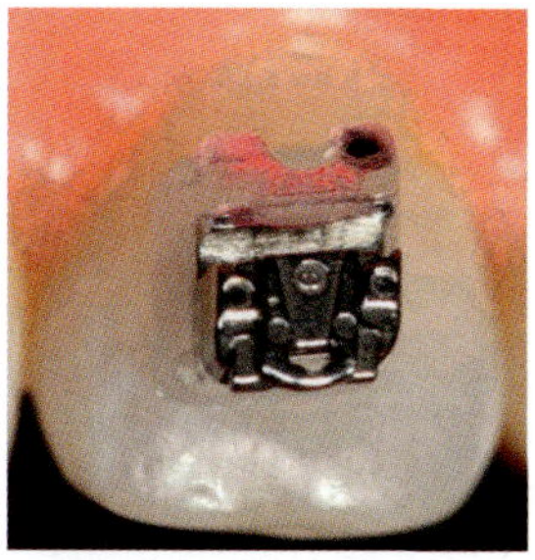

Fig. 1.14 The third-generation Damon bracket. (Reproduced with permission from Bock et al.[2])

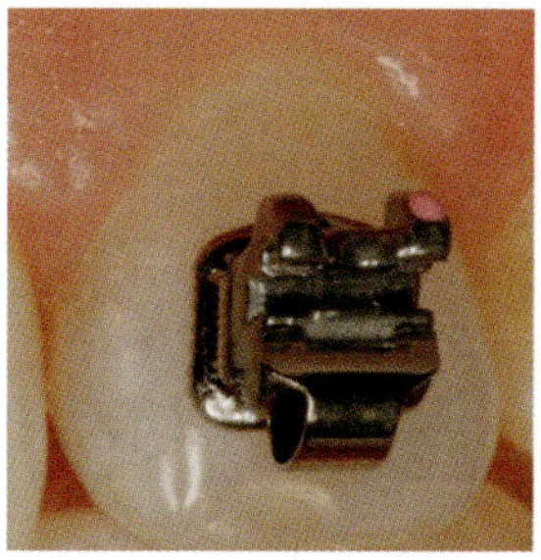

Fig. 1.15 The In-Ovation R bracket. (Reproduced with permission from Bock et al.[2])

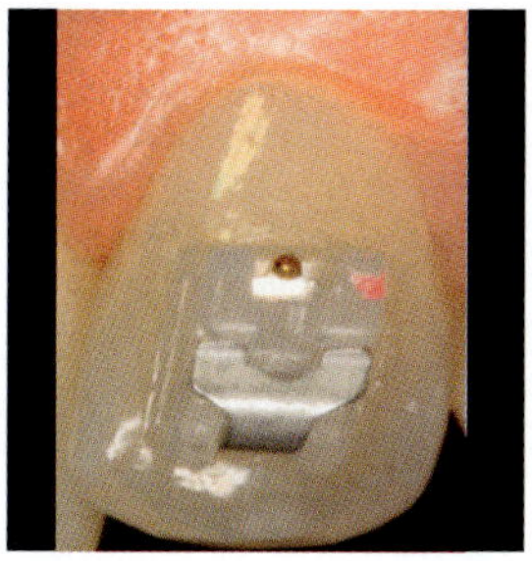

Fig. 1.16 The In-Ovation C bracket.

The 21st Century

The Opal bracket, marketed as the "most comfortable bracket in the world," was introduced by Abels in 2004 (**Fig. 1.17**). It was made completely of translucent acrylic. However, due to its mechanical properties with regard to force translation, abrasion resistance, the locking mechanism, as well as frequent discoloration it did not meet the high expectations raised for it.[2] All of the above characteristics were due to the use of acrylic as the bracket material. In 2007 a metal bracket based on the same principle, the Opal M (**Fig. 1.18**) was introduced but it has also disappeared from the market since.

The design of the passive SmartClip bracket (2004) (**Fig. 1.19**) is based on a completely different approach to ligature-free ligation. It does not have any movable locks or doors. The archwire is held in place with two NiTi clips that are mounted on the outside of the tie-wings. Ligation and removal of the archwires is achieved by elastic deformation of the clips. This bracket has also been available in an esthetic version (Clarity SL) since 2007 (**Fig. 1.20**). The body of the bracket is ceramic, but it has a stainless steel slot to reduce friction. It is also engineered with a predetermined fracture line point to facilitate debonding.

In 2005, another self-ligating active twin bracket, the Quick bracket, was introduced (**Fig. 1.21**). An esthetically improved version (QuicKlear) has been available since 2008 (**Fig. 1.22**).

The Vision LP bracket (**Fig. 1.23**), a relatively small metal twin bracket, was also introduced in 2005. The NiTi clip is opened with a rotational movement towards the gingiva. It has been available in Europe since 2007.

An alternative locking mechanism was introduced in 2008 in the Discovery SL bracket (**Fig. 1.24**). This is a passive metal bracket in which the locking mechanism is hinged open towards the gingiva. The bracket is very small and comparatively flat. It has been promoted as the smallest self-ligating bracket available today.

A number of other systems are also commercially available, but are beyond the scope of this book. More than 14 different types of self-ligating bracket were developed during the 70-year history of self-ligating brackets in 2003.[27]

NOTE

There have been numerous recent developments, demonstrating that there is growing interest in self-ligation: Self-ligating brackets are available today even for lingual orthodontics.

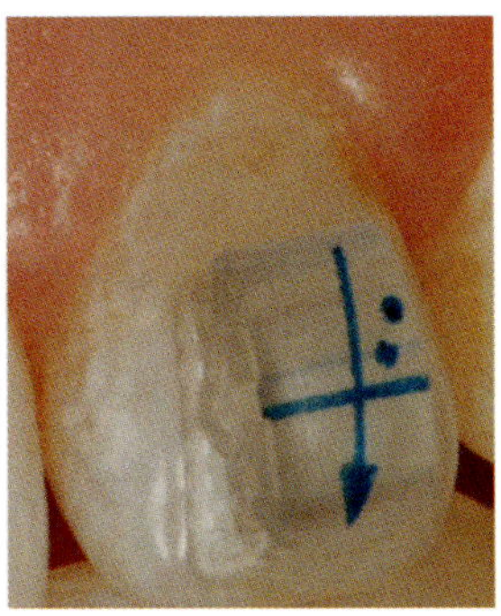

Fig. 1.17 The Opal bracket. (Reproduced with permission from Bock et al.[2])

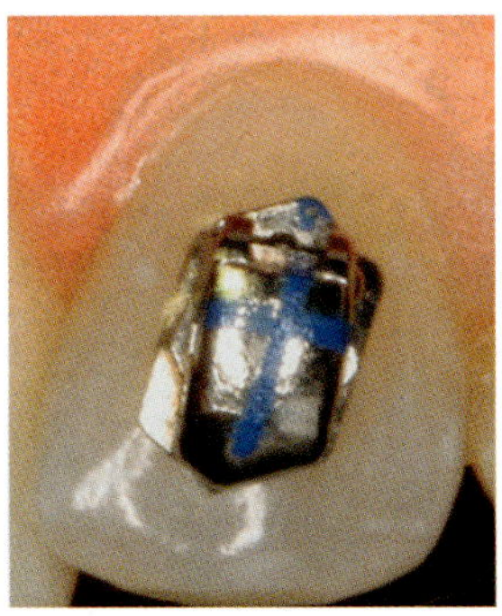

Fig. 1.18 The Opal M bracket.

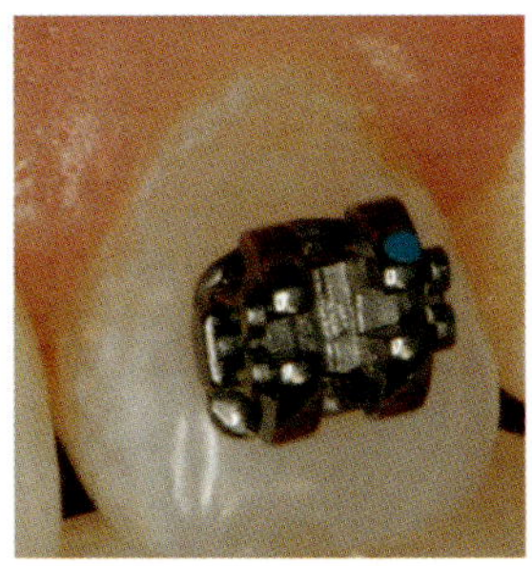

Fig. 1.19 The Smart clip bracket. (Reproduced with permission from Bock et al.[2])

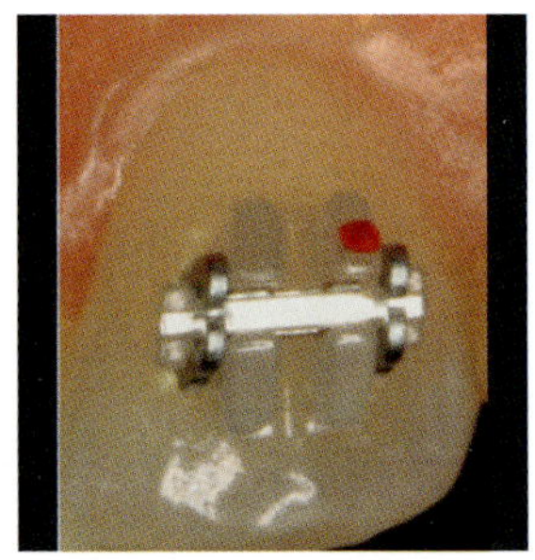

Fig. 1.20 The Clarity SL bracket.

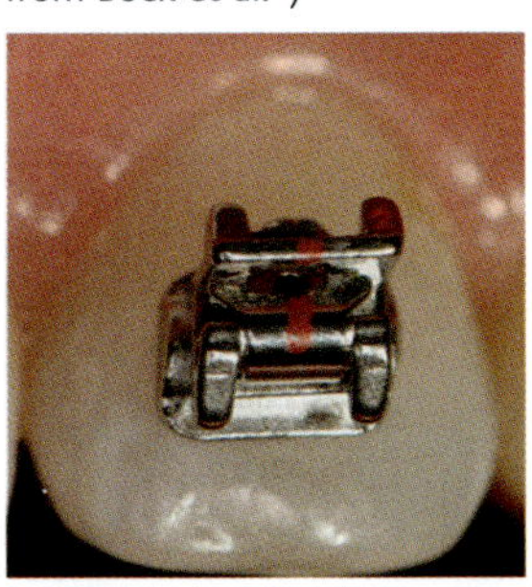

Fig. 1.21 The Quick bracket. (Reproduced with permission from Bock et al.[2])

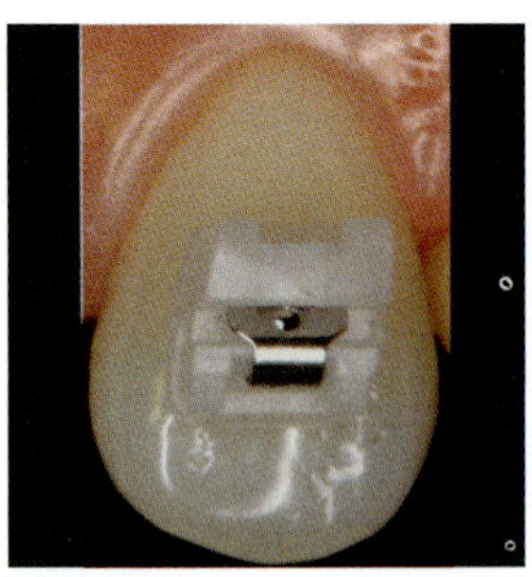

Fig. 1.22 The Quick C bracket.

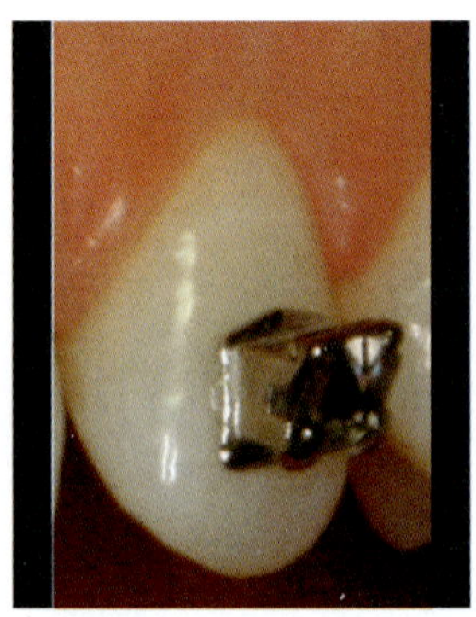

Fig. 1.23 The Vision LP bracket.

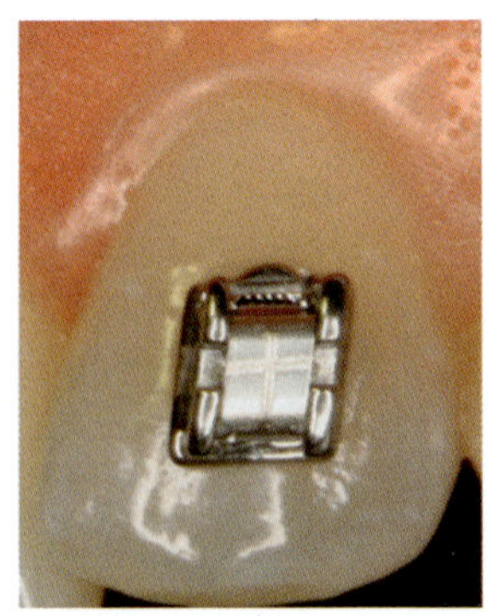

Fig. 1.24 The Discovery SL bracket.

Expectations and Reality

NOTE

The most important advantages that self-ligating brackets are expected to provide are:

1. Reduced friction
2. Shorter overall treatment time
3. Longer intervals between visits
4. Reduced chairside time[14,17,21,26]

More and more 'ligature-free' bracket systems have been introduced that claim to offer improved and more efficient treatment, particularly during leveling and alignment (**Table 1.1**). Another proposed advantage is the ability to reduce the forces acting on the teeth, which supposedly improve patient safety by reducing adverse effects such as root resorption resulting from high force levels. Other advantages claimed include reduced patient discomfort.[1] Previous in-vitro studies have shown that active systems are associated with slightly greater friction than passive ones. However, active self-ligating brackets are slightly better at dealing with rotation and torque.[7,26,27] Further details comparing active and passive self-ligation brackets are provided in Chapter 2. The effectiveness of distalization for class II treatment due to reduced friction is another advantage that has been claimed for self-ligating systems.[8,28] However, scientific proof that self-ligating brackets have improved friction characteristics in comparison with standard brackets is still lacking.[3,4] An investigation by Fuck et al.[7] showed on the contrary that conven-

Table 1.1 A selection of self-ligating brackets developed between 1935 and 2008

Year	Developer/company	Name	Ligation principle	Design
1935	Stolzenberg	Russell	Passive	Metal
1972	Wildman/Ormco	EdgeLok	Passive	Metal
1973	Sander/Forestadent	Mobil-Lock	Passive	Metal
1980	Hanson/Strite Industries	SPEED	Active	Metal
1986	Plechtner/A-Company	Activa	Passive	Metal
1994	Heiser/Adenta	Time	Active	Metal
1996	Damon/A-Company	Damon	Passive	Metal
1997	Voudouris/GAC	In-Ovation	Active	Metal
1998	Wildman/Ormco	TwinLock	Passive	Metal
1999	Damon/A-Company/Ormco	Damon 2	Passive	Metal
2002	Voudouris/GAC	In-Ovation R	Active	Metal
2004	Abels/Ultradent	Opal	Passive	Aesthetic
2004	3 M Unitek	SmartClip	Passive	Metal
2004	Damon/Ormco	Damon 3	Passive	Aesthetic
2005	Adenta	Flair	Active	Metal
2005	Forestadent	Quick	Active	Metal
2005	American Orthodontics	Vision LP	Passive	Metal
2007	Abels/Ultradent	Opal M	Passive	Metal
2007	GAC	In-Ovation C	Active	Aesthetic
2007	3 M Unitek	Clarity SL	Passive	Aesthetic
2008	Dentaurum	Discovery SL	Passive	Metal
2008	Forestadent	QuicKlear	Active	Aesthetic

tional twin brackets with "loose" steel ligatures are associated with the least friction in comparison to self-ligation. However, elastic elements and tight steel ligatures are routinely used for treatment with twin brackets, so that the friction characteristics of self-ligation can be expected to be beneficial for this type of treatment. Some clinical studies have shown that the overall treatment time is significantly shorter with self-ligating brackets.[6,11,15] The locking mechanisms of self-ligating brackets are not subject to biological degradation, as elastomeric ligatures are, and in this case intervals between routine checkups can sometimes be increased. Most self-ligating brackets are very small, and this should make cleaning easier and hence reduce the risk of demineralization. Avoiding elastomeric ligatures may also further reduce the risk of plaque retention.[21] Some authors have also claimed that patient comfort is improved, as there are fewer hooks and ligatures that irritate the lips or cheeks.

NOTE

Small self-ligating brackets and completely tooth-colored brackets are now also commercially available that may be able to satisfy patients' esthetic requirements.

It is difficult to provide a comprehensive and balanced overview of the advantages of self-ligation systems compared to conventional ligation, due to the complexity and sheer numbers of self-ligating systems that are on the market today (**Table 1.1**). It is also often difficult to scientifically verify the advantages that bracket manufacturers claim for their products. The following two chapters therefore focus on the science behind self-ligation and self-ligating brackets.

REFERENCES

1. Berger JL. The influence of the SPEED bracket's self-ligating design on force levels in tooth movement: a comparative in vitro study. Am J Orthod Dentofacial Orthop 1990;97(3):219–228
2. Bock F, Goldbecher H, Stolze A. Klinische Erfahrungen mit verschiedenen selbstligierenden Bracketsystemen. Kieferorthopädie 2007;21(3):157–167
3. Bourauel C, Höse N, Keilig L, et al. Friktionsverhalten und Nivellierungseffektivität selbstligierender Bracketsysteme. Kieferorthopädie 2007;21(3):169–179
4. Bourauel C, Husmann P, Höse N, Keilig L, Jäger A. Die Friktion bei der bogengeführten Zahnbewegung. Inf Orthod Kieferorthop 2007;39:18–26
5. Byloff FK. Das Speed-System – Eine Behandlungsphilosophie mit selbstligierenden Brackets. Inf Orthod Kieferorthop 2003;35:45–53
6. Eberting JJ, Straja SR, Tuncay OC. Treatment time, outcome, and patient satisfaction comparisons of Damon and conventional brackets. Clin Orthod Res 2001;4:228–234
7. Fuck LM, Wilmes B, Gürler G, Hönscheid R, Drescher D. Friktionsverhalten selbstligierender und konventioneller Bracketsysteme. Inf Orthod Kieferorthop 2007;39:6–17
8. Garino F, Garino GB. Distalization of maxillary molars using the speed system: a clinical and radiological evaluation. World J Orthod 2004;5(4):317–323
9. Hanson GH. The SPEED system: a report on the development of a new edgewise appliance. Am J Orthod 1980;78(3):243–265
10. Hanson GH, Berger JL. Commonly Asked Questions About Self-ligation and the Speed Appliance. Cambridge, Ontario: Strite Industries Ltd.; 2005
11. Harradine NW, Birnie DJ. The clinical use of Activa self-ligating brackets. Am J Orthod Dentofacial Orthop 1996;109(3):319–328
12. Harradine NWT. Self-ligating brackets and treatment efficiency. Clin Orthod Res 2001;4:220–227
13. Henao SP, Kusy RP. Evaluation of the frictional resistance of conventional and self-ligating bracket designs using standardized archwires and dental typodonts. Angle Orthod 2004;74(2):202–211
14. Kapur R, Sinha PK, Nanda RS. Frictional resistance of the Damon SL bracket. J Clin Orthod 1998;32(8):485–489
15. Maijer R, Smith DC. Time savings with self-ligating brackets. J Clin Orthod 1990;24(1):29–31
16. Matasa CG. Moderne Klebebrackets und die Probleme, die sie verursachen können. Inf Orthod Kieferorthop 1997;29:193–207
17. Pizzoni L, Ravnholt G, Melsen B. Frictional forces related to self-ligating brackets. Eur J Orthod 1998;20(3):283–291
18. Renfroe EW. Edgewise. Philadelphia: Lea & Febiger; 1975
19. Schoebel H, Thedens K. Das Damon-System. Darstellung der Technik in Verbindung mit einem Patientenbericht. Kieferorthopädie 2007;21(3):191–202
20. Sergl HG. Festsitzende Apparaturen in der Kieferorthopädie. Munich: Hanser Verlag; 1990:73–75
21. Shivapuja PK, Berger J. A comparative study of conventional ligation and self-ligation bracket systems. Am J Orthod Dentofacial Orthop 1994;106(5):472–480
22. Sonnenberg B, Göz G. Die Entwicklung der festsitzenden Apparatur. Teil 1 – Historischer Überblick 1728–1878. zm 2002;92(12):80–82
23. Sonnenberg B, Göz G. Die Entwicklung der festsitzenden Apparatur. Teil 2 – Historischer Überblick 1906–1980. zm 2002;92(13):84–86
24. Sonnenberg B, Göz G. Die Entwicklung der festsitzenden Apparatur. Teil 3 – Bracketentwicklung. zm 2002;92(14):82–84
25. Stolzenberg J. The Russell attachment and its improved advantages. Int J Orthod Dent Children 1935;9:837–840
26. Thorstenson GA, Kusy RP. Comparison of resistance to sliding between different self-ligating brackets with second-order angulation in the dry and saliva states. Am J Orthod Dentofacial Orthop 2002;121(5):472–482
27. Voudouris JC, Kuftinec MM, Bantleon H-P, et al. Selbstligierende Twin-Brackets (Teil I) – Ist weniger mehr? Inf Orthod Kieferorthop 2003;35:13–18
28. Voudouris JC, Kuftinec MM, Bantleon H-P, et al. Selbstligierende Twin-Brackets (Teil II) – Klinische Anwendung. Inf Orthod Kieferorthop 2003;35:19–26
29. Ward G. Fauchard's influence on orthodontic technics. J Am Dent Assoc 1964;69:695–696
30. Gottlieb EL, Wildman AJ, Hice TL, Lang HM, Lee IF, Strauch EC Jr. The Edgelok bracket. J Clin Orthod 1972;6(11):613–623, passim

Materials

Bjoern Ludwig and Bettina Glasl

2

Recent advances in fixed appliance treatment in orthodontics are based on a combination of applied knowledge and the use of materials relating to that knowledge. For self-ligation, the applied knowledge consists of the generally transferable skills involved in diagnosis and treatment. The hardware consists of brackets, archwires, and bands, which are used for treatment with conventional fixed appliances. All of the approaches used in self-ligation are identical to those used for general treatment with conventional fixed appliances.
Fixed appliance treatment is easier when straight-wire techniques are used, and auxiliary elements are often useful. The basic principles, however, are the same for self-ligation as in conventional orthodontics—for example, bracket placement is of paramount importance for good finishing. Inadvertent errors in bracket placement can be compensated for either by repositioning the brackets or by using first-, second-, or third-order bends. Self-ligation does not confer any advantages in this respect.

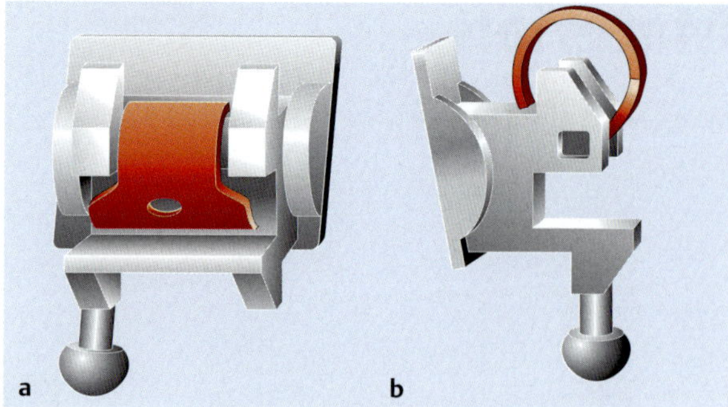

Fig. 2.1 a, b The general design of a self-ligating bracket.

Self-Ligating Brackets

Like ordinary fixed appliances, a self-ligating bracket consists of a bracket base and a body containing slots and tie-wings (**Fig. 2.1**). The difference between conventional and self-ligating brackets lies in the way in which the archwire is engaged in the slot. In self-ligation, the bracket itself contains a clip or other mechanism, which is used instead of either elastic or metal ligatures.
Just like conventional brackets, self-ligating brackets really only serve one function: they are the junction between the element generating the force (wire or auxiliary) and the tooth—so that they are simply a means to an end. The use of self-ligating brackets has given rise to a number of treatment philosophies, which are believed to offer significant advantages over ordinary ligation. However, it is important to remember that the tooth is not aware of how the force is being applied to it—whether it is by self-ligation or ordinary ligation.
A number of challenges that apply to traditional brackets also apply to self-ligating brackets: the fit of the bracket base to the tooth, the precision of the archwire slot, etc. There are few differences between self-ligation and ordinary ligation, as the method of production for the two systems is identical. Depending on how self-ligating brackets are manufactured, there may be a number of technical issues with the locking mechanism, which are described in greater detail in the section on "Rotation and Friction" below.
An ideal self-ligating bracket should have the following characteristics:

- Anatomically appropriate curvature of the bracket base including retention and undercut
- Marking of the vertical and horizontal axis
- An appropriately designed layout for good bracket positioning
- The bracket should be identifiable for each individual tooth (color coding or laser engraving)
- Hooks should be available for the application of elastics
- Precise slot dimensions (either 0.018 or 0.022)
- Robust self-ligating mechanism
- Twin tie-wings for engaging elastic chains or elastic modules
- Additional auxiliary slots

Bracket Base

The bracket base connects the bracket to the tooth and therefore must have retentive elements such as mesh, undercuts, or other retentive features which allow for good band strength. The adhesive enters the undercuts and allows mechanical retention, which should be resistant to everyday masticatory forces on the one hand, but should still be capable of being debonded without damaging the enamel surface on the other.

Shape of the Base

An ideal base should follow the curvature of the respective tooth surface for a good fit. This should enable the operator to place the bracket securely in the appropriate position on the tooth without rocking. A poorly fitting base can result in unprecise torque, angulation, and rotation once the full-sized wire is completely engaged. In order to produce an appropriately fitting bracket base, the manufacturer needs to pay attention to a number of factors.
The buccal surfaces of individual teeth show only very minor anatomical variations. An anatomically preformed bracket base is ideal and will fit well in the majority of cases. A precisely fitting base needs to take into account both the occlusal–gingival and also the mesiodistal curvature of the tooth surface. This is a challenge from the manufacturing point of view as a tooth surface is not built with a uniform curvature and a single radius like a circle, where a bracket can be positioned anywhere on the surface with equally good results. A tooth surface has many diverse radii and curvatures, depending on the location on the surface—and this applies to both the occlusal–gingival and mesiodistal directions (**Fig. 2.2**).

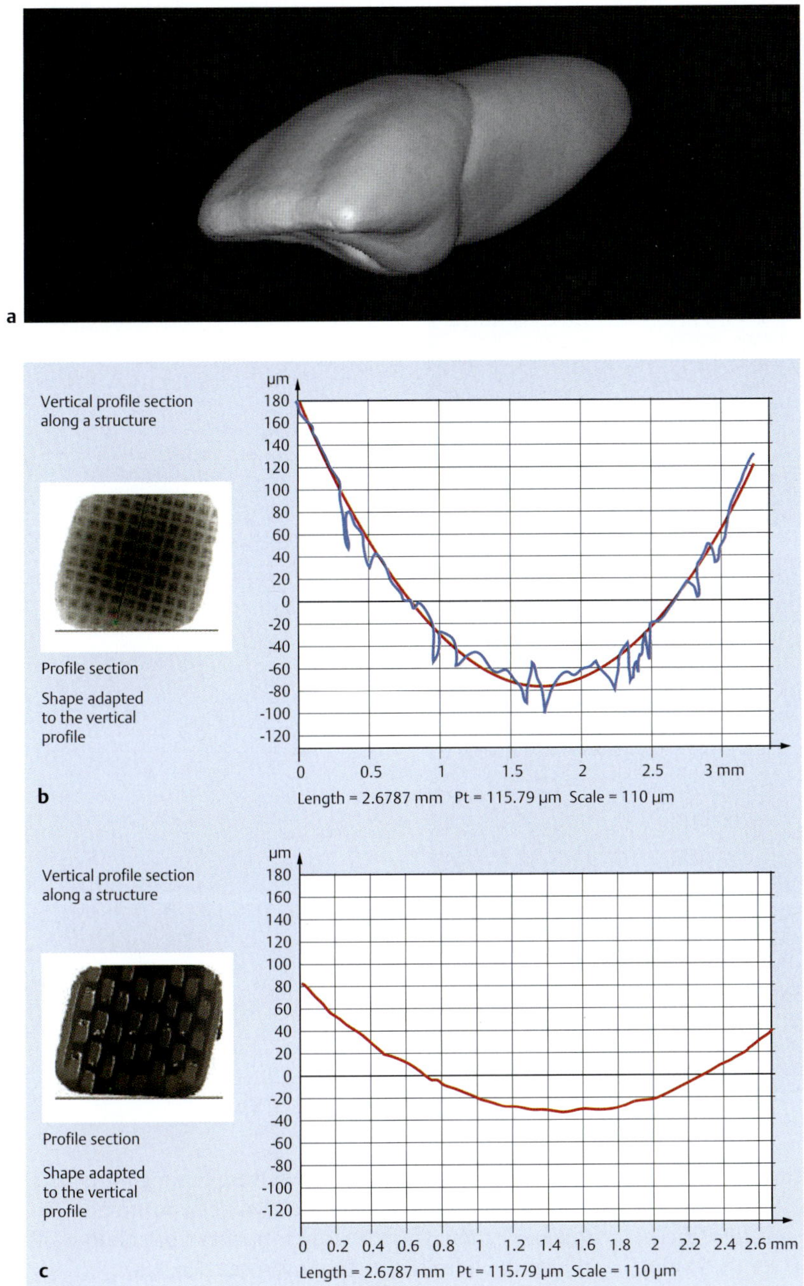

Fig. 2.2a–c This three-dimensional scan of an incisor shows that the buccal surface has multiple different radii instead of a uniform curvature (**a**). The surface curvature differs in both horizontal and vertical directions. In practical terms, this means that the radius of the incisor decreases from mesial to distal, whilst it increases in the occlusal–gingival direction. The three-dimensional scan of a bracket designed to fit on a central incisor (**b**) shows that its base is quite curved (vertical section). This incongruence leads to poor fitting on the tooth surface, which has to be compensated for with composite material. A different bracket base (**c**) shows improved bonding characteristics by adhering more closely to the results of the tooth-shape analysis. Comparison of the two bracket bases illustrates the differences between the curvatures of different brackets (**b, c**).

The importance of the congruence of the bracket base and the surface of the tooth has been known for a long time. Most manufacturers now offer brackets that have different surface characteristics with increased or decreased convergence. These convergences were originally determined by cross-sectional analysis of teeth that were cut in order to measure the curvature. It was therefore only possible to obtain a small number of convergences per analyzed tooth; due to the intense labor involved, the sample size per tooth type was usually small. Despite this, the results from the original studies are still often used in the manufacturing of bracket bases even today. Modern three-dimensional reconstructions of tooth surfaces are nowadays used in computer models and this method allows better correlation of the bracket base with the actual surface of the teeth, due to the increased number of teeth that can be analyzed and averaged (**Fig. 2.3**). Some manufacturers use this technique to design and construct their bracket bases and therefore claim to produce better-fitting bracket bases than others, but it is important for the bracket base to be manufactured in such a way that the data obtained can be used in a meaningful way. This is most likely to be possible with metal injection molding (MIM) or ceramic injection molding (CIM). Both of these techniques allow the individualized and fitted shape to be transferred when the bracket is

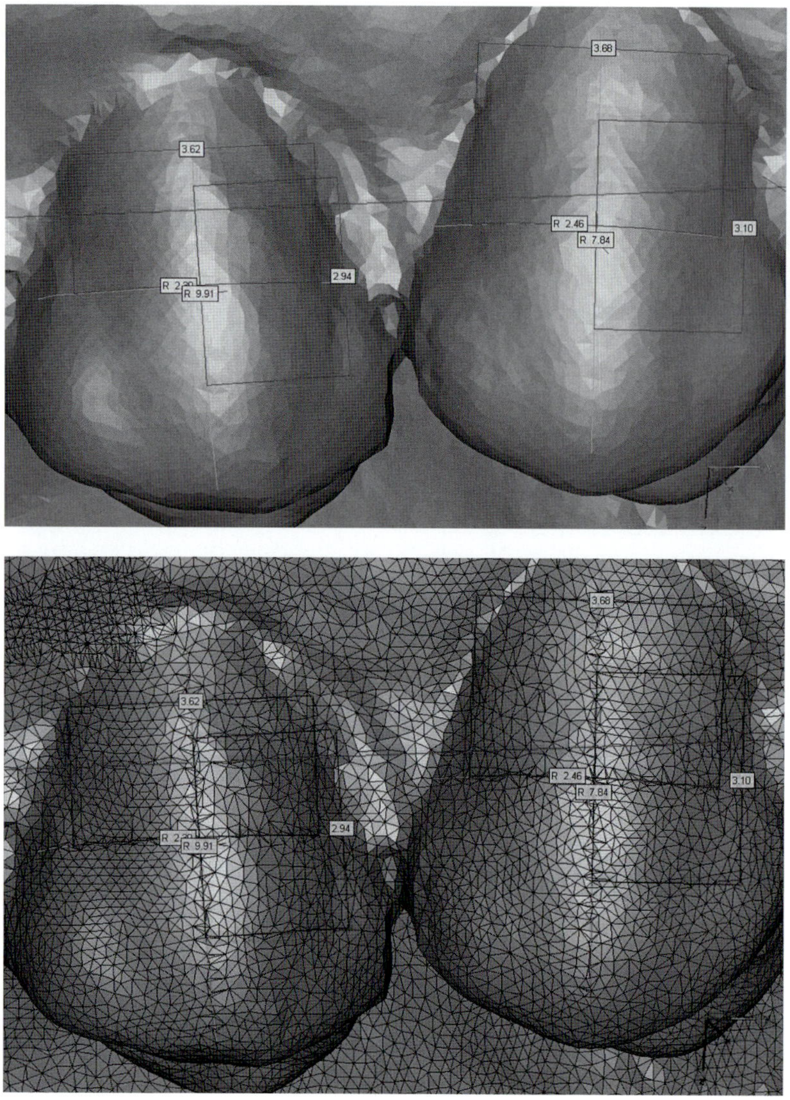

Fig. 2.3a, b Three-dimensional scanning makes it possible to collect morphological data for a large number of individual teeth and allows precise analysis of surface characteristics. Average values are calculated from this data and can help improve bracket base designs.

produced. A number of bracket manufacturers produce a bracket base from premanufactured plates, which are then bent into the desired shape. In a separate step, this bracket base is then connected to the bracket itself (see the section on “Bracket Body” below). It is not possible to produce the ideal surface characteristics that a bracket should have using these techniques. This is due to the very small size of the bracket base, resistance to deformation by the metal itself, and manufacturing issues with the application of forces to the small surfaces.

NOTE

Mismatches between the bracket surface and the tooth have to be compensated for by the adhesive, which may lead to poor bracket positioning and in turn result in incorrect tooth positioning.

Positioning errors can also result from canting the bracket or from migration of the bracket between positioning and polymerization. This may lead to poor slot orientation and in turn to undesired tooth movement (**Fig. 2.4**).

Bond Strength

The ideal orthodontic bracket adhesive should have two main properties: on the one hand, it should ensure a sufficient bond strength to be able to withstand the everyday stresses of mastication and manipulation. On the other hand, it should also allow easy removal of the bracket without damage to the enamel. As these two properties are diametrically opposed, orthodontic adhesives compromise by trying to deliver an adequate bond strength for most clinical situations—neither too strong nor too weak.

Most studies would agree that the minimum bond strength necessary for orthodontic treatment is in the

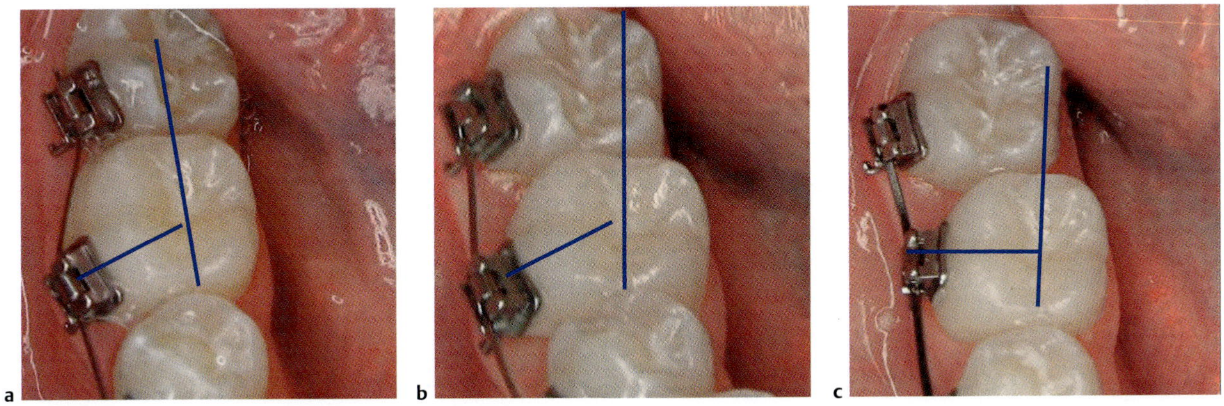

Fig. 2.4a–c The bracket on tooth 46 has been poorly positioned in the horizontal direction. After insertion of a rectangular wire, the poor positioning of the bracket is fully revealed. This can be treated by compensatory bending of the archwire or repositioning of the bracket on the tooth.

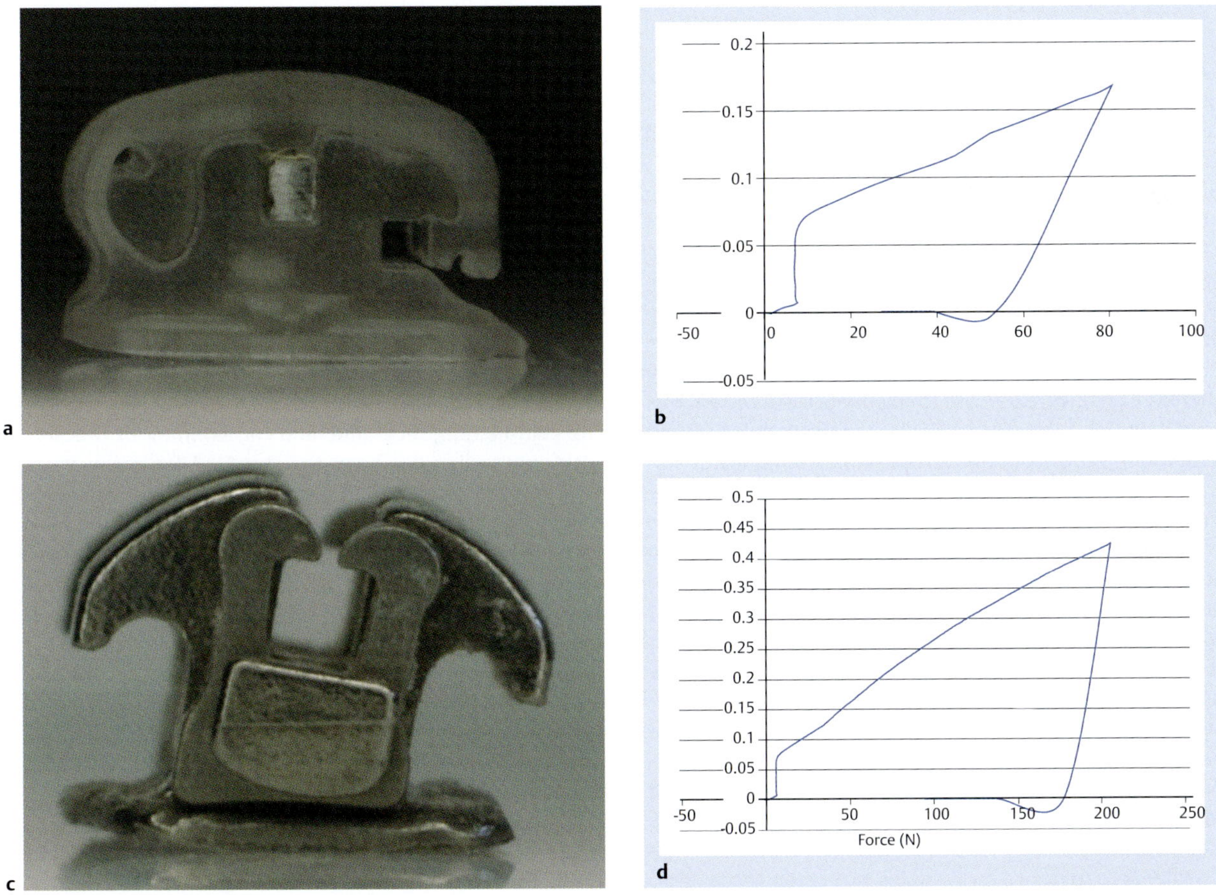

Fig. 2.5a–d Bond strength of an Opal and a SmartClip bracket undergoing the shear test in a universal testing machine (Zwick, Ulm).

a, b Bracket: Opal; manufacturer: Ultradent; adhesive system: Opal prime, Opal bond. The bracket base is 21.14 mm^2, the average shear bond strength is 4.2 MPa, and the majority of the adhesive stays on the tooth.

c, d Bracket: SmartClip; manufacturer: 3 M Unitek; adhesive system: transbond XT; bracket base:12.4 mm^2; average shear bond strength 10.19 MPa. The majority of the adhesive stays on the tooth.

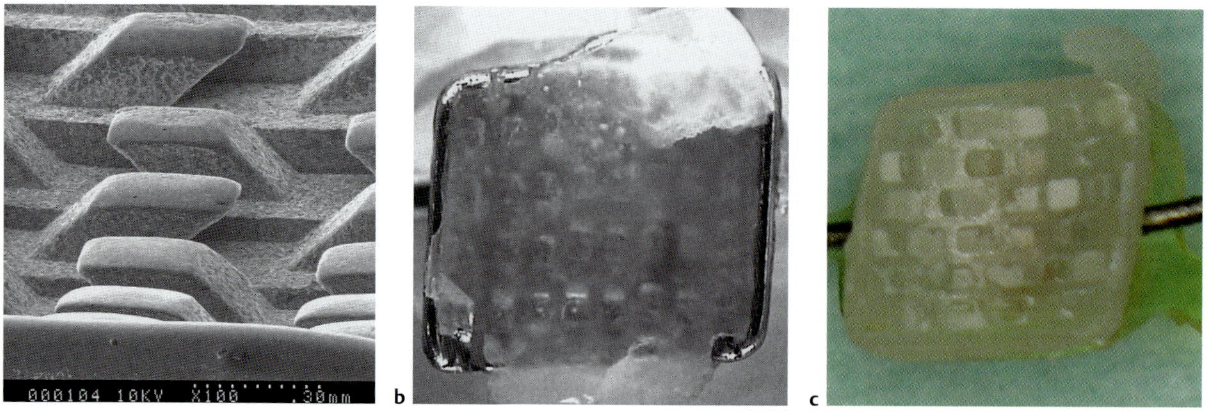

Fig. 2.6a–c The patented interlocking bracket base of a Quick SL bracket (**a, b**) compared to the base of a ceramic QuicKlear bracket (**c**). The undercuts of the metal bracket base lead to secure retention of the adhesive. On debonding, the vast majority of the composite material remains on the metal bracket base; only very little composite is left on the tooth surface; the opposite happens on a ceramic bracket.

range of 8–10 MPa.[8,15] More frequent bracket failures can be expected if the bond strength values are below this. At retention values above 20 MPa, there is a greater risk of enamel fracture on debonding.[12,15]

The Opal bracket (Ultradent) had a shear bond strength of only 4 MPa when the adhesive suggested by the manufacturer was used (**Fig. 2.5**). This was insufficient to withstand everyday stresses and strains.[4] Other brackets have a retention strength of more than 20 MPa, and these values are similar to those used in restorative dentistry. Brackets that produce retention values of that order may therefore pose a greater risk to the integrity of the enamel on debonding.[4] As a general rule, the weak point during debonding shifts from the bracket-adhesive (at lower values) to the adhesive–tooth interface.[1,3,15]

There is an extensive literature on the shear bond strength of brackets, but it is difficult to compare the different studies. Even in studies that use similar brackets and adhesives, the results are often not comparable, as there are too many variables that are not standardized—such as different teeth (bovine or human), the thickness of the adhesive, the direction and type of force application (torsion or shear force), and so forth. The German Institute for Standardization (DIN) recommends a standard methodology for testing the shear bond strength of adhesives for orthodontic attachments (DIN 13990), which could lead to the standardization of research findings if it was internationally accepted.

NOTE

The most important factors that affect the bond strength are the adhesive used, the chairside workflow, and the quality of the retention surface.

The bond between the bracket base and the adhesive can be obtained in a number of ways. For metal brackets, it is usually mesh, laser-etching, or other retentive elements that provide the undercuts necessary for mechanical retention. In addition, for ceramic brackets chemical retention is usually achieved through silane coupling. Generally, the bracket base should come with a retentive pattern that allows the adhesive to sit in the undercuts, creating a tight mechanical connection between the bracket base and the tooth. With metal injection molding, a number of bracket bases can be created in this way, some better than others (**Fig. 2.6**).

The acid-etching technique and the bonding of brackets with composites has been the standard for many years now. A more recent trend using self-etching primers improves workflow and time efficiency by up to 60%, as claimed by some manufacturers. Having fewer steps in the process means fewer potential mistakes during enamel conditioning, which should improve treatment outcome (**Fig. 2.7**). Self-conditioning primers contain acidic hydrophilic monomers, which etch the surface of the teeth and at the same time apply a very thin coating of unfilled composite (primer). A number of investigations have shown that although none of the currently available self-etching primers achieve the same depth of action as 35% phosphoric acid, comparable shear strengths result.[2,7,8,22] However, due to the reduced penetration depth, the fracture point on debonding is typically located at the enamel–adhesive interface, which means that less composite residue is left on the tooth surface.[3,15] The advantages of self-etching primers in orthodontics are the reduced surface erosion they cause during conditioning and the enamel proximity of the fracture point on debonding, and factors that make this primer attractive in the clinical setting.[1,2]

Bracket Body

The body of the bracket consists of the tie-wings and the bracket slot, but in the case of self-ligating brackets, it also houses the ligation mechanism. It is therefore challenging to keep the overall size of a self-ligating bracket small but strong enough to withstand everyday stresses without distorting. Depending on the manufacturer's preferences, bracket frames can either be produced in one piece or can be assembled from various parts using laser welding or soldering (**Fig. 2.8**). The latter technique—assembling bracket bodies from a number of components—can lead to spontaneous disassembly during treatment, and there is an increased tendency for corrosion to develop between the parts. There may also be a tendency for plaque to accumulate on the adjoining structures.

Self-ligating bracket bodies can be classified into either a tie-wing design or a block design. The former is the classic twin design, and with self-ligation it is accompanied by a locking mechanism. The four tie-wings allow additional modules such as elastic chains to be attached over the archwire if needed. Brackets in the block design group do not allow additional elements to be attached over the archwire, and the body is simply used as the retention mechanism for the self-ligating complex (**Fig. 2.9**). However, it is still possible with this design to use elastic thread or chain by placing it under the archwire, which in turn will hold the auxiliaries in place. The disadvantage of this approach is that attaching and removing the auxiliaries is relatively cumbersome, as it requires removal of the wire at each appointment.

Either colored markers or laser etching are commonly used to identify the bracket and proper positioning (**Fig. 2.10**). Color coding is easier and quicker to read than laser engraving, but the latter lasts longer and is more resistant to wear. These markings are also used with conventional brackets, but with most self-ligating brackets both the vertical axis and the horizontal bracket slot are covered by the self-ligating mechanism, making it sometimes difficult to identify the ideal bracket position. Some manufacturers counter this by adding additional horizontal and vertical markings on their brackets.

NOTE

Some self-ligating brackets (e.g., Discovery SL) do not have the bracket slot in the middle of the bracket, and it is very important to remember this during bracket placement.

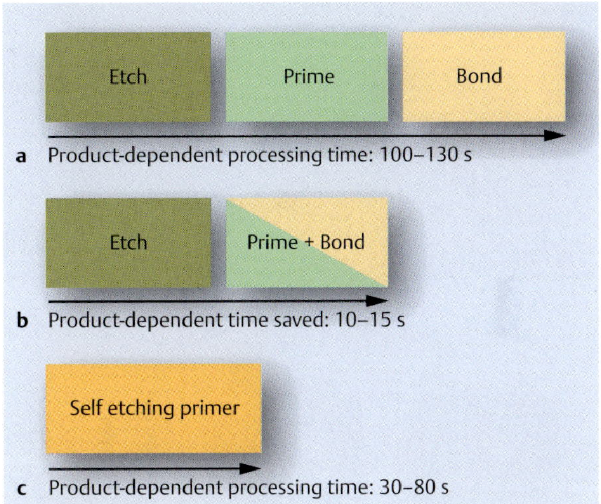

Fig. 2.7 a–c The workflow with a multiple-component adhesive in comparison with single-step applications of self-conditioning primers.
a Product-dependent processing time: 100–130 s.
b Product-dependent processing time: 115–120 s.
c Product-dependent processing time: 30–80 s.

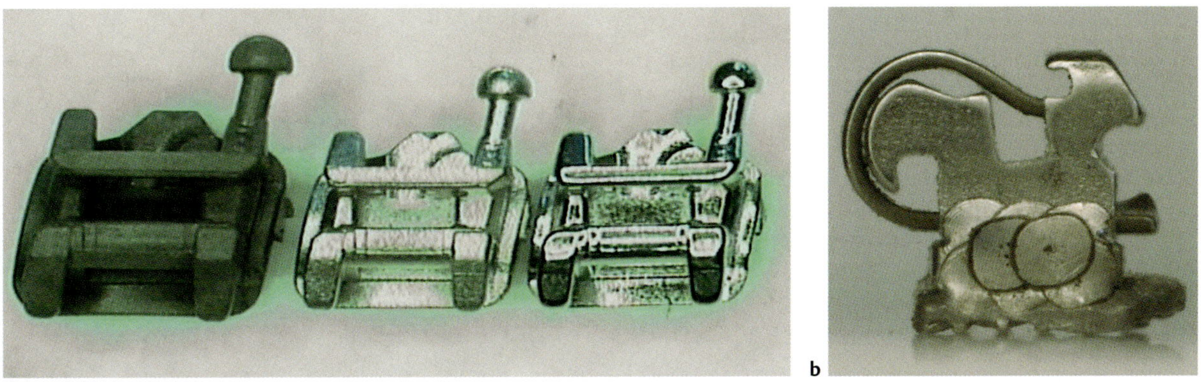

Fig. 2.8 a, b Manufacturing processes for brackets.
a A sintered bracket made in a single-step casting (Quick, Forestadent). This complex production method leads to optimized material properties. The deciding factor for good bracket quality is precise sintering of the bracket, which entails a process-related 20% reduction in volume.
b Multiple-component brackets with weld spots (SPEED, Strite Industries Ltd.). Separation of the base and the body during treatment is a possibility.

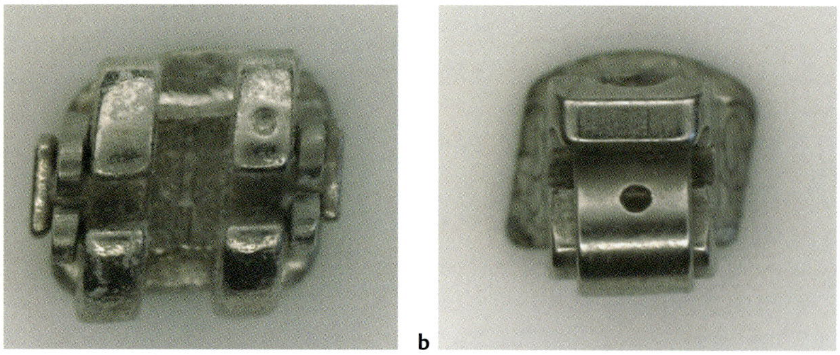

a b

Fig. 2.9a, b The bracket can be designed in a classic twin design with bracket wings like a conventional bracket (**a**, SmartClip, 3 M Unitek), or it can be designed as a compact block (**b**, Speed, Strite Ltd).

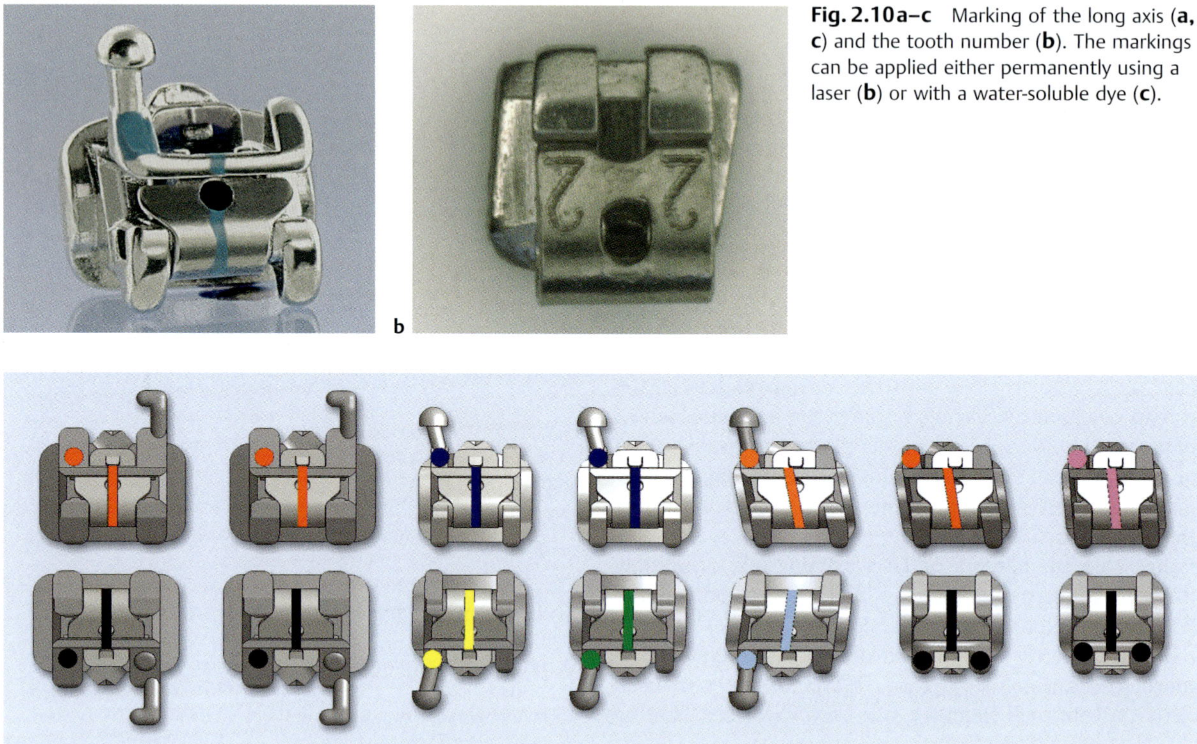

a b c

Fig. 2.10a–c Marking of the long axis (**a**, **c**) and the tooth number (**b**). The markings can be applied either permanently using a laser (**b**) or with a water-soluble dye (**c**).

Slot

As in conventional brackets, the bracket slot is of the utmost importance in a self-ligating bracket, especially with the straight-wire using a preadjusted appliance. By appropriately deflecting the archwire, the slot translates the three-dimensional information from the bracket prescription onto the tooth:

- First-order information: inset, outset, rotation
- Second-order information: angulation
- Third-order information: torque

APPLICATION

Checklist

1. Inset, outset (in/out)
   - The distance of the bracket slot from the surface of the tooth
   - Easily identifiable in an occlusal view
   - The shape of the arch at the occlusal level
2. Angulation
   - Horizontal inclination of the slot relative to a plane perpendicular to the vertical axis (anterior teeth, including carines)
   - The sagittal inclination of the slot relative to a plane perpendicular to the vertical plane (posterior teeth)
3. Torque
   - Inclination of the bracket base to the vertical slot plane (for torque-in-face brackets)

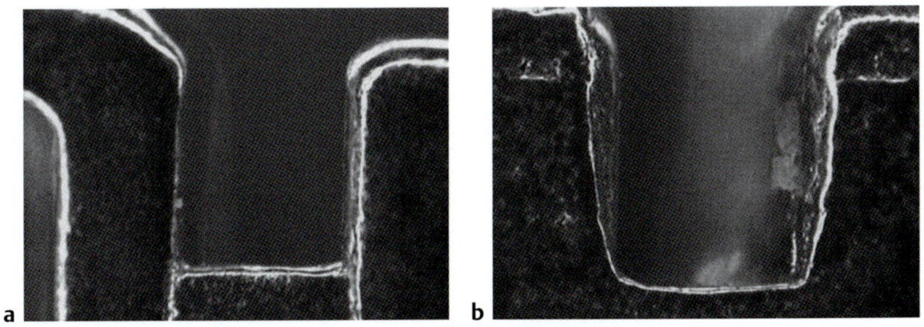

Fig. 2.11 a, b Differences in the quality of the slot, depending on the production method. The actual shape and size of the bracket slot have a major impact on the precision of the bracket and the forces that are translated from the archwire to the tooth.
a A high-quality bracket with well-defined edges.
b A poorly manufactured bracket slot with uneven surfaces and inconsistent dimensions.

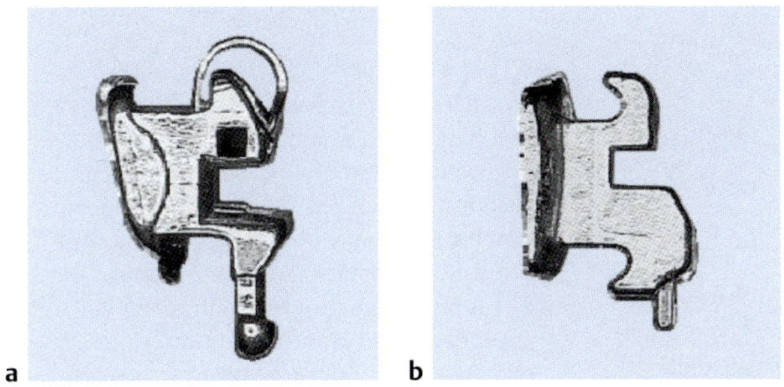

Fig. 2.12 a, b Slot design exemplified on the mesial and distal aspects of the bracket.
a Enlarged slot entry.
b Sharply angulated slot entry.

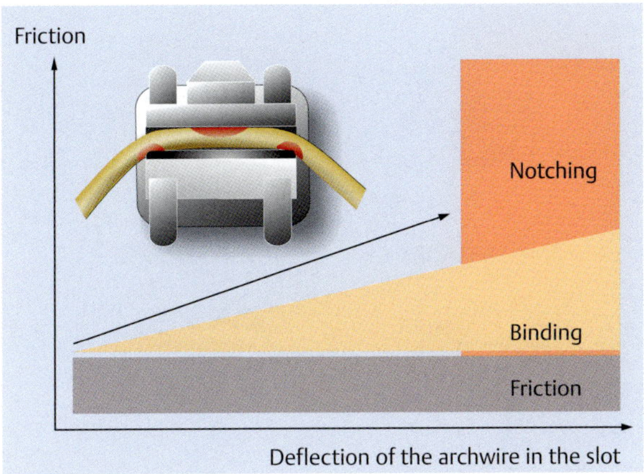

Fig. 2.13 The phenomenon of binding and notching. Even a straight archwire sliding through the bracket slot will undergo some friction. The friction increases if the wire is deflected (binding). Depending on the severity of the misalignment between the archwire and bracket, the archwire can be permanently deformed at the bracket corners (notching).

As in conventional brackets, the precision and inclination of the slot are important factors, as they determine how the force is translated onto the tooth and how the tooth will respond in terms of movement in the three spatial planes. The size of the slot depends on the technique used; it can be either 0.018 or 0.022 inches high and is always 0.028 inches deep. However, the manufacturing process is never absolutely precise, and variations from this nominal value do occur. In Germany, the permitted tolerance of bracket slots has been established by the German Institute for Standardization (DIN 13971-2). In countries that do not have a comparable standard, the degree of tolerance depends on the various manufacturers' quality standards. Additional slot properties such as surface quality, adherence to standard values, and the configuration of the slot openings are important parameters and can vary widely between manufacturers (**Fig. 2.11**). Overall, the quality of the slot depends mainly on the way the brackets are manufactured. The most precise method is milling, followed by the MIM technique. Brackets that are cast have the poorest dimensional consistency.
Small things can often make a great difference for clinicians, and an item that is frequently overlooked is the configuration of the slot openings (**Fig. 2.12**). To avoid notching and binding of archwires in the bracket slot during insertion, some manufacturers slightly round off the archwire slot on the mesial and distal aspects, creating a funneled opening that facilitates the insertion of full-sized archwires.

Friction

Friction (i.e., the resistance to free movement provided by the archwire in the bracket slot) should ideally be reduced during leveling and alignment, as well as during sliding mechanics. If the archwire wire is deformed substantially during the initial treatment phase, binding and notching may occur. In such cases, the wire typically assumes a point contact within the bracket slot at three sites—the corners of the slot on one side, and the slot surface on the other (**Fig. 2.13**). As the deflected wire tries to resume its original shape, it begins to bind in the slot, which increases friction. If a large amount of deflection takes place, the wire deformation can become permanent, especially at the sharp edges of the mesial and distal ends of the bracket slot, where the wire can literally become notched. At the extremes, the friction can become so great that tooth movement is all but halted. Binding and notching can be reduced using sophisticated slot design (**Figs. 2.14** and **2.15**). Rounding off the mesial and distal ends of the bracket slot increases the amount of contact between the archwire and the surface area of the bracket slot and thus reduces binding and eliminates the risk of notching the archwire.

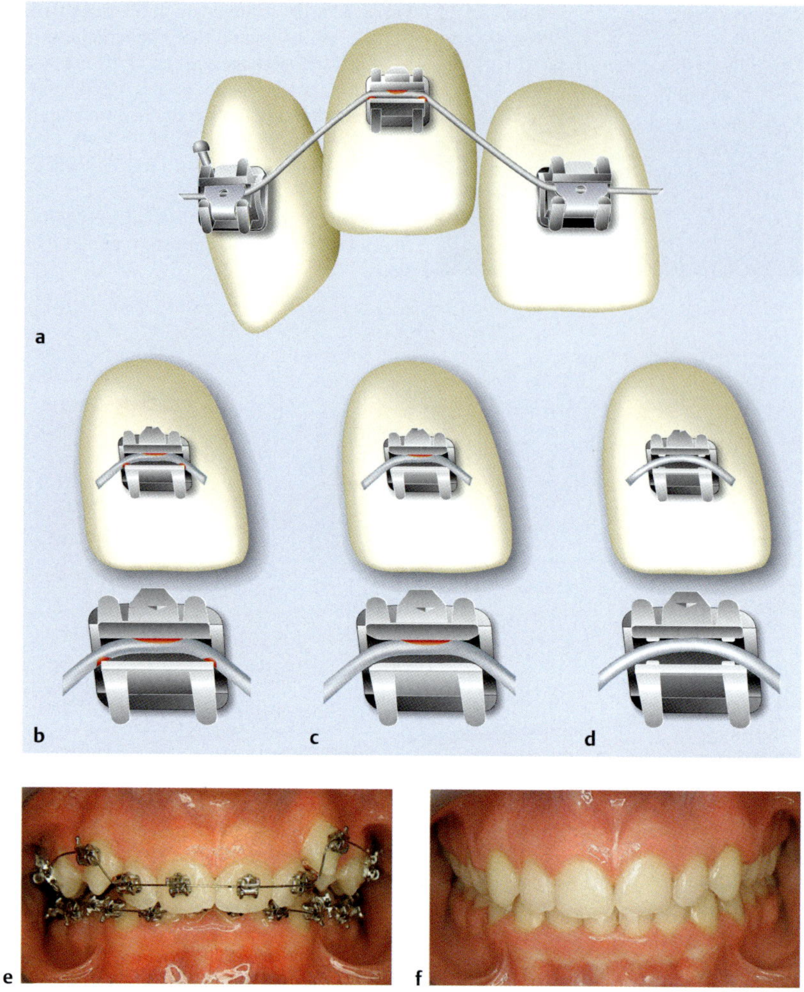

Fig. 2.14a–f Impact of the slot design on binding and notching, based on the amount of archwire deflection.
a Initial situation.
b Slot ends with sharp right angles (horizontal level): the ligated archwire will have contact with the bracket slot at three sites (binding). As the forces on the archwire exceed the elastic capabilities of the archwire, plastic deformation results (notching).
c Beveled slot entrance (horizontal level): due to the rounding of the bracket slot, pressure peaks and notching are averted. Friction, mainly from binding at the opposite wall, remains.
d Four-point contact at the slot entry (horizontal level). To reduce the effects of binding and notching, some brackets have four contact points incorporated into their design, such as the Quick SL bracket (Forestadent), which guide the wire through the slot and avoid direct contact with the slot boundaries.
e, f A typical treatment situation, with a significant need for leveling and aligning. Full engagement of all teeth, which is possible with modern superelastic archwires, will deflect the wire considerably, increasing the likelihood of binding and notching.

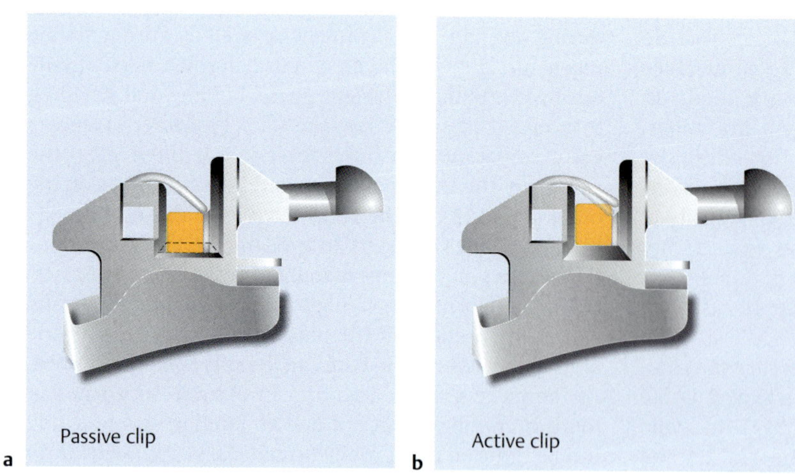

Fig. 2.15a, b Controlled torque application in extraction cases. To reduce friction and maintain torque control on the anterior segments, a bidimensional technique can be used. Using 0.018 slot brackets in the anterior segments, a 0.022 slot bracket in the posterior segment, and an 0.018 × 0.025 SS working wire, it is possible to close spaces with the wire, maintaining full torque control at the incisors and simultaneously allowing the wire to slide freely in the larger slot of the posterior segments. For self-ligation, the Time bracket (Adenta) is available with two slot dimensions. The Quick-SL bracket is available with a passive and active clip instead.

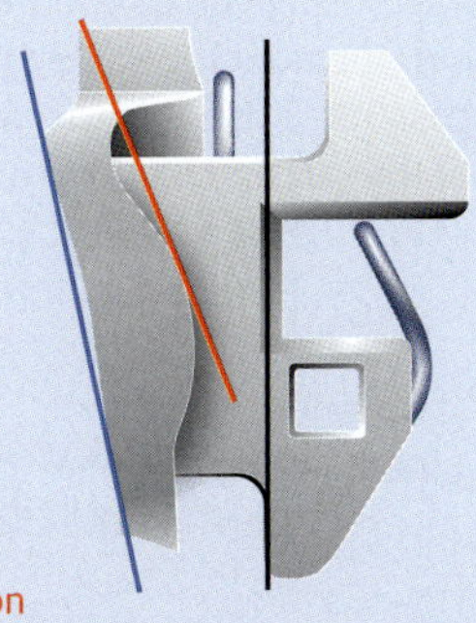

a MBT prescription

1|1	2|2	3|3	4|4	5|5	6|6	7|7
+17°	+10°	-7°	-7°	-7°	-9°	-9°
-6°	-6°	-11°	-17°	-22°	-26°	-10°
1|1	2|2	3|3	4|4	5|5	6|6	7|7

b Roth prescription

1|1	2|2	3|3	4|4	5|5	6|6	7|7
+12°	+8°	-2°	-7°	-7°	-14°	-14°
-1°	-6°	-10°	-17°	-22°	-30°	-30°
1|1	2|2	3|3	4|4	5|5	6|6	7|7

Fig. 2.16a, b Roth and McLaughlin, Bennett and Trevisi (MBT) bracket prescriptions. In the MBT system, the torque values for the upper incisors (11 and 21) are 17° (red line). The Roth value is 12° (blue line).

Torque

Tooth movement in the buccal–lingual direction, protrusion and retrusion, and also extrusion and intrusion of single teeth are all applications that require torque control. Full-sized archwires achieve the maximum torque expression. The main differences between bracket prescriptions lie in the torque values. Brackets using either Roth or MBT prescriptions are widely used (**Fig. 2.16**). Other bracket prescriptions have been introduced by a number of practitioners such as Andrews, Rickets, Hilgers, Burstone, Hasund, and Alexander. Full torque expression depends on a number of factors, some of which can be controlled by the operator and some of which cannot. When all of these variables are taken into account, it becomes questionable whether the different torque values in the various prescriptions are of real clinical importance, particularly when it is considered that torque loss is often due to variations in:

- Slot quality
- Archwire quality
- Dimensions of the surface of the tooth
- Bracket positioning

These issues may be more important than the bracket prescription itself. A number of manufacturers follow DIN standard 13971, which determines the tolerances of the slot and archwire dimensions.

Torque Loss (Slop)

DIN standard 13971 allows a slot tolerance of 0.04 mm; this means that the slot width can vary between 0.56 mm and 0.61 mm (equivalent to 0.022 inches and 0.024 inches, respectively). For rectangular archwires, a tolerance of 0.01 mm is acceptable. This means that even when acceptable standards are met, there is still a certain amount of play between the archwire and the slot—also known as "slop."
For example, 0.022 slot system archwires with a size of 0.016 × 0.022 will have no significant torque expression (**Table 2.1**). It is necessary to use archwires that completely fill the slot so that useful torque expression can be achieved (**Figs. 2.17** and **2.18**).

Table 2.1 Torque loss (slop) with different rectangular archwires. The table includes the maximum and minimum permissible slot dimensions and shows the theoretical slop of both traditional rectangular and modern hybrid archwires. Values greater than 45° reflect complete torque loss, which means that despite insertion of a rectangular wire, the tooth experiences no torque. Values around 22.5° thus reflect a 50% torque loss.

Slot	Archwire size								
0.61 mm (0.024 in)		0.016 × 0.016	0.016 × 0.022	0.016 × 0.025	0.017 × 0.025	0.018 × 0.022	0.018 × 0.025	0.019 × 0.025	0.021 × 0.025
	Hybrid		**48°**	33°	26°	24°	21°	16°	3°
	Rectangular	**63°**	18°	16°	12°	12°	10°	7°	1°
0.56 mm (0.022 in)									
	Hybrid			**45°**	35°	40°	30°	24°	11°
	Rectangular		25°	22°	17°	18°	15°	11°	5°

Archwire production also incorporates other tolerances not mentioned above. A number of commercially available rectangular archwires, for example, show that the edges are rounded to various degrees. The reason for this lies in the production of the wires. In most instances, the wires are 'rolled' into shape using the raw material which has a round cross-section. Introducing the edges is technically challenging and cost-intensive. This is why a number of commercially available archwires are 'rounded' and have ill-defined edges (**Figs. 2.19** and **2.20**).

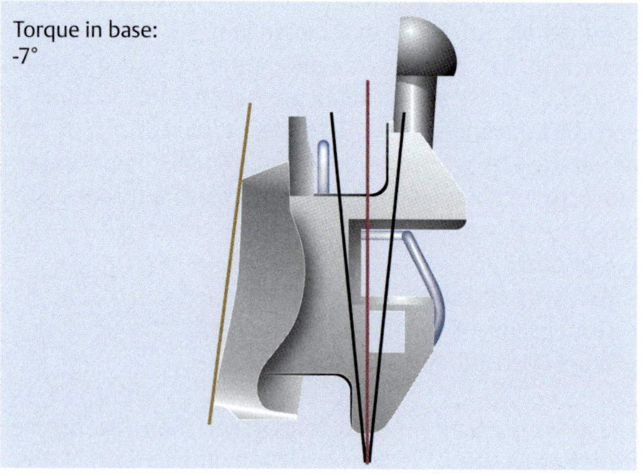

Fig. 2.17 Torque and slop in a 0.022 slot. For the maxillary premolars, the MBT and Roth values are identical at −7°. DIN standard 13971 allows a torque play of 12–17° when engaging a 0.017 × 0.025 archwire in a 0.022 slot system. This means a torque loss of approximately 33 %.

NOTE

The two criteria for assessing the quality of an archwire are its dimensional precision and the execution of the edges.

DIN 13971 does not allow precise definition of the edges (at exact right angles); this is to minimize the likelihood of injury. The minimum radius permitted by the standard is 0.03 mm.

However, expressing torque becomes increasingly difficult with increased rounding of the archwire edges. This may be more important for some self-ligating brackets than for others. The SmartClip (3 M Unitek), for example, relies on wires with rounded edges, known as hybrid wires, for larger wire sizes for ligation purposes. Without rounded edges, it would be very difficult to engage larger rectangular wires into the bilateral clips. Poor torque ex-

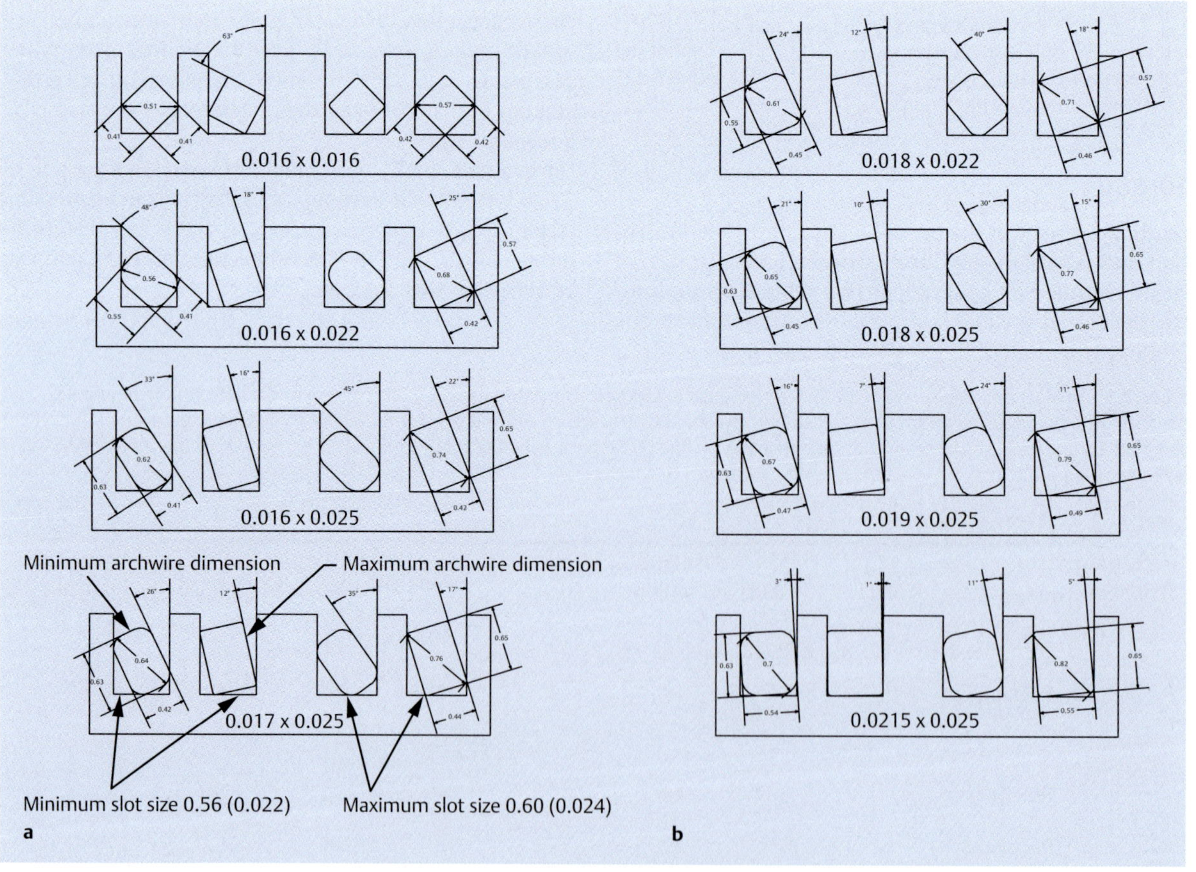

Fig. 2.18a, b Torque loss relative to archwire dimensions 0.016 × 0.016 to 0.021 × 0.025 in a 0.022 slot. Only a rectangular wire that fills the slot can express maximum torque; a rectangular wire of 0.021 × 0.025 has 1° of freedom.

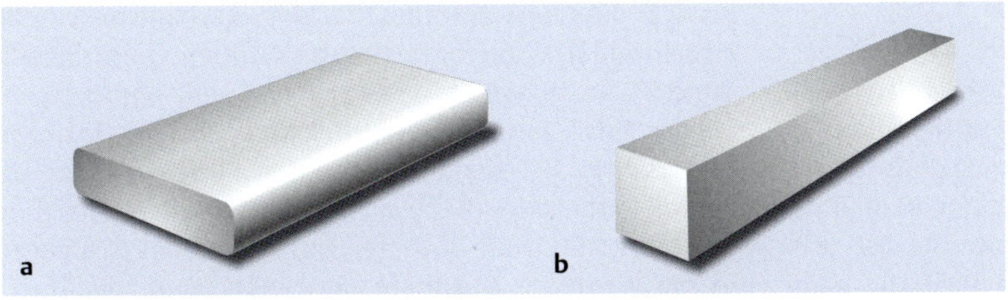

Fig. 2.19a, b The degree of rounding of the archwire edges varies tremendously between manufacturers.

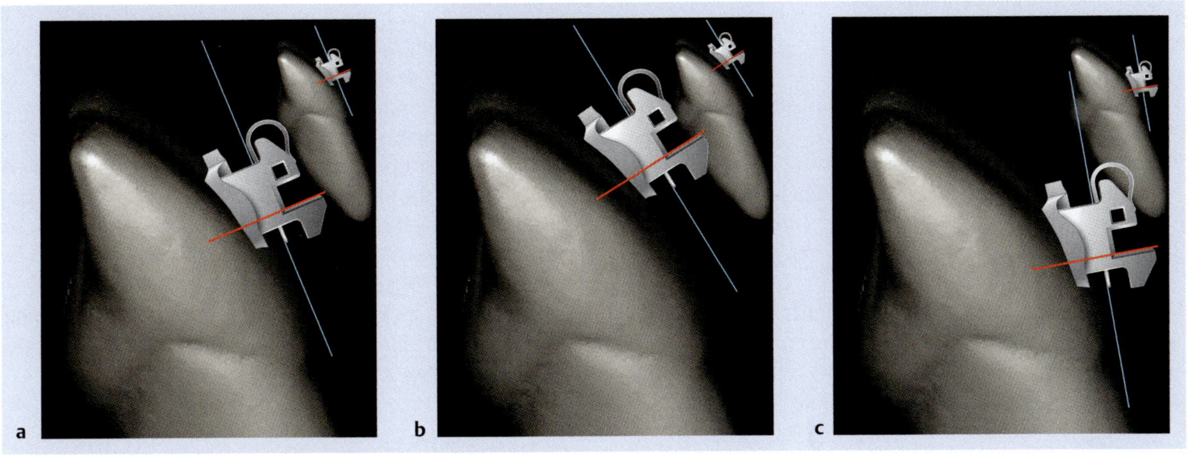

Fig. 2.20a–c The effect of bracket positioning on slot orientation. The orthodontic literature usually gives values of 4.5 mm (± 0.5 mm) distance between the slot and the incisal edge. If the bracket position is altered by ± 1 mm, for example, the resulting slot orientation will be considerably different. This will have a substantial impact on the torque values expressed.

a Centered position.
b The bracket is moved 1 mm incisally.
c The bracket is moved 1 mm gingivally.

pansion may therefore be due to wire engineering and the associated issues of transferring torque onto the teeth.

Torque Errors Due to Erroneous Bracket Positioning

There is significant controversy in the literature regarding the ideal position of a bracket on a tooth. A number of authors use a fixed distance from the incisal edge to determine the ideal place for bracket positioning. Other authors recommend what is known as selective bracket placement, which means that the bracket positioning will be modified based on the existing malocclusion. The aim is that selective placement of the brackets in the occlusal or gingival direction can be used to improve the biomechanics and help with bite opening or bite closure during the leveling phase. As mentioned above, teeth do not have a universally uniform surface curvature. This, in combination with selective bracket positioning, can lead to significant variation of torque expression from the intended prescription (**Fig. 2.20**).

Torque Errors Due to the Variation of Tooth Morphology

The morphology of the tooth surface plays an important part in bracket positioning. The more a tooth is rounded and the less the congruence there is between the bracket base and the tooth, the more frequently problems can occur regarding the consistency of bracket placement. When there is a significant difference between the curvature of the bracket base and the tooth, rocking of the bracket on the tooth may occur. These inconsistencies will need to be compensated for by the adhesive, but this means that the bracket may not be positioned in its intendend position, which in turn can have a significant effect on torque expression (**Fig. 2.20**).

Auxiliary Slots

Some brackets have additional slots to the main archwire slot, known as auxiliary slots (**Fig. 2.21**). For these slots to be useful, they should be of minimum dimensions such as 0.016 × 0.016 (Quick SL, SPEED, and In-Ovation R) or 0.018 × 0.018 (Opal). The additional slots allow the use of a second force system, which can be useful if the main slot is already engaged (**Fig. 2.22**). An additional slot is particularly useful for:

- Derotation of severely rotated teeth; a very thin flexible wire can be used for this
- Alignment of ectopic or severely displaced teeth using “piggyback” archwires
- Avoidance of reactive forces during segmental techniques when using auxiliary springs (anchorage)

Clips, etc.—SL Mechanics

With normal ligation techniques, either elastomeric or metal ligatures engage the archwire in the bracket slot. In self-ligation, this is achieved by the locking mechanism. A number of variations are available. Some slide in a vertical direction, and these locking mechanisms can be either rigid (Damon) or flexible (In-Ovation, Quick, SPEED, Time 2), i.e. active or passive. A different approach involves “lids,” as used in the Discovery SL and Opal systems. Other self-ligating methods use clips that are attached to the sides of the twin bracket, such as SmartClip and Clarity SL. None of these ligation methods is superior in every respect, and there are a number of advantages and disadvantages that relate to functionality and the individual clinical situation (see Chapters 3 and 8). It is generally rather difficult to allocate their advantages and disadvantages to individual systems, as a number of the perceived beneficial characteristics depend on the operator’s preferences rather than on a scientific evaluation of the system’s properties. However, it is important to remember that for all self-ligation systems, it is the locking mechanism itself that is the sensitive part of the bracket and that there is a learning curve associated with the successful use of self-ligation.

The philosophies and design used in the locking mechanism divide the systems into two main categories—active and passive (**Fig. 2.23**).

Active Systems

The active clip is manufactured either from cobalt-chrome or nickel–titanium. It can force the archwire into the bracket slot in a spring-like fashion, which already occurs with fully active clips at relatively small wire sizes. Some manufacturers market their clips as semiactive or interactive (**Fig. 2.24**). In these cases, the clip becomes active only once the archwire reaches a certain size. Before that, there is no active contact between the wire and the clip.

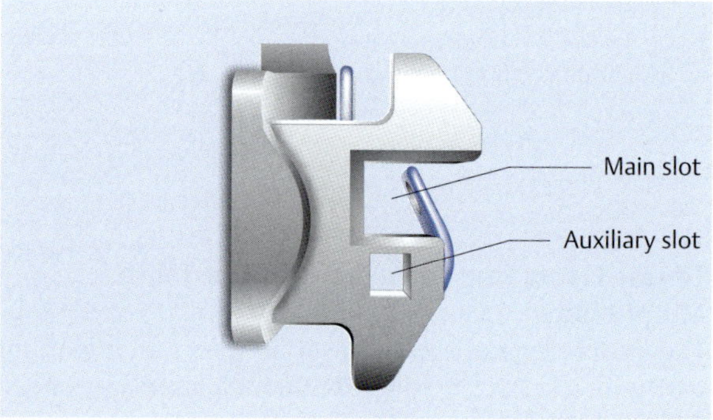

Fig. 2.21 The SL bracket with an auxiliary slot.

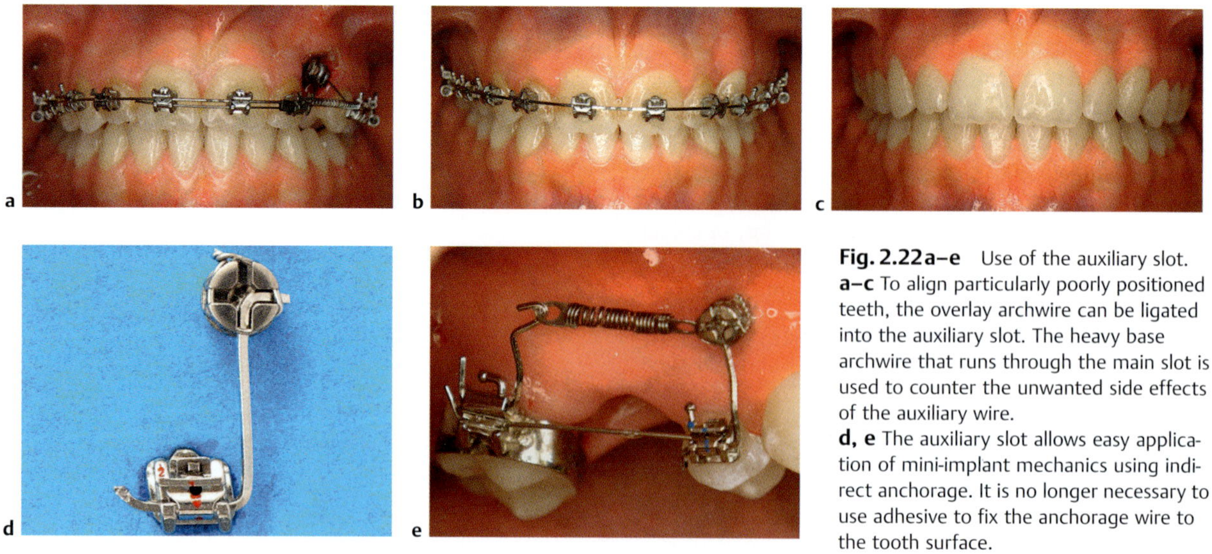

Fig. 2.22a–e Use of the auxiliary slot. **a–c** To align particularly poorly positioned teeth, the overlay archwire can be ligated into the auxiliary slot. The heavy base archwire that runs through the main slot is used to counter the unwanted side effects of the auxiliary wire. **d, e** The auxiliary slot allows easy application of mini-implant mechanics using indirect anchorage. It is no longer necessary to use adhesive to fix the anchorage wire to the tooth surface.

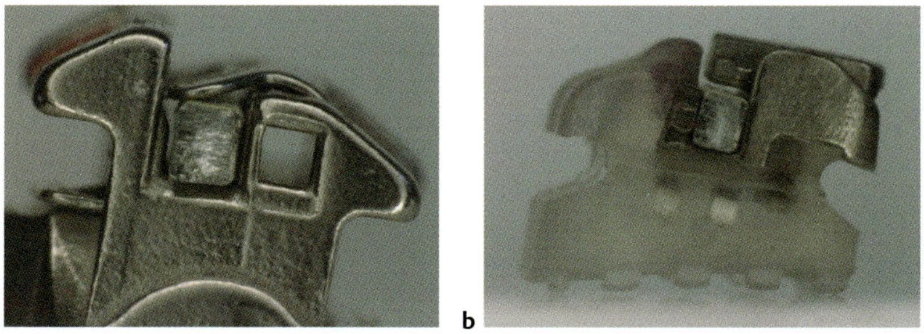

Fig. 2.23 a, b There are two methods of locking the bracket slot with SL brackets.
a Active system: archwires with specific dimensions are actively pressed into the bracket slot by a clip.
b Passive system: the slot is covered with a lid or a slider, which is stiff and does not exert active forces on the archwire.

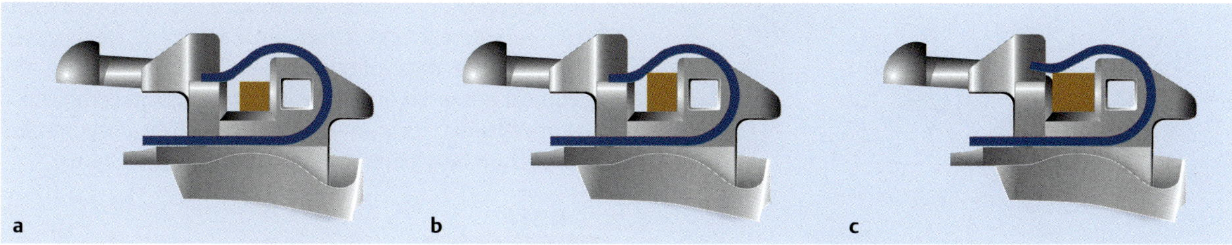

Fig. 2.24 a–c The working principle of an active clip during the insertion of archwires of various dimensions: 0.016 × 0.022 (**a**), 0.017 × 0.025 (**b**), and 0.021 × 0.025 (**c**). The clip becomes active only when larger, slot-filling archwires are used.

NOTE

Interactive clips are identical to passive clips for small archwire sizes.

Passive Systems

In a passive system, a rigid lid or bolt-like locking mechanism holds the slot shut. This effectively turns the bracket into a tube. No active force is exerted by the locking mechanism on the archwire itself. The presumed advantage of passive systems is reduced frictional resistance of the archwire, but this has only been demonstrated in in-vitro tests.[14] The disadvantage of a passive system lies in their different biomechanical properties. The passive clip is thought to have disadvantageous properties leading to inferior rotational and torque control. The manufacturers of passive systems have responded to this by developing specific archwire sizes for the passive systems and have attempted to improve the torque and rotational control of their brackets with variations in the cross-section (e.g., 0.014 × 0.025).

Rotation and Friction

Rotation

It is mainly the mesial–distal size of the archwire slot and the width of the locking mechanism that affect the rotational control of a bracket. The narrower the bracket, the less efficient the rotational control of the tooth. With conventional bracket systems, the distance to the tie-wings determines the efficiency of a bracket's derotational characteristics. Single-wing or solid brackets are less effective for rotational control compared to tie-wing brackets. The same principle applies to self-ligating brackets. Narrow clips provide less support for the archwire and therefore lead to less rotational control of the tooth (**Fig. 2.25**). This needs to be taken into account when choosing a self-ligating bracket. On the other hand, the advantage of narrow brackets, apart from the improved esthetics, is a longer working distance of the archwire, which increases its efficiency. A narrow-bodied bracket can therefore be advantageous in cases with severe crowding.

Friction

Friction is an important factor in tooth movement. About half of the forces applied to teeth are lost to frictional resistance[9,10]. One of the original ideas behind self-ligation was to reduce this frictional resistance by avoiding elastomeric and wire ligatures altogether. A number of studies, mainly experimental, have investigated the frictional characteristics of self-ligating brackets and compared them with conventional brackets. The results ranged from showing a significantly reduced frictional component to the exact opposite—increased friction.[6,14,21] No final conclusions can be drawn, due to the lack of standardization between the tests and the very varied study designs used. In addition, there are difficulties with transferring the findings of in-vitro studies into clinical scenarios, which are far more complex.[11,13,17] The following data are from our own investigations, which are based on in-vitro studies. We tested self-ligating brackets in a three-point investigation (**Figs. 2.26** and **2.27**). The frictional resistance was measured with a number of dif-

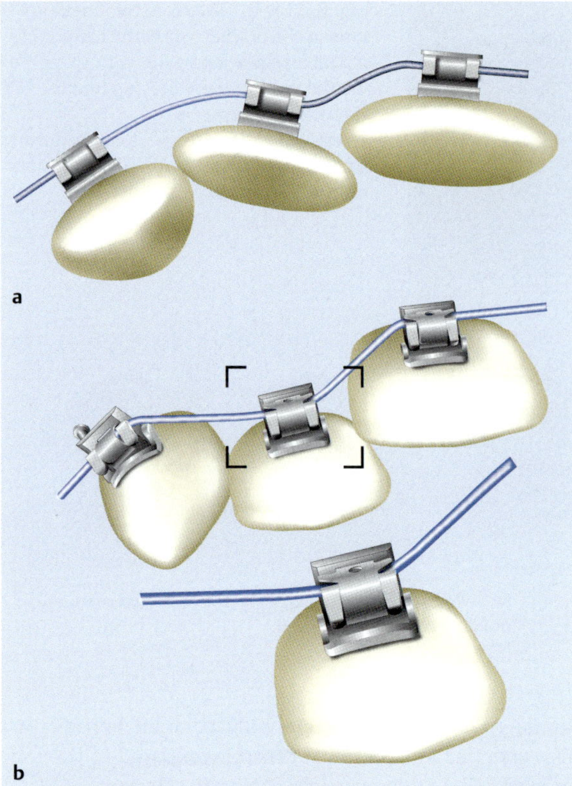

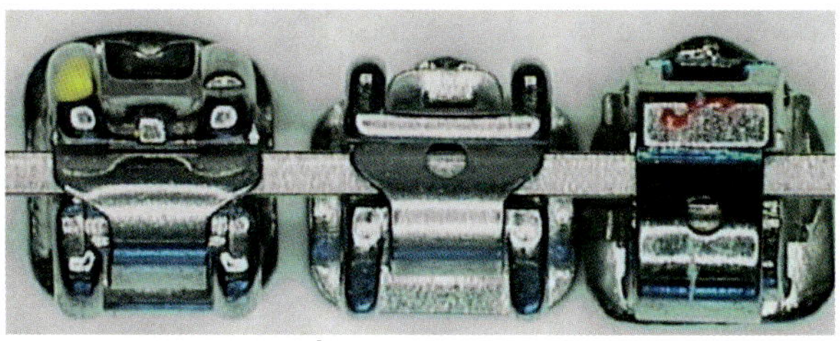

c d e

Fig. 2.25 a–e Active clips are very helpful for derotating teeth if they are designed with increased flexibility and increased mesiodistal dimensions. Some clips are designed with increased width at the slot level (**c, d**), as opposed to a narrow clip (**e**). If the clip becomes narrower again after leaving the slot level, springiness is increased at the extensions (**d**). However, a rigid lock results if the width remains constant after leaving the slot level and the entire clip locks (**c**).

ferent archwire sizes. The selection of the archwires was determined by the stage of treatment (superelastic wires starting at 0.012 for initial leveling to 0.018 × 0.025 for the latter stages of leveling and initial torquing). The resulting friction can be explained by interference between the following components:

- Material used for the archwire
- The ligation method
- Slot sizes and dimensions
- Slot surface characteristics[5]

This set-up cannot claim to simulate intraoral characteristics completely, and it has some inherent weaknesses. However, the data obtained give an indication of the technical potential of self-ligating brackets in comparison to conventional techniques, and they allow a preliminary comparison between different self-ligating systems.

NOTE

The locking mechanisms of self-ligating brackets have to withstand repeated opening and closing as well as everyday masticatory stresses.

The possible wear and tear on the locking mechanism that occurs after repeated opening and closing during archwire changes, and also the chemical challenges that occur in the oral cavity, should also be emphasized.[16] Probably the most common cause of defects in locking mechanisms is unduly increased stress placed on the mechanism by the operator; this is more often than not caused by inappropriate opening of the self-ligating mechanism (**Fig. 2.28**). We have tested a self-ligating bracket by simulating chewing in order to obtain an indication of whether the locking mechanism in self-ligating brackets is more likely to fail due to the occlusal load or due to inappropriate operating techniques. To do this, we subjected a self-ligating bracket (**Fig. 2.29 a**) to the Regensburg chewing simulator for one million cycles, equivalent to approximately 4 years' wear and tear.[18] No fractures occurred during this simulated usage. Finite-element analysis was used to simulate stresses and strains caused by repeated opening and closing of self-ligating mechanisms (**Fig. 2.29**), the variables included in the model were stiffness, springiness, strength, and resilience.

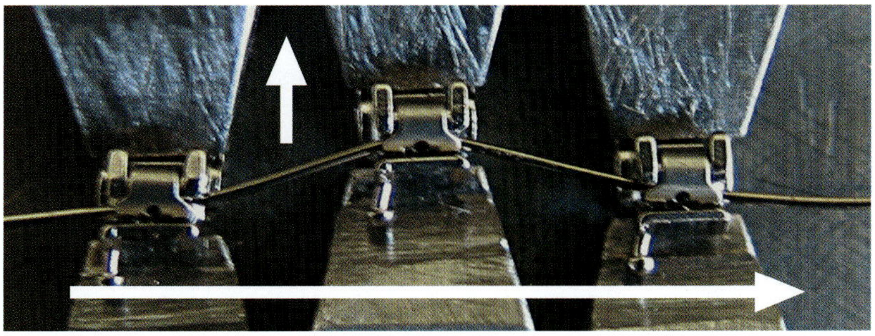

Fig. 2.26 A three-point experimental trial to measure friction. The central bracket can be moved vertically in increments. When the archwire is pulled horizontally, an initial threshold has to be overcome before the wire starts sliding. The forces required to move the archwire through the bracket slots are measured.

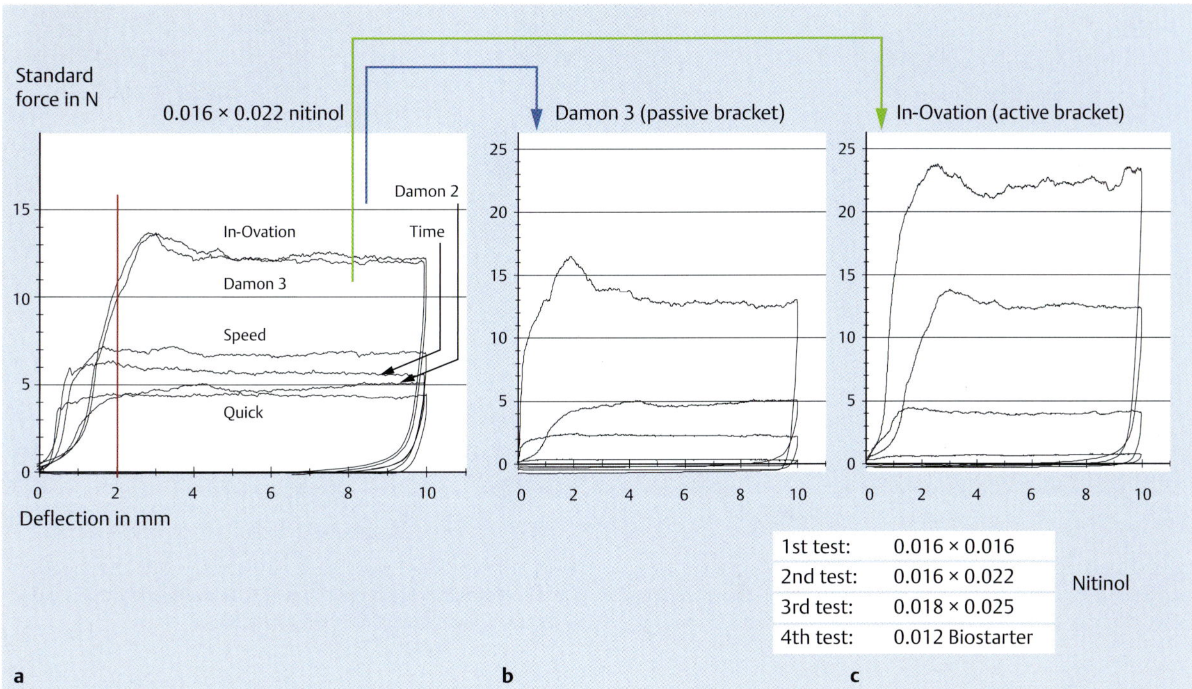

Fig. 2.27 a–c Friction in current SL brackets using a rectangular NiTi wire (0.016 × 0.022) (**a**). The force levels measured for different brackets begin to differ only after more than 2 mm deflection of the wire. When this particular experimental design is used, a passive (Damon 3, Ormco) and an active bracket (Innovation, GAC) show the highest values for four different archwire dimensions (**b, c**).

ERRORS AND RISKS

There are no standardized test designs for studying the frictional characteristics of self-ligating brackets. One should therefore be very cautious in interpreting the findings of ex-vivo studies.

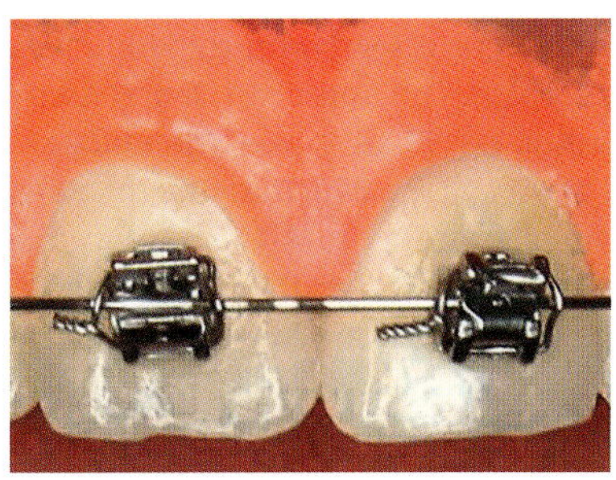

Fig. 2.28 The brackets' self-ligating mechanism failed due to poor handling by the operator. Functional overload due to masticatory forces can be ruled out, as these brackets are positioned on the maxillary incisors. If the self-ligating brackets have tie-wings, conventional ligation can replace self-ligation.

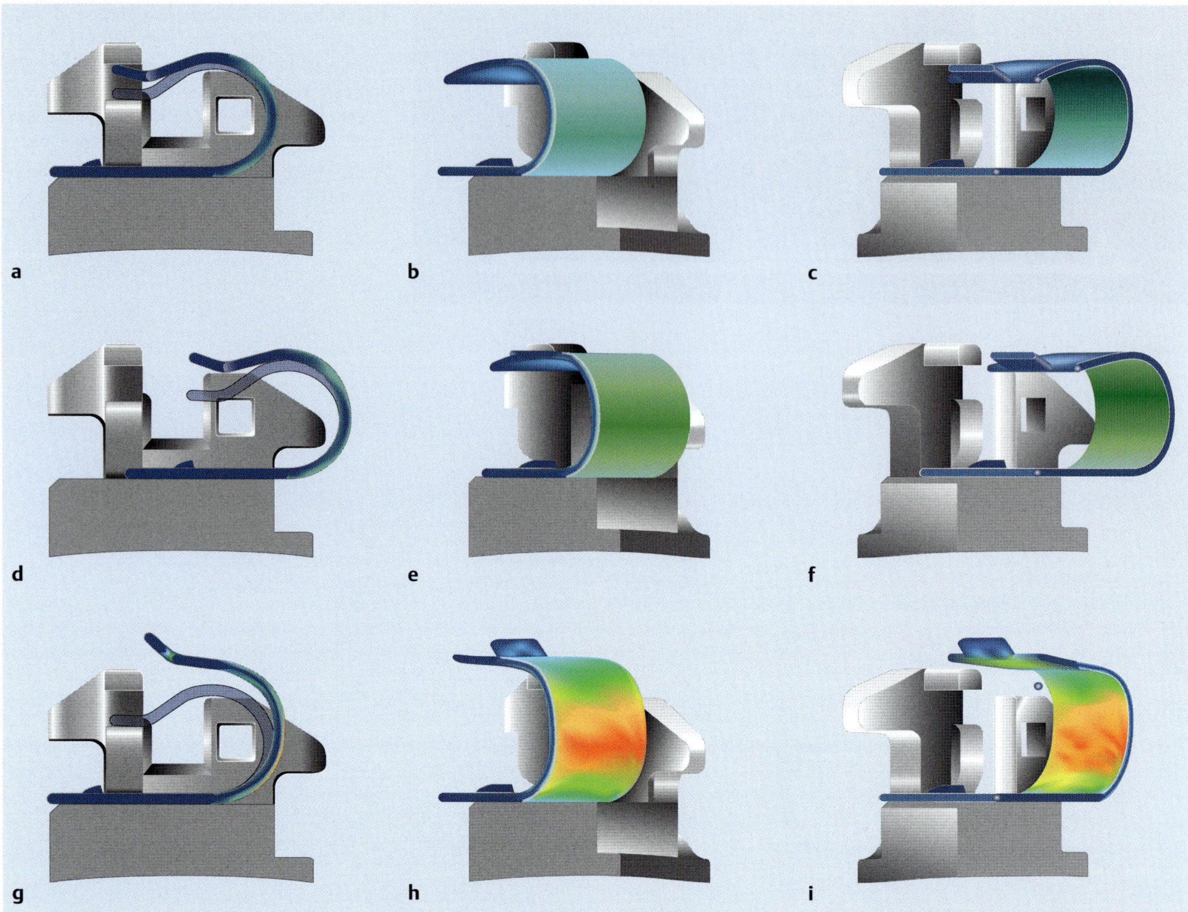

Fig. 2.29a–i Finite-element modeling analysis, illustrating stresses and strains at the self-ligating clips on opening. Green coloring shows that the deformation is within the elastic range of the clip (**a–f**). Yellow and red areas show overloading, with subsequent plastic deformation or fracture (**g–i**). The overloading was caused by opening the clip further than intended.

Archwires

Three metal alloys that are clinically relevant as archwire material are nickel–titanium, titanium–molybdenum alloy (TMA or beta-titanium), and stainless steel. Again, there is currently no standardized methodology for establishing the elastic properties of these materials, and manufacturers' claims and subsequent research on this topic are therefore difficult to compare. The American Dental Association (ADA) specification no. 32 advocates the unilaterally supported beam approach, in which a straight wire with a set length (1 inch according to ADA specification no. 32) is deflected up to 90°, and either the required force or the resulting bending moment is measured. This methodology may not be ideal, particularly in relation to the mechanical properties of wires made of nitinol (a substance named after the alloy components nickel and titanium, NiTi, and the institution that developed it, the Naval Ordinance Laboratory in White Oak, Maryland, USA). This is why the bilaterally supported beam approach is preferred in engineering (**Fig. 2.30**). But a number of variations exist even for this, particularly with a view to standardizing the exact fixation of the wires in the testing equipment. A typical force deflection diagram is shown in **Fig. 2.31**.

NOTE

Steel archwires are rigid and are mainly used during the space closure stage of orthodontic treatment.

Flexible wires made of nickel–titanium alloys can have both superelastic and thermoelastic properties. The terminology applying to these properties has not been standardized in the literature, and manufacturers' information and research studies can therefore be difficult for the practicing clinician to interpret. Generally, thermoelasticity refers to the property of NiTi to change phases based on temperature: the martensite phase exists at lower temperatures and the austenite phase at higher temperatures. An archwire that has been deformed, within limits, in the martensitic phase will resume its original shape in the austenitic phase. This is known as the "memory effect" of NiTi, and while it is theoretically

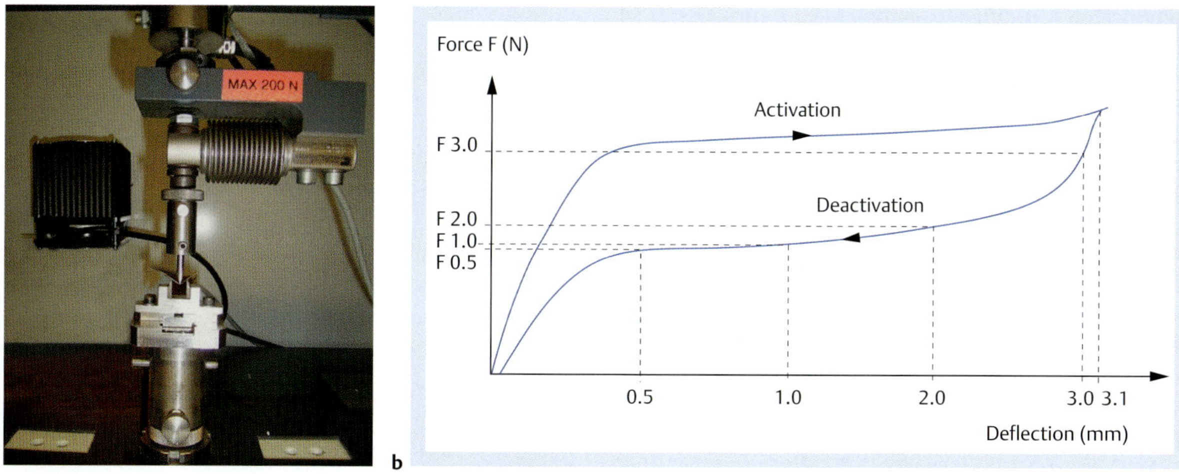

a b

Fig. 2.30 a, b A test apparatus (**a**) designed to measure force and deflection for orthodontic archwires (**b**).

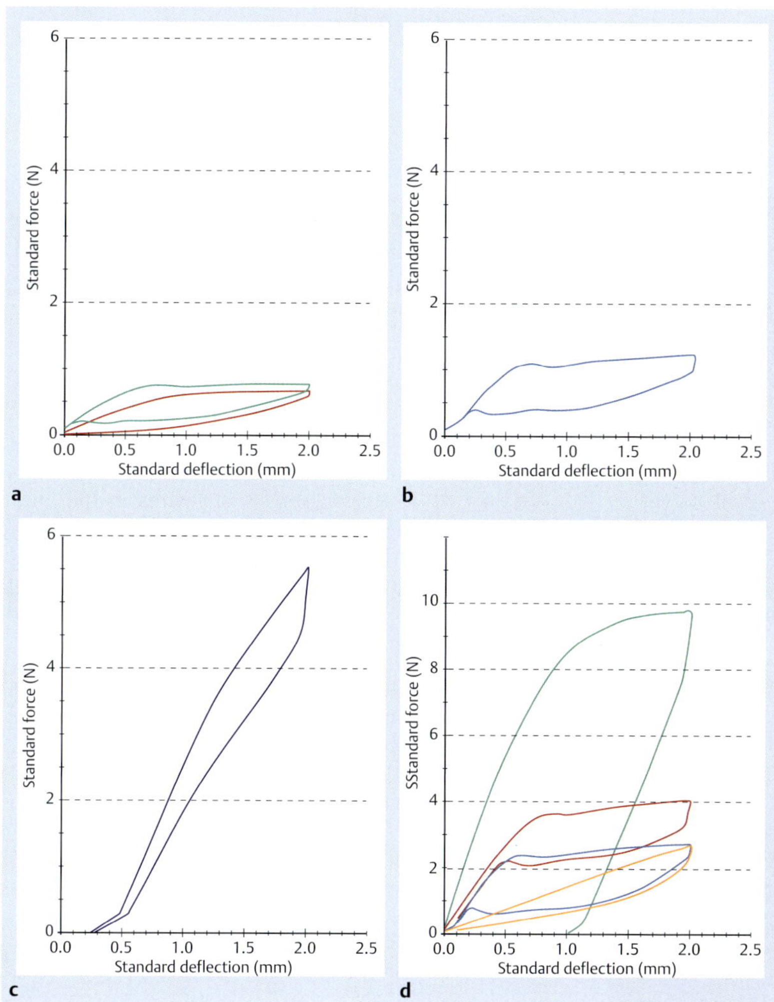

Fig. 2.31 a–d Typical force/deflection diagrams for the following wires.
a 0.016 SE NiTi at 25°C and 37°C.
b 0.016 × 0.016 SE.
c 0.016 × 0.016 stainless steel.
d Stainless steel, rectangular SE nitinol, 0.016 × 0.022 Twist Flex, SE nitinol in comparison. Green, stainless steel; red, rectangular SE; blue, Twist Flex; yellow, SE NiTi.

quite useful, it is difficult to implement in practice in an orthodontic treatment protocol, as the transition to the austenite phase occurs immediately after the wire enters the warmer oral cavity.

Superelasticity usually refers to the property the alloy exhibits in the transition from the austenite phase to the martensite phase when tension is applied to the wire, creating what is known as "tension-induced martensite" (TIM). This state is not stable and will immediately convert back to the austenite phase, and the original shape associated with that phase, when the tension is released. The orthodontically interesting phenomenon occurring here is not only that the wire resumes its original shape, but that it does so at lower force levels than were required to deform the wire (hysterisis) (**Fig. 2.30b**).

In clinical practice, however, we often observe that superelastic archwires do undergo plastic deformation, depending on the quality and composition of the NiTi alloy (**Fig. 2.32**).

The friction of an archwire in the bracket slot is also determined by its surface characteristics. Microscopic investigations have demonstrated the variations seen in the surface structure of different archwires (**Fig. 2.33**).

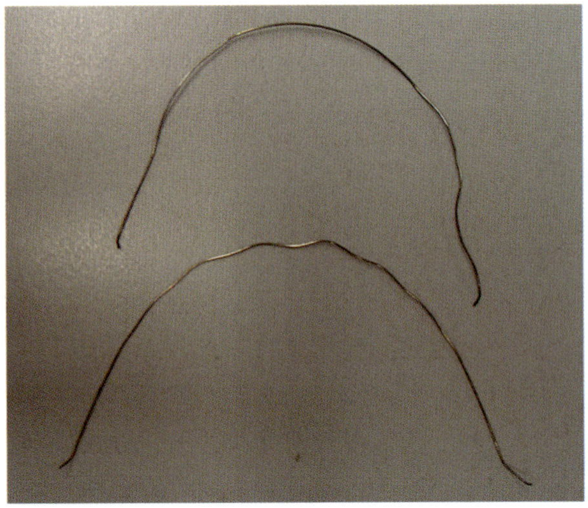

Fig. 2.32 The superelastic archwires shown were removed after 6 weeks of ligation because treatment did not progress as expected. The archwires underwent permanent deformation, and consequently no tooth movement occurred.

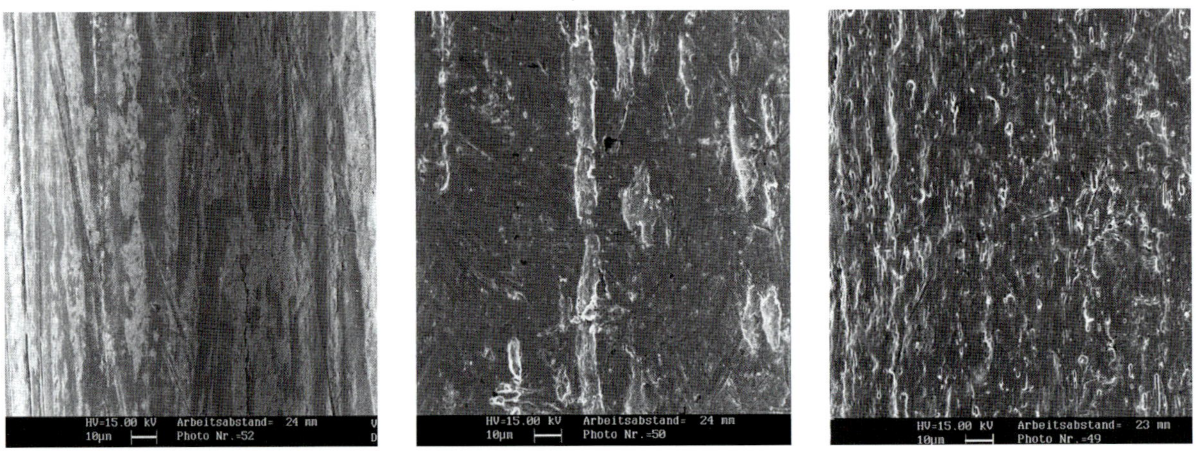

a

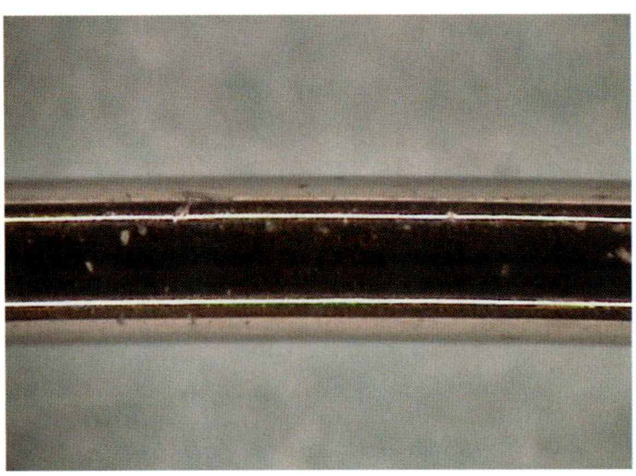

b

Fig. 2.33a, b
a Scanning electron microscopy shows differences in surface qualities between different elastic archwires. Rough surfaces increase the friction and require greater force levels for tooth movement.
b Macroscopic view of an SE NiTi archwire (0.012 Biostarter, Forestadent)

Archwire Sequence

One proposed advantage of self-ligating systems lies in their reduced friction, so that at least on a theoretical basis, fewer archwires are required for leveling and alignment. The authors mainly use the following wires (**Fig. 2.34**):

- 0.012 NiTi SE
- 0.016 NiTi SE
- 0.016 × 0.022 NiTi SE
- optional: 0.016/0.018 SS or 0.016 × 0.022 TMA (I do not use TMA a lot, apart from finishing)
- 0.018 × 0.020 NiTi SE
- optional: for space closure/opening depending on the anchorage/torque requirements:
- 0.018 × 0.025 SS/0.019 × 0.025 SS
- 0.021 × 0.025 NiTi SE Biofinisher

With the more pronounced plateau differences between austenite and martensite in high-quality alloys such as Sentalloy™ (GAC) or HANT™ (3 M Unitek), a further reduction in the total number of archwires is possible. A moderately crowded dentition could therefore be treated with the following sequence:

- 0.018 Sentalloy
- 0.018 × 0.025 Sentalloy
- 0.017 × 0.025 stainless steel or 0.019 × 0.025 stainless steel

Archwire Shape

NOTE

The arch shape is less important for the leveling and alignment of the teeth than the quality and resilience of the archwire.

In our own three-dimensional analysis of scanned diagnostic orthodontic models, we showed that industrially prefabricated archwire shapes only fit approximately 80% of patients treated in terms of shape, width, and curvature (**Fig. 2.35**). However, even with identically shaped archwires, the final treatment results may be entirely different in terms of the arch shape from one patient to another.

NOTE

An ideal arch shape in the wire will not necessarily lead to a similarly shaped arch after the completion of orthodontic treatment.

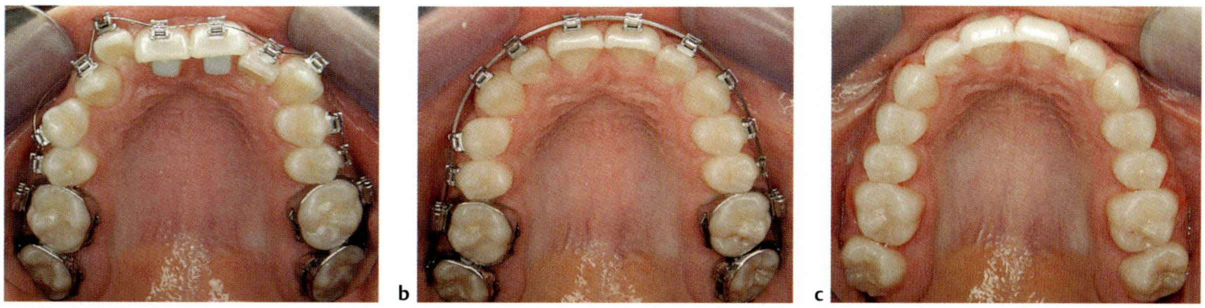

Fig. 2.34a–c Leveling and alignment of the arch with the following archwire sequences:
a 0.012 SE (see figure), 0.016 SE, 0.016 stainless steel, 0.016 × 0.022 titanium–molybdenum alloy (TMA).
b 0.018 × 0.025 SE (see figure), optional 0.019 × 0.025 stainless steel.
c The final result.

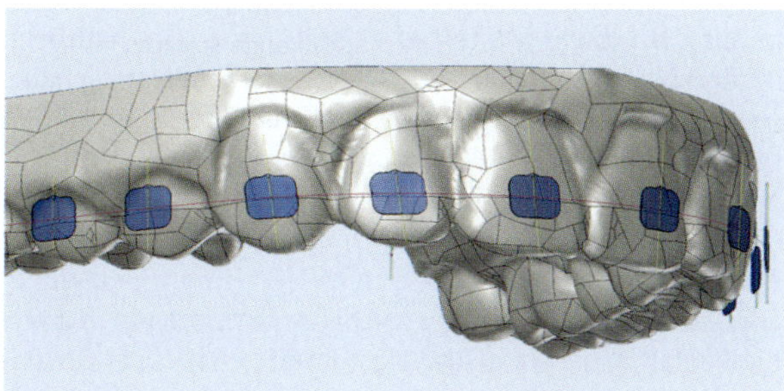

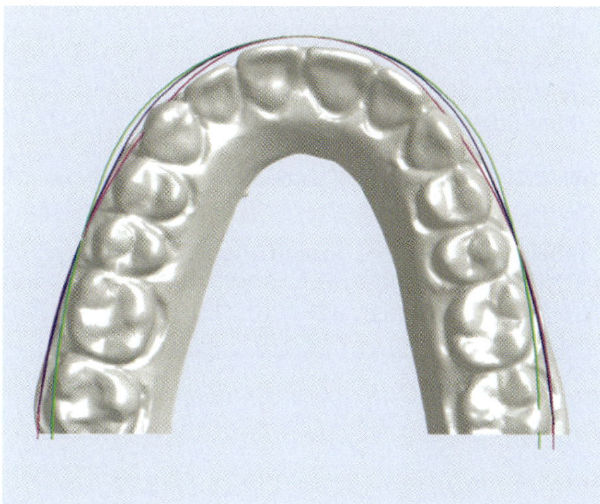

Fig. 2.35a, b
a The brackets and archwires are placed in their ideal positions in this virtual set-up.
b The final result in a three-dimensional scan. Blue, the arch form achieved; green, the archwire that was actually used; pink, a different arch form that could have been used (Eurosmile).

The reason for the inability to shape the dental arches may involve patient-related factors. The forces created by the archwire, which are translated to the teeth via the bracket, only determine the direction of movement. The final result varies depending on the quality and quantity of the bone surrounding the teeth and on the patient's metabolism.

Stainless-steel archwires can be customized based on the patient's individual needs, with elaborate bends using pliers such as hollow chop pliers. For elastic and particularly superelastic archwires, the Sander Memory-Maker can be used (with an electric current running through the archwires to change their shape without altering their physical characteristics). If the patient's arch shape is very different from the arch delivered by the manufacturer, the latter can be adjusted to fit the patient's needs. It may be useful to trace the original arch shape onto an acetate sheet and store it in the patient's chart for future adjustments. This will eliminate the need for plaster casts to be present at every appointment. Printing out an occlusal view to scale and score it in the patient's chart is possible when digital models are used, or if cone-beam computed tomography was carried out.

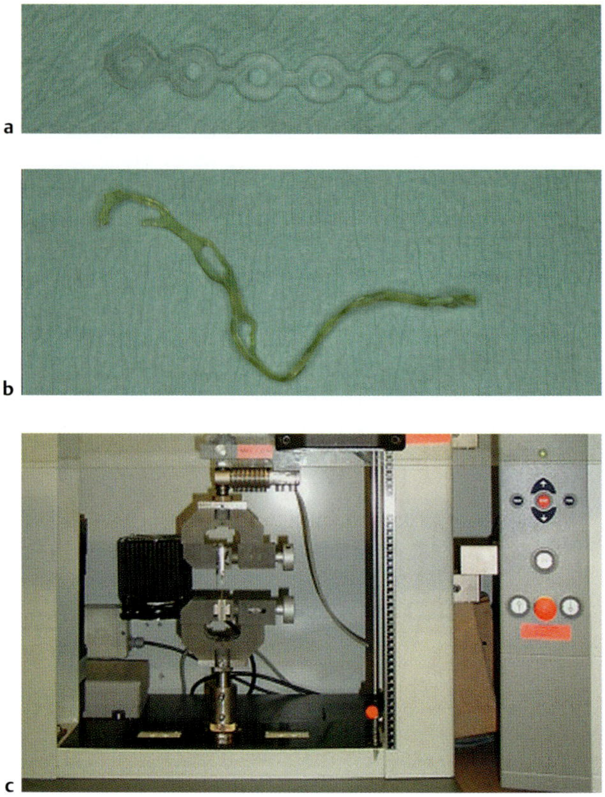

Fig. 2.36a–c A force/deflection study of elastic chains with clinically relevant extension in artificial saliva.
a, b The elastomeric chain before and after 4 weeks.
c The experimental set-up for testing elastomeric chains with clinically relevant extension in artificial saliva.

Auxiliaries

Conventional brackets and archwires are not always able to achieve all the desired tooth movements, and auxiliaries are therefore often necessary in clinical practice. Modern bracket and archwire combinations allow longer intervals between orthodontic review appointments. The operator should therefore be aware that there are significant differences in the quality of auxiliaries. Auxiliaries are efficient if they can exert a low force on the teeth that is active over a long period of time. The auxiliaries should also be easy to ligate. The most important auxiliaries in orthodontics are:

- Elastic chains
- Open or closed NiTi coil springs
- Segmental archwires
- Uprighting springs
- Intrusion and leveling springs
- Space-Jet
- Rotation springs or rotation wedges
- Mini-implants

Table 2.2 Tension testing of elastic chains with clinically relevant extension in artificial saliva

Product	Product length (mm)	Length after 24 h extension and 24 h relaxation (mm)	Elongation in %
1	16.1	16.9	5.0%
2	12.8	13.4	4.7%
3	19.2	20.2	5.2%

Elastics

Elastic chains are the most commonly used auxiliary for space closure. It is important to remember that the environment in the oral cavity (i.e., with humidity, warmth, functional stress, and an abrasive chemical milieu) will lead to a decline in the elastic properties very rapidly after the initial application (**Fig. 2.36a, b**). These parameters were tested as shown in **Table 2.2**.

In our own study, we tested elastic chains that had been immersed in artificial saliva (37°C). The elastic chains were stretched to twice their original length, which is a realistic simulation of a clinical scenario. The tension was held constant for 24 hours, and after a further 24 hours we measured the increase in the length of the elastic chain. After only 1 day, an increase in the length of the chain of approximately 5%, was seen. This in turn means that the molecular structure of the elastomeric chain was permanently changed. Elastomer chains should conform with the EN ISO 21606:2007 standard for "Elastomeric Auxiliaries for Use in Orthodontics" (**Fig. 2.36c**).

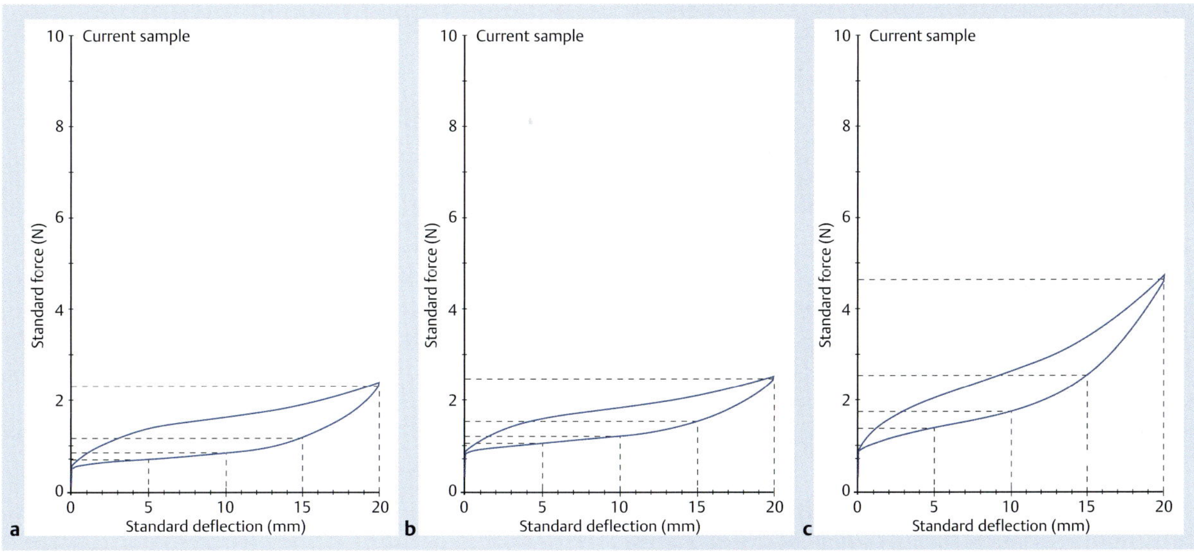

Fig. 2.37a–c Force/deflection diagrams of NiTi springs (8 mm long) with forces of 80 g (**a**), 125 g (**b**), and 175 g (**c**).

NiTi Coil Springs

Most contemporary coil springs are made of a nickel titanium alloy. The advantage of nickel titanium is its prolonged action and the fact that it is less affected by intraoral conditions than elastomers (**Fig. 2.37**). Nickel titanium is superior to stainless steel, as it delivers a consistent force over a large activation range and maintains its activation over longer time intervals.

NOTE

Based on Newton's third law of motion, springs always work in two directions, as every force produces an equal and opposite reactive force. Loss of anchorage (unwanted tooth movement) can be prevented by using auxiliaries such as headgear, transpalatal arches or mini-implants that are coupled to the anchorage segment, preventing unwanted tooth movement there (**Fig. 2.22**).

Additional auxiliaries such as the Sander uprighting spring, the Space-Jet, and other devices traditionally used in the segmented-arch approach can be easily combined with contemporary treatment approaches to increase treatment efficiency (**Fig. 2.38**). Additional information on the use of these auxiliaries is given in Chapter 8.

REFERENCES

1. Amm EW, Hardan LS. BouSerhal JP, Glasl B, Ludwig B. Shear bond strength of orthodontic brackets bonded with self-etching primer to intact and pre-conditioned human enamel. J Orofac Orthop 2008;69(5):383–392
2. Arhun N, Arman A, Sesen C, Karabulut E, Korkmaz Y, Gokalp S. Shear bond strength of orthodontic brackets with 3 self-etch adhesives. Am J Orthod Dentofacial Orthop 2006;129(4): 547–550
3. Attar N, Taner TU, Tülümen E, Korkmaz Y. Shear bond strength of orthodontic brackets bonded using conventional vs one and two step self-etching/adhesive systems. Angle Orthod 2007;77(3): 518–523
4. Azezullah F, Glasl B, Ludwig B, Kopp P. Experimental study of adhesive stability of esthetic brackets in debonding. Poster presented at the 83rd Congress of the European Orthodontic Society, Berlin, 11–17 June 2007
5. Bourauel C, Höse N, Keilig L, Reimann S, Rahimi A, Jäger A. Friktionsverhalten und Nivellierungseffektivität selbstligierender Bracketsysteme. Kieferorthopädie 2007;21:169–179
6. Bourauel C, Husmann P, Höse N, Keilig L, Jäger A. Die Friktion bei der bogengeführten Zahnbewegung—eine Übersicht. Inf Orthod Kieferorthop 2007;39:18–26
7. Cal-Neto JP, Carvalho F, Almeida RC, Miguel JA. Evaluation of a new self-etching primer on bracket bond strength in vitro. Angle Orthod 2006;76(3):466–469
8. Cehreli ZC, Kecik D, Kocadereli I. Effect of self-etching primer and adhesive formulations on the shear bond strength of orthodontic brackets. Am J Orthod Dentofacial Orthop 2005;127(5):573–579, quiz 625–626
9. Drescher D, Bourauel C, Schumacher HA. The loss of force by friction in arch-guided tooth movement. [Article in German] Fortschr Kieferorthop 1990;51:99–105
10. Drescher D, Bourauel C, Schumacher HA. Frictional forces between bracket and arch wire. Am J Orthod Dentofacial Orthop 1989;96(5):397–404
11. Drescher D, Bourauel C, Thier M. Application of the orthodontic measurement and simulation system (OMSS) in orthodontics. Eur J Orthod 1991;13(3):169–178

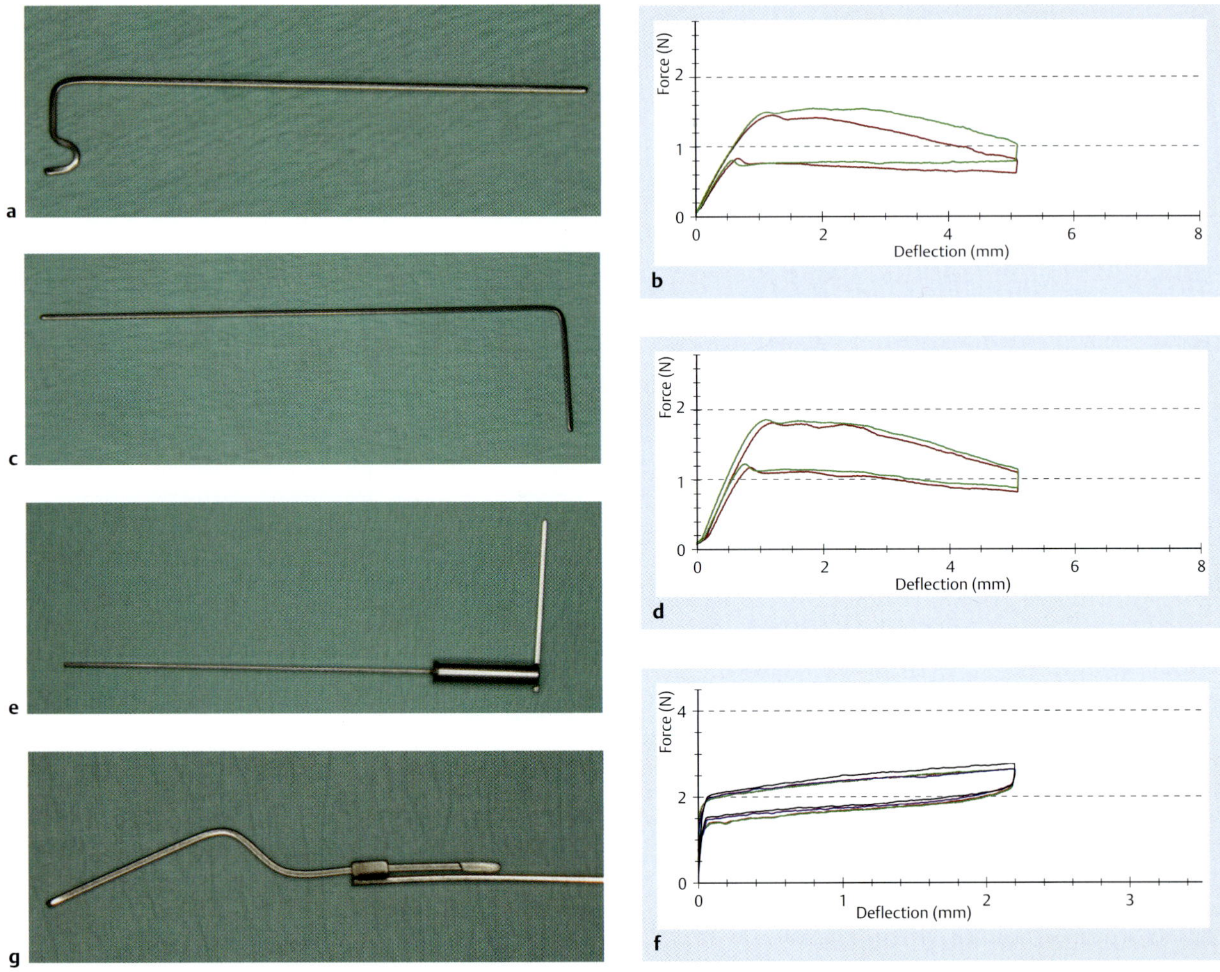

Fig. 2.38 a–g A leveling spring (**a, b**), derotating spring (**c, d**), and Space-Jet (**e, f**) in force/deflection diagrams. An uprighting spring is also shown (**g**).

12. Fritz UB, Diedrich P, Finger WJ. Self-etching primers—an alternative to the conventional acid etch technique? J Orofac Orthop 2001;62(3):238–245
13. Fuck LM, Drescher D. Force systems in the initial phase of orthodontic treatment—a comparison of different leveling arch wires. J Orofac Orthop 2006;67(1):6–18
14. Fuck LM, Wilmes B, Gürler G, Hönscheid R, Drescher D. Friktionsverhalten selbstligierender und konventioneller Bracketsysteme. Inf Orthod Kieferorthop 2007;39:6–17
15. Holzmeier M, Schaubmayr M, Dasch W, Hirschfelder U. A new generation of self-etching adhesives: comparison with traditional acid etch technique. J Orofac Orthop 2008;69(2):78–93
16. Pandis N, Bourauel C, Eliades T. Changes in the stiffness of the ligating mechanism in retrieved active self-ligating brackets. Am J Orthod Dentofacial Orthop 2007;132(6):834–837
17. Reicheneder CA, Baumert U, Gedrange T, Proff P, Faltermeier A, Muessig D. Frictional properties of esthetic brackets. Eur J Orthod 2007;29(4):359–365
18. Rosentritt M, Leibrock A, Lang R, Behr M, Scharnagl P, Handel G. Regensburger Kausimulator – Apparatur zur Simulation des Kauorgans. Materialprüfung 1997;39:77–80
19. Sernetz F. Physikalische und technische Eigenschaften von Drähten für die Kieferorthopädie und Orthodontie – Teil 4 (Ni-Ti-Legierungen). Quintessenz Zahntech 1999;25:885–894
20. Sernetz F. Physikalische und technische Eigenschaften von Drähten für die Kieferorthopädie und Orthodontie – Teil 2 (Biegung und Torsion). Quintessenz Zahntech 1999;25:569–574
21. Tecco S, Festa F, Caputi S, Traini T, Di Iorio D, D'Attilio M. Friction of conventional and self-ligating brackets using a 10 bracket model. Angle Orthod 2005;75(6):1041–1045
22. Vicente A, Bravo LA, Romero M, Ortíz AJ, Canteras M. Shear bond strength of orthodontic brackets bonded with self-etching primers. Am J Dent 2005;18(4):256–260

Bracket Systems

Heiko Goldbecher

3

Basic Principles

A large number of different self-ligating bracket (SLB) systems are available on the market today. The properties of an individual system depend on the materials used for the bracket, as well as on the ligation mechanism. Usually, SLBs are divided into two main categories: active and passive. Theoretically, no force is exerted by the clip itself when the archwire is ligated in passive systems (**Fig. 3.1**). However, the clip in active systems is designed to actively "press" the wire into the bracket slot upon locking of the mechanism (**Fig. 3.2**). Some manufacturers additionally subdivide the systems into semiactive or interactive locking mechanisms. In these, archwires are not actively forced into the slot until the wire has reached a certain dimension. The proposed advantage of passive systems lies in the reduction of friction.[1,2] However, to date, an actual reduction of friction between the archwire and bracket has only been confirmed in in-vitro experiments.[3] The alleged advantage of reduced friction in passive systems comes at the expense of inferior biomechanical properties; the lack of active ligation often reduces rotational and torque control in passive SLBs. The manufacturers therefore offer different archwire sequences and dimensions for the systems: rectangular archwires with small dimensions and high elasticity, such as a 0.014 × 0.025 superelastic wire, are introduced early on in the treatment to fill the slot as much as possible.[4] The aim is to rapidly progress to thicker archwires, ideally completely filling the slot early on in the treatment so that all of the preprogrammed values are transferred to the teeth as soon as possible.

NOTE

Using either traditional tie-wing brackets in combination with elastomeric or steel ligatures or SLBs with an active locking mechanism leads to active engagement of the wire into the slot. Given appropriate slot and bracket dimensions, this allows outstanding rotational and torque control. However, wires with very rounded edges provide less torque control, regardless of how well they are engaged (**Fig. 3.3**).

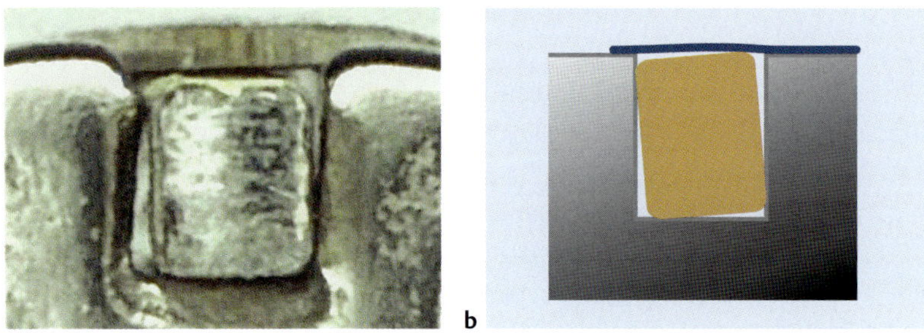

a b

Fig. 3.1 a, b
a The passive Discovery SL bracket (Dentaurum) with a 0.021 × 0.025 NiTi archwire. The archwire is passive in the bracket slot. Full torque expression and rotational control are only achieved when a maximum-sized archwire is used. The torque loss is mainly caused by the rounded archwire edges.
b A combination of a passive self-ligation system and rounded archwire edges results in a 5° torque loss even when a 0.021 × 0.025 archwire is used.

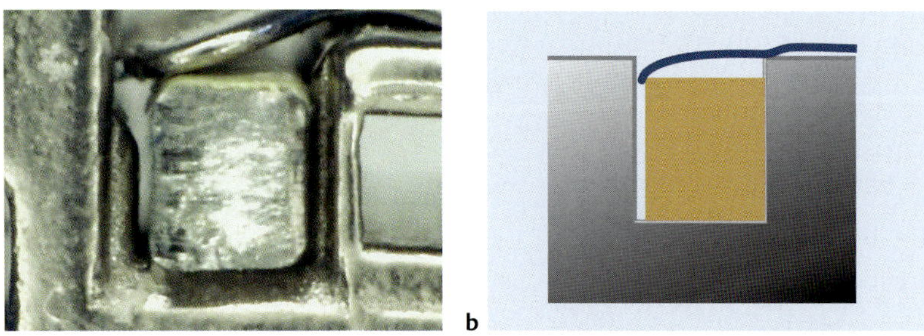

a b

Fig. 3.2 a, b
a The active Quick 2 bracket (Forestadent) with a 0.021 × 0.025 NiTi archwire. Here the wire is actively pressed into the bracket slot. Even before the slot is completely filled by the archwire, torque and rotational control are well established by the active clip.
b The clip actively presses the archwire into the slot. For a 0.022 slot system, torque is expressed starting with a wire size of 0.017 × 0.025.

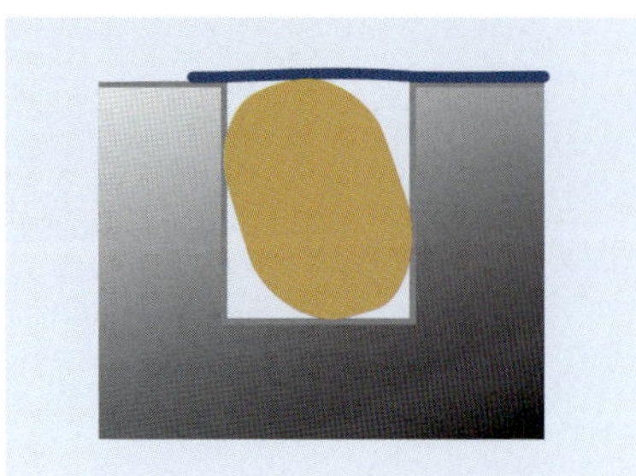

Fig. 3.3 Rounded edges facilitate ligation of large archwires, but decrease torque control.

The Various Self-Ligating Bracket Systems

This section provides a detailed look at the most popular self-ligating bracket systems and a direct comparison of widely used esthetic (**Table 3.1**) and metal bracket (**Table 3.2**) systems. An overview of the different manufacturers is also provided (**Table 3.3**).

Damon 3

The Damon 3 bracket (**Figs. 3.4** and **3.5**) is a passive system. The locking mechanism consists of a rigid sliding door with guiding grooves or rails. The bracket base and part of the body consist of acrylic. Opening of the bracket requires a special instrument and is in a caudal direction (i.e., occlusal for the upper jaw and gingival in the lower jaw). On delivery, the bracket is open.

Advantages

Although some discoloration may be observed (**Table 3.1**), it is generally thought that this bracket maintains esthetic properties for a long time in clinical practice. The learning curve for the operator is short, allowing precise bracket positioning after only a short initial phase. Generally, rotational and torque control are sufficient, as long as the manufacturer's recommended archwire sequence is adhered to. Elastomeric chains can be fitted under the archwire.

Disadvantages

Oral hygiene is difficult, and professional dental cleaning should be recommended with this bracket—this applies particularly to smokers. Due to the poor abrasion characteristics of the acrylic part of the bracket, it is often not possible to use elastic chains or steel ligatures on top of the archwire. When rectangular wires with dimensions such as 0.020 × 0.020 or greater are used, the sensitive locking mechanism may not work well or may actually be damaged during operation, particularly when there are food residues or plaque in the bracket. Composite removal may be an issue; most of the composite bonding material will stay on the tooth at debonding, increasing the chair time for removal of the adhesive.

Indications

In the authors' opinion, the Damon 3 system represents an acceptable compromise between esthetics and functionality. The bracket is quite small, and its use is therefore not recommended for severely rotated teeth or teeth that will need significant torque control (**Fig. 3.6**). It is a suitable bracket for patients with increased esthetic requirements and good oral hygiene.

Contraindications

Not indicated for use of Chlorhexidine rinse, Meridol, nicotine, coffee, and red wine, as well as some other foodstuffs (such as turmeric) can lead to early discoloration of the brackets.

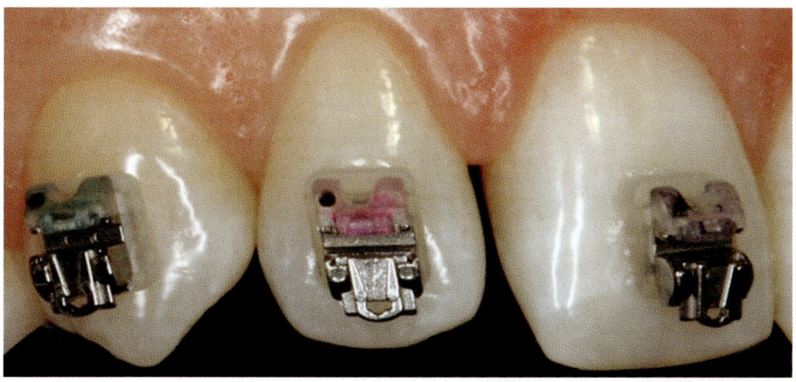

Fig. 3.4 A Damon 3 bracket after opening. The bracket is identified by color coding. The lateral edges of the bracket serve as orientation for positioning parallel to the long axis.

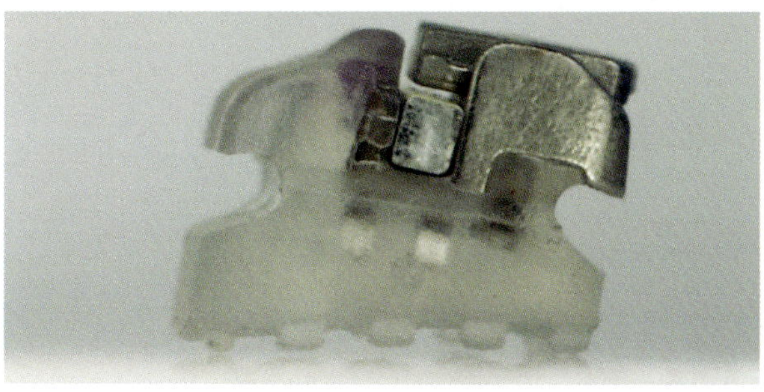

Fig. 3.5 A Damon 3 bracket with a 0.021 × 0.025 facially coated (esthetic) NiTi archwire. The archwire almost completely fills the bracket slot, which allows full application of the torque and rotational moments. Due to the rigidity of the locking mechanism, this archwire is often difficult to ligate in a clinical scenario.

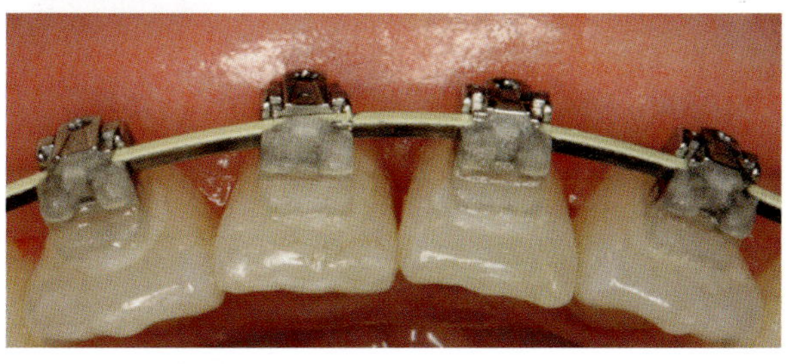

Fig. 3.6 The typical rotational issues that are commonly found in passive self-ligating systems are seen on tooth 41 here. The bracket's rigid clip cannot be closed on a 0.021 × 0.025 wire; steel ligatures cannot be applied. The acrylic tie-wings of this bracket are abraded.

In-Ovation R (GAC)

The In-Ovation R (**Figs. 3.7–3.9**) is an active bracket system. It has a well-defined and contoured bracket base, the body resembles the classic twin design. The base is connected to the body of the bracket by laser welding. The clip itself is a chromium–molybdenum alloy. Opening of the bracket occurs from gingival to occlusal and requires a specific tool, which can alternatively be replaced with a similarly shaped explorer.

Advantages

The In-Ovation R bracket is easy to place, easy to open and close, and has good rotational and torque control properties. Elastic chains can be placed over or under archwires.

Disadvantages

This is a metal bracket and therefore does not meet the highest esthetic requirements. In addition, archwire sizes of 0.018 × 0.018, in the 0.022 system and above may sometimes lead to difficulties in opening or closing the bracket. It is therefore of the utmost importance not to progress to the next wire size until the current wire has become passive.

Indications

Even severe crowding can be readily treated using In-Ovation R brackets. Also, good torque control can be achieved with rectangular archwires (larger than 0.020). The In-Ovation R bracket is manufactured to a high standard and has a relatively robust ligation mechanism, so that it can be recommended for novices wishing to gain experience with self-ligating brackets.

Contraindications

The In-Ovation bracket should not be used in patients with known allergies to chromium–molybdenum or nickel.

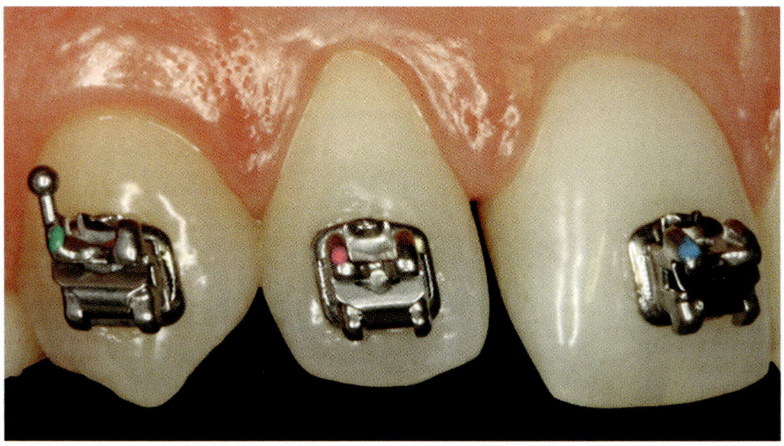

Fig. 3.7 In-Ovation R with a closed bracket slot. The bracket is identified by color coding. The lateral edges of the bracket serve as orientation for bracket positioning parallel to the long axis.

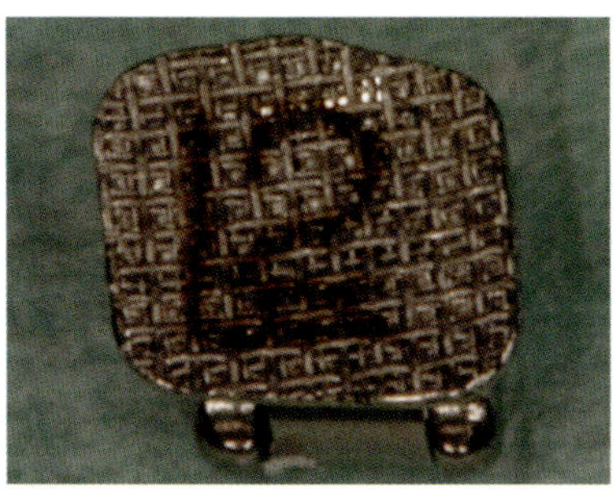

Fig. 3.8 Brackets can also be identified by markings on the base.

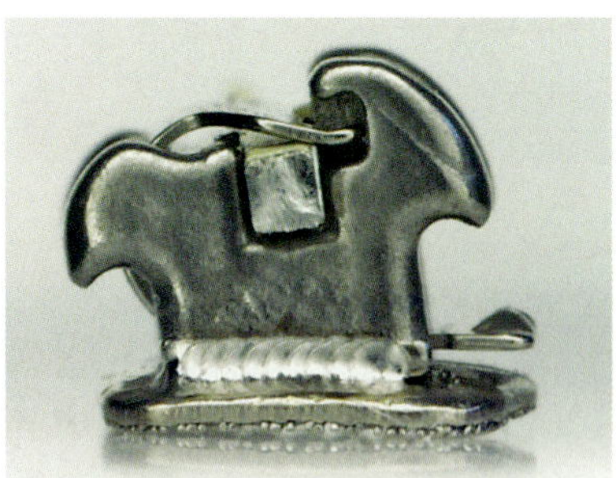

Fig. 3.9 In-Ovation R with a facially coated (esthetic) 0.021 × 0.025 NiTi wire. The archwire is actively pushed into the slot and hence allows maximum torque and rotational control. The elastic clip allows easy ligation even of full-sized archwires.

In-Ovation C (GAC)

The In-Ovation C is an active ceramic bracket (**Figs. 3.10–3.12**). The bracket base of this nicely contoured bracket and the twin body are produced in one piece using a ceramic injection molding technique. The clip has been treated so it has a matt appearance, which is advantageous from an esthetic point of view (**Table 3.1**). The bracket is somewhat larger than its metal counterpart (In-Ovation R). The bracket can be opened from the gingival direction using a specially designed tool and it is available for all teeth except for the molars and lower premolars. The company offers tubes for the lower premolar attachments that are made from the same ceramic material. However, these tubes fracture easily on insertion or removal of thicker archwires.

Advantages

The bracket is easy to position, easy to open and close, and is even better at correcting rotations and transferring torque values than the In-Ovation R bracket. Elastomeric chains are easily placed over or under the archwires. The manufacturer claims that due to the solid manufacturing process, it is possible to reuse the bracket (for the same patient) once the bracket base has been cleaned with a sandblaster, and this can be advantageous when repositioning brackets.

Disadvantages

The clip itself is not of quite the same quality as its metal counterpart (In-Ovation R). Chromium–molybdenum alloys cannot be easily covered with rhodium, and the manufacturer therefore chose to use a different material, which is not as flexible. Bracket debonding can be challenging due to the size of the bracket base and the bracket material—it is better carried out by the dentist/orthodontist rather than by assistants or dental auxillaries/therapists, to prevent possible enamel damage. Removal of the bracket and the remaining composite can be time-consuming, particularly if the bracket fractures and/or large amounts of composite are left behind.

Indications

Thanks to its size and mechanical characteristics, this bracket can be used universally. Tooth movement in large rectangular wires (> 0.020) is possible and allows good torque control. The In-Ovation C bracket is well-made and can be recommended for novices and experts.
Due to the increased bracket size, there may be potential issues with bracket placement in severely crowded cases. Enamel abrasion of the incisal edges of the upper front teeth has been observed in patients with class I or class II malocclusions and deep bites.

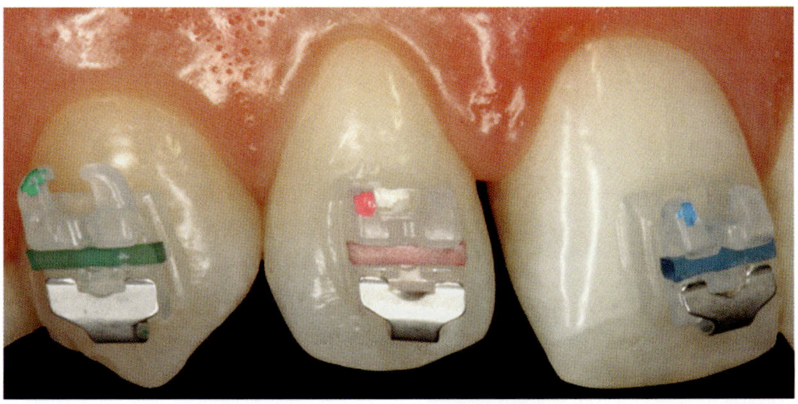

Fig. 3.10 In-Ovation C opened, with a rubber protector for the archwire slot. Bracket identification is simple due to the easily visible color coding. The lateral edges of the bracket serve as orientation for positioning along the long axis of the tooth.

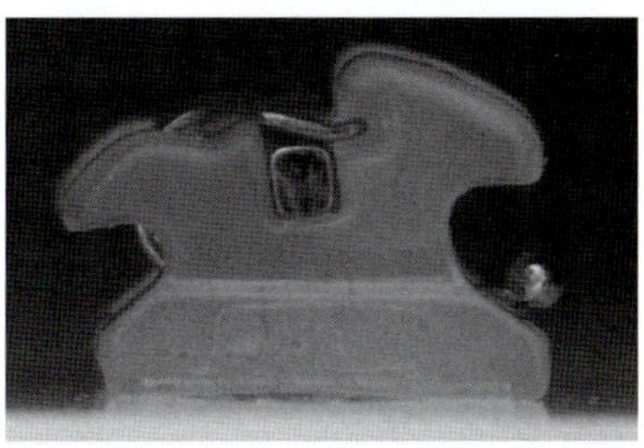

Fig. 3.11 In-Ovation C with a facially coated (esthetic) 0.021 × 0.025 NiTi archwire. The archwire is actively pushed into the bracket slot and thus translates the torque and rotational moments well. The clip is elastic and allows easy ligation of full-sized archwires.

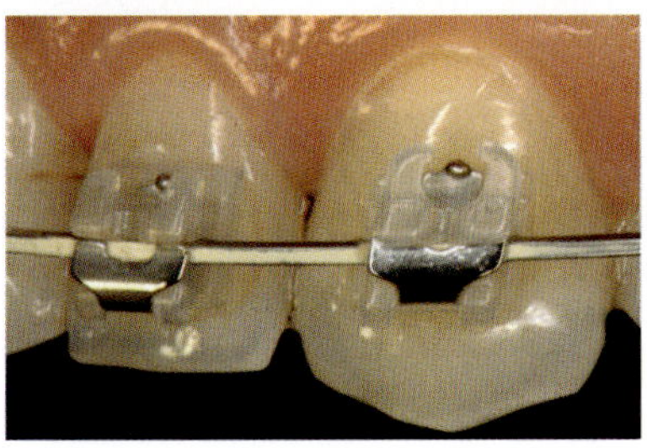

Fig. 3.12 In-Ovation C after 6 months of use. The coating of the archwire and the bracket clip have been almost completely lost.

Opal (Ultradent)

The Opal bracket (**Figs. 3.13–3.15**) is a passive bracket. It consists of a translucent fiber-reinforced composite polymer. It has a smooth and rounded one-piece design with an integrated lid mechanism for self-ligation. Opening occurs with a special instrument from the incisal direction.

Advantages

The Opal bracket is very smooth and gentle on the soft tissues and is initially highly esthetic (**Table 3.1**). It is reasonably easy to position and has very easy to read, good markings.

Disadvantages

Bracket loss is a common occurrence. In addition, opening of this bracket can be difficult and elastomeric chains are difficult to place. Cleaning of the brackets is best undertaken by a hygienist or other dental health-care professional. In our opinion, the bracket discolors easily. We cannot recommend this bracket if rotational or torque control are major issues.

Indications

Opal brackets can be recommended for short treatment durations of 6–9 months. Correction of smaller rotations and mild crowding is easily carried out. This bracket is esthetic in the initial phases and can be recommended for patients with high esthetic requirements, good oral hygiene, and good dietary control, ideally avoiding foodstuffs that discolor the brackets easily (such as red wine and other discoloring agents such as turmeric).

Contraindications

This bracket cannot be recommended for patients with severe crowding. It also has a number of disadvantages for patients with generously spaced dentitions. As mentioned above, the bracket discolors easily, particularly when substances such as chlorhexidine, turmeric, or red wine are used regularly or if the patient is a smoker. Removal of residual composite after debonding can be time-consuming, and this needs to be borne in mind.

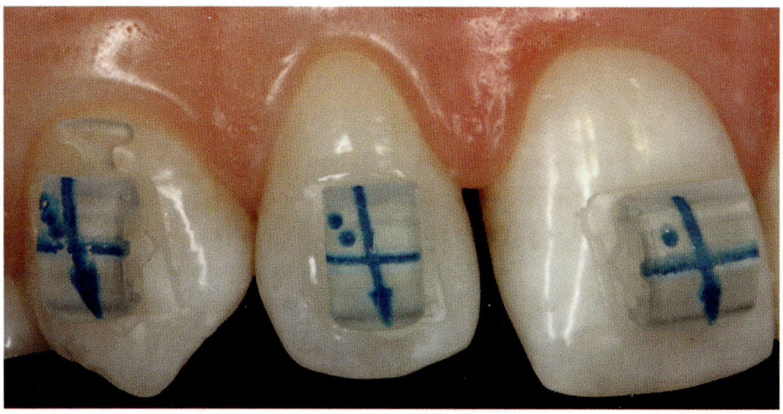

Fig. 3.13 The Opal bracket closed. Color markings allow identification of the bracket. Positioning of the bracket on the tooth is made easy by the markings on the bracket clip.

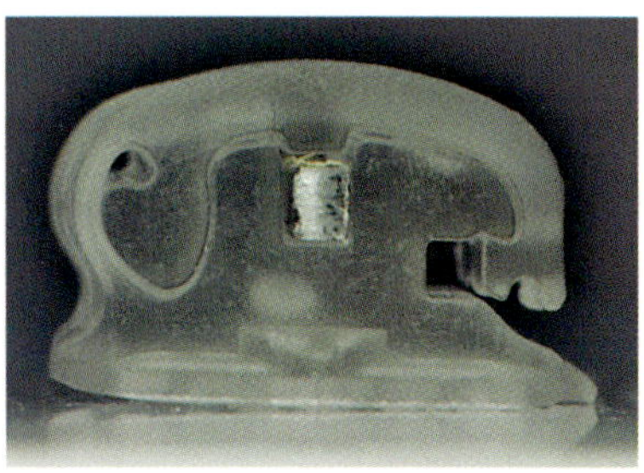

Fig. 3.14 Opal with a facially coated (esthetic) 0.021 × 0.025 NiTi archwire. The archwire is passively held in the slot. The material properties of the acrylic bracket do not allow good torque expression and rotational control. The clip can be closed easily; the clip presses the wire into the bracket slot.

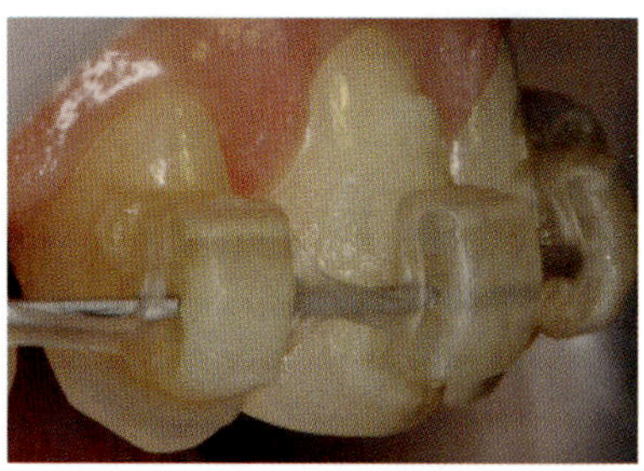

Fig. 3.15 The composite material discolors easily, depending on the patient's dietary habits. Elastomeric ligatures can be used, but these are difficult to apply.

Opal M (Ultradent)

The Opal M bracket is a passive bracket (**Figs. 3.16–3.18**) and is produced using the metal injection molding technique (MIM). The molding is followed by sintering. The bracket is very smooth, as the edges are nicely rounded, and it has a "lid" that covers the slot. Opening is from the incisal, using a specially designed instrument.

Advantages

The Opal M bracket is very smooth and very gentle on the soft tissues. Like its esthetic counterpart, it is easy to position due to the marking on the face of the lid. Elastic chains can be positioned easily due to a modified design.

Disadvantages

Opening of the mechanism can be challenging. Apart from that, the bracket appears larger than its actual size due to its shape and surface properties.

Indications

This bracket can be recommended for patients with very sensitive soft tissues. Due to its size and physical characteristics, it can be used for all types of malocclusion; rotational and torque control of the teeth are good for a passive bracket.

Contraindications

Potential issues mainly involve esthetic concerns; due to its metallic surface, the bracket appears very dark in the patient's mouth and it may therefore not meet the highest esthetic requirements.

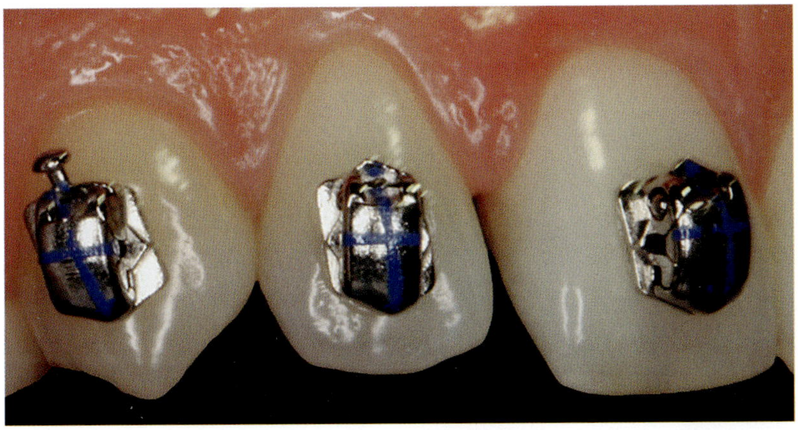

Fig. 3.16 Opal M closed. Bracket identification is easy and similar to the acrylic Opal bracket.

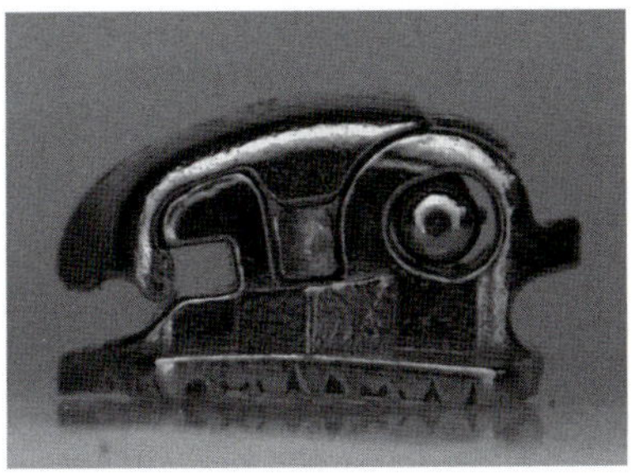

Fig. 3.17 Opal M with a facially coated (esthetic) 0.021 × 0.025 NiTi archwire. The archwire is held passively in the bracket slot. The clip is easy to close even when full-sized archwires are used, as the clip forces the wire into the bracket. Stainless-steel and elastomeric ligatures can be easily used. The auxiliary slot is clearly visible.

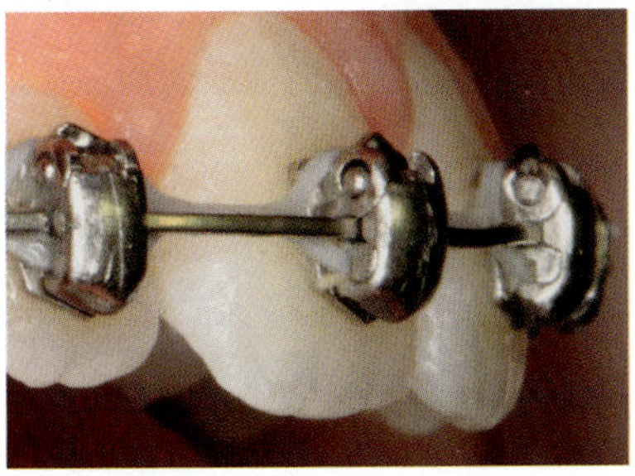

Fig. 3.18 In contrast to the Opal bracket, Opal M allows easy application of elastomeric ligatures over or under the archwire.

Quick 2 (Forestadent)

The Quick bracket (**Figs. 3.19–3.21**) is an active bracket. It is a one-piece construction using metal injection molding (MIM), followed by sintering. The elastic clip is made from a chromium–molybdenum alloy. This bracket can be opened with a specially designed instrument either from the gingival or labial aspects.

Advantages

The Quick bracket is easy to position. The seating is very similar to that of a conventional twin bracket and can be easily carried out even by operators with little or no experience with self-ligating brackets. The bracket is clearly marked, which aids orientation, and the clip mechanism is easy to operate. Rotational and torque control are very good, and placement of elastomeric chains is easy. Even very thick archwires (0.021 and above) can be ligated. It also has an additional 0.016 × 0.016 auxillary slot.

Disadvantages

The disadvantages of this bracket are mainly esthetic; as with all metal brackets, it may not meet patients' highest requirements.

Indications

This is a small, solid, metal bracket that can be used in patients with severe crowding in whom rotational control is paramount. Torque control is good, as even archwires larger than 0.020 can be ligated. This bracket can be recommended for novices in self-ligation. The additional auxiliary slot improves the bracket's versatility.

Contraindications

These are mainly esthetic and if patients have any known allergies to the metals used to produce the bracket.

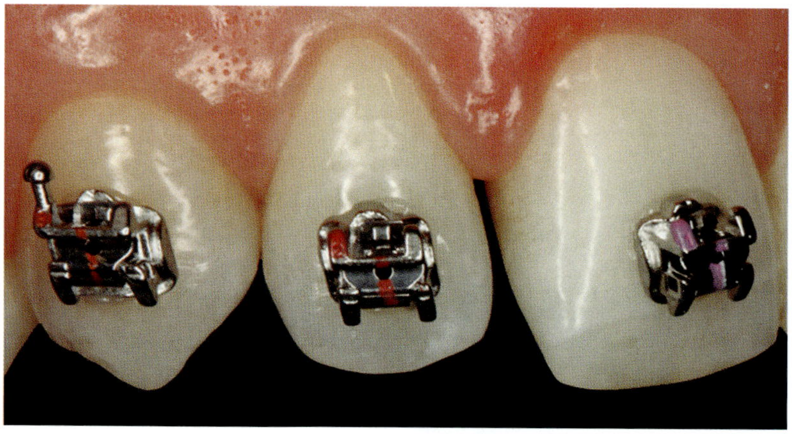

Fig. 3.19 Quick 2 closed; identification and orientation of the bracket are easy due to color coding.

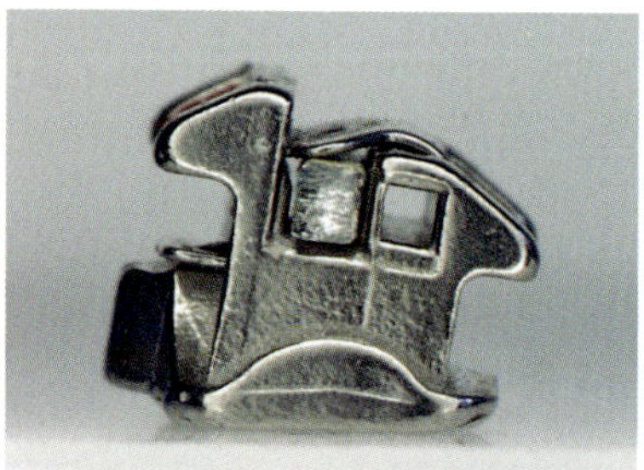

Fig. 3.20 Quick 2 with a facially coated (esthetic) 0.021 × 0.025 NiTi wire. The archwire is actively pressed into the bracket slot and thus allows full expression of torque and rotational control. Ligation of full-sized archwires is easily possible, due to the elasticity of the clip. This bracket has an additional archwire slot for auxiliaries (0.016 × 0.016).

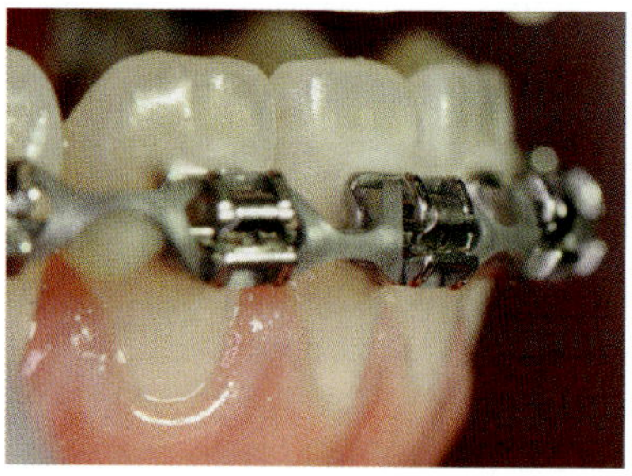

Fig. 3.21 Elastomeric chains can be easily placed under or over the archwire due to the bracket's twin-wing design.

SmartClip (3 M Unitek)

The SmartClip bracket is a passive system and the bracket basically consists of a traditional twin bracket. The bracket has two clips laser-welded to it, which are mesial and distal to the tie-wings. There are no movable parts such as lids or locks. The mechanism itself consists of two nickel–titanium clips that open automatically once the archwire is dislodged in the buccal–lingual direction. Special instruments are available to facilitate ligation and disengagement of the archwire (**Figs. 3.22–3.24**).

Advantages

The SmartClip bracket is easy to position on the tooth; its main characteristics are those of a normal twin bracket. No additional training or experience is necessary to position it well. Rotational control and torque control are excellent as long as the appropriate wires are used to their full size. The markings on the brackets are good, and elastic chains are very easy to place. As the SmartClip bracket does not use any locking mechanisms, oral hygiene is easily maintained. The bracket can also be converted into an active bracket by ligating traditional ligatures to the tie-wings in the later stages of treatment, when greater control of tooth movement is required. The bracket is delivered precoated with 3 M's Transbond™ Plus adhesive, and each bracket is individually packaged in a small container with a sealed lid. This facilitates stock-keeping and increases the consistency of the bonding results, as it prevents contamination of the bracket base and variations in the adhesive application.

Disadvantages

Insertion and removal of the thick archwires can be problematic and can lead to debonding of brackets and/or cause discomfort for the patients. The manufacturer recommends using a number of small archwires in some situations instead of using one full-sized or large wire. Larger rectangular wires are also available as hybrid wires to facilitate ligation—but this may be associated with the previously described potential disadvantage of loss of torque control.

Indications

This bracket has good leveling and alignment properties.

Contraindications

The bracket should not be used in patients with known allergies to the metals used. It may also not be ideal for very sensitive patients, as the insertion and removal of archwires may cause discomfort—although this can be minimized with proper technique.

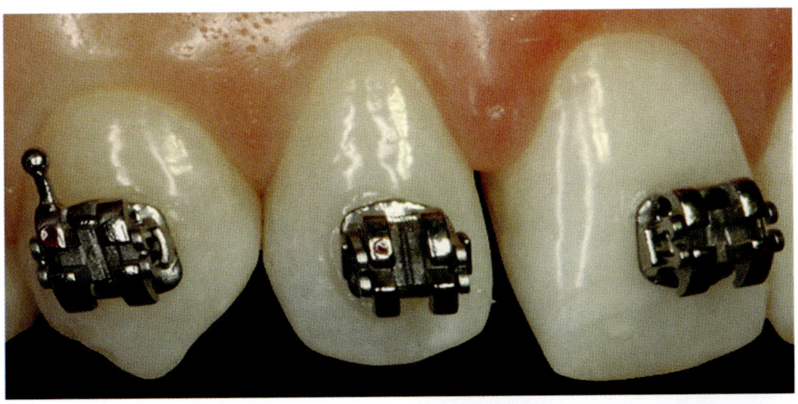

Fig. 3.22 SmartClip. Color coding allows bracket identification. These brackets can be positioned relatively easily in comparison with other self-ligating brackets; they still have a vertical groove that allows easy positioning of the bracket along the long axis.

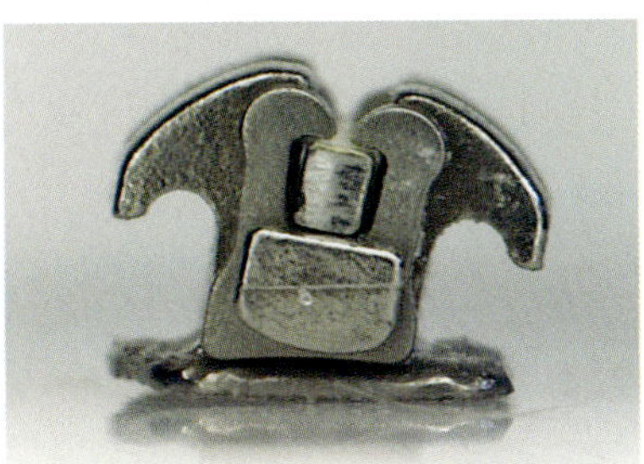

Fig. 3.23 SmartClip with a facially coated (esthetic) 0.021 × 0.025 NiTi wire. The archwire is passively held in the slot, but ligation of full-sized archwires can be difficult due to the elastic clip design. When coated esthetic archwires are used, the coating is often lost during initial ligation.

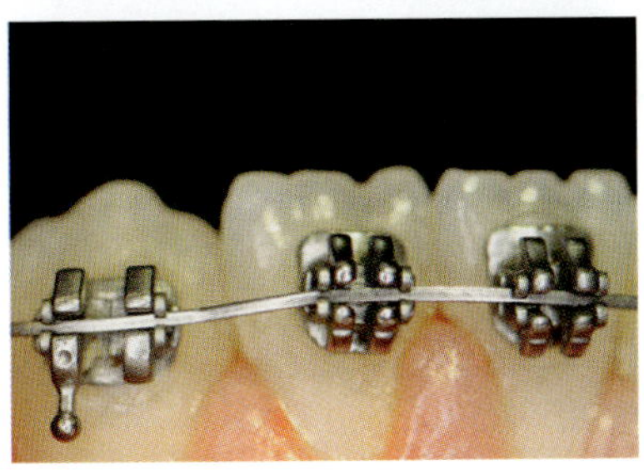

Fig. 3.24 Detailed view of a 0.021 × 0.021 NiTi archwire in a SmartClip bracket in the lower jaw. Although this is a passive system, the rotational control is generally good, as the clips are positioned lateral to the tie-wings. However, rectangular archwires are often difficult to ligate. 3 M offers beveled archwires, but these do not always allow full torque expression (see **Fig. 3.3**).

Clarity SL (3 M Unitek)

The Clarity SL bracket (**Figs. 3.25** and **3.26**) is a passive system that consists of a ceramic body. This has a metal slot incorporated in the ceramic base to improve the frictional characteristics. As in the SmartClip bracket, the self-ligating mechanism consists of a NiTi clip that is fixed to the mesial and distal aspects of the twin bracket. Special tools are available for inserting and removing archwires.

Advantages

The Clarity SL bracket can be placed in the same way as its conventional-ligation counterpart. No additional training or experience are necessary. Rotational and torque control are excellent. The markings on the bracket are easy to recognize and elastomeric chains can be easily placed. Cleaning is easy for the patient, as there are no additional mobile parts such as lids or other locking mechanisms. Debonding is relatively convenient for a ceramic bracket, due to an intentional weak spot at which the bracket fractures when the proper debonding technique is used. Like the SmartClip bracket, it is individually packaged and precoated with adhesive.

Disadvantages

Ligation and removal of very rigid and heavy archwires can be uncomfortable for the patient. We would recommend using the instruments designed for this purpose to avoid breakage of the clips during ligation or removal of archwires. The coating of tooth-colored esthetic archwires may be compromised on ligation. This bracket cannot be reused for repositioning or repairs, as it has a predetermined fracture point along the vertical axis of the bracket, which was designed to facilitate bracket removal on completion of orthodontic treatment.

Indications

Quick and effective leveling and alignment, as well as the proposed frictional characteristics, are the advantages of this bracket. It is also esthetically pleasing, as most of the metal parts are hidden behind the archwire. The esthetics of the bracket may be slightly compromised during the initial stages of alignment. The clip may be quite visible on rotated teeth.

Contraindications

This bracket cannot be recommended for very sensitive patients, as the ligation and removal of archwires can cause discomfort, especially on the lower incisors. It is also not recommended to use esthetically coated archwires of the first generation as the clip may damage the esthetic coating of the archwire on ligation. Cases with high torque requirements may also present difficulties, as the hybrid wires used for larger sizes fall short of regular rectangular wires with sharp edges.

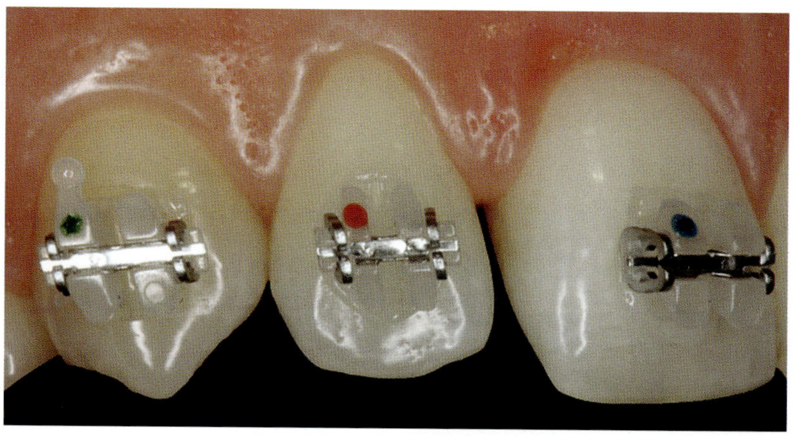

Fig. 3.25 In the Clarity SL bracket, identification is by color coding. This bracket has a metal slot to reduce friction. The metal slot partly hides the vertical groove of the bracket and can make positioning more challenging than for its metal counterpart.

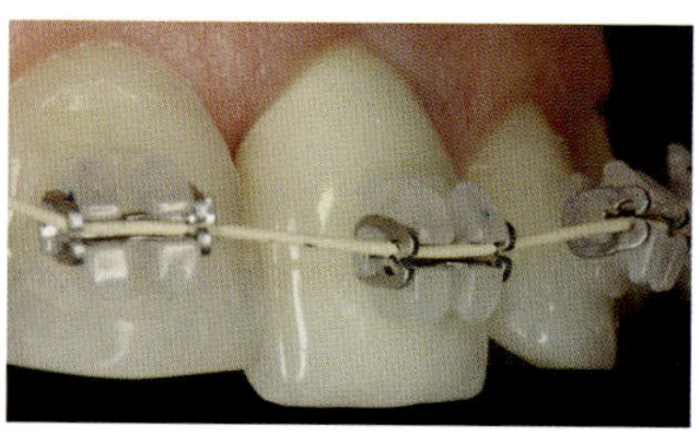

Fig. 3.26 Clarity SL with a coated esthetic 0.014 NiTi archwire. The archwire is passively held in the slot. The clips can make it difficult to ligate full-size archwires. As seen in this image, the coating of esthetic archwires is already lost on initial ligation of the wire.

Speed (Strite Industries, Ltd.)

The Speed bracket (**Figs. 3.27–3.30**) was the first active self-ligating bracket on the market. The bracket base is well contoured. It is welded to the body. Opening occurs from gingival to occlusal for both upper and lower arches, and a customized tool is recommended for this.

Advantages

The bracket is small, and after a short training period it can be positioned easily and precisely. Despite the small size, it is easy to open and close. This bracket has an auxillary slot that can be very useful.

Disadvantages

Due to its size, the bracket does not allow the same rotational and torque control of teeth in comparison with other self-ligating brackets. Elastomeric chains can only be positioned under the archwire. The bracket is too small and lacks tie-wings to allow chain placement over the archwire and bracket. Using rectangular wires with sizes larger than 0.020 × 0.020 can lead to difficulties with the opening and closing mechanism, particularly in the lower premolar area.

Indications

The advantage of this bracket lies in its comparatively small size and is suitable for the treatment of severe crowding, although the final rotational control can sometimes be less than ideal. It is also one of the least expensive self-ligating brackets currently on the market.

Contraindications

Lingual torque control of premolars in the lower jaw is not always easy with this bracket. Ligation of heavy stainless steel wires can be difficult (archwires larger than 0.020). The precision of the bracket slot and the general bracket quality is not of the same standard as that of many other self-ligating brackets.

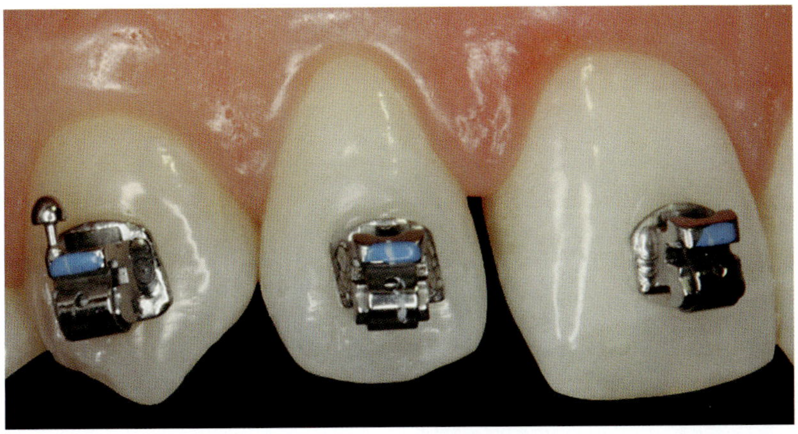

Fig. 3.27 Speed is an active self-ligating bracket. Color coding identifies the arches, but not the individual teeth. Bracket identification is therefore difficult.

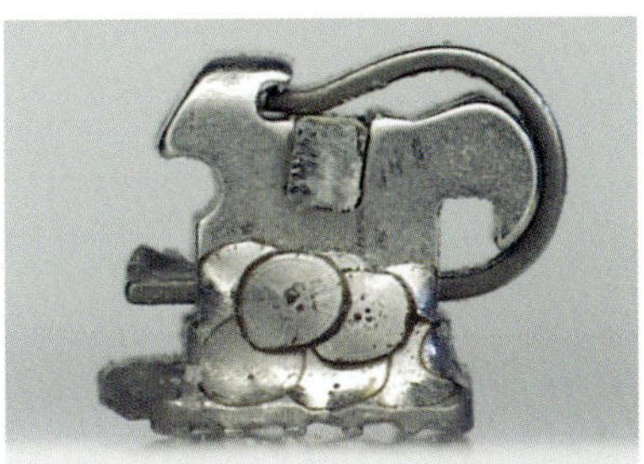

Fig. 3.28 A Speed bracket with a facially coated esthetic 0.021 × 0.025 NiTi archwire. The wire is actively held in the slot. Due to the very narrow and small bracket design, torque and particularly rotational control are often poor. The convenient auxiliary archwire slot is clearly visible in this image.

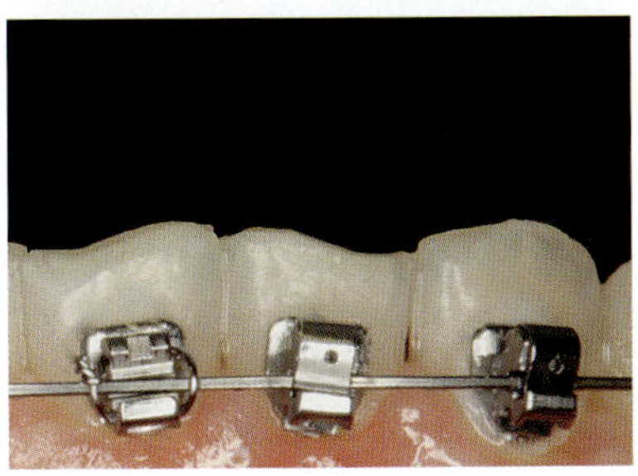

Fig. 3.29 If the clip fails due to material fatigue or technique errors (center bracket), the clip can be removed and the wire can be tied in with a steel or elastomeric ligature (left bracket).

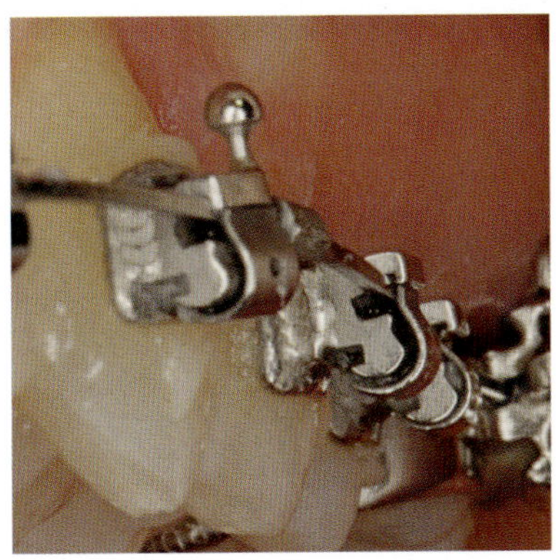

Fig. 3.30 On teeth 23 and 24, the archwire is not engaged in the bracket slot but in the retentive groove for the clip. The clip can still be closed, but it may permanently distort due to the overload.

Time 2 (American Orthodontics)

The Time 2 bracket (**Figs. 3.31** and **3.32**) is an active system with a base and body produced in one piece using the MIM technique. The bracket can be opened with a special tool that is introduced labially, so that the mechanism can be hinged gingivally. The bracket is closed with a specifically designed tool.

Advantages

The Time 2 bracket is easy to position and this does not require extensive additional expertise. The markings are easy to read, and it is easy to open and close. The bracket itself is quite large and may offer good rotational control if the locking mechanism shuts tight.

Disadvantages

Due to the size of the bracket, its esthetic qualities are poor. Elastomeric chains get stuck in the closing mechanism. The locking mechanism itself does not always translate the forces of the clip to the archwire, and rotational and torque control can therefore be difficult. It is often advantageous to use a steel ligature in theses cases.

This is the first bracket in this comparison in which the clip opens on a hinge in the direction in which the active wire pushes. This means that in cases of severe rotation, the force of the wire can lead to opening of the bracket, which then disengages the wire.

Indications

The Time 2 bracket is a large, solid metal bracket, and ligation of heavy archwires (larger than 0.020) is possible. It is a good self-ligating bracket that is well suited for novices in this field.

Contraindications

The bracket is not ideal for patients with small teeth, allergies to any of the alloy components, or high esthetic requirements. Rotational control can be challenging.

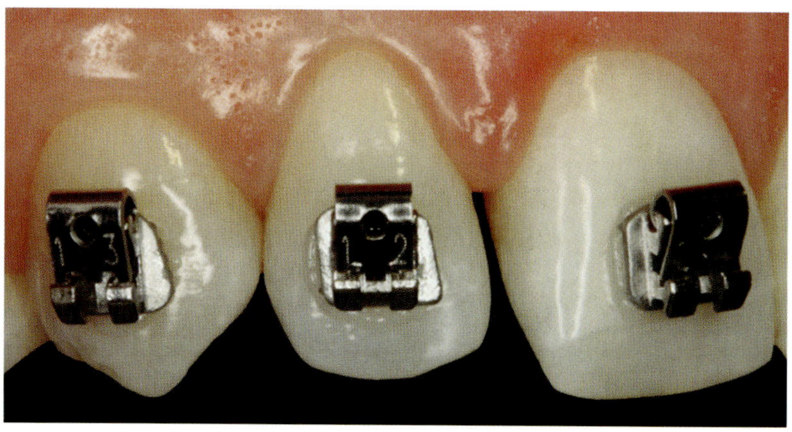

Fig. 3.31 Time 2 is an active bracket. Permanent laser etching allows identification of the bracket. The long axis is not marked.

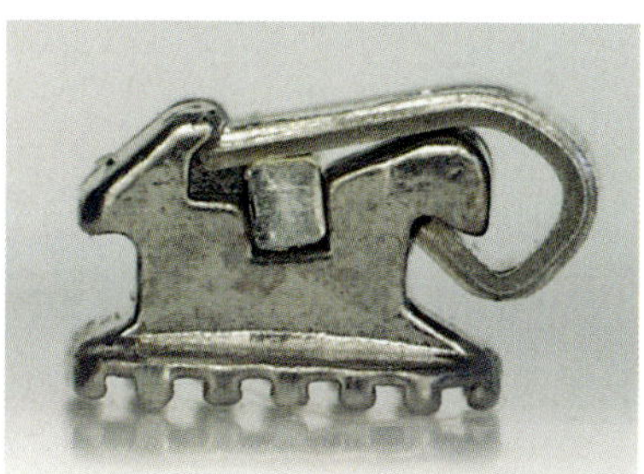

Fig. 3.32 Time 2 with a facially coated esthetic 0.021 × 0.025 NiTi archwire. The wire is actively pressed into the slot. Torque and rotation are often poorly translated to the teeth due to lack of tension. Stainless-steel and elastomeric ligatures can be used to overcome these shortcomings.

Time 3 (American Orthodontics)

The Time 3 bracket (**Fig. 3.33**) is a smaller version of the Time 2 bracket. The bracket base and the body are produced with the MIM technique. This bracket is also opened using a special tool that is introduced labially. It is opened by hinging the door gingivally. The same instrument is used to close the bracket.

Advantages

Opening and closing the Time 3 bracket requires very little additional training to position. The markings are easy to identify.

Disadvantages

Elastomeric chains may interfere with the locking mechanism. The tension exerted by the clip is often not sufficient for full torque and rotational control.

Indications

The Time 3 bracket is a solid medium-sized bracket that allows ligation of even very thick rectangular archwires (larger than 0.020). It can be recommended for novices in the field.

Contraindications

This bracket should not be used for patients who have known allergies to the alloy components of the bracket or high esthetic requirements.

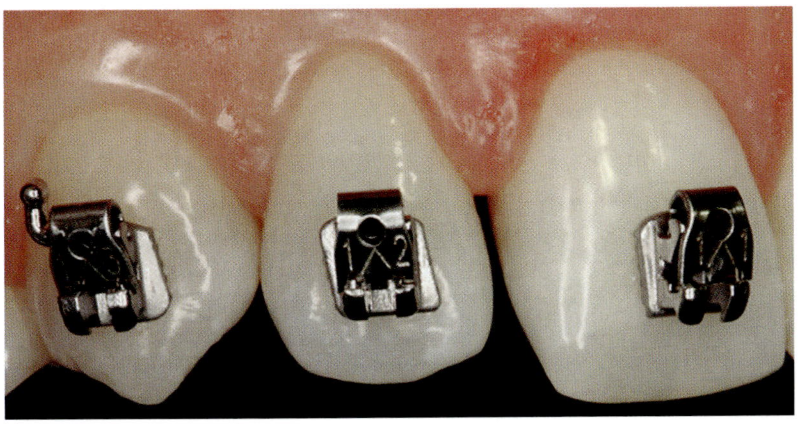

Fig. 3.33 Time 3 bracket. Laser etching allows identification of the bracket. The long axis is not marked.

Vision LP (American Orthodontics)

The Vision LP (**Figs. 3.34** and **3.35**) is an active system with tie-wings. The base and body are produced using the MIM sintering technique. This bracket can be opened with a special instrument or a dental probe. The brackets are opened, again rotating around a gingival hinge, from occlusal to gingival. The bracket can be closed either with a special instrument or by finger pressure.

Advantages

The Vision LP bracket is easy to position. Due to the greater thickness of the brackets, they can debond somewhat more easily than other self-ligating brackets, particularly in the lower jaw. The markings on the bracket are unobtrusive and the bracket is relatively easily opened and closed.

Disadvantages

The tension exerted between the locking mechanism and the archwire is sometimes not strong enough for full rotational and torque control (as described above in the description of the Time 2 bracket). Additional steel ligatures, which can be tied around the tie-wings, may be helpful.

Indications

The Vision LP bracket is a solid, medium-sized metal bracket that allows easy ligation of very heavy archwires (larger than 0.020). Positioning and opening/closing are relatively easy, and the bracket can be used even by novices in self-ligation.

Contraindications

Due to the quite large cavity in the locking mechanism, food debris and plaque can easily become trapped under the archwire. It is often advisable to open the brackets and have the bracket slot cleaned by a professional hygienist, auxiliary, or therapist.

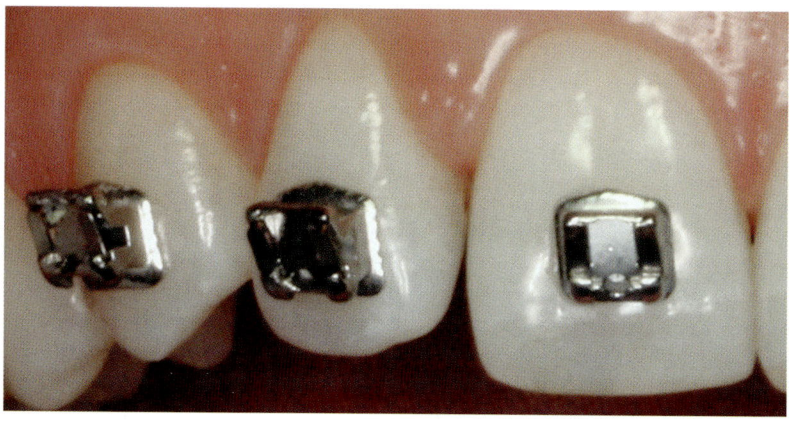

Fig. 3.34 Vision LP bracket. Color coding allows bracket identification. The long axis is not marked.

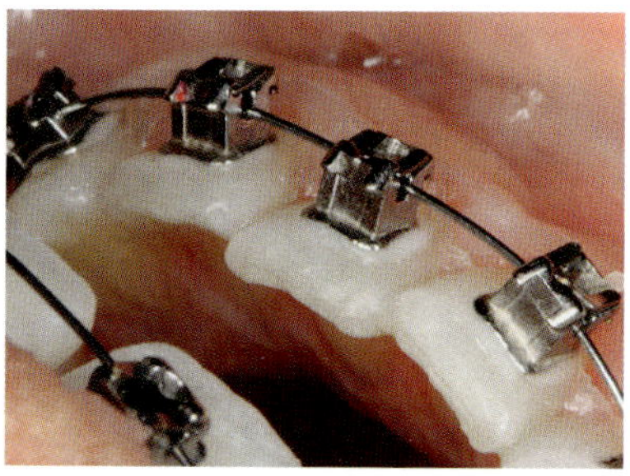

Fig. 3.35 The high-profile construction of the mandibular brackets increases the likelihood of premature contacts with the upper arch which can lead to bracket failure.

Discovery SL (Dentaurum)

The Discovery SL bracket (**Figs. 3.36–3.38**) is a passive system with tie-wings and a well-contoured base. The bracket base and body are produced using the MIM sintering technique. It has a door that serves as an opening/closing mechanism with a hinge, and the mechanism is operated with a special tool in an incisal–gingival direction.

Advantages

The Discovery SL bracket has easily identifiable markings, the well-contoured base allows easy positioning and secure bonding. It has a very smooth surface that does not irritate the soft tissues easily. The tie-wings allow it to be handled in the same way as a regular twin bracket if necessary. Because of its small size, its esthetic qualities are good for a metal self-ligating bracket.

Disadvantages

Opening and closing of the bracket requires some training, as the mechanism appears very small. Rotational and torque control are hence not always ideal, due to the mesiodistal width of the bracket and the direction in which the door opens. However, additional elastomeric ligatures can easily be used to overcome this. Due to the space underneath the clip, however, food and plaque can accumulate.

Indications

The Discovery SL system is a relatively small self-ligating bracket that allows ligation of heavy rectangular archwires (larger than 0.020). Again, this is a good bracket for novices in the field to gain experience in self-ligation.

Contraindications

These brackets should not be used in patients who have known allergies to the metals used to produce the device. The hinge doors may open and disengage the wire. The wires that are too large are chosen too early during the treatment, or if rotations are too severe. This is similar to the problem reported with the Time bracket series.

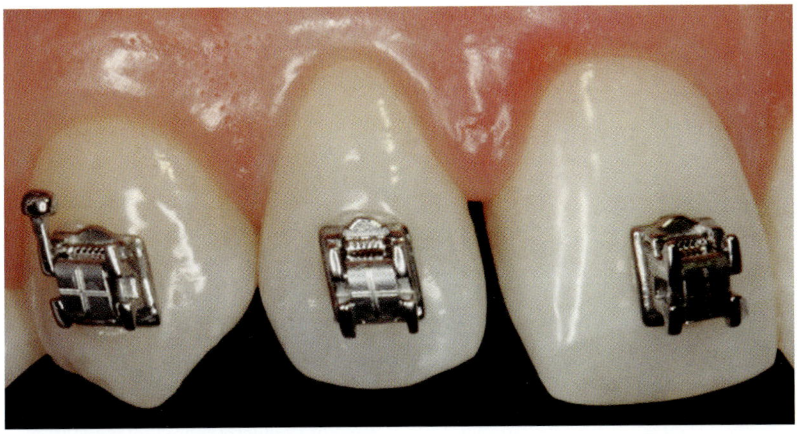

Fig. 3.36 Discovery SL. Permanent laser-etched markings help with the horizontal and vertical positioning of the bracket on the tooth.

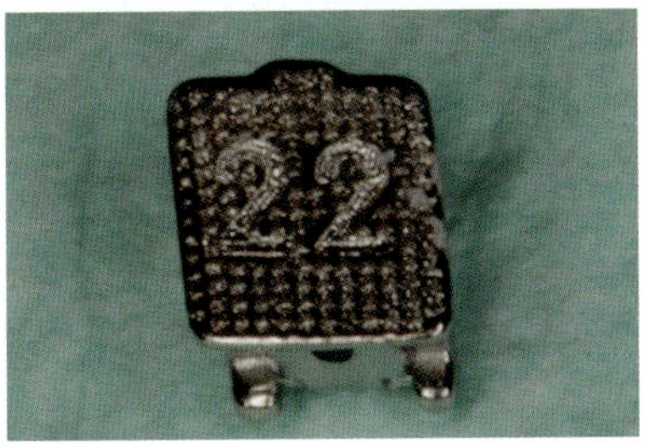

Fig. 3.37

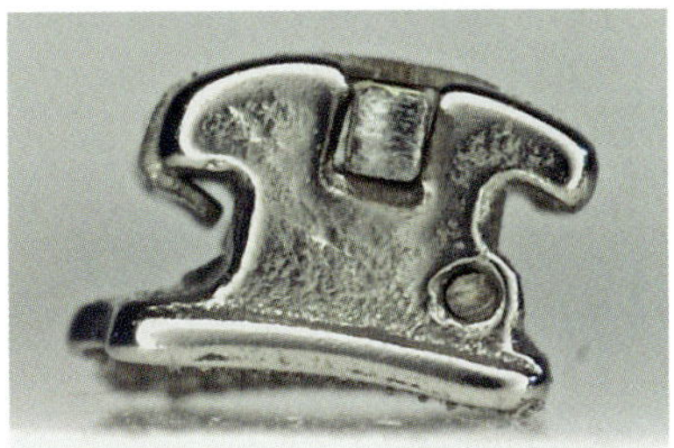

Fig. 3.38

Fig. 3.37 Bracket identification by permanent laser etching on the bracket base.

Fig. 3.38 Discovery SL with a facially coated esthetic 0.021 × 0.025 NiTi archwire. The archwire is engaged passively. Stainless-steel ligatures can be used to ligate the wire.

Table 3.1 A comparison of esthetic self-ligating brackets

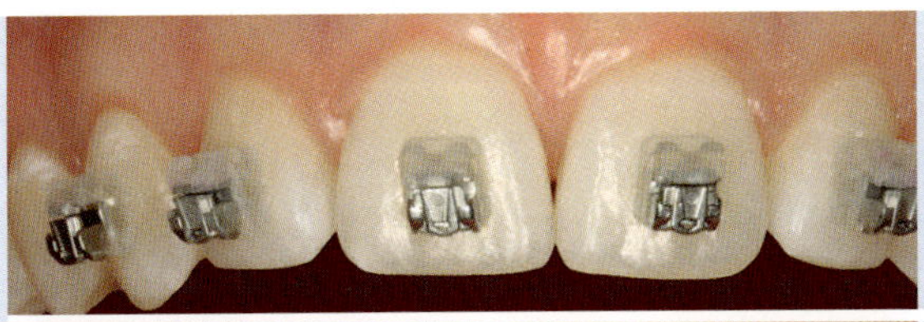	**Damon 3 (Ormco)** + Available for all teeth; useful for narrow teeth – Sometimes poor rotation and torque control, marked abrasion of the acrylic possible
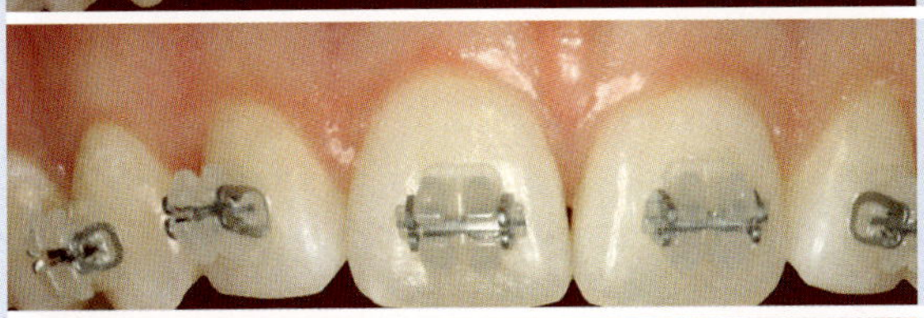	**Clarity SL (3 M Unitek)** + Hygiene easily maintained, even for narrow teeth; discoloration-resistant ceramic – Clips can damage coated esthetic archwires; difficult ligation of larger archwires
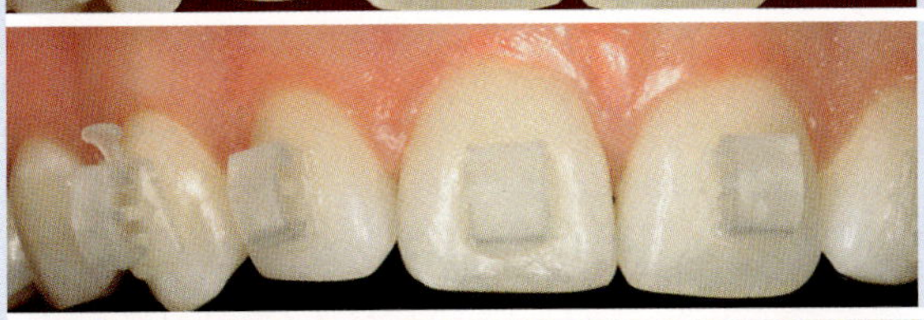	**Opal (Ultradent)** + Good patient comfort at lips and cheeks – Discolorations of acrylic, sometimes poor rotation and torque control
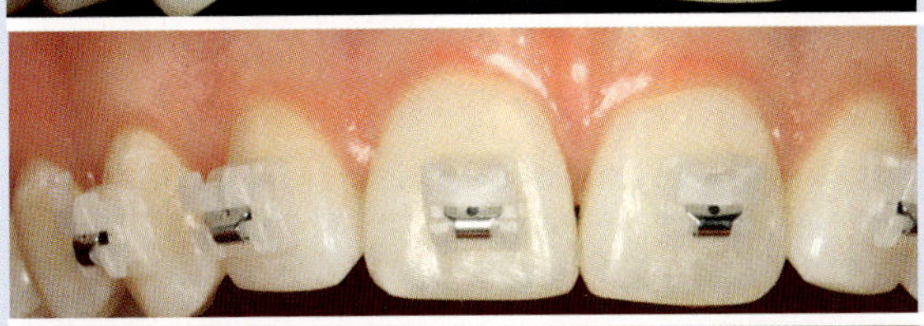	**QuicKlear (Forestadent)** + Discoloration-resistant ceramic; good mechanical properties; resilient clip – Visible clip (more so than for In-Ovation C)
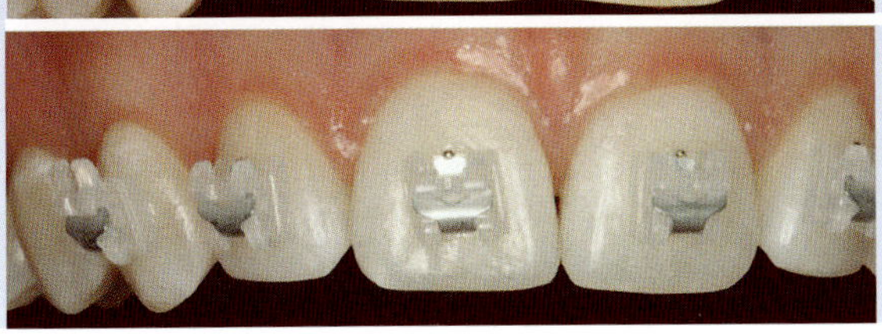	**In-Ovation C (GAC)** + Discoloration-resistant ceramic; good mechanical properties; best combination of esthetics and function – Clip not as resilient as QuicKlear

Table 3.2 A comparison of metal self-ligating brackets

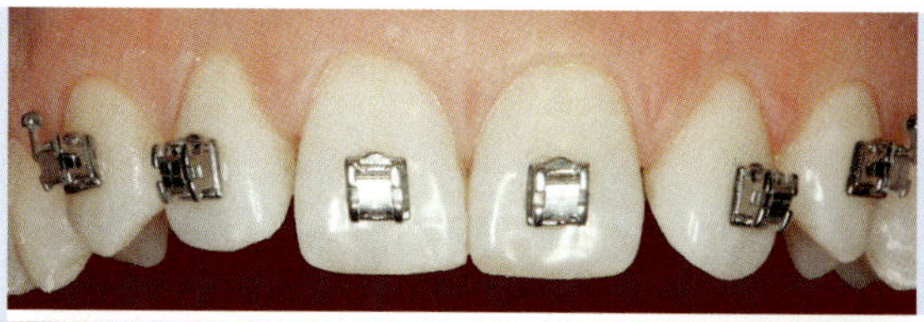	**Discovery SL (Dentaurum)** + Very small, low-profile, lip- and cheek-friendly surface – Due to size and ligation principle (passive), sometimes poor rotation and torque control
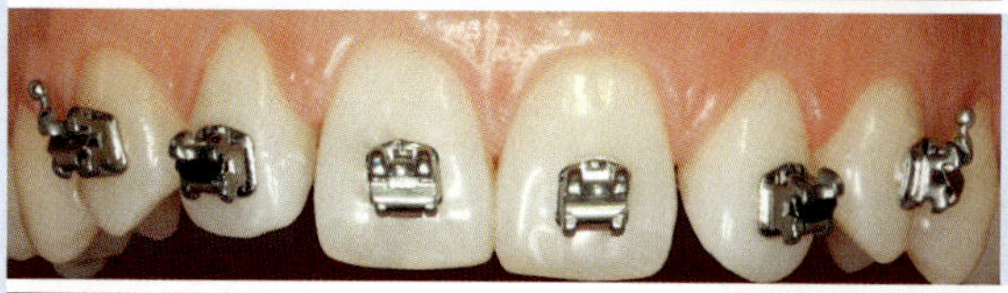	**In-Ovation R (GAC)** + Very good rotation and torque control; small, smooth-running door – Initial irritation of lips and cheeks possible due to surface properties
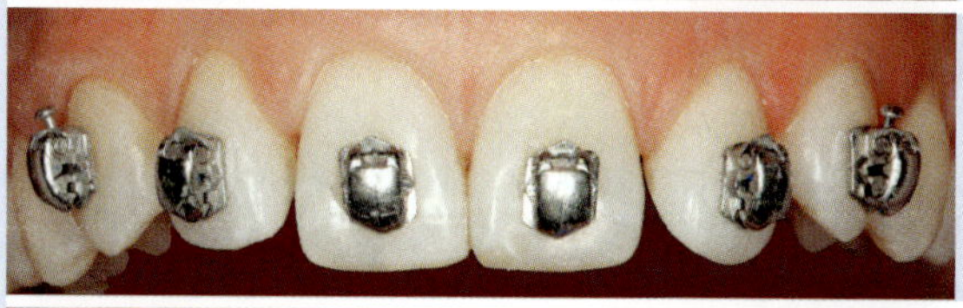	**Opal M (Ultradent)** + Smooth surface, due to ligation characteristics (passive): – shortcomings in rotation and torque control, elastomeric chain can get caught
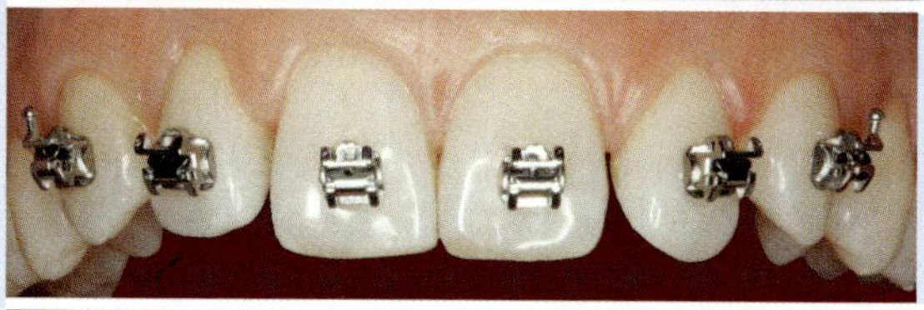	**Quick 2 (Forestadent)** + Very good rotation and torque control; small, precise and smooth-running mechanism – Initial irritation of lips and cheeks possible due to surface properties
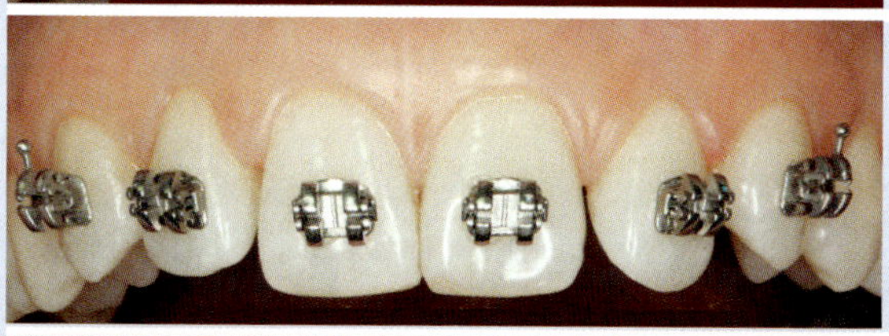	**SmartClip (3 M Unitek)** + very good rotation control, bonding like "regular" twin-bracket – poor torque control, discomfort during ligation of archwires
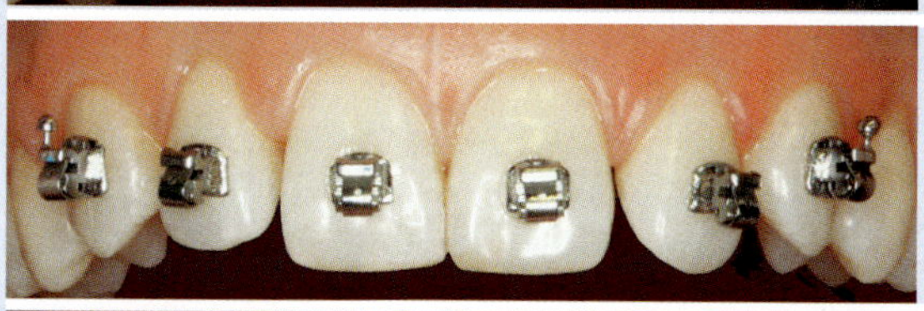	**Speed (Strite Industries)** + Very small; inexpensive; locking mechanism is easy to operate but seizes easily – Due to the small size: poor rotation control, moderate manufacturing quality, binding of archwires possible
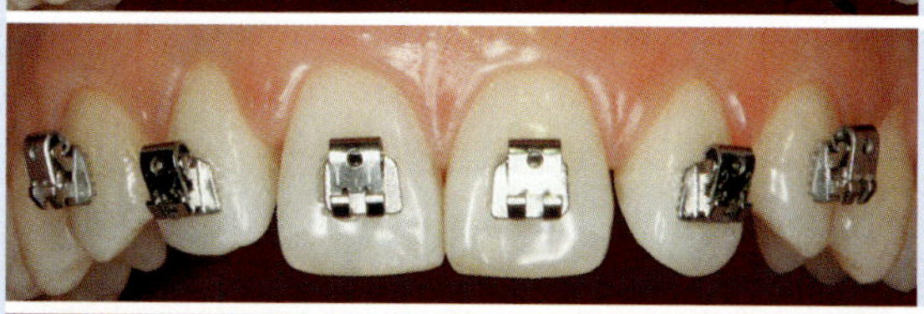	**Time 2 (American Orthodontics)** + Easy to bond, easy application of elastic chains – Due to poor tension of clip: rotation and torque control resemble a passive bracket, elastic chains can get caught
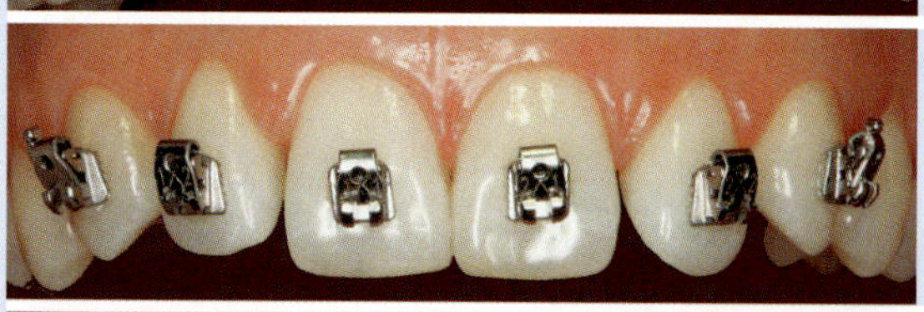	**Time 3 (American Orthodontics)** + Easy to bond, easy application of elastic chains – Due to poor tension of clip: rotation and torque control resemble a passive bracket, elastic chains can get caught
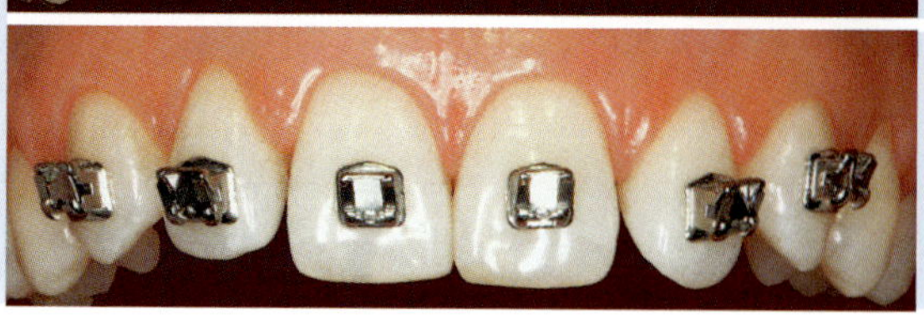	**Vision LP (American Orthodontics)** + Smooth-running mechanism; easy application of elastic chains – Passive bracket with sometimes poor rotation and torque control; high profile; bonding requires practice

Table 3.3 Overview of currently available self-ligating brackets, arranged by material and product name

Bracket Name	Manufacturer	Lock Principle	Type	Material	Available From/since	To	Further information available at …
Self-ligating brackets—metal							
Autonomy SL	Ortho-byte	Passive	Mobile clip	Metal	2006		www.ortho-byte.com
Carriere LX	OrthoOrganizer	Passive	Vertical slider	Metal	2007		www.orthoorganizers.com
Damon 1	Ormco	Passive	Vertical slider	Metal	1996	1999	
Damon 2	Ormco	Passive	Vertical slider	Metal	1999	2005	
Damon MX	Ormco	Passive	Vertical slider	Metal	2007		www.ormco.com
Discovery SL	Dentaurum	Passive	Hinge door	Metal	2008		www.dentaurum.de
Flair	Adenta	Active	Mobile clip	Metal	2005		www.adenta.de
In-Ovation R	GAC	Active	Mobile clip	Metal	1997		www.gacinovation.com
Opal M	Ultradent	Passive	Hinge door	Metal	2007		www.opalorthodontics.com
Praxis Glide	Lancer	Passive	Vertical slider	Metal			www.lancerortho.com
Protect	PT China	Passive	Mobile clip	Metal	2008		
Quick	Forestadent	Active	Mobile clip	Metal	2005	2007	
Quick 2.0	Forestadent	Active	Mobile clip	Metal	2007		www.forestadent.de
SmartClip, first-generation	3 M Unitek	Passive	Static clip	Metal	2004	2006	
SmartClip, second-generation	3 M Unitek	Passive	Static clip	Metal	2006		http://solutions.3 m.com/wps/portal/3m/en_us/ orthodontics/unitek/
Speed	Strite Industries	Active	Mobile clip	Metal	1976		
SureSeries Self-Ligating	Denrum	Passive	Vertical slider	Metal	2007		www.denrum.com.cn
SWLF Synergy R	Rocky Mountain	Passive	Convertible lid	Metal	2007		www.rmortho.com
T3	American Orthodontics	Active	Mobile Clip	Metal			www.americanortho.com
Tenbrook Axis	Ortho Classic	Passive	Rotating slider	Metal	2008		www.orthoclassic.com
Time	Adenta	Active	Mobile clip	Metal	1994		www.adenta.de
Time 2	American Orthodontics	Active	Mobile clip	Metal			www.americanortho.com
Vision LP	American Orthodontics	Passive	Mobile clip	Metal	2007		www.americanortho.com
Self-ligating brackets—tooth-colored							
Clarity-SL	3 M Unitek	Passive		Ceramic	2007		http://solutions.3 m.com/wps/portal/3 m/en_us/orthodontics/unitek/
Clippy C	Tomy	Passive	Mobile clip	Ceramic	2007		www.tomyinc.co.jp
Damon 3	Ormco	Passive	Vertical slider	Acrylic + metal	2005		www.ormco.com
In-Ovation C	GAC	Active	Mobile clip	Ceramic	2007		www.gacinovation.com
Opal	Ultradent	Passive	Hinge door	Acrylic	2004	2008	
Oyster 2.0	Gestenco	Passive	Hinge door	Acrylic			www.gestenco.com
QuicKlear	Forestadent	Active	Mobile clip	Ceramic	2008		www.forestadent.de
Self-ligating brackets—lingual							
Clippy L	Tomy	Passive	Mobile clip	Metal			www.tomyinc.co.jp
Evolution	Adenta	Active	Mobile clip	Metal			www.adenta.com
In-Ovation L	GAC	Active	Mobile clip	Metal			www.gacinovation.com
Phantom	Gestenco	Passive	Hinge door	Composite			www.gestenco.com
2 D Bracket	Forestadent	Active	Static clip	Metal			www.forestadent.de
2 D Bracket, third-generation	Forestadent	Active	Static clip	Metal	2008		www.forestadent.de

Treatment

Manufacturers of self-ligating bracket systems claim that these systems have a number of advantages over conventional ligation, such as that treatment can be achieved more quickly and more effectively, and that the brackets in combination with the recommended archwires exert lower forces and there is consequently less risk of root resorption. Self-ligation is also thought to allow better oral hygiene and cause less discomfort during treatment. A number of these claims are discussed below in greater detail, focusing particularly on the following claims:

1. Chairside time is shorter for each appointment.
2. Overall treatment time is shorter.
3. Self-ligating brackets are more hygienic and easier to keep clean.
4. There are longer intervals between adjustments, so that fewer adjustments are necessary.
5. The dental practice is able to work with fewer staff.

Shorter Chairside Time

It is essential to have appropriate and well-established reference standards to test the theory that self-ligating brackets lead to reduced chairside time. The authors used the German health-insurance schedule (BEMA 2004), which standardizes the payments dentists receive for itemized dental services, as a basis for assessment. This assessment was based on the following procedures: bonding time for straight-wire brackets; teeth etched and primed separately; elastomeric elements used to ligate the archwires. The time values used for the calculations assumed that the average operator needed the following amount of time per procedure:

1. Approximately 3 minutes for placement of a bracket
2. Approximately 9 minutes for placement and cementing of a band
3. Approximately 9 minutes for an archwire change (removal and placement of a new wire)
4. About 1 minute to remove a bracket or band (per bracket and band)

NOTE

The times mentioned above do not include preparation time, such as time for cleaning surfaces or giving the patient instructions (on oral hygiene, etc.). The focus is therefore exclusively on the time the doctor spends with the patient.

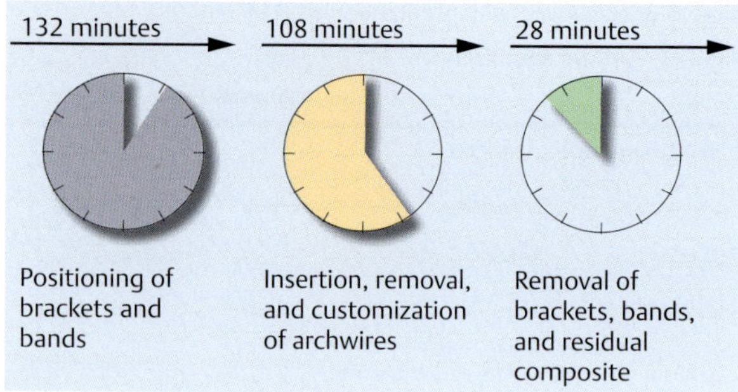

Fig. 3.39 Total chairside time

Using the above data, the average chair times for orthodontic treatment were:

- Bonding: 60 minutes (20 minutes × 3)
- Band placement and cementing: 72 minutes (8 × 9 minutes)
- Archwire change: 108 minutes (12 × 9 minutes; assuming that 12 visits are necessary)
- Remove bands and brackets: 28 minutes (28 × 1 minute)

The average chairside time thus adds up to 268 minutes (**Fig. 3.39**). Only an experienced operator would be able to achieve these times reliably. The above data are used for reference purposes only; no attempt is made here to discuss the validity of the data.

Bonding of Brackets

There is little scope for shortening the bonding time required for self-ligating brackets in comparison with a normal ligation system. It might in fact be argued that due to the physical characteristics of the brackets, as well as the ligation mechanism involved, the bonding time may actually increase rather than decrease. It is more likely that the chairside time could be reduced by using different primers and etching techniques (for example, using a self-etching primer), rather than self-ligating brackets. One could also consider using indirect bonding, which may be able to reduce the chairside time by up to 30 minutes. However, this requires complex and costly laboratory techniques. It is difficult to determine whether the 30 minutes saved during bonding are lost due to the time required for laboratory production of the model used to bond the brackets. Also, an additional impression may need to be taken. However, self-etching primers do reduce chairside time, as it is no longer necessary to remove the phosphoric acid and have a drying step before application of the bond, and the time reduction should be approximately 15 minutes per patient. It has to be taken into consideration, however, that slightly lower bond strengths are obtained with self-etching primers in comparison with the conventional phosphoric acid and bond technique.

NOTE

Self-ligating brackets do not confer any advantage during the bonding procedure. Time savings could potentially be made using indirect bonding techniques and/or with self-etching primers.

Ligation of Archwires

A number of manufacturers claim that less chairside time is required for removing and ligating archwires. We are not aware of any study that confirms this. A direct comparison between self-ligation and standard brackets showed similar times for both methods.[5] However, it is important to remember that changing the elastomeric modules has to be undertaken by an experienced operator. There may be one other potential advantage with self-ligating systems: the operator can open and close the self-ligating brackets easily without any assistance. For efficient and speedy archwire changes using conventional elastomeric modules, it is best to have an assistant handing the modules to the operator. Another advantage may be that self-ligating brackets usually ensure full engagement of the wire, as the locking mechanisms would otherwise not shut properly. This can be important if wire changes are done by less experienced operators who have yet to learn how to spot partially disengaged wires.

It is also worthwhile mentioning that not all bracket-archwire combinations are advisable or indeed possible.[6] The Damon system, for example, works with a rigid locking mechanism. This can make it difficult to ligate thicker rectangular wires, and occasionally it is difficult to open or close the clip. The manufacturer recommends specific archwire sequences to avoid these potential issues (**Fig. 3.40**).

The same also applies for 3 M's SLBs. For example, it is not possible to engage a 0.017 × 0.025 Turbo-NiTi (Ormco) in a SmartClip or Clarity SL bracket (**Fig. 3.41**). In general, it is uncomfortable for patients who are being treated with these brackets to use wires that are larger than 0.021 × 0.021 (NiTi or stainless steel).

A shorter procedure time with SLBs is only evident in comparison with ligating an entire arch using steel ligatures.[7]

NOTE

Even an experienced operator may find it challenging to complete an archwire change in both upper and lower arches in less than 9 minutes, the basic value established by health insurance companies in Germany for reimbursement to dentists (BEMA).

Another important aspect of the treatment is often not mentioned by the manufacturers—i.e., the possibility of using elastomeric chains. There are significant differences between self-ligating bracket systems in this respect. Some systems do not even allow silicone or elastomeric chains to be used under or over the archwire. Bracket systems with a very rounded design may make it very challenging for elastic chains to be used at all (**Fig. 3.42**). Elastomeric chains interfere with the locking mechanism of some self-ligating systems. This applies in particular to the Discovery SL bracket (Dentaurum), the Time 2 and Time 3 brackets (American Orthodontics), and the Flare bracket (Adenta). Other self-ligating brackets make it difficult, if not impossible, to ligate silicone elastomeric chains on top of the archwire. The Speed bracket, for example, has no retention for attaching a chain on top of the archwire. Some composite-based materials with poor abrasion characteristics (e.g., Damon 3) may lose their capacity to engage an elastomeric chain (**Fig. 3.43**). Removing the archwires can also be difficult in patients with significant calculus accumulation, which is often more pronounced in adult patients. Passive brackets (such as Damon) can be particularly difficult to open and close (**Fig. 3.44**) in such cases. Some manufacturers recommend using vinegar or 37% phosphoric acid to overcome the blockage of the system. "Airflow" and "sandblasting" have also been recommended. Any of the above methods would certainly eliminate any potential advantages of self-ligation over conventional ligation.

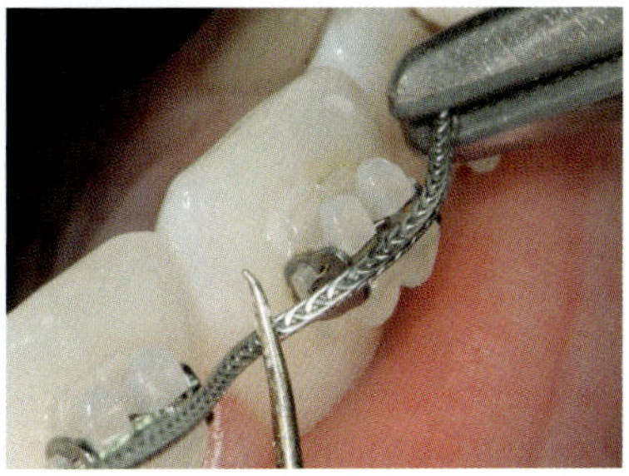

Fig. 3.40 Failure to engage a braided 0.017 × 0.025 Turbo-NiTi into a Clarity SL bracket.

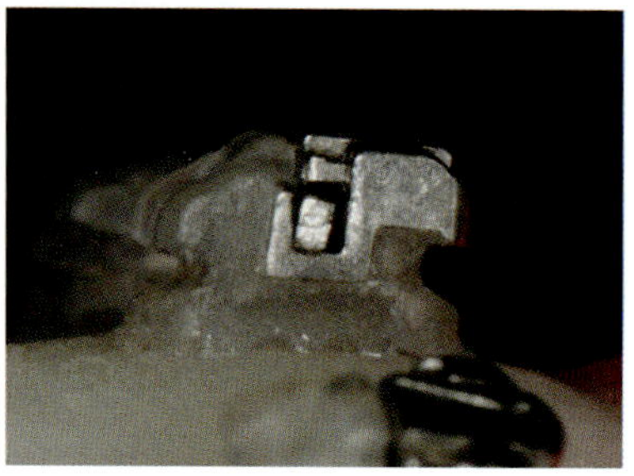

Fig. 3.41 A 0.014 × 0.025 NiTi archwire in a Damon 3 bracket. These archwire sizes are used to improve torque and rotational control of passive self-ligating brackets.

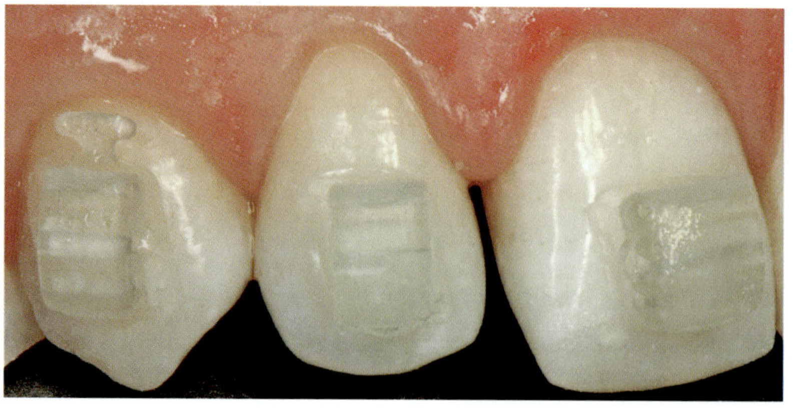

Fig. 3.42 Opal Bracket (Ultradent). The nicely rounded surface of the bracket makes this bracket easy to tolerate. However, it provides little undercut for the application of elastomeric ligatures or chains.

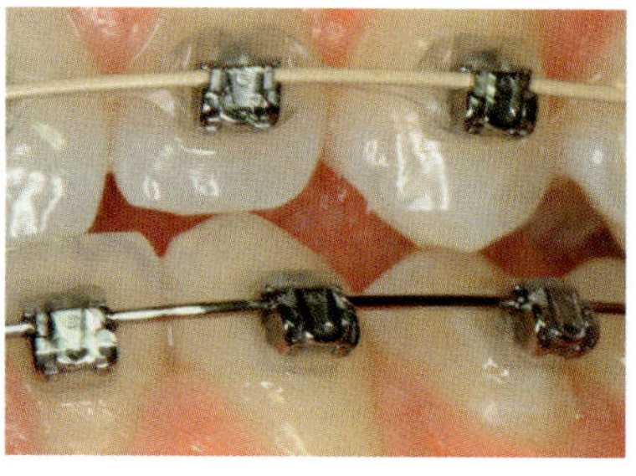

Fig. 3.43 Damon 3 brackets after 12 months of use. Abrasions on the acrylic incisal tie-wings make them unusable in the lower jaw.

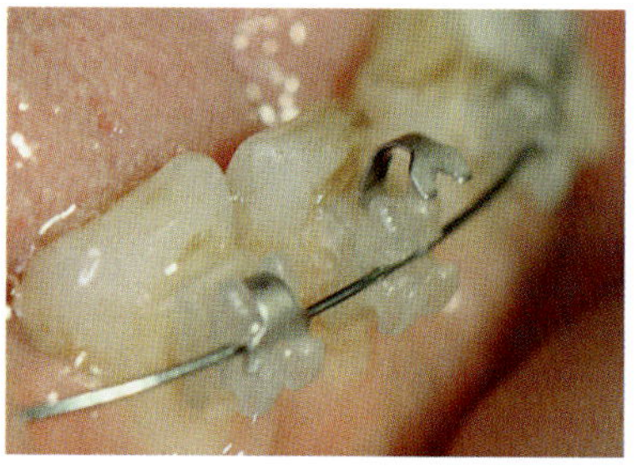

Fig. 3.44 Innovation C bracket (GAC). Inappropriate handling led to permanent deformation of the bracket clip. After removal of this clip, the bracket can still be used with a conventional elastic or steel ligature.

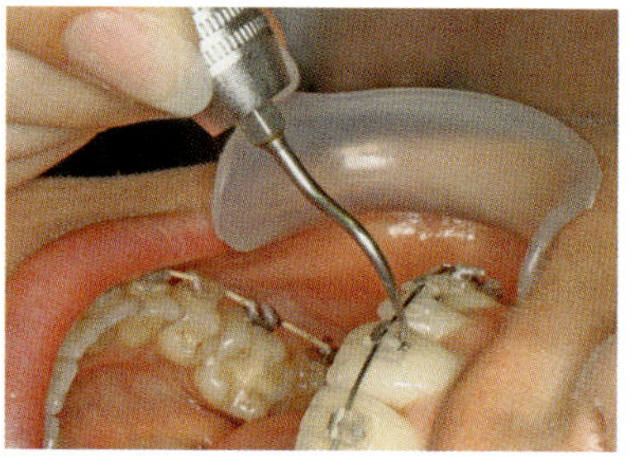

Fig. 3.45 An ultrasonic cleaner can be a valuable auxiliary tool to open self-ligating brackets once the mechanisms have become difficult to open; this is often due to accumulation of calculus or food debris.

CLINICAL PEARL

Ultrasound cleaning devices can be used to reestablish the mechanism used in self-ligating brackets, particularly in patients with increased calculus accumulation (**Fig. 3.45**). Ceramic brackets may fracture when using ultrasound cleaning devices.

NOTE

It is unlikely that there is any time-saving in comparison with conventional ligation during ligation or removal of archwires using a self-ligation system. However, fewer staff may be needed, as the ligation and removal of archwires can be carried out by a single operator rather than with a four-handed technique, which requires two operators. It needs to be borne in mind that chairside time may occasionally be prolonged due to mechanical problems associated with the opening and closing of self-ligating brackets.

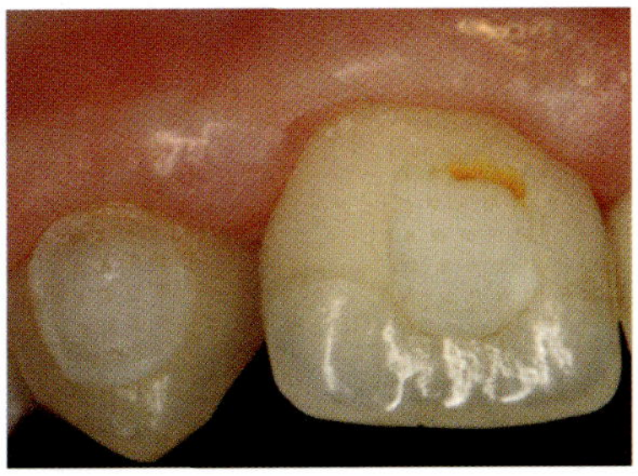

Fig. 3.46

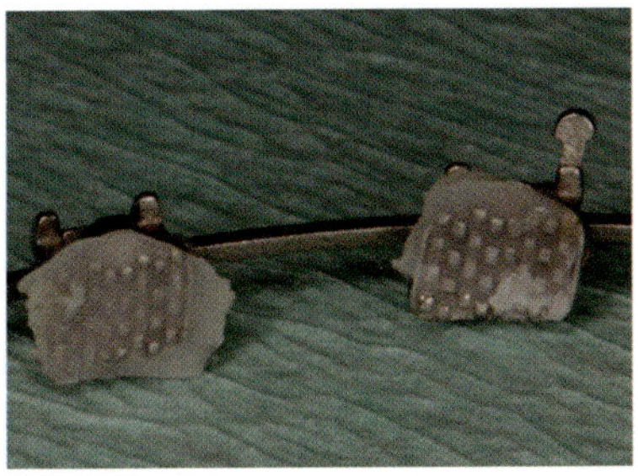

Fig. 3.47

Fig. 3.46 Composite residues on the patient's tooth after removal of a Damon 3 bracket. Removal of the composite requires significant chairside time and may cause discomfort to the patient. The bracket pad on tooth 11 was not fully coated with composite, leading to plaque accumulation on the mesiogingival aspect.

Fig. 3.47 Very little composite removal was required after debonding. The bracket base of this Quick 2 bracket retained virtually all the composite.

Debonding of the Fixed Appliances

There are significant differences when debonding brackets, because manufacturers pursue one of two goals: brackets such as Damon 3 and Opal usually leave a large amount of composite on the tooth on debonding (**Fig. 3.46**). The advantage claimed for this is that it reduces the vulnerability of the enamel on debonding, which occurs at the bracket–adhesive interface, with no risk to the enamel. However, the operator needs to remember that removing any residual composite is time-consuming and may also be traumatic to the tooth.

NOTE

Additional time may have to be spent to remove residual composite when using some of the self-ligating systems.

In an ideal situation, the operator would like the bonding agent to be completely attached to the bracket after debonding, so that the cleaning-up process is shortened or even eliminated (**Fig. 3.47**). However, this type of approach could lead to enamel fractures in rare cases, as the debonding would occur at the adhesive–enamel interface.

NOTE

Using self-ligating brackets does not reduce the treatment time on debonding in comparison with normal ligation. In fact, some self-ligating brackets create a significant disadvantage if all the composite is left on the tooth surface at debonding.

Repairs

The need for regular repairs of self-ligating brackets has been significantly reduced in the last few years. This is due to improved manufacturing techniques, and improved engineering based on clinical experience which have made the systems more robust.

However, the picture is not homogeneous across the whole range of self-ligating brackets. For example, the Damon 3 bracket often shows significant abrasion of the tie-wings after some use (**Fig. 3.48**). This does not affect the mechanical properties of the bracket in terms of rotational and torque control, as the wire-bearing metal portion of the bracket is not affected by the abrasions. Loss of the acrylic tie-wings, however, leads to reduced functionality for auxiliaries such as power chains or steel ligatures. It is interesting to note that the passive systems in particular often need steel ligatures to fully engage a wire, correct rotations, and transfer maximum torque (**Figs. 3.49** and **3.50**). The same also applies to the Damon 3 metal bracket, where issues with rotational and torque control have been reported.[8] One advantage of the full metal version is the increased stability of the stainless-steel tie-wings, which can now be used reliably for retention of elastic chains or steel ligatures.

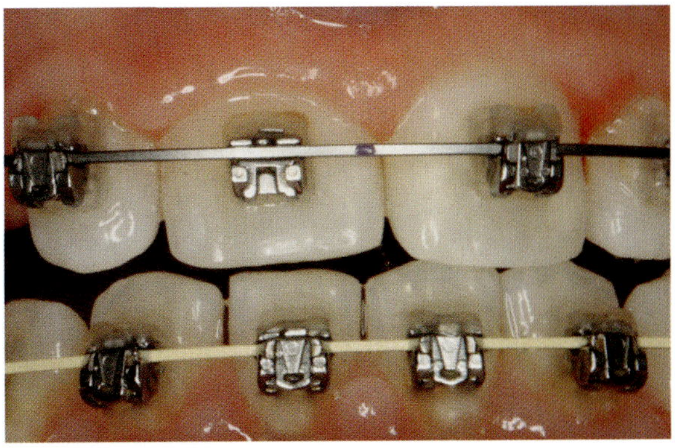

Fig. 3.48 While abrasions and discolorations on a Damon 3 bracket are almost always noticeable after some time, the loss of clips is a rare occurrence (tooth 11).

Another reason for repairs may be bracket loss (i.e., failure between the adhesive and the bracket base, or between the adhesive and tooth surface). Recent years have seen tremendous improvements in this field, thanks to advanced bracket base designs, better adhesives, and conditioning agents. Bonding has become easy and intuitive with most brackets. However, when acrylic self-ligating brackets such as the Opal system are used, the procedure is different and it becomes important to adhere strictly to the manufacturer's instructions. It is recommended in particular that a primer should be placed on the bracket base and on the preconditioned (preetched) enamel surface. The adhesive is then added and subsequently light-cured. Any additional conditioning, such as sandblasting of the bracket base or additional time for bracket primer, does not improve the failure rates. The use of self-etching primers is not recommended for Opal brackets.

In case of bracket loss, we have found that active self-ligating brackets are easier to repair than passive self-ligating brackets. The active self-ligating brackets often tolerate slight changes in the bracket positioning after the repair, while passive systems often will not (**Fig. 3.51**).

NOTE

Passive self-ligating systems have a rigid locking mechanism, which may require reduction of the archwire size or use of an archwire material with greater elasticity following repositioning of a lost bracket.

NOTE

The chair time is generally not reduced when self-ligating brackets are used. The only noticeable advantage of using self-ligating brackets in relation to chair time is the ability to change archwires without needing an assistant (two-handed dentistry in contrast to four-handed dentistry). This potential advantage can amount to approximately 108 minutes in the overall treatment time. The assistant can then be used for other tasks, such as oral hygiene instruction, etc. However, this has to be seen in the light of other unknown factors that may occur when self-ligating brackets are used, such as their different mechanical properties.

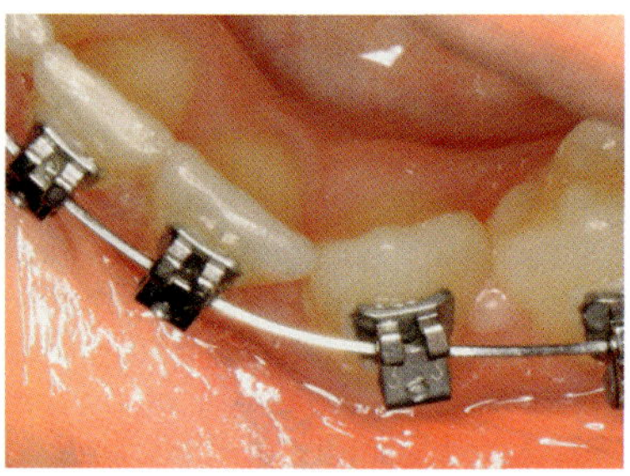

Fig. 3.49 Poor rotational control on tooth 33. The clip was damaged.

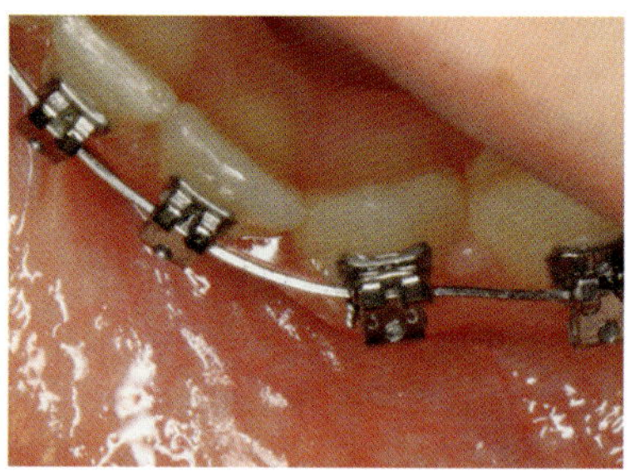

Fig. 3.50 Improved rotational control due to use of a steel ligature in a Time 2 bracket (American Orthodontics).

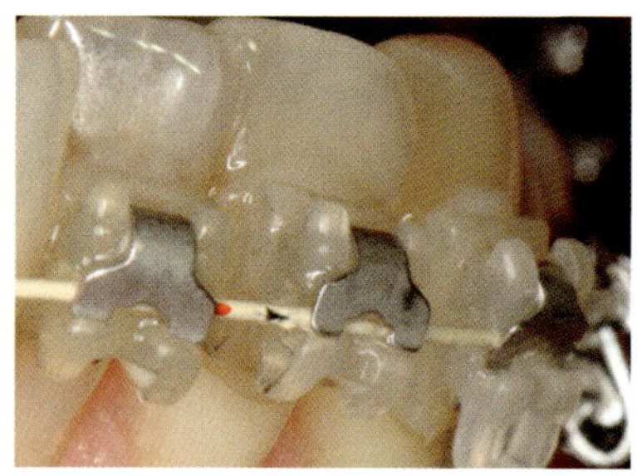

Fig. 3.51 A clip with some elasticity can be very useful when brackets have been repositioned or replaced; it is not always necessary to step back to a smaller archwire. The clip on this Innovation C bracket is stretched to its limits, however.

Reduction of Overall Treatment Time

In general, the overall orthodontic treatment time consists of two components—active treatment (movement of the teeth with appliances) and the retention phase.

Active Treatment

The active treatment is often subdivided into the following categories:

- Leveling and alignment
- Space closure and correction of molar relationship
- Detailing and finishing

Treatment data for 350 well-documented cases provided the basis for the following observations.

Leveling and alignment. Self-ligating systems showed significantly faster tooth movement during the leveling and aligning phase (**Fig. 3.52**). The reason for this is probably the reduced friction of the self-ligating system in comparison with conventional ligation. The main movements during this phase of treatment are extrusion of teeth and tipping of the crowns. These movements can be achieved readily and easily, as clinical experience shows.[9–11] One of the fastest and most efficient movements in orthodontics is the extrusion of teeth, but tipping of teeth can also be achieved quickly and efficiently. With conventional ligation, elastomeric or metal ligatures prevent free sliding of the archwire through the bracket slot, which is essential for efficient tooth movement. This is generally not observed with self-ligating brackets. It is worth remembering, however, that similar results can be obtained by using conventional brackets with loosely tied steel ligatures, and investigations by Fuck et al.[3] appear to confirm this. The study compared the frictional characteristics of a number of self-ligating brackets and compared them with conventional brackets, which had archwires tied either using elastomeric or stainless steel ligatures. It was found that self-ligating brackets have reduced frictional characteristics in comparison with classic brackets with elastomeric ligatures. However, the investigation also demonstrated that the frictional characteristics of self-ligating brackets were similar to those of conventional brackets using loose steel ties for ligation. It is important to remember that the time required for archwire change (9 minutes), the standardized value used in the health-insurance system in Germany, is based on using elastomeric modules rather than stainless-steel ties. It is used as the standard reference value here, as it applies to 90% of orthodontic patients in Germany (**Fig. 3.53**).

NOTE

Elastomeric ligatures may reduce the speed of tooth movement during leveling and alignment. Self-ligating brackets have similar frictional characteristics to conventional brackets with loose stainless-steel ties. Some in-vitro studies have confirmed that all self-ligating systems show better frictional characteristics in comparison with conventional brackets and elastomeric ligatures.

The effectiveness of leveling and alignment, however, depends not only on the bracket system, but also on the archwires used. The most important factor is not necessarily the dimension of the archwire, but rather the force that is translated from the bracket to the tooth, as shown by Pandis et al. in 2007.[12] Another very important factor affecting the efficiency of tooth movement is the surface characteristics of the archwires themselves.[13,14] Manufacturers are already developing archwires that have reduced frictional characteristics.

NOTE

It is not necessarily the bracket or the archwire alone, but rather the combination of the two, that plays an important role in the efficiency of leveling and alignment of the dentition.

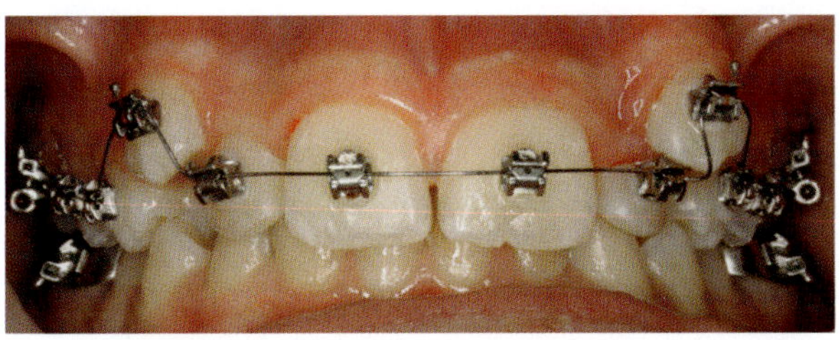

Fig. 3.52 Quick 2 bracket system. The advantages of self-ligating brackets become clear in the leveling and alignment phase. Assuming there is sufficient space in the arch, alignment of the upper canines can be expected within 3 months and without proclination of the upper labial segment.

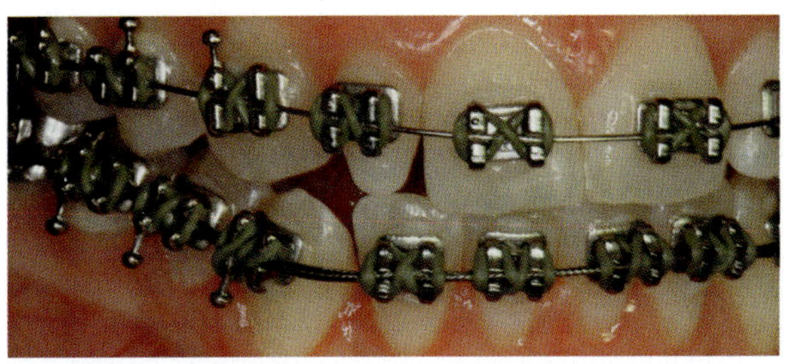

Fig. 3.53 The BEMA sets the standard of care for about 90% of all patients in Germany and assumes the use of elastomeric ligatures as a standard.

An unwanted side effect of using self-ligating brackets, particularly in nonextraction cases, is nonocclusion in the buccal segments, tending towards a scissors (Brodie) bite. It is not entirely clear why this happens. We recommend changing the archwires around for such cases, so that the upper archwire is used in the lower jaw and the lower archwire is used in the upper jaw (**Fig. 3.54**). It appears that the cause of this nonocclusion is rooted in the jaw(s). During the alignment of the upper jaw in the first step of treatment, a tipping movement occurs, in which the upper premolars and molars are moved buccally. One often notes the "hanging" palatal cusps of the upper premolars and molars. In the lower jaw, however, the teeth are initially moved lingually, resulting in the tendency for a Brodie bite to develop. These side effects can best be explained by the biomechanical effects of leveling the curve of Spee in the straight wire technique, which tends to tip the maxillary buccal segments buccally and the mandibular buccal segments lingually. This tendency may be explained by the differential thickness of the buccal and lingual cortical plates of the respective alveolar processes.

CLINICAL PEARL

To avoid the potential negative side effect of labial tipping of the upper buccal segment and lingual tipping of the lower buccal segment during the leveling and alignment phase, we recommend exchanging the upper archwire to the lower jaw and the lower archwire to the upper jaw (**Fig. 3.54**).

Space closure and finishing. In our retrospective analysis of treated cases, we did not observe any advantage for self-ligating brackets for either of the above treatment phases.[15,16] However, it is interesting to note that the differences in the self-ligating group were quite large. The determining factors here were the material characteristics as well as the production quality of the brackets. Most problems occurred in the group of the acrylic-based brackets. We found that the Opal bracket was the least useful for most indications; we were unable to produce good tip and torque values with it (**Fig. 3.55**). It was very difficult to use elastomeric chains for space closure or to stabilize teeth in a particular position.

Another important issue is resistance to abrasion in composite brackets. The Damon 3 bracket was not very resistant to abrasion. While it did not show significant failure rates and delivered good torque expression, we found that there was a considerable amount of abrasion between the contacts of the upper dentition and the lower brackets (**Fig. 3.56**). It appears that size, material characteristics, and manufacturing had a noticeable impact on the biomechanical properties and thus indirectly on the treatment time. From the sample, we drew the following conclusions:

- Active systems express better rotational control than passive ones (**Table 3.4**).
- The smaller the brackets, the poorer their mechanical properties in terms of rotation and torque control.
- The less expensive the brackets are, the less well made they generally are, and this has an impact on the mechanical properties of the bracket (**Fig. 3.57**)
- Archwire sequences suggested by the manufacturers are tailored to fit particular bracket systems, and changing the sequences may be disadvantageous in terms of treatment duration and the quality of the final result.

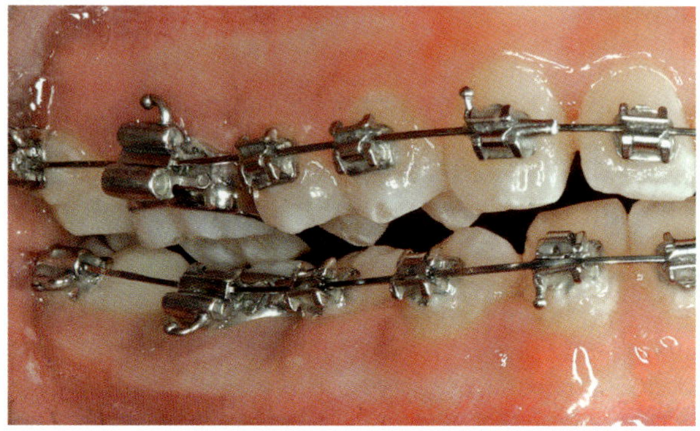

Fig. 3.54 Tendency toward buccal crossbite (scissors bite, Brodie bite). To remedy this situation, we recommend using an upper archwire for the lower jaw and a lower archwire for the upper jaw.

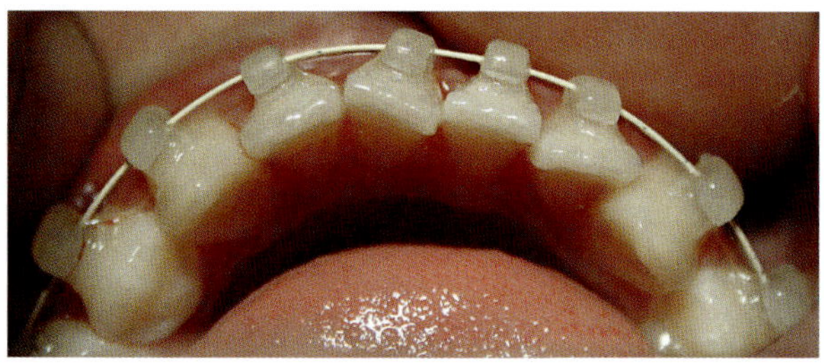

Fig. 3.55 The material properties of Opal brackets are poor: the archwire is engaged in the bracket slots without any activation, and yet the teeth are still rotated. Thicker archwires may be able to improve the situation. However, the elastic properties of the bracket do not always allow full rotational control.

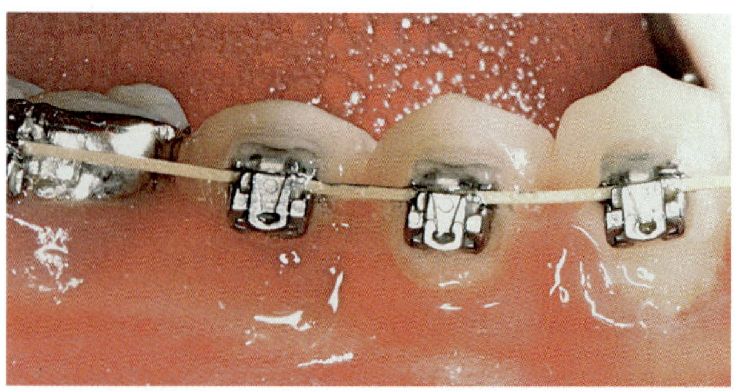

Fig. 3.56 Strong abrasions on the acrylic tie-wings of an Ormco bracket are clearly visible. However the clip mechanism is not affected.

NOTE

While all self-ligating brackets perform better during the leveling and alignment phase than conventional ligation, for space closure and detailing the bracket quality and size play a more important role than the method of ligation used.

To achieve all the potential advantages of self-ligating brackets, one sometimes has to resort to auxiliaries such as anterior bite planes (**Fig. 3.58**). Using these auxiliaries can be advantageous, as they disocclude the dentition and have the potential to reduce bond failures in deep bites. Treatment mechanics can also be applied at lower force levels, and class II correction may be facilitated as interdigitation no longer hinders the correction of the buccal segments.

Retention

The retention of the occlusion can be achieved in many different ways. Some practices use a gnathologic positioner or Osamu retainers for this. Very good results can also be achieved with functional appliances, but these have to be meticulously adjusted for full effect. It is also often advisable to use bonded retainers to maintain the alignment of the labial segments in particular. Some authors also recommend occlusal adjustment of the dentition to improve the stability of the orthodontic result. As a general rule, we would recommend that the more significant the changes in tooth position and occlusion, the more sophisticated the longer the retention regime should be. However, this will depend not only on the characteristics of the original malocclusion, but also on patient expectations.

Table 3.4 Reduced rotational control with passive brackets

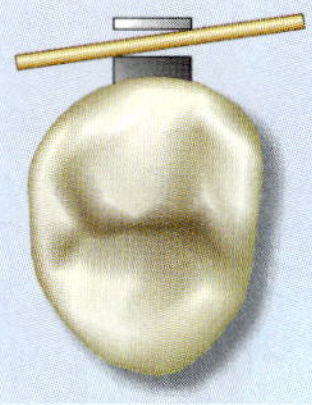	Loss of rotational control of about 10° due to the narrow design of the bracket when a 0.016 archwire is used
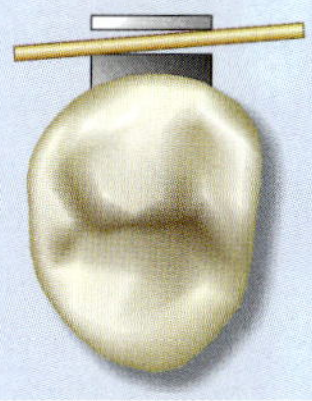	Loss of rotational control of only about 6°, due to the wider design of the SmartClip bracket when a 0.016 archwire is used
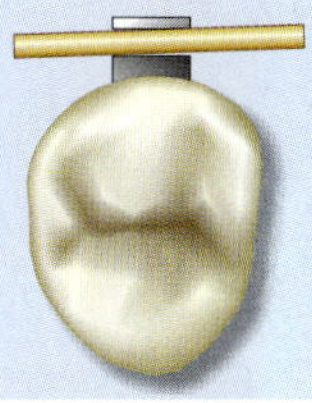	Loss of rotational control of about 4°, due to the narrow design of the bracket when a 0.019 × 0.025 archwire is used
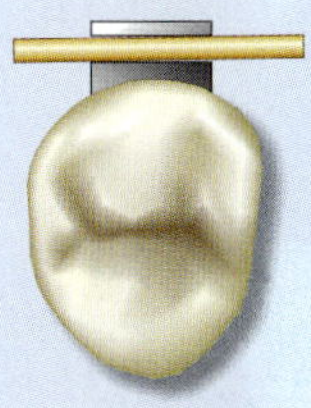	Loss of rotational control of only about 2°, due to the wider design of the SmartClip bracket when a 0.019 × 0.025 archwire is used

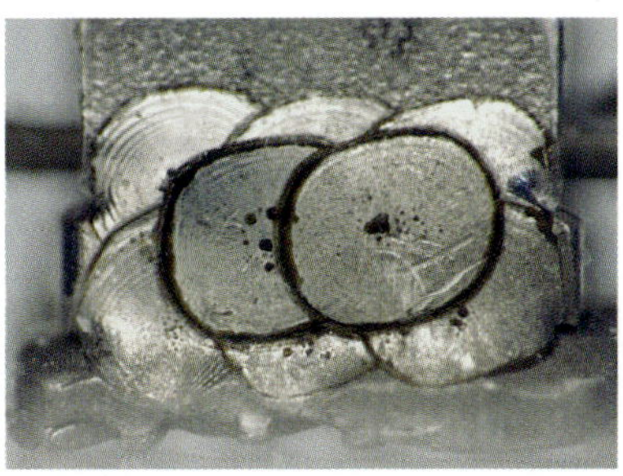

Fig. 3.57

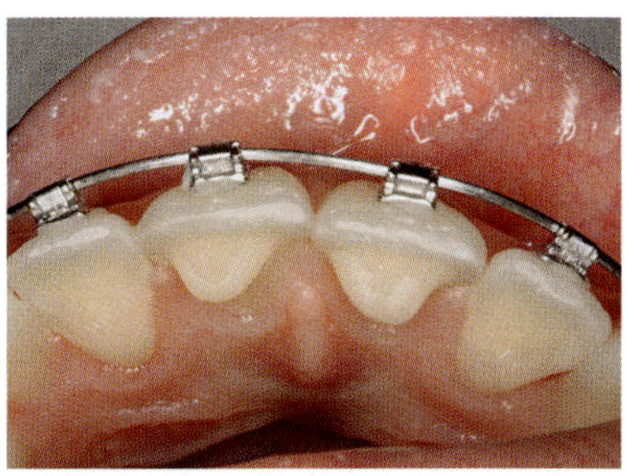

Fig. 3.58

Fig. 3.57 Detailed view of a Speed bracket before insertion. The two-piece design of this bracket is clearly visible.

Fig. 3.58 Anterior bite plane.

NOTE

The overall treatment time with self-ligating fixed appliances and the retention period after treatment are not reduced when compared to conventional ligation. Although we can confirm that leveling and alignment may be slightly more efficient with self-ligating systems, we did not observe any shortening of the overall treatment time; indeed, some tooth movements may take longer when self-ligating systems are used. We would also suggest that the retention phase is likely to be longer with self-ligation, particularly if a nonextraction approach is used.

Oral Hygiene of Self-Ligating Brackets

Most orthodontic practices use elastomeric rings made of polyurethane and/or silicone for ligation of conventional bracket systems. It is well known that these retain plaque, and it has therefore been suggested that self-ligating brackets have an advantage over elastomeric systems (**Figs. 3.59–3.66**).

For comparison, our study used the bracket-plaque index as well as the orthodontic plaque index, the sulcus bleeding index, and the approximal plaque index. We also investigated the amount of plaque and food remnants left after the removal of fixed appliances. Our study did not come to clear conclusions; some of the bracket systems allowed impaction of food debris in the bracket slots and around the bracket. Before and after scaling the brackets, we weighed the wet and dry mass of the plaque and food remnants in an ultrasonic bath. The results showed that it is not the plaque accumulation around the bracket itself, but rather compressed plaque and food debris that had accumulated in the recesses of the self-ligating mechanism that characterizes each individual bracket system. This is particularly visible in brackets that use a trapdoor mechanism. It was therefore more noticeable in the Opal and Opal M (Ultradent), Discovery SL (Dentaurum), Time and Vision LP (American Orthodontics) and ODS (Flare)

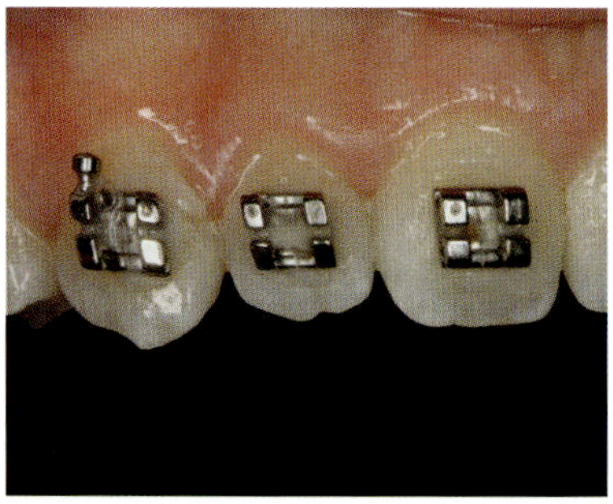

Fig. 3.59 Brackets after the removal of steel ligatures and removal of the archwire. Regardless of the ligation philosophy and type of ligature used, due to their complex design, all orthodontic brackets have undercuts that allow plaque accumulation.

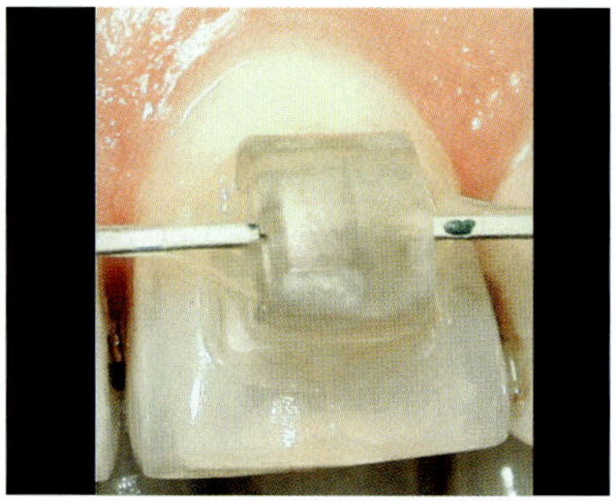

Fig. 3.60 A closed Opal bracket in a patient with good oral hygiene.

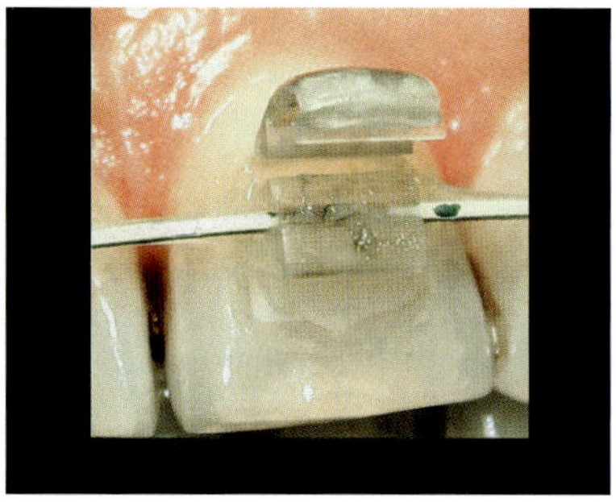

Fig. 3.61 An open Opal bracket in the same patient. Plaque accumulation is not completely avoided when a self-ligating bracket is used; the plaque is confined to the inside of the clip mechanism.

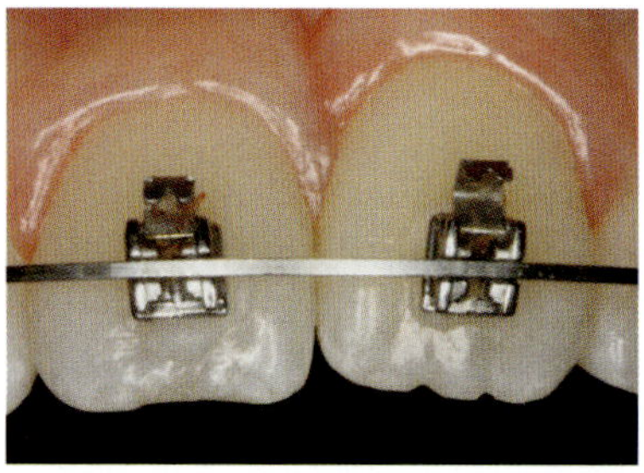

Fig. 3.62 Once unlocked, this Discovery SL bracket reveals food debris that has accumulated under the hinge door of the bracket. It can now be easily cleaned.

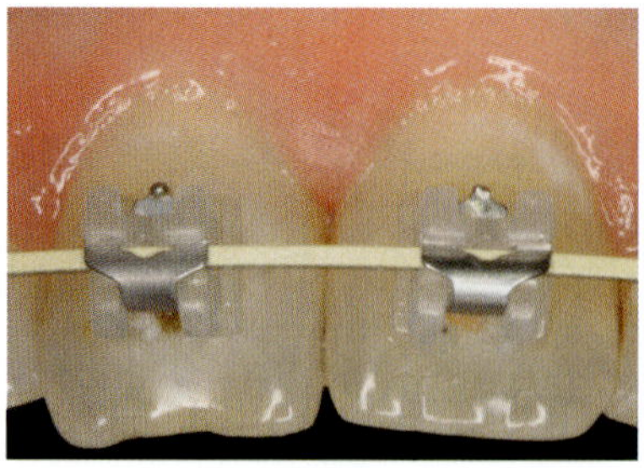

Fig. 3.63 Food debris in an Innovation C bracket. Systems with sliding clips usually conceal the impacted food and make cleaning and removal of the debris difficult.

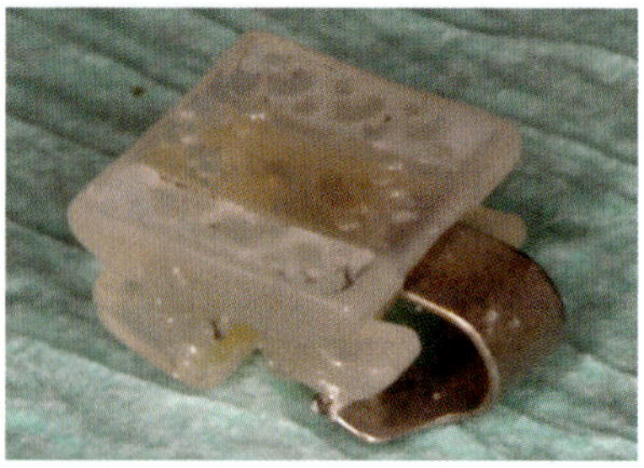

Fig. 3.64 An Innovation C bracket after removal. Food debris in the bracket slot can be seen through the bracket base.

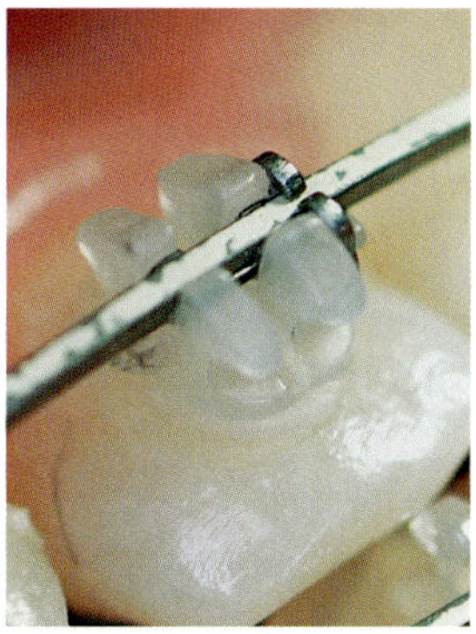

Fig. 3.65

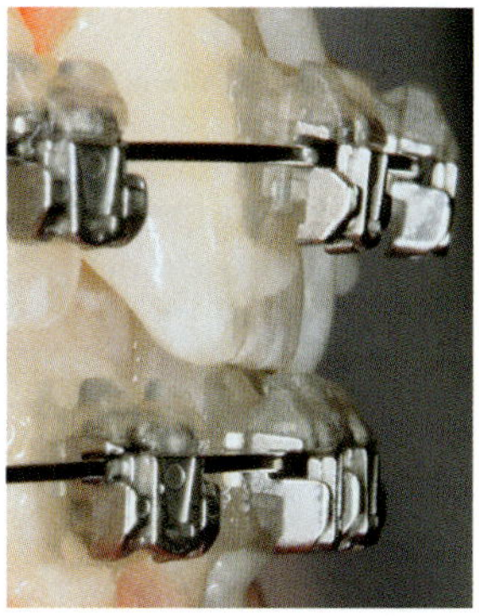

Fig. 3.66

Fig. 3.65 A Clarity SL bracket. This bracket is very smooth and does not have the undercuts that are often associated with self-ligating brackets and allow food debris to accumulate.

Fig. 3.66 A Damon 3 bracket. In patients with good oral hygiene, self-ligating brackets should result in fewer review appointments.

systems. However, this seems to be a more or less severe problem with SLBs in general.

The exceptions were the Clarity SL and SmartClip brackets (3 M Unitek). In both of these brackets, the archwire is attached via NiTi clips on either side of the tie-wings. There are no additional cavities on the Clarity SL or SmartClip brackets (**Fig. 3.65**) that would allow plaque accumulation. It is virtually impossible for food debris to become trapped in this type of bracket, as there is no locking clip or door integrated in the system. Routine oral hygiene instructions as recommended for all patients with fixed appliances are adequate to keep these braces sufficiently clean. It is worth noting that the additional clip on either side of the bracket does occasionally lead to plaque accumulation around the clip.

Overall, we reached the following conclusions regarding plaque accumulation with self-ligating brackets:

- The bracket system itself is not the most important predisposing factor for plaque accumulation. There is more variability between patients than between ligation systems.
- Because of their complex structure, self-ligating brackets have "hollow" areas and recesses that allow for plaque accumulation.
- Oral hygiene in patients with self-ligating brackets is similar to that in patients with conventional bracket systems using steel ligatures.
- In normal bracket systems, plaque accumulation occurs on the surface of the bracket (i.e., the elastomeric ligatures). In self-ligating systems, the plaque accumulation is more concentrated on the inside of the SLB locking mechanism.
- The more complex the self-ligating mechanism, the more recesses there are and the greater the tendency for plaque to accumulate.
- Composite (plastic) brackets accumulate more plaque than ceramic or metal brackets.
- In comparison with conventional brackets using elastomeric rings, oral hygiene is better with self-ligating brackets, but the use of elastomeric chains negates this effect.

NOTE

Oral hygiene in patients wearing self-ligating brackets does improve slightly in comparison with conventional brackets ligated with elastomeric ligatures. However, individual variations in patients' oral hygiene play a greater role than the bracket type used.

Longer Intervals between Adjustments

The elastomeric elements used for conventional ligation lose their elasticity relatively quickly. Most of the elastics lose about a third of their initial force within the first 3 days, as described in the previous chapter in the section on "Auxiliaries." Further force decay is much reduced, however. It is generally accepted that after 4–6 weeks, the ligation becomes ineffective and force levels tend towards zero. For this reason, and because of bacterial colonization, it is generally recommended to change the elastomeric elements every 6–8 weeks.

It can therefore be concluded that due to the absence of force decay in the ligating mechanism with self-ligating brackets, the intervals between control or check-up appointments can be made longer. It is important to remember that in general, the patient's oral hygiene has to be adequate to allow for this. The length of the interval between appointments also sometimes depends on when the intended tooth movements were achieved, and when archwire changes become necessary, it is not always desirable to leave long intervals between visits. Typically, these advantages are observed during the initial phase of leveling and alignment and in the subsequent space closure phase.

NOTE

Generally, self-ligating brackets show little or no "wear and tear" on the ligation mechanism and may therefore allow for longer intervals between routine orthodontic visits. It is important to remember that the patient's oral hygiene has to be adequate.

Reduction of Staff

The use of self-ligating brackets can lead to fewer staff being needed, as it is possible to use two-handed instead of four-handed dentistry. The time saved for the second assistant is approximately 6 minutes per archwire change. However, these time gains are sometimes difficult to translate into effective savings in staffing levels. Restructuring of tasks between individual staff members is sometimes necessary.

NOTE

It is generally thought that self-ligating brackets can lead to a reduction in the numbers of staff needed in an orthodontic practice. Reassigning of tasks undertaken by staff members can be considered, potentially making office operations more efficient.

Summary

All the evidence from our sample indicates that ligature-free systems (**Tables 3.1** and **3.2**) have distinct advantages and disadvantages. No single specific bracket system was unequivocally superior to any of the other systems. The findings did not confirm any significant reduction in chairside time, although fewer staff may be needed when self-ligation is used, as the operator may be able to work without assistance. Generally, longer intervals between appointments can be considered with the self-ligation approach (given appropriate oral hygiene). The leveling and alignment phase of treatment may also be shortened, although this has been discussed controversially in the literature. However, self-ligating brackets are more expensive than conventional ones. Using self-ligation also requires a change in practice routine for efficient use, and it may be necessary to acquire additional instruments such as the opening tools. Some operators may wish to use loupes or other visual aids to facilitate treatment. The decision on which system to use must be taken carefully after weighing up all the advantages and potential disadvantages of a particular system, as these are often associated with particular treatment concepts.

NOTE

On balance, it can be concluded that self-ligating systems have some advantages over conventional ligation; however, there are a large number of factors that may have an impact on the individual performance of any particular system.

REFERENCES

1. Damon DH. The Damon low-friction bracket: a biologically compatible straight-wire system. J Clin Orthod 1998;32(11):670–680
2. Harradine NW. Self-ligating brackets: where are we now? J Orthod 2003;30(3):262–273
3. Fuck LM, Wilmes B, Gürler G, Hönscheid R, Drescher D. Frictional behavior of self ligating brackets in comparison to conventional brackets. Inf Orthod Kieferorthop 2007;39:1–12
4. Pandis N, Strigou S, Eliades T. Maxillary incisor torque with conventional and self-ligating brackets: a prospective clinical trial. Orthod Craniofac Res 2006;9(4):193–198
5. Harradine NW. Self-ligating brackets and treatment efficiency. Clin Orthod Res 2001;4(4):220–227
6. Turnball NR, Birnie DJ. Treatment efficiency of conventional vs self ligating brackets: effects of archwire size and material. Am J Orthod Dentofacial Orthop 2007;131(3):395–399
7. Berger JL, Byloff FK. The clinical efficiency of self-ligated brackets. J Clin Orthod 2001;35(5):304–308
8. Badawi HM, Toogood RW, Carey JPR, Heo G, Major PW. Torque expression of self-ligating brackets. Am J Orthod Dentofacial Orthop 2008;133(5):721–728
9. Eberting JJ, Straja SR, Tuncay OC. Treatment time, outcome, and patient satisfaction comparisons of Damon and conventional brackets. Clin Orthod Res 2001;4(4):228–234
10. Miles PG, Weyant RJ, Rustveld L. A clinical trial of Damon2 versus conventional twin brackets during initial alignment: is there a difference? Angle Orthod 2006;6:480–485
11. Miles PG. SmartClip versus conventional twin brackets for initial alignment: is there a difference? Aust Orthod J 2005;21(2): 123–127
12. Pandis N, Eliades T, Partowi S, Bourauel C. Forces exerted by conventional and self-ligating brackets during simulated first- and second-order corrections. Am J Orthod Dentofacial Orthop 2008;133(5):738–742
13. Neumann P, Bourauel C, Jäger A. Corrosion and permanent fracture resistance of coated and conventional orthodontic wires. J Mater Sci Mater Med 2002;13(2):141–147
14. Iwasaki LR, Beatty MW, Randall CJ, Nickel JC. Clinical ligation forces and intraoral friction during sliding on a stainless steel archwire. Am J Orthod Dentofacial Orthop 2003;123(4):408–415
15. Miles PG. Self-ligating vs conventional twin brackets during en-masse space closure with sliding mechanics. Am J Orthod Dentofacial Orthop 2007;132(2):223–225
16. Fleming PS, DiBiase AT, Sarri G, Lee RT. Efficiency of mandibular arch alignment with 2 preadjusted edgewise appliances. Am J Orthod Dentofacial Orthop 2009;135(5):597–602

II Treatment

Diagnosis

Bjoern Ludwig and Bettina Glasl

4

Sound diagnosis is the prerequisite for good treatment planning, whether self-ligating brackets are used or not. The summary of the diagnostic findings will lead to a more or less comprehensive problem list, and for every problem on that list, there should be at least one treatment option. This list will determine the scope of potential corrective measures and will lead to the development of a detailed treatment plan, addressing not only the patient's chief concern, but ideally all the points on the problem list. The treatment plan should constitute a step-by-step road map for the patient's future treatment and it will determine the appliances required to achieve the ultimate treatment goal.

Good diagnosis usually depends on the availability of orthodontic records, including a number of standard items and specialized examinations. It is very important to remember that legal obligations may vary from country to country and that local regulations need to be borne in mind when reading this chapter.

This is not a textbook on orthodontic diagnosis per se. This chapter is intended to highlight the difficulties in the decision-making processes that practitioners face every day, and it is designed to elaborate on the different diagnostic tools available in contemporary orthodontics. The chapter also outlines the future potential of the digital planning methods available; treatment simulation techniques are likely to become readily available may prove very useful for treatment planning as well as patient education.

Digital records (including radiographs, study models, and two-dimensional or three-dimensional photographs) are now widely available and are likely to become the standard for orthodontic practitioners. Computers can be used to run dental practices more efficiently, and a large number of dedicated software programs are available for running orthodontic offices. Many software solutions consist of practice management programs with integrated diagnostic capabilities (such as ViewPoint; Ortho2 Ltd., Ames, Iowa). Some companies offer dedicated software that can either be purchased separately or in packages (such as Dolphin Management and Dolphin Imaging; Dolphin Imaging and Management Solutions Ltd., Chatsworth, California) and even offer patient education programs (such as Dolphin Aquarium). The latest innovation in orthodontic software was introduced by Ortho2. Its new management software package, Edge, is the first orthodontic management package that is "cloud-based." This means that data are no longer stored on an expensive server in the orthodontic office, but are kept remotely in a secure data storage center. The cloud application eliminates the need for backups and downtime while updating the software. Edge Imaging is included with the management system, and patient education software is also available for the package. Onyx Ceph (Image Instruments Ltd., Chemnitz, Germany), is a dedicated software program that has been developed for orthodontic diagnosis only. The advantage of purchasing a purely diagnostic software tool lies in the availability of updates that are independent of the management software at an orthodontic practice, which may occasionally cause 'downtimes' unless cloud-based computing is used. Onyx Ceph is the program used by the present authors and it is also used for the illustrations in this chapter.

Using digital diagnostic software allows the operator to switch between various cephalometric analyses at the click of a button. This means the orthodontist is no longer restricted to one diagnostic tool (such as a particular type of cephalometric analysis) or philosophy. Once an image or a model has been digitized, it can be analyzed in many different ways, and it is possible to combine measurements from different analyses to customize the diagnostic approach.

Standard Diagnostic Tools in Orthodontics

Standard orthodontic records may consist of study models, radiographs (orthopantomogram and lateral cephalogram, where indicated), as well as photographic records. Most of these records are regarded as an orthodontic standard, as they are usually required for comprehensive diagnosis and treatment planning. Although intraoral photographic documentation is not compulsory in many countries, we find that it is often very helpful; magnification of photographic records may highlight issues that are difficult to detect in a visual intraoral examination or from analysis of the study models. It is often an examination of photographic records that highlights clinical issues (such as bracket positioning or achievement of three-dimensional tooth movements) that are not observed during routine clinical examinations.

NOTE

Further diagnostic imaging may involve additional radiographs, such as:

- Periapical, upper and/or lower standard occlusal radiographs
- Posteroanterior cephalometric analyses (PA cephs)
- Cone beam computed tomography (CBCT)
- Magnetic resonance imaging (MRI)

Cone-beam tomograms or dental CTs provide good modeling of the three-dimensional structure for analysis and exact positioning of the teeth (**Fig. 4.1**). They can also be used for three-dimensional reconstructions of the facial skeleton (**Fig. 4.2**). However, it is important to remember that radiation protection is paramount, and it is often possible to ascertain the exact positioning of teeth using clinical observations and/or conventional radiographs on two different spatial planes.[1,5,6,7,8] MRI scanning in orthodontics is rare, but can be particularly useful in cases where conventional x-ray imaging fails, such as detailed

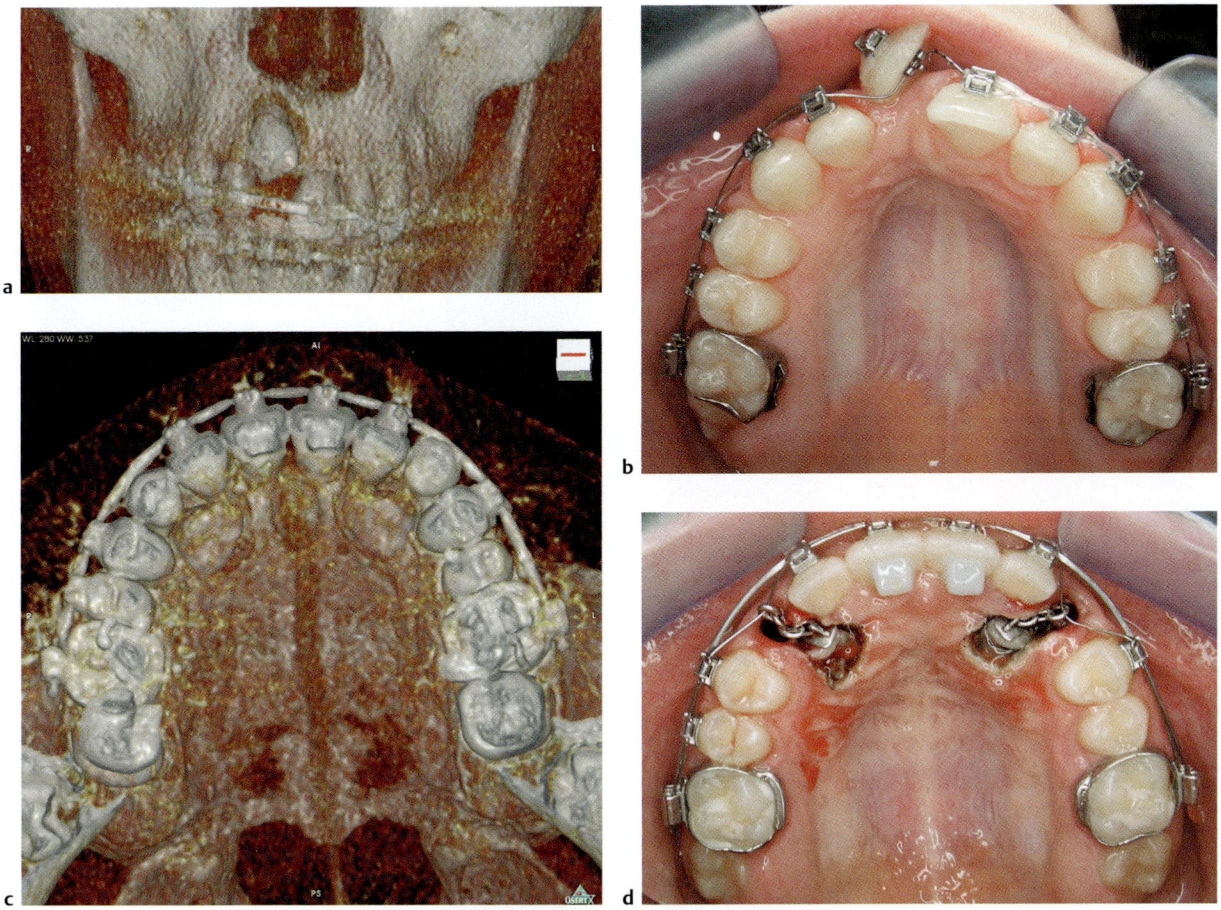

Fig. 4.1 a–d Dental cone-beam computed tomography (CBCT) with three-dimensional reconstruction for diagnostic purposes.
a, b A displaced tooth 11.
c, d Impacted canines.

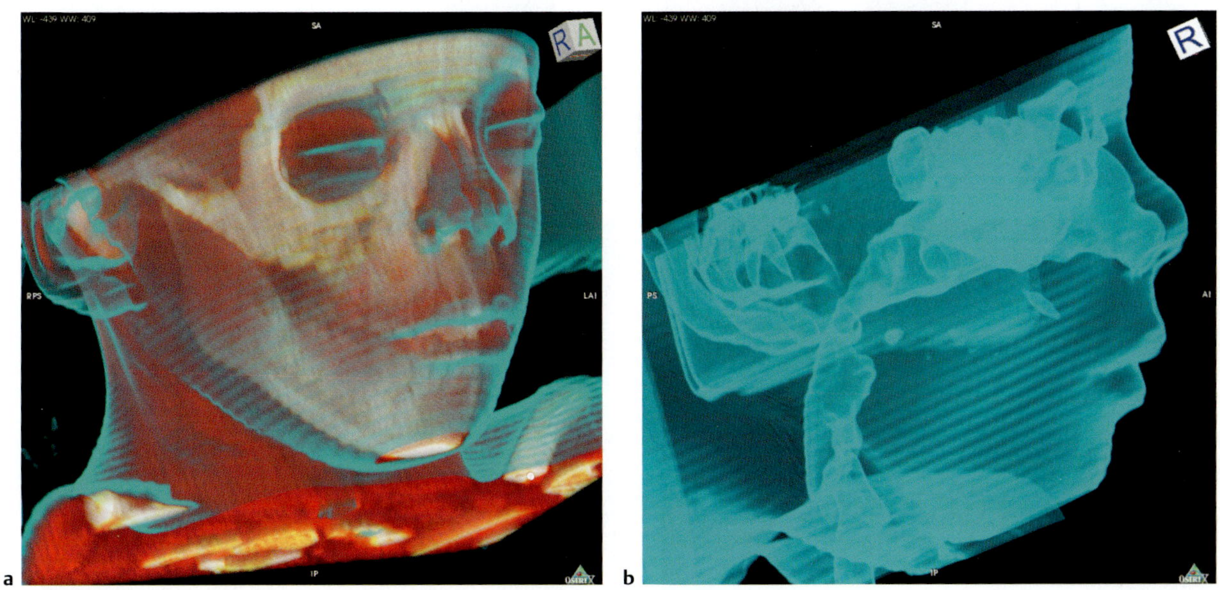

Fig. 4.2 a, b Reconstruction of the posterior airway.

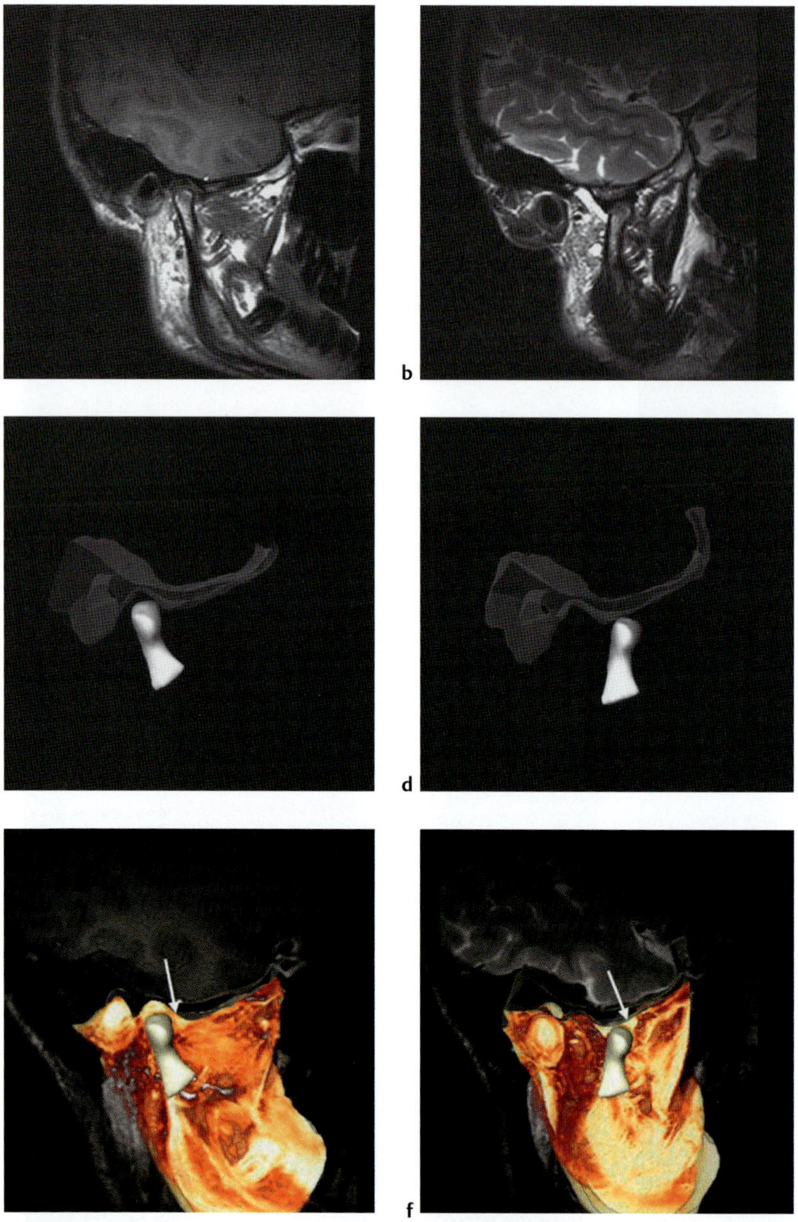

a b c d e f

Fig. 4.3 a–f Three-dimensional reconstruction of magnetic resonance images for improved visualization of articular disk displacement. The raw scan (**a, b**) was modified using Amira 4.0 (Mercury Computer Systems) to focus on the condyle (**c, d**) as well as allowing visualization of the articular disk and the surrounding muscles (**e, f**). The conventional tomographic images remain readily available for comparative purposes.[2–4] The images were kindly provided by Prof. Kober and Prof. Kinzinger.

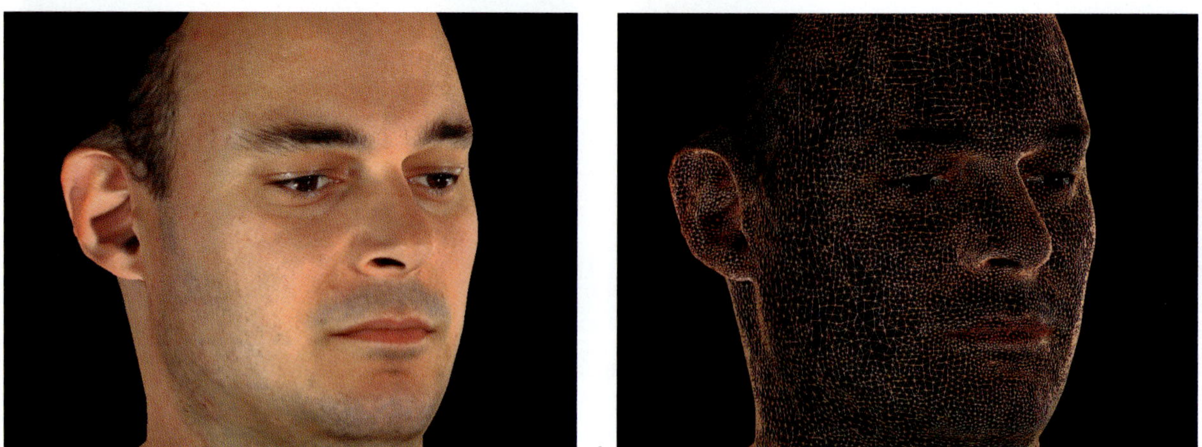

a b

Fig. 4.4 a, b Three-dimensional reconstruction of the facial soft tissues after optical scanning of the facial contours (FaceScan 3 D).

imaging of soft-tissue structures. The present authors use magnetic resonance imaging (MRI) as an additional technique for precise diagnosis of temporomandibular joint disorders and occasionally for presurgical assessment and planning of potential treatments, particularly lower jaw surgery (**Fig. 4.3**). Occasionally, interdisciplinary care may be necessary for patients affected by periodontal disease, for example. Further diagnosis of preexisting diseases or conditions may also be indicated. Other developments in optical three-dimensional imaging techniques can also be expected, such as FaceScan 3 D (GF Messtechnik Ltd., Berlin, Germany, 3D-Shape Ltd., Erlangen, Germany), which do not expose the patient to ionising radiation and allow three-dimensional digital data analysis of the patient's profile and soft tissues (**Fig. 4.4**).

Diagnosis and Treatment Planning

The treatment records for one patient are used here as an example of the advanced diagnostic facilities provided by systems such as Onyx Ceph (Image Instruments Ltd., Chemnitz, Germany). The treatment of most of the cases presented in subsequent chapters was planned using the methodology described below.

An 18-year-old patient presented for an orthodontic evaluation. She had undergone previous orthodontic treatment involving removal of two upper first premolars to align the upper canines. Post-treatment records following the first orthodontic treatment showed a left-sided unilateral crossbite as an initial sign of maxillary deficiency. In addition, she had a reduced overjet and overbite, which was at risk for worsening with further growth given the patient's class III tendency. The current records showed a bilateral crossbite and anterior edge-to-edge relationship as a result of the previous treatment and additional craniofacial growth.

The patient's chief complaint was a protruding chin, which was accentuated by a maxillary deficiency. After initial decompensation, it became clear that the underlying class III malocclusion should ideally be treated with an orthognathic approach (**Fig. 4.5**: **21, 22**).

After superimposition of the cephalogram and the clinical photograph, a prediction tracing was obtained with a "visualized treatment objective" (VTO). Analysis of the three-dimensional models allowed further planning in this case.

Case Study 4.1 (Fig. 4.5)

Patient: F. K., female, age 18.

Diagnostic records: models, panoramic radiograph, lateral cephalometric radiograph, intraoral/extraoral photographs.

Main findings: class III malocclusion due to mandibular excess and relapse after previous orthodontic treatment, combined with residual craniofacial growth.

Treatment aims: combined orthodontic surgical treatment to improve the profile and the stability of the treatment result.

Appliances: self-ligating brackets, Hybrid RPE (see p. 135).

Archwire sequence: 0.012 round wire, superelastic; 0.016 round wire, superelastic, 0.016 × 0.022 superelastic, 0.018 × 0.025 superelastic and 0.019 × 0.025 stainless-steel archwires.

Alternative treatment strategy: opening of spaces in the upper jaw for later replacement of the previously extracted upper first pre-molar teeth (14 and 24), or alternatively extraction of two corresponding premolars in the lower jaw for further dental compensation.

Active treatment time: 11 months.

Retention: three-dimensional retention.

1
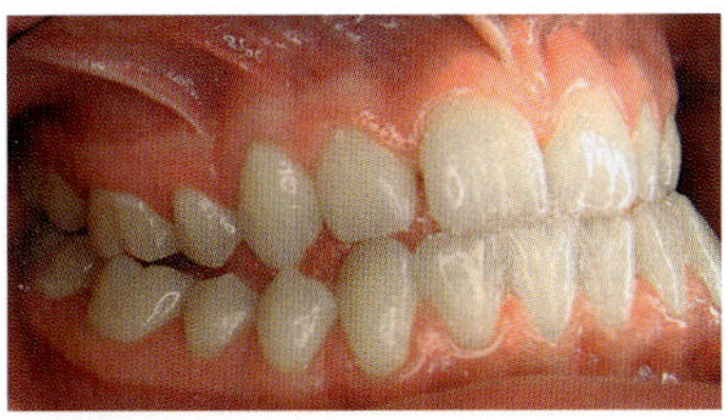
2
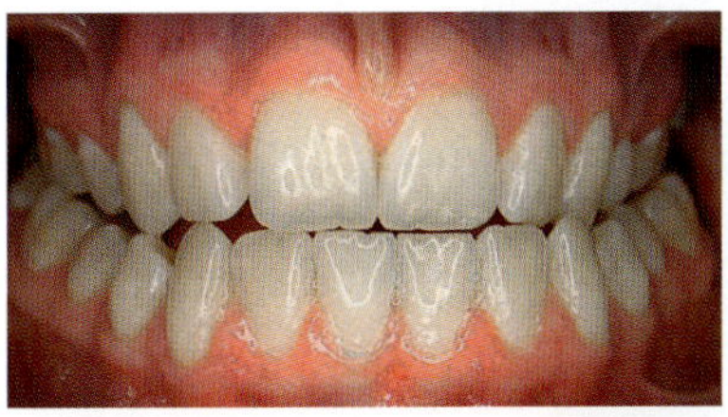
3
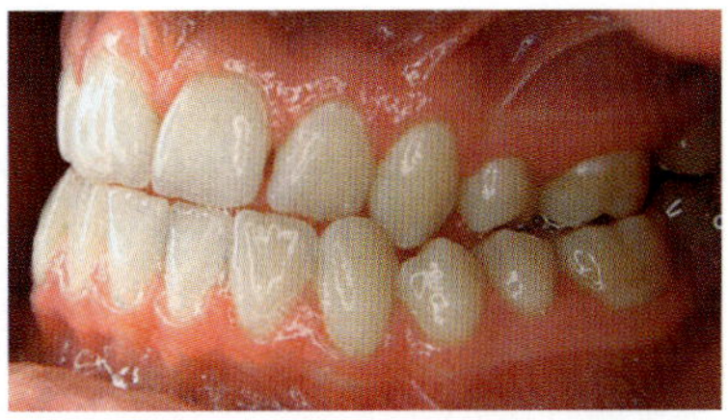
4
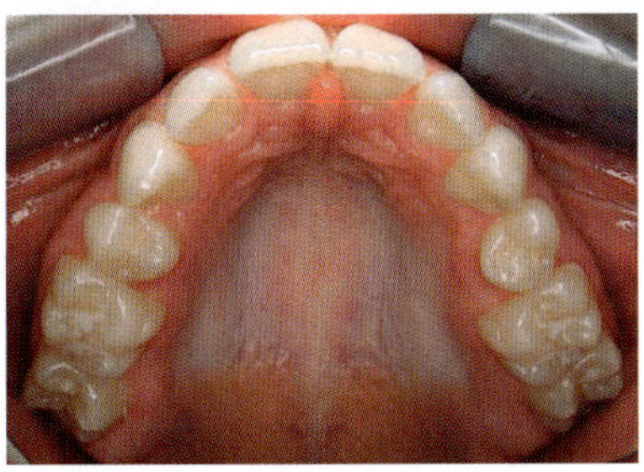
5
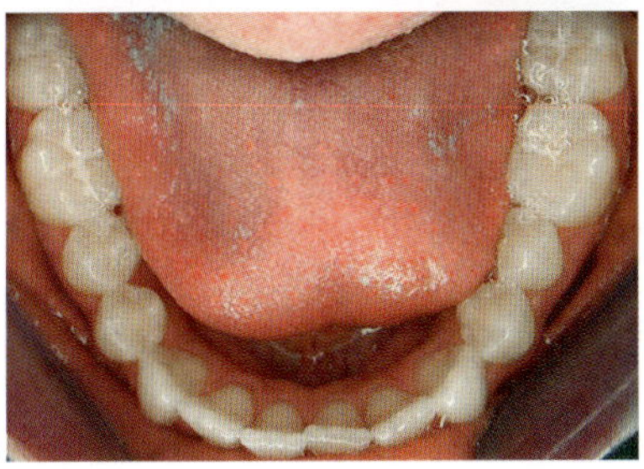

Fig. 4.5 **1–5** Condition after orthodontic treatment of several years' duration. The treatment involved removal of 14 and 24.

Errors and risks:
It might be prudent to consider a nonextraction approach for the upper jaw when planning treatment for growing patients with a class III malocclusion on a class III skeletal base. Particularly when undertaken in the upper jaw, extractions only often lead to poor treatment outcomes. Maxillary extractions alone are generally not indicated for class III cases.

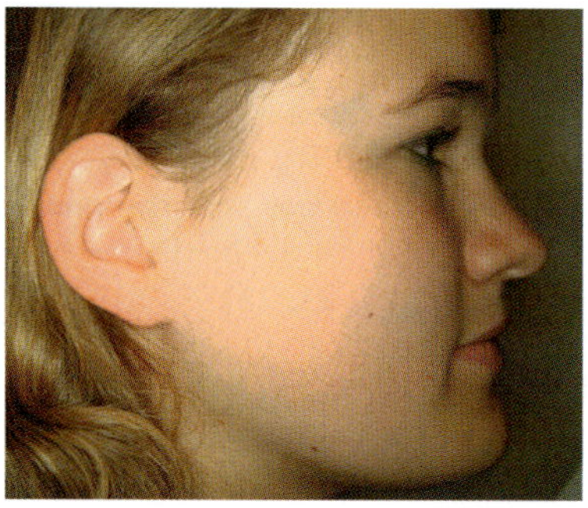
6

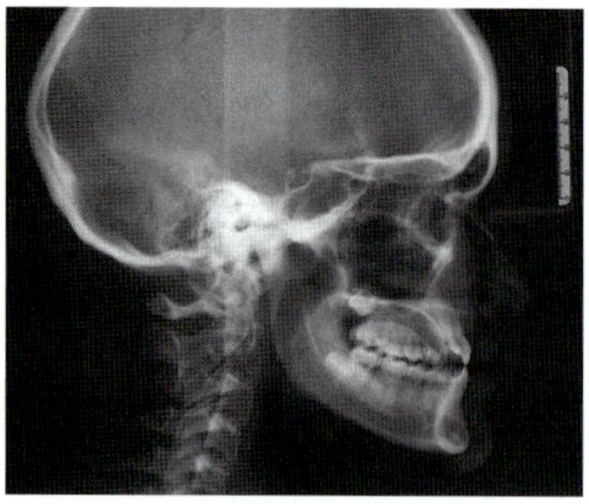
7

6, 7 Both the profile picture and cephalometrics show a hypoplastic and retruded maxilla, combined with mandibular prognathism.

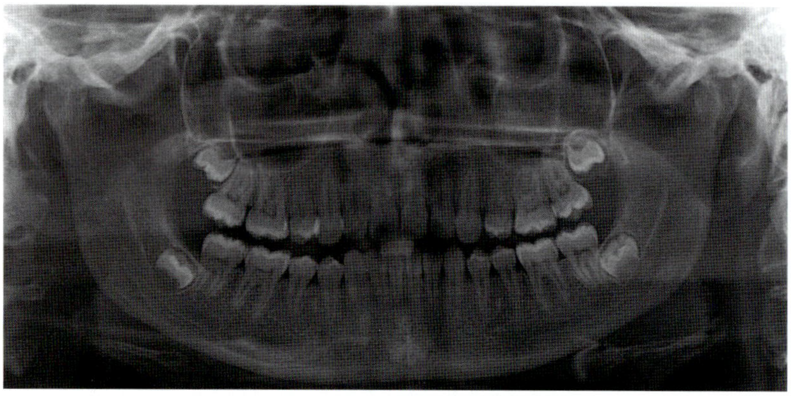
8

8 The panoramic radiograph shows shortened and pipette-shaped roots on the incisors and premolars in particular; all wisdom teeth are present.

Errors and risks:
The reduced root length and pipette-shaped roots indicate an increased risk of root resorption during orthodontic treatment.

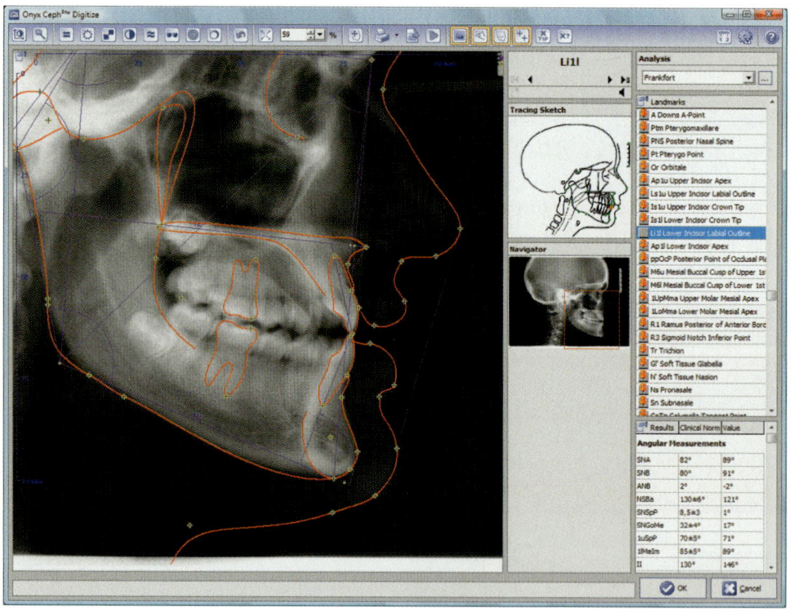
9

9 Cephalometric analysis reveals a class III malocclusion and a low maxillary–mandibular plane angle. Digital cephalometry allows easy use of a number of analyses and comparison between them. Cephalometric landmarks for further analysis can be easily added.

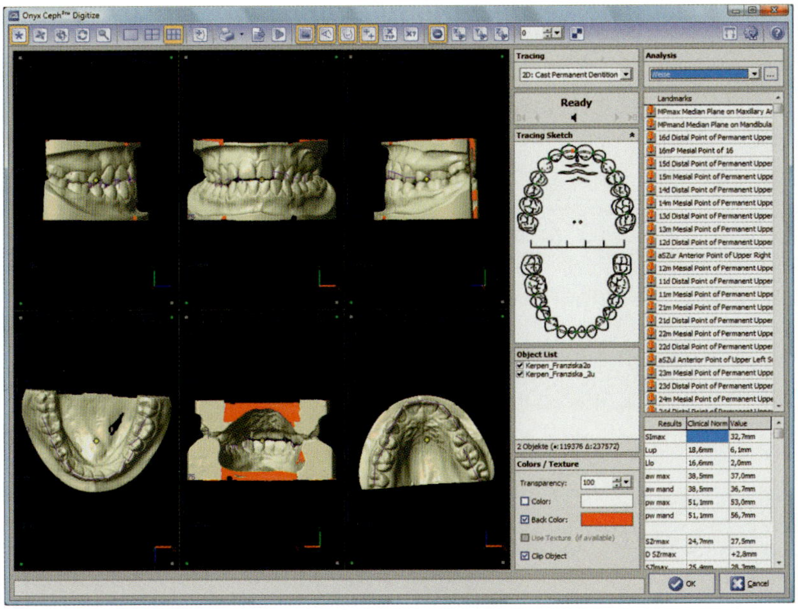

10

10 Space analysis using a digital three-dimensional computer-aided analysis of the study models. The plaster models were scanned and measured digitally. The software helps to assess the space requirements for alignment.

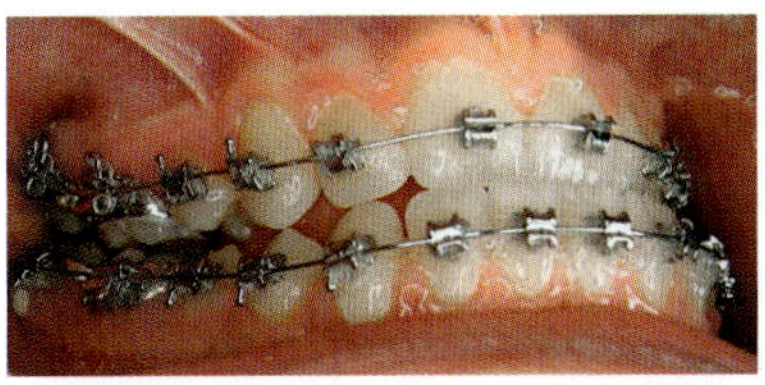

11

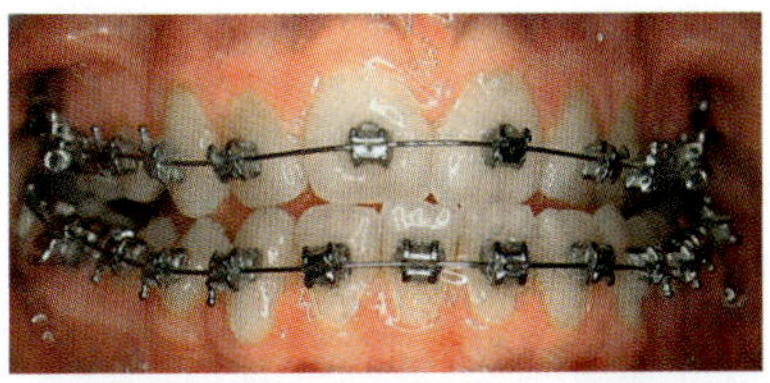

12

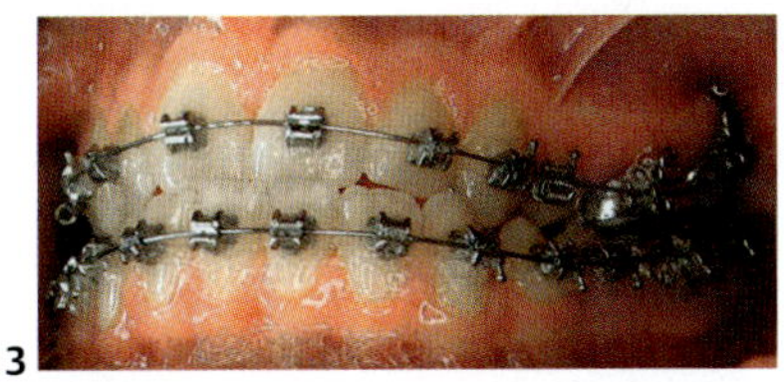

13

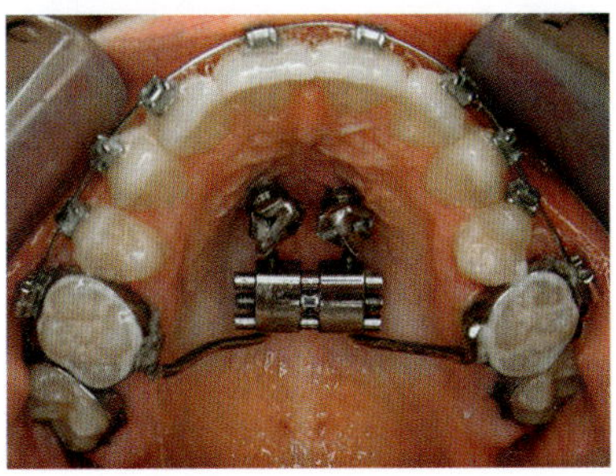

14

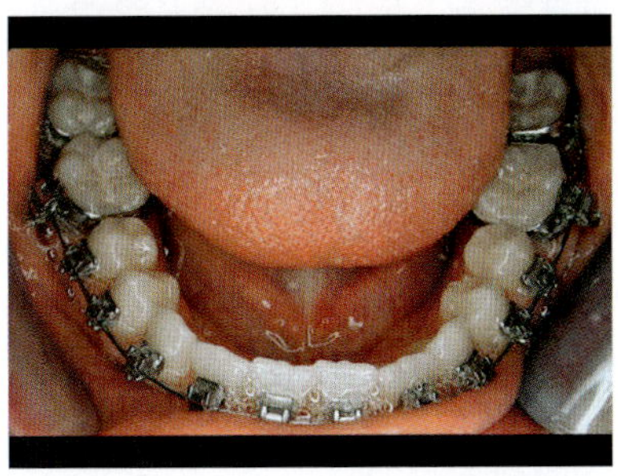

15

11–15 Skeletally supported rapid palatal expansion (see also Chapter 8). Self-ligating brackets are used to align the teeth.

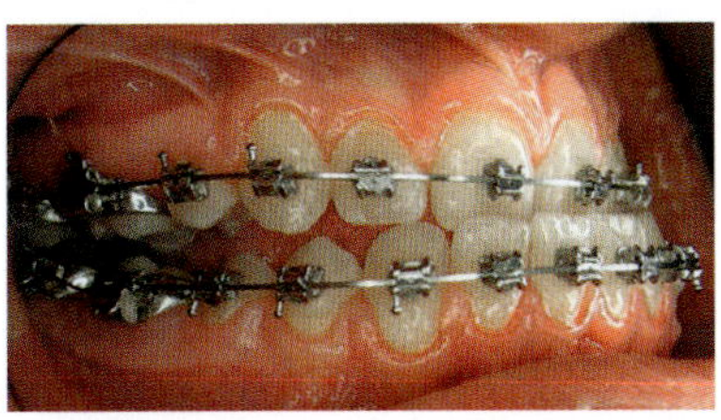

16

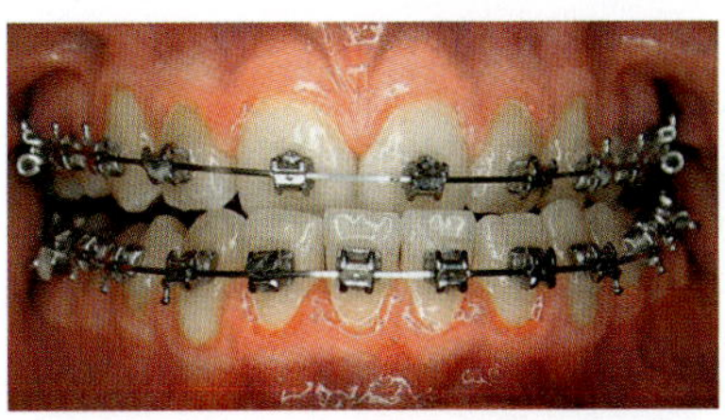

17

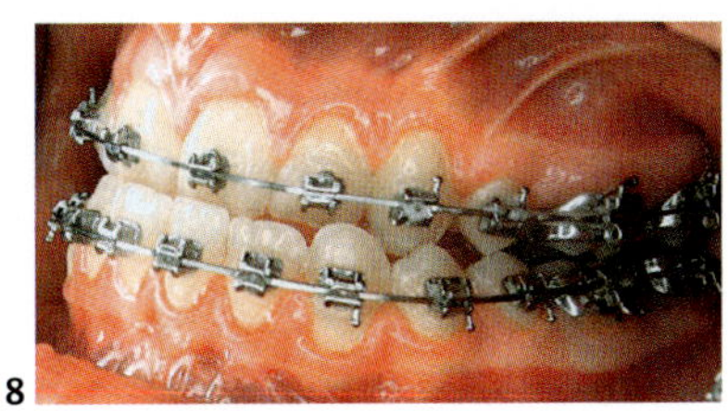

18

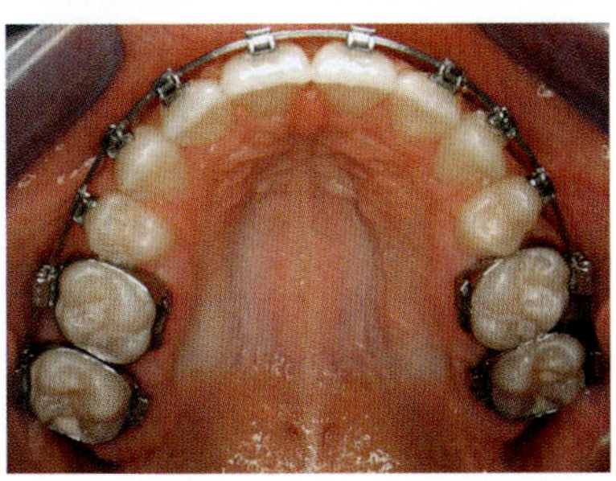

19

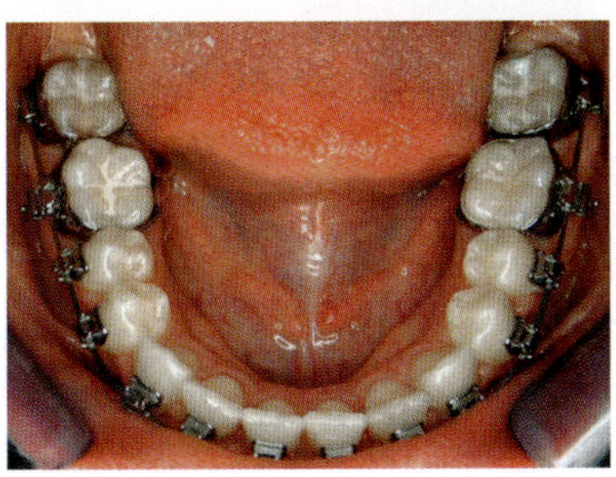

20

16–20

Errors and risks:
Decompensated occlusion just prior to orthognathic surgery; it is often difficult to fully appreciate the extent of the underlying skeletal discrepancy before decompensation has taken place.

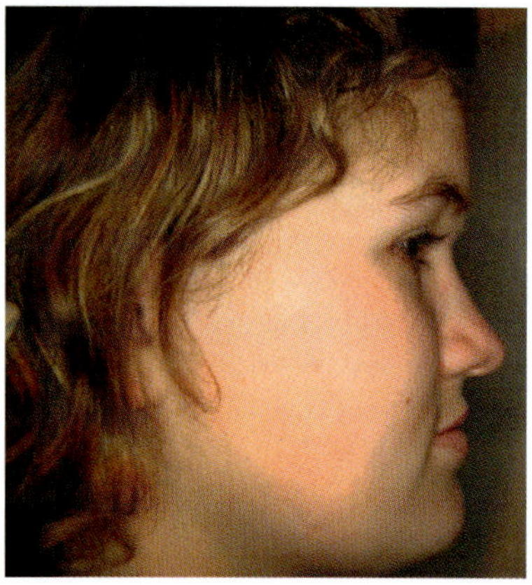

21

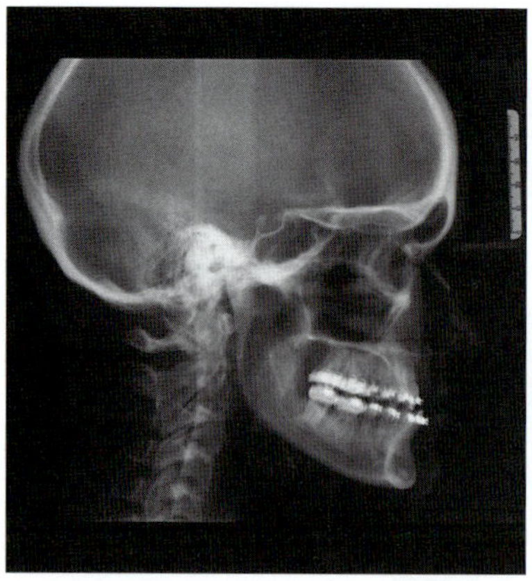

22

21, 22 Lateral cephalometric view of the patient after presurgical decompensation. The underlying class III skeletal base is now fully revealed.

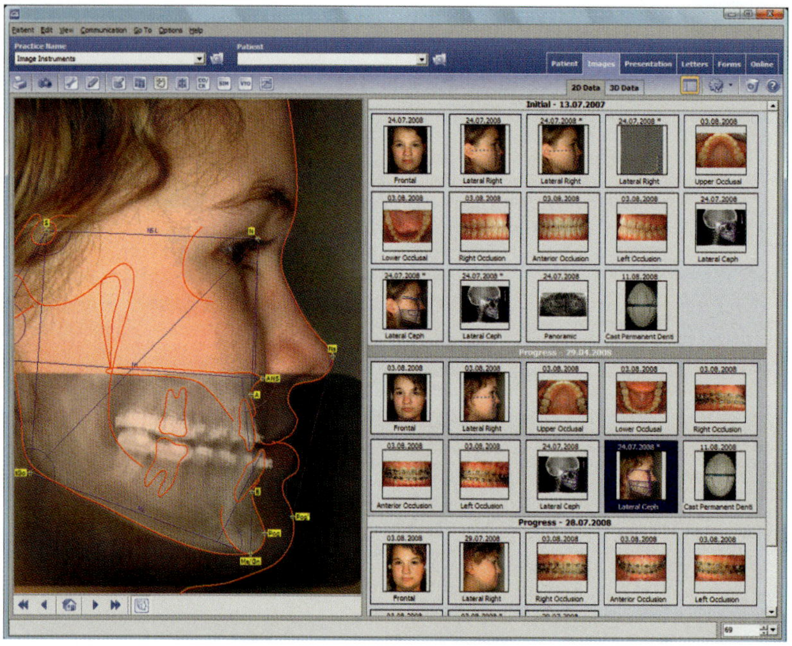

23

23–26 Surgical prediction tracing by means of computer-aided superimposition of the lateral photograph and lateral cephalometric view. This can sometimes be helpful to establish whether single-jaw or bimaxillary osteotomy is indicated, and it also helps establish the best esthetic parameters for the surgical outcome. It is an extremely helpful tool for communication between the multidisciplinary team (orthodontist and maxillofacial surgeon) and the patient.

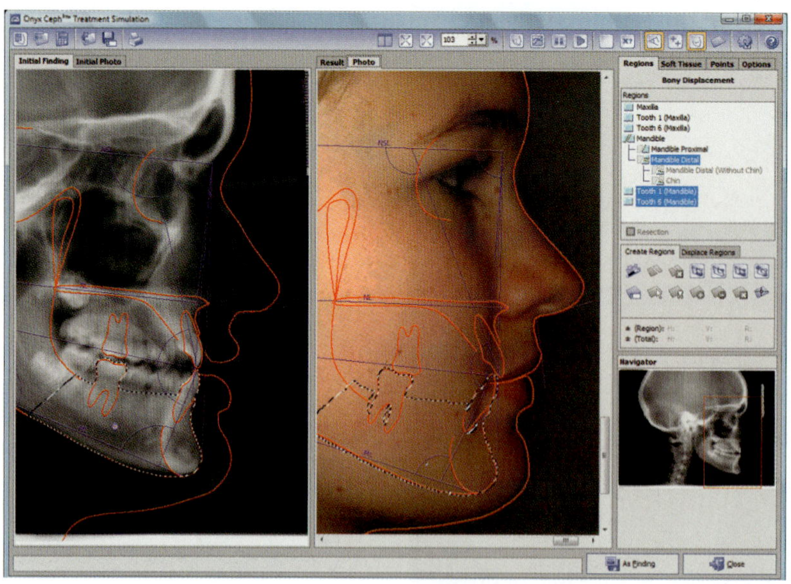

24

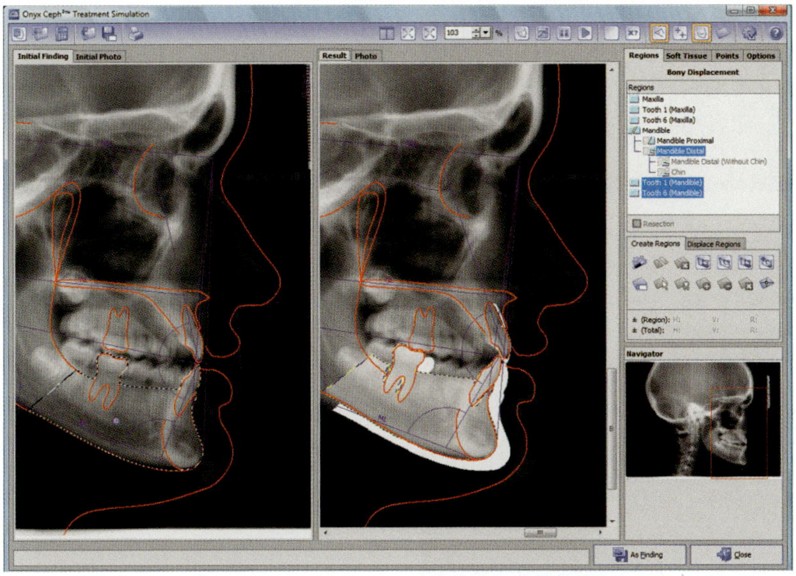

25

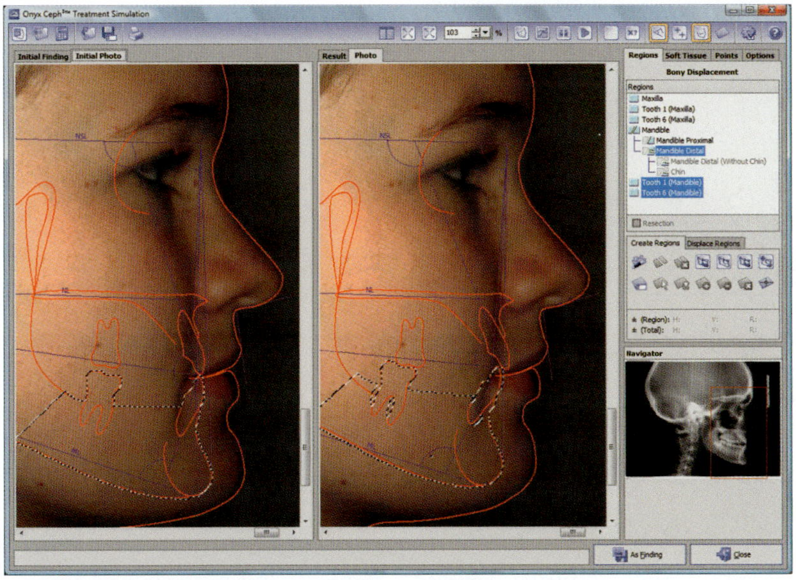

26

25–26 Continued

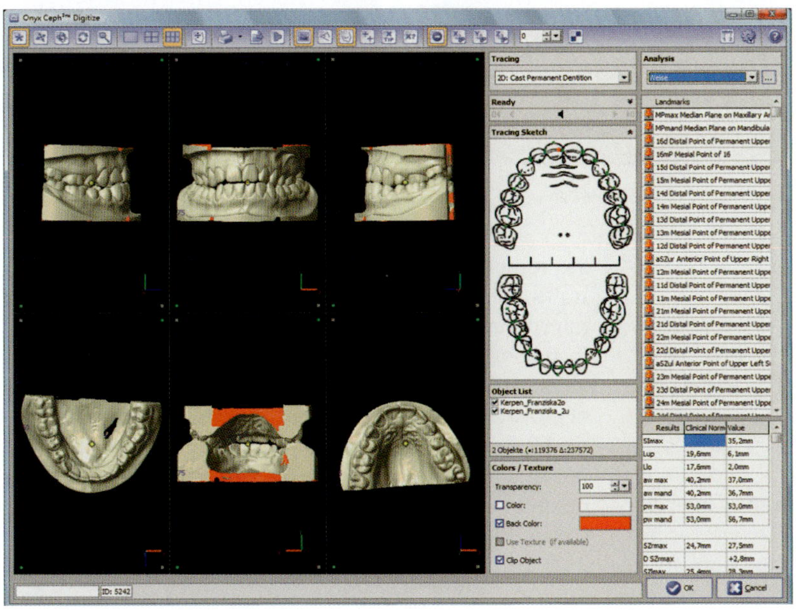

27

27 Digital analysis of the preoperative diagnostic models. The arch coordination is usually difficult to determine clinically; digitized three-dimensional analysis of the study models can facilitate this task and is therefore helpful in assessing the outcome of presurgical orthodontics.

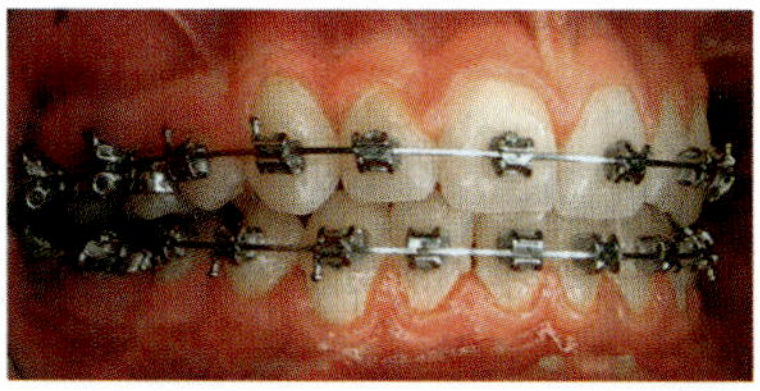
28
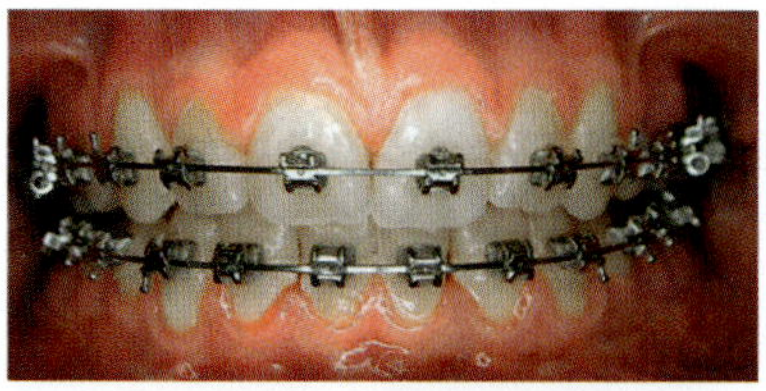
29
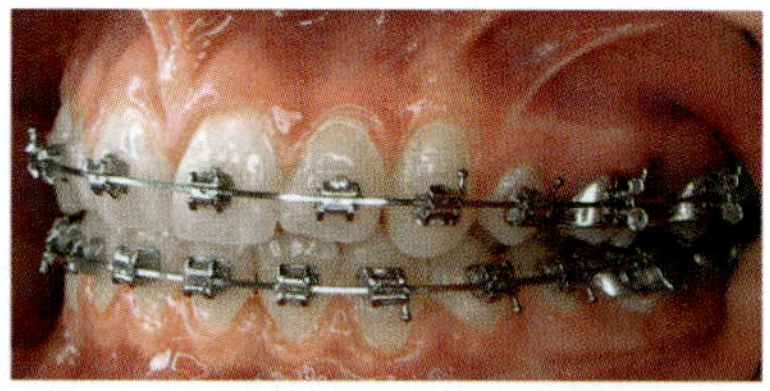
30

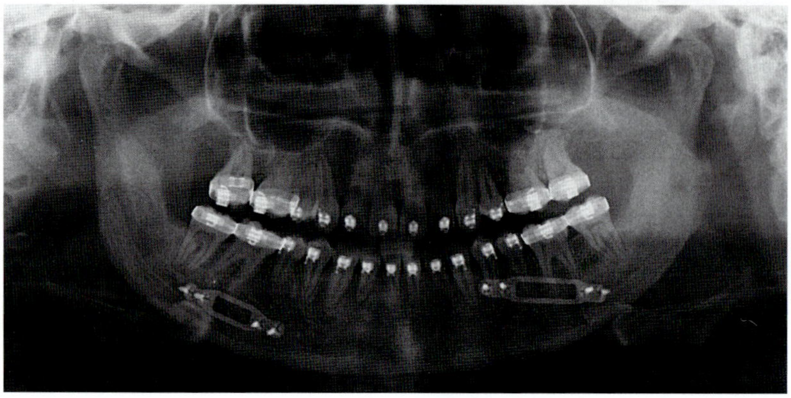
31

28–31 Postoperative situation images.

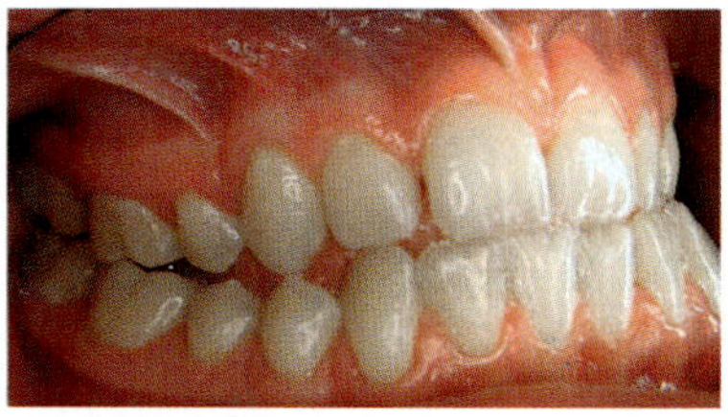
32
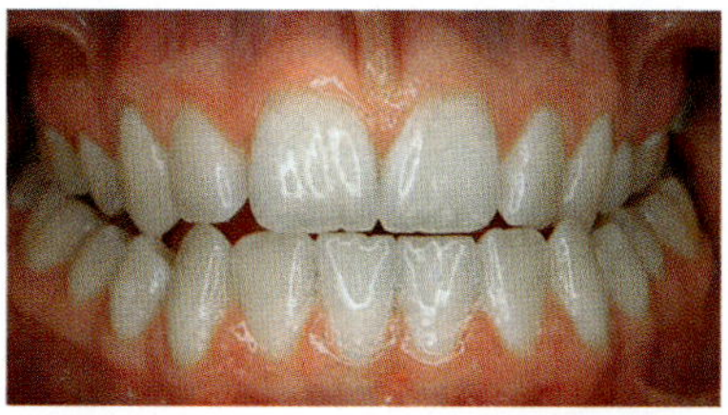
33
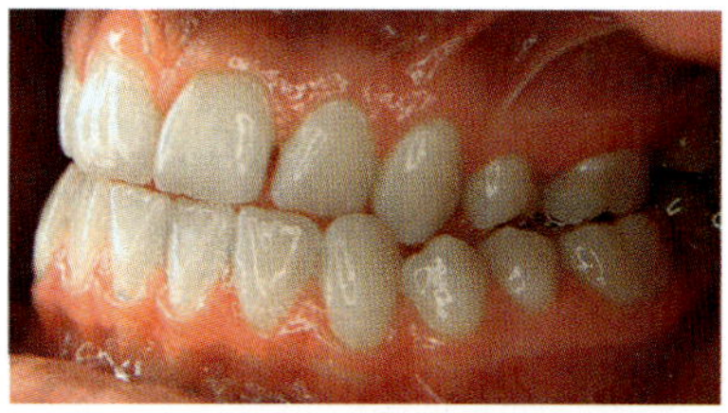
34
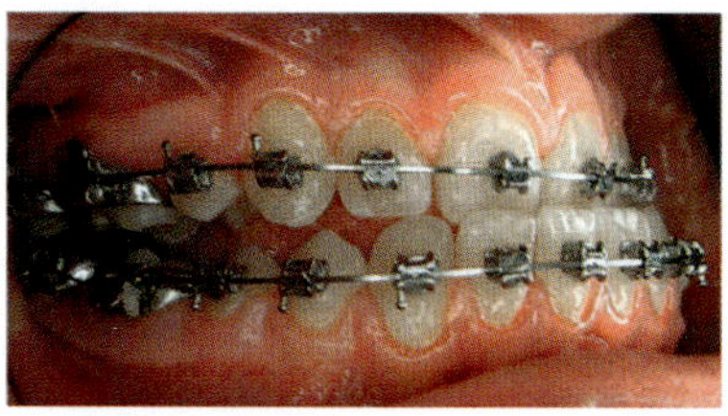
35
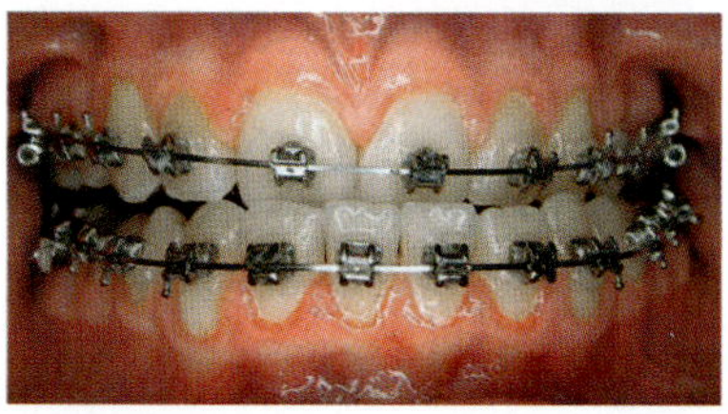
36
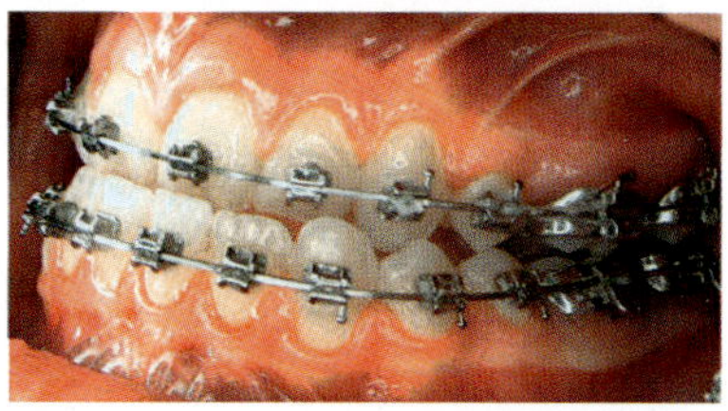
37
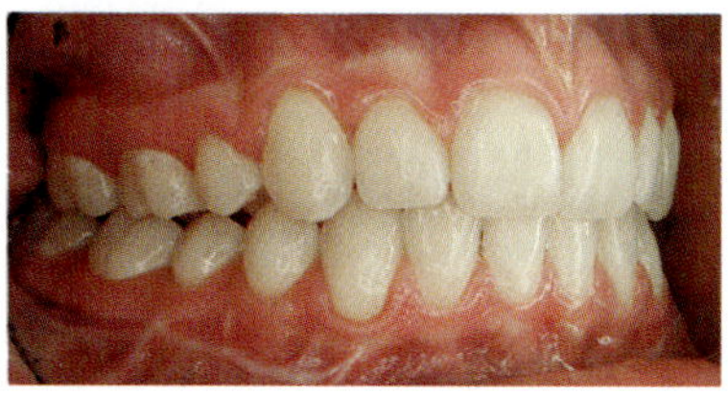
38
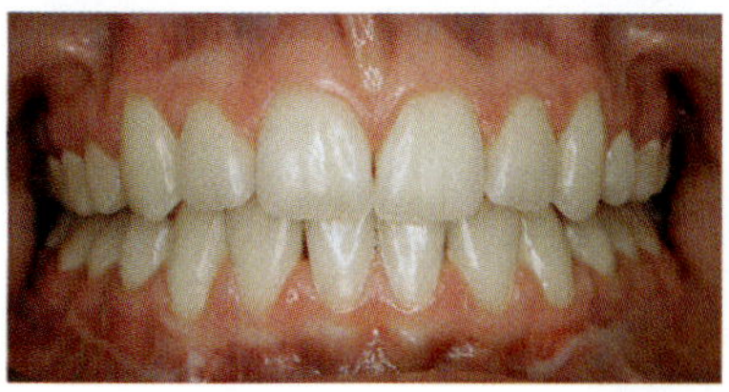
39
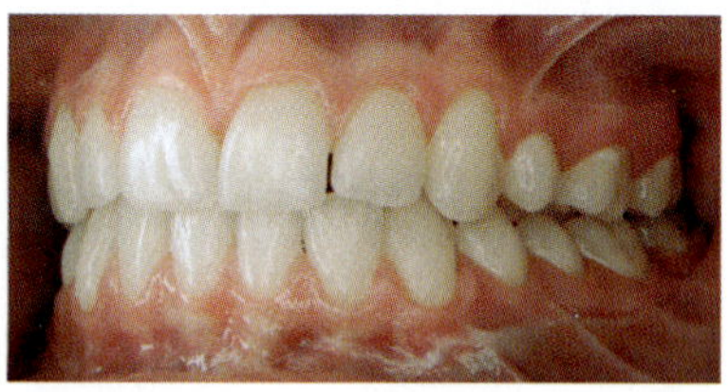
40

32–40 Intraoral views before treatment (top row), preoperatively (middle row), and 1 year in retention (lower row).

CLINICAL PEARL

There is no evidence that the removal of osteosynthesis plates following orthognathic surgery is beneficial for the patient (unless the plates are infected), and the patient needs to be informed of this.

After extensive orthodontic treatment as well as interdisciplinary treatment, involving orthodontics, we recommend collecting full records before the fixed appliances are removed. The treatment example shown here illustrates the value of appropriate diagnosis, which includes interpretation of previous orthodontic treatment. Unfortunately, it is still difficult to predict growth for individuals with any precision, either in terms of the amount of growth or the timing. Growth subsequent to orthodontic treatment may jeopardize an excellent orthodontic outcome; it is important to be aware of potential signs of unfavorable growth to ideally avoid treatment outcomes such as the one illustrated in this case.

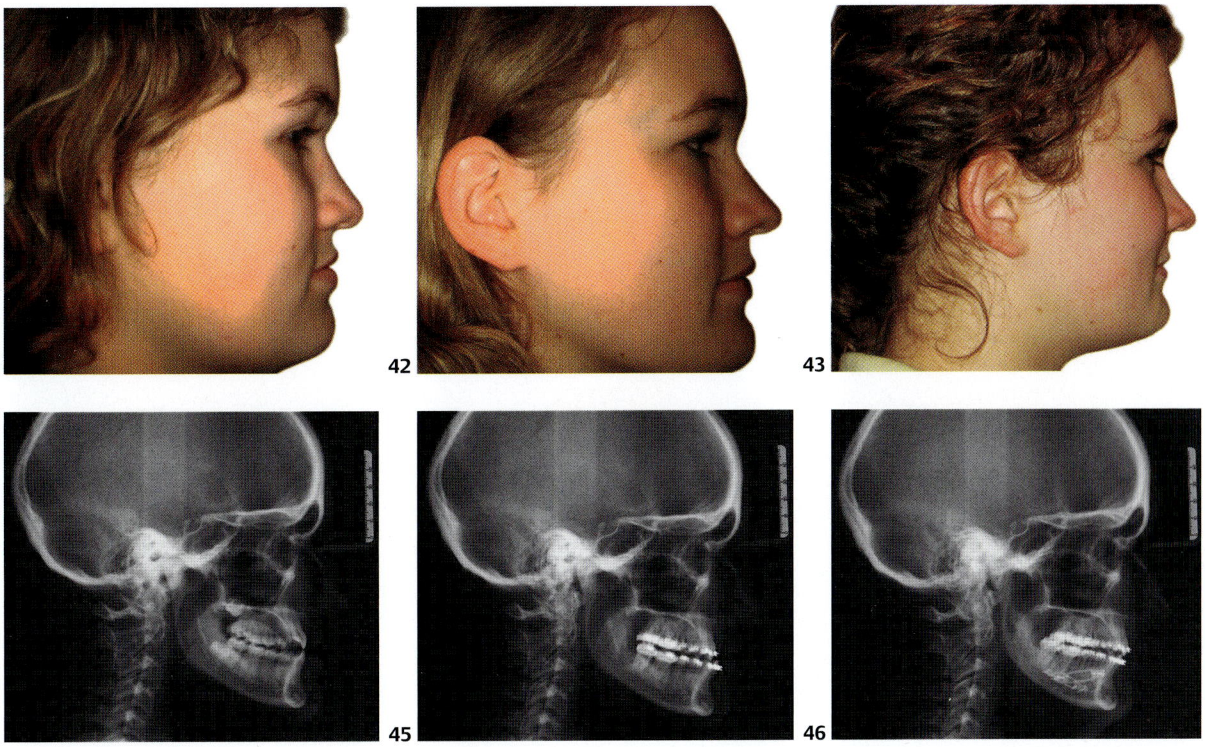

41–46 Profile view and lateral cephalometric views before treatment (left), preoperatively (middle), and postoperatively (right).

Additional Diagnostic Tools

As pointed out in Chapter 3, self-ligating brackets are not necessarily more hygienic than conventional bracket systems. Good oral hygiene cannot always be taken for granted even when self-ligating brackets are used. It is therefore particularly important to keep the patient's periodontal condition in mind before and during orthodontic treatment, whether self-ligating brackets are used or not. Monitoring oral hygiene with plaque markers and the various periodontal screening indices may become necessary in patients with poor oral hygiene or unstable periodontal conditions.

Orthodontic treatment of patients affected by periodontal disease is discussed in greater detail in Chapter 5.

REFERENCES

1. Kiefer H, Lambrecht JT, Roth J. Dose exposure from analog and digital full mouth radiography and panoramic radiography. [Article in German] Schweiz Monatsschr Zahnmed 2004;114(7):687–693
2. Kinzinger G, Kober C, Diedrich P. Topography and morphology of the mandibular condyle during fixed functional orthopedic treatment—a magnetic resonance imaging study. J Orofac Orthop 2007;68(2):124–147
3. Kober C, Hayakawa Y, Kinzinger G, et al. An approach for three-dimensional rendering of the mandibular disc based on high-resolution MR images. Int J CARS 2006;1(Suppl 1):405–406
4. Kober C, Hayakawa Y, Kinzinger G, et al. 3 D-visualization of the temporomandibular joint with focus on the articular disc based on clinical T1-, T2-, and proton density weighted MR images. Int J CARS 2007;2:203–210
5. Lemkamp M, Filippi A, Berndt D, et al. Diagnostic possibilities of digital volume tomography. [Article in French, German] Schweiz Monatsschr Zahnmed 2006;116(6):645–650
6. Ludlow JB, Davies-Ludlow LE, Brooks SL, Howerton WB. Dosimetry of 3 CBCT devices for oral and maxillofacial radiology: CB Mercuray, NewTom 3G and i-CAT. Dentomaxillofac Radiol 2006;35(4):219–226
7. Ludlow JB, Davies-Ludlow LE, Mol A. Dosimetry of recently introduced CBCT units for oral and maxillofacial radiology. 16th Int Congress of Dentomaxillofacial Radiology, Peking, China; 2007
8. Ritter L, Neugebauer J, Mischkowski RA, et al. Dreidimensionale Bildgebung in der Zahnmedizin – Aktuelle Trends und Techniken. Z Oral Implant 2007;3:86–95

Oral Hygiene

Heiko Goldbecher and Jens Bock

5

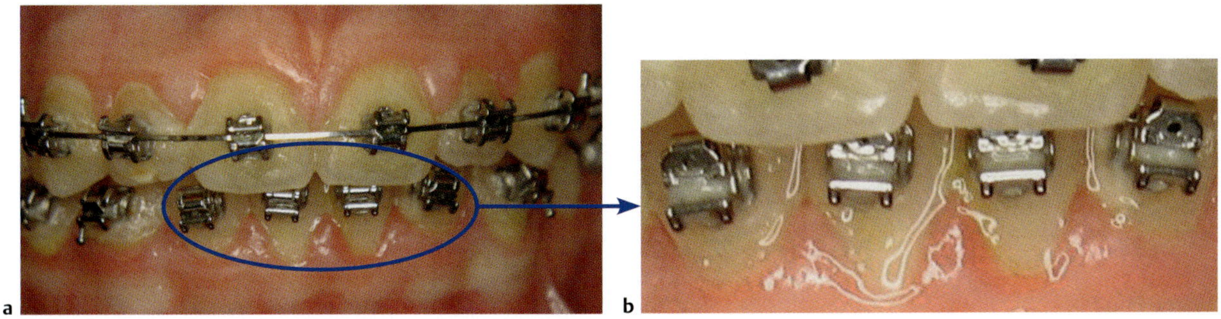

Fig. 5.1 a, b Plaque accumulation around self-ligating brackets. Due to the mechanical complexity and surface characteristics of self-ligating brackets, the risk of plaque accumulation around the brackets is increased. This becomes particularly visible in patients with poor oral hygiene and when a bracket has been opened.

This chapter focuses on the basic principles of periodontology and preventive dentistry as they relate to oral hygiene in patients wearing fixed appliances, with special emphasis on self-ligating brackets.

Basics

Dental decay (caries), gingivitis, and periodontitis can be regarded as infectious diseases in the wider sense. A combination of numerous etiological factors plays a role in the pathology, but contrary to popular belief, genetic predisposition appears to be of minor importance. The level of oral hygiene appears to be the major cause of the above diseases. Fixed-appliance treatment is very likely to induce plaque, and it is therefore extremely important that the patient's oral hygiene should be of the highest possible standard. It is therefore advisable for patients to use the services of a professional oral hygienist to achieve the best possible level of oral hygiene.

NOTE

Plaque is primarily found in the retentive areas around the bracket base, and within a short period of time—sometimes less than a month—it may cause permanent decalcification, which ultimately leads to caries if left unattended.

It is widely known that after fixed appliances have been fitted, a bacteriological shift occurs in the oral cavity toward an increase in anaerobic, cariogenic bacteria. The same also applies to the use of self-ligating brackets, which often have larger undercuts and recesses than the traditional tie-wing brackets and therefore provide greater potential for plaque retention (**Fig. 5.1**). Demineralization around the bracket is a significant risk associated with fixed-appliance treatment in general. It is well known that in patients with poor oral hygiene, caries may develop within weeks of fixed appliances being fitted.[9] Although in ideal conditions, remineralization of initial lesions can be achieved, the damage is often irreversible.[4,11,12] Remineralization is rarely seen and can only occur if the patient's oral hygiene is of the highest possible standard. Regular general check-up visits with a dental hygienist or general dental practitioner are often the best way of achieving this. However, once the initial lesions have become established, and even if all the above favorable conditions are subsequently met, the patient may still progress from decalcification to carious lesions.

Symptoms and Etiology of Caries

Caries is a disease of the dental hard tissues, with a high prevalence and incidence in adults. Carious disease is characterized by several phases, involving progression, stagnation, and remission. The more advanced stages of the disease are diagnosed clinically and may range from small initial lesions to open cavities.

Active incipient caries is characterized by an "initial white spot" (**Fig. 5.2a**). This is often without loss of continuity in the dental surface. The surface of the affected area appears matt and is rough on probing. This is diagnostically different from the inactive initial carious lesion, which has the typical appearance of a smooth, shiny surface, often associated with a brown spot (**Fig. 5.2b**). Both active and inactive initial caries can progress further to create irreversible loss of tooth substance.

The development and progression of carious lesions is characterized by a number of very diverse and variable factors. The combination of an increased number of pathogens, the presence of low-molecular-weight carbohydrates, and adequate residence time creates an environment in which tooth decay is likely to occur. In physiological conditions and good oral health, the oral cavity is colonized by a relatively stable flora, in terms of the quality and quantity of bacteria. However, this sensitive balance can easily be disturbed by various factors.

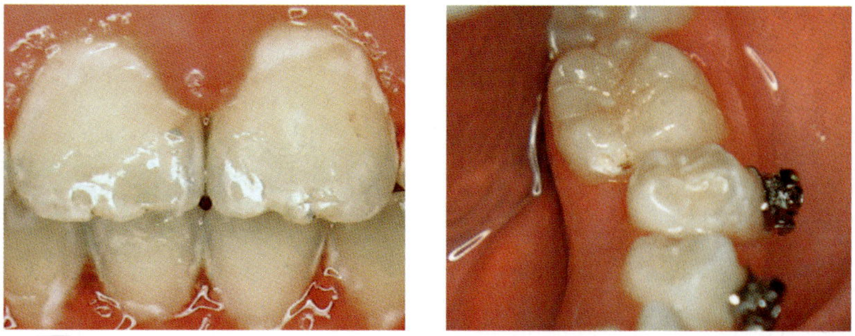

Fig. 5.2a, b Carious lesions on the teeth due to demineralization. Demineralization occurs to an acid environment. Initial carious lesions will appear when the balance between demineralization and remineralization tips toward the former.

a Typical decalcification due to plaque accumulation: this was due to poor oral hygiene around the brackets. Probing of the surface on the decalcified areas shows softened enamel.

b After widening of the interdental space with an elastic separator, a carious lesion becomes visible, which partly consists of a remineralized lesion (brown spot), while the majority consists of an active lesion (chalky white area). The pigmentation of brown spots takes place over several years as a result of the encapsulating coloring agents in the demineralized, porous enamel surface.

NOTE

Inappropriate oral hygiene and poor nutrition result in an increase in plaque, with a subsequent increase in pathogens.

The addition of glucose and saccharose (low-molecular-weight carbohydrates) to the diet leads to an increase in the bacterial turnover of sugars into organic acids. This is associated with a decrease in the pH level in the oral cavity, which in turn induces demineralization of the dental hard tissues. The critical pH level below which demineralization occurs is between 5.2 and 5.7.[8]

Epidemiology of Caries

The incidence and prevalence of caries are assessed using the decayed, missing, and filled teeth (DMFT) index. The results of a German study conducted in 2005 show that there was a significant reduction in DMFT during the 8-year study period. In comparison with the corresponding 1997 study, the DMFT declined from 1.7 to 0.7 teeth (58.8%) for 12-year-olds, and 70.1% of 12-year-olds and 46.1% of 15-year-old patients had a completely healthy dentition. The most important factors for reducing caries appear to be regular visits to the general dentist and provision of fissure sealants. Conversely, nearly 80% of all carious teeth were seen in 26.8% of the 15-year-olds. A significant reduction in caries in adults was observed for the first time (16.1% in 1997 versus 14.5% in 2005).[10]

Gingivitis and Periodontitis

Gingivitis and periodontitis are caused by bacterial colonization of the periodontal tissues. In etiological terms, the great majority of patients affected by periodontal disease also have increased plaque accumulation. The progression of the disease can be influenced by a number of factors and hormonal changes, medication, and symptoms of systemic diseases can all play a contributory role. Progression from chronic and long-standing to very aggressive disease may occur. A distinction is also made between localized disease (no more than 30% of the surfaces of the teeth affected) and generalized disease (more than 30% of the surfaces of the teeth affected).

NOTE

Gingivitis is characterized by typical signs of infection—reddening, swelling, and bleeding on probing (**Fig. 5.3**). It is prevalent in all age groups and social classes.[10]

Progressive periodontal disease usually leads to further attachment loss, which is characterized by an increase in probing depth. To allow international comparisons, the use of the World Health Organization's Community Periodontal Index (CPI) is recommended.

NOTE

The risk of periodontal disease increases with the patient's age.

a 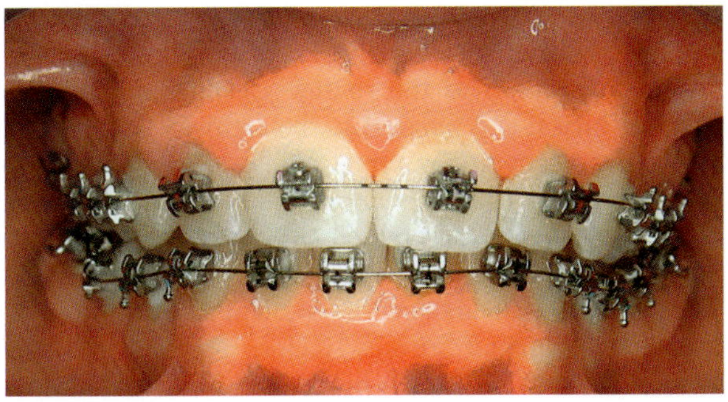 b 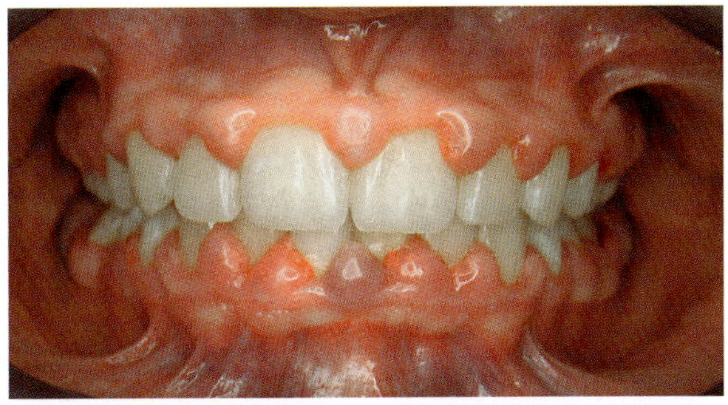

Fig. 5.3a, b Gingivitis, accompanied by the typical symptoms. The lower labial segment is often particularly affected, as it is difficult to maintain good oral hygiene in the tight spaces between the brackets. Gingival hyperplasia becomes quickly established after placement of fixed appliances and poor oral hygiene. The above images show the condition during orthodontic treatment (**a**) and following removal of the fixed appliances (**b**).

While gingivitis has a prevalence of 80% in children and adolescents, the prevalence of periodontitis in children is markedly lower than in adults. However, the epidemiological study mentioned above showed that 12.6% of all 15-year-olds have moderate periodontal disease and 0.8% have severe periodontal disease.[10] In the 35–44-year-old age group, who are increasingly seeking orthodontic treatment, a large proportion of patients have periodontal disease. More than half of the patients enrolled in the epidemiological study mentioned had a CPI of 3 (medium severity) and 20.5% were suffering from a severe form of periodontal disease. In comparison with the 1997 study, there was an increase of 26.9% in the overall prevalence.[10]

Hygiene Approaches for Fixed-Appliance Treatment

Prophylactic Measures

Bonding

Oral hygiene is more difficult after fixed appliances have been fitted. Efforts to maintain a patient's oral health should therefore start at the bonding appointment. Removing excess composite around the brackets, which may contribute to plaque accumulation, is as important as sealing the tooth surface surrounding the brackets with fluoride varnishes or other protective agents. A new generation of sealants that gradually release fluoride are a promising development. Although they provide only a very thin covering of the tooth surface, these sealants allow complete polymerization, which is not inhibited by oxygenation. Two of the more widely used products are manufactured by Reliance Orthodontics (Maximum Cure and Pro Seal). The products are reinforced with filler particles and consequently offer good abrasion resistance against everyday wear and tear (such as brushing teeth). According to the manufacturer, the sealing of the surrounding surface area should last for at least 2 years and possibly even longer. Even after 2 years, there is still residual resin on the tooth surface in up to 70% of cases. Reports in the literature[1,5] have shown that this system provides an equivalent bond strength to that of conventional adhesive systems and that remineralization of the dental enamel from the sealant's reserve has a protective effect against caries.[7,14]

The operator should carefully remove the adhesive material in the vicinity of the bracket (**Fig. 5.4**) to allow oral hygiene. Particularly in the area near the gingivae, residual composite can rapidly lead to accumulation of food debris and consequent overgrowth of the gingivae.

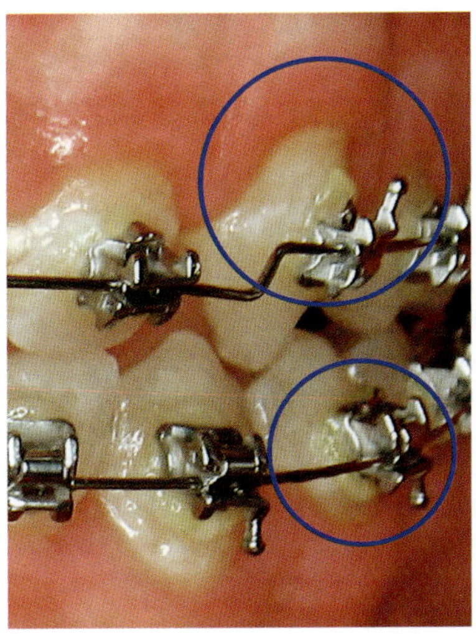

Fig. 5.4 Surplus bonding material that was not removed immediately after bonding. The excess adhesive is discolored and has contributed to plaque accumulation. Good cleaning has been hindered by the surplus bonding material, particularly in the vicinity of the gingiva.

CLINICAL PEARL

Bonding agents that incorporate a light-sensitive dye are colored before setting and thus make it easier for the orthodontist to remove excess composite (**Fig. 5.5**).

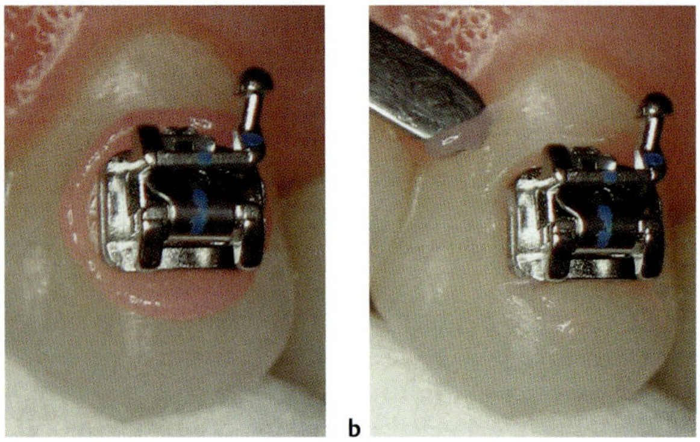

Fig. 5.5a, b After the bracket has been positioned on the tooth surface (**a**) the excess adhesive is clearly visible due to the added color and can be removed easily (**b**).

Active Tooth Movement

After fixed appliances have been fitted, plaque undergoes qualitative and quantitative changes, and there is a noticeable increase in *Streptococcus mutans*. Bearing in mind the etiology and pathogenesis of carious and periodontal disease, the orthodontist should coordinate prophylactic measures specifically during orthodontic treatment with fixed appliances. Important measures include the following:

- Instruction and motivation for the patient to practice good oral hygiene
- Patient education on the etiology of caries and periodontal disease
- Dietary counseling
- Regular maintenance by dental hygienists, with professional cleanings and consultations
- Topical fluoride applications
- Use of fluoride-containing materials
- Chemical plaque control

In a review of the extensive literature, Chadwick et al.[3] concluded that there is no single approach to oral hygiene that can be recommended. However, it is possible to significantly reduce the amount of decalcification by using fluoride-containing varnishes and/or sealants, fluoride-containing gels, or fluoride-containing mouth rinses (**Fig. 5.6**).

Maintaining good oral hygiene is complex and time-consuming for patients receiving treatment with fixed appliances. In addition to the routine cleaning of all tooth surfaces incisal and gingival to the archwire, it is particularly important to pay attention to cleaning the interdental spaces. Patients therefore need to be instructed in depth on hygiene requirements with orthodontic fixed appliances on the day the appliances are placed. It is advisable to use aids such as V-shaped bristled toothbrushes, interdental brushes (such as TePe®), and single tufted brushes (**Fig. 5.7**). A number of studies have confirmed that for most patients, the time spent on brushing teeth is significantly less than the recommended time. It is therefore very important, particularly when considering treatment periods lasting several years, to monitor oral hygiene regularly and ideally support patients in their efforts to keep the teeth clean by encouraging regular visits to the hygienist, for example.

NOTE

In addition to daily use of fluoride-containing toothpaste, we also recommend either a daily or weekly fluoride mouth rinse. Local fluoride applications can also be used, and fluoride-containing salt can be used as an adjunct to the above measures.

Effective oral hygiene can also be achieved with an electric toothbrush. These can basically be divided into systems that have a rotating or oscillating head and sonic systems (**Fig. 5.8**). For systems with rotational or oscillating heads, patients can purchase special heads designed for fixed-appliance treatment.

Some studies have reported that sonic-based systems are superior in comparison with the rotational or oscillating

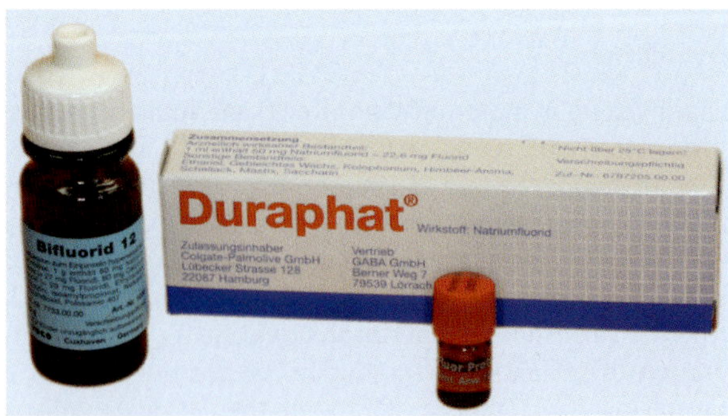

Fig. 5.6 Self-polymerizing fluoride varnishes to prevent demineralization and decalcification:
Bifluorid 12 (Voco): NaF, CaF_2; 55,900 ppm
Duraphat (GABA): NaF; 22,600 ppm
Fluor Protector (Ivoclar, Vivadent): Fluorsilan; 1000 ppm

systems,[9,13] but it remains to be seen whether these findings will be validated in subsequent studies. However, it is very important to remember that regular control visits and careful explanations are often the best way of keeping patients motivated and ensuring the best possible oral hygiene, regardless of which type of toothbrush is used. The peculiarities of the mixed and early permanent dentition in particular often require a very intensive oral hygiene regimen (**Fig. 5.9**). There is an increased incidence of caries during this period, as self-cleaning of the teeth is significantly reduced and good cleaning, particularly of the molars, can be difficult during their emergence. In addition, food retention and plaque accumulation may occur under residual opercular mucosa that partially covers the erupting teeth. Poor positioning of the teeth relative to the adjacent dentition can also give rise to carious lesions.

NOTE

The fissures on the first and second molars are particularly susceptible to the development of carious lesions.

Apart from the genetically predetermined fissures of the first and second molars, their prolonged eruption time is an additional factor that promotes increased plaque accumulation. Newly erupted teeth are generally more susceptible to decay, as the posteruptive maturation of the enamel (with a reduction in the water content and an increase in crystal size) is only completed after several months or years after exposure to the oral cavity. Final resistance to acid-based demineralization is only established after the completion of this maturation process. In addition, malaligned teeth can increase the incidence of periodontal disease and caries, particularly in adults.[6]

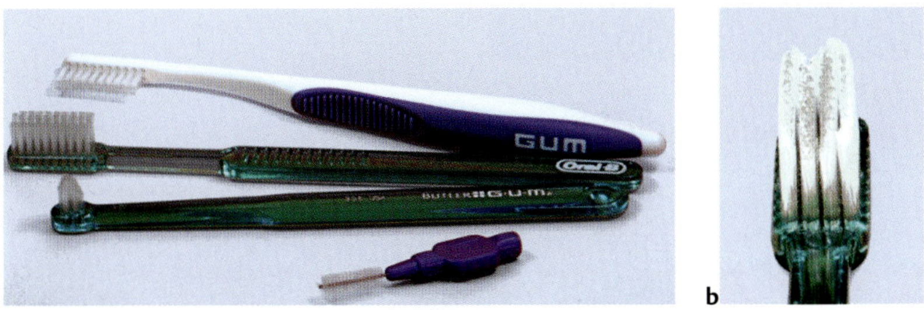

Fig. 5.7 a, b Various cleaning aids that may be useful during orthodontic treatment.
a Various toothbrushes: tufted brushes, interdental brushes.
b A V-shaped toothbrush, with better access around fixed appliances.

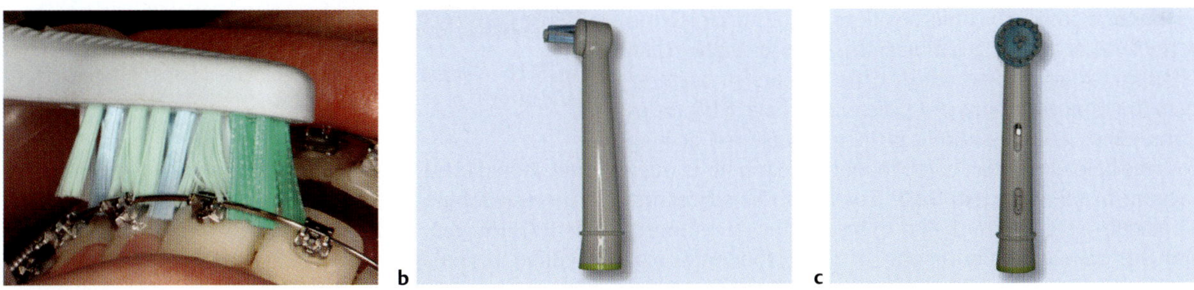

Fig. 5.8 a–c Electric toothbrushes.
a Ultrasonic brush (Sonicare/Philips).
b, c Several brush attachments for rotating and oscillating electric toothbrushes (Ortho Care Essentials/Oral B).

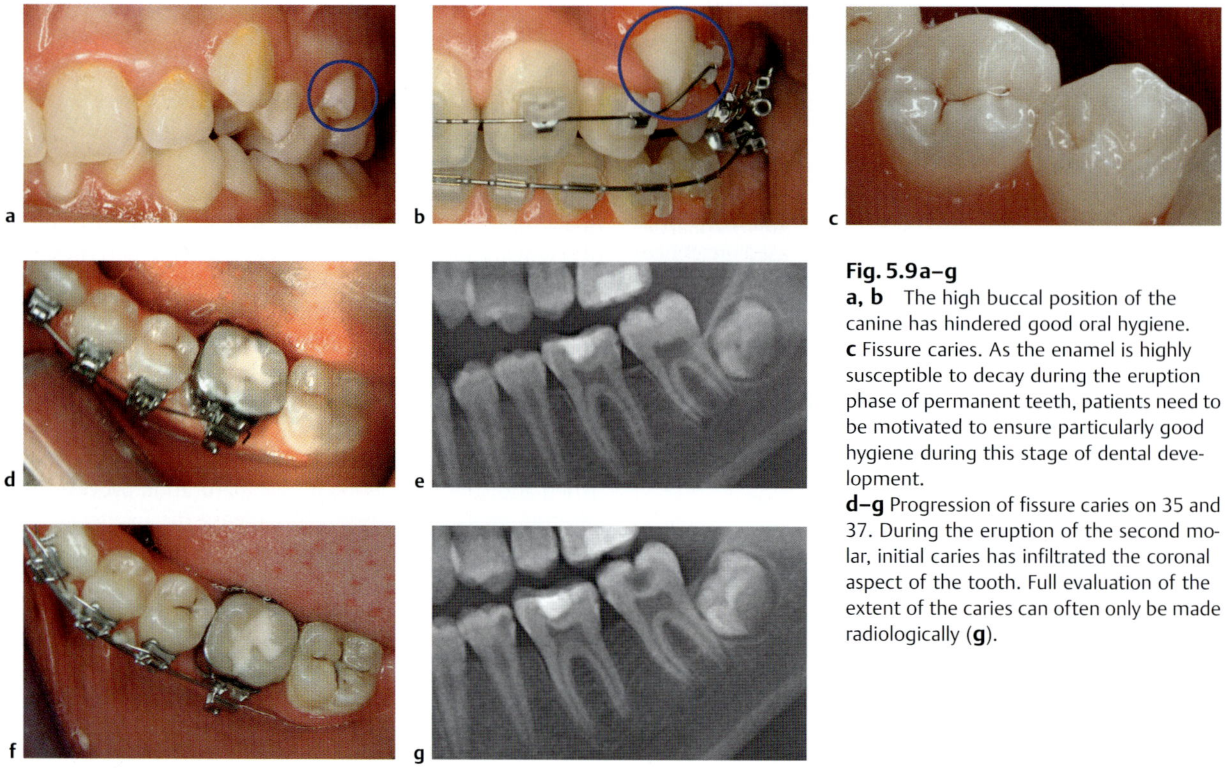

Fig. 5.9a–g
a, b The high buccal position of the canine has hindered good oral hygiene.
c Fissure caries. As the enamel is highly susceptible to decay during the eruption phase of permanent teeth, patients need to be motivated to ensure particularly good hygiene during this stage of dental development.
d–g Progression of fissure caries on 35 and 37. During the eruption of the second molar, initial caries has infiltrated the coronal aspect of the tooth. Full evaluation of the extent of the caries can often only be made radiologically (**g**).

Active Measures

When a high incidence of caries has been noted, or a predilection to developing caries or simple gingivitis has been diagnosed, appropriate measures must be considered to prevent exacerbation or development of more serious oral pathology. Chlorhexidine can be administered in the form of a rinse, gel, or varnish. At doses higher than 100 ppm, chlorhexidine reduces the number of bacteria. Even low concentrations of 1 ppm or less have a bacteriostatic effect. Chlorhexidine can be administered at high dosages before the start of orthodontic treatment using a vacuum-formed tray (**Fig. 5.10**). For this to be successful, all plaque—soft and hard—has to be previously removed, and this should ideally be part of the orthodontic oral hygiene regimen. Ideally, patients should receive chairside demonstrations on how to use the soft splints. They are applied after the teeth have been appropriately cleaned, and 2–3 cm of chlorhexidine gel is placed in the tray and distributed evenly. The splint should then be worn for approximately 10 minutes in the evening, after the evening meal and following thorough oral hygiene. This should be continued for at least 14 days, and the treatment outcome should be documented.

Patients requiring more intensive treatment can also benefit from using highly concentrated chlorhexidine varnishes, which are applied to areas where oral hygiene is difficult, such as the interdental spaces and fissures, and around the gingival margin. A small reservoir is applied and should ideally be left for approximately 5–15 minutes. The residual gel is then removed with a rubber cup. Biodent (Nijmegen, Netherlands) offers a varnish that is embedded in sandarac resin and is available in two different forms, under the trade name "EC 40" in a 35% concentration or as "BioC" in a 20% concentration. It is designed for particularly gentle application around the gingival margin. High-quality intraoral photography and regular assessment using oral hygiene indices such as the Approximal Plaque Index (API) and Sulcus Bleeding Index (SBI) make it possible to document treatment progress and help objectify the treatment results. It is important to have policies in place if oral hygiene is insufficient (as indicated by objective standards such as the various oral hygiene indices), so that the patient is appropriately warned and informed that the fixed appliances may have to be removed before the completion of treatment if oral hygiene standards deteriorate.

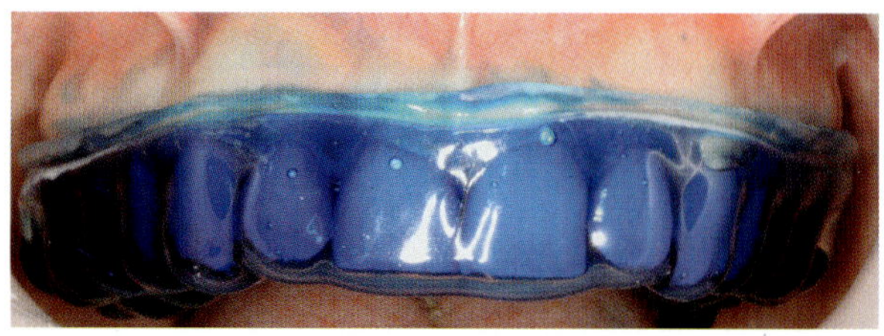

Fig. 5.10 Clinical use of a vacuum-formed tray containing chlorhexidine gel.

NOTE

Good orthodontic records also include documentation of oral hygiene (such as plaque retention, bleeding on probing, and probing depth) as well as previous caries.

Oral hygiene can be improved by patient education and plaque indicators are often very helpful (**Fig. 5.11**). After documentation of the findings and instructions on good oral hygiene, a number of professional aids for cleaning deposits on the teeth can be considered, for example, an ultrasonic scaler (**Fig. 5.12**) for hardened plaques, polishing paste or intraoral sandblasters such as the Prophy-Jet (**Table 5.1**).

ERRORS AND RISKS

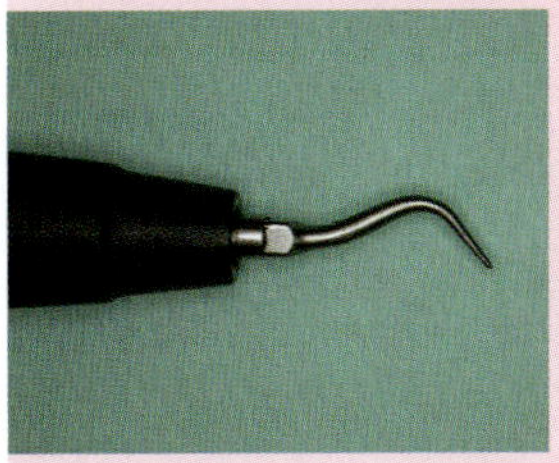

Fig. 5.12 Ultrasonic scalers, as shown here (SMS) should only be used cautiously with self-ligating bracket systems. The bracket mechanism may be damaged during the scaling process, and inadvertent bracket loss is also possible.

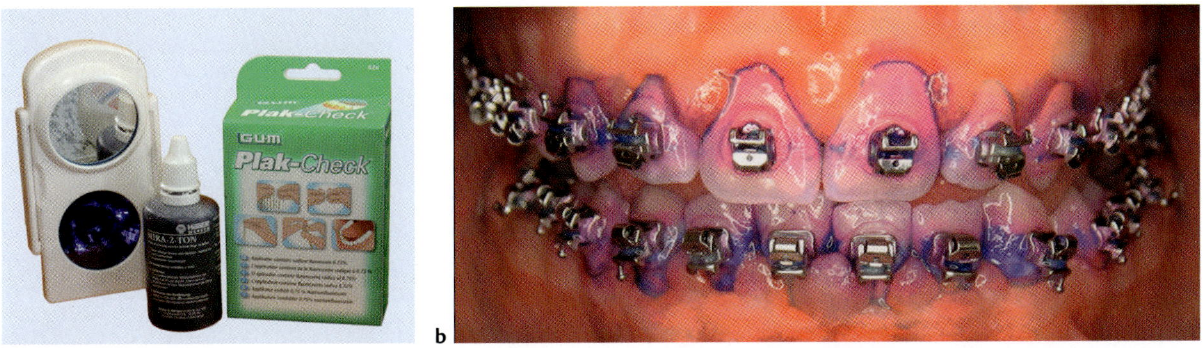

Fig. 5.11 a, b

a Plaque indicators: MIRA-2-Tone (Hager and Werken) and Plak-Check (GUM). Under ultraviolet illumination, Plak-Check reveals plaque with a yellow color.

b The MIRA-2-Tone indicators differentiate between nature and new plaque. Plaque more than 3 days old appears blue, while pink coloring indicates plaque that is less than 3 days old.

Table 5.1 Standard procedures for chairside care during fixed-appliance treatment: a clinical example for enhanced plaque control

To be undertaken at every visit

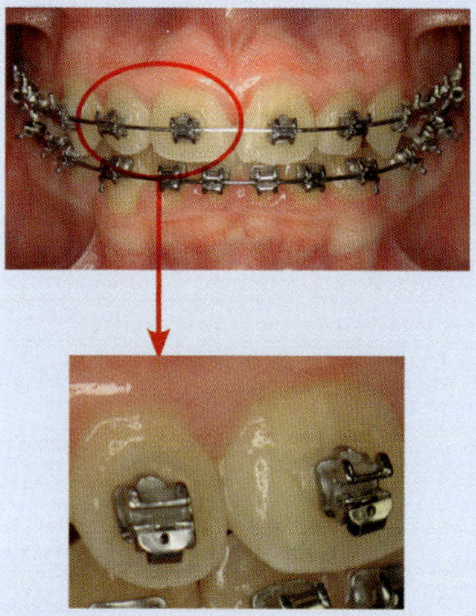

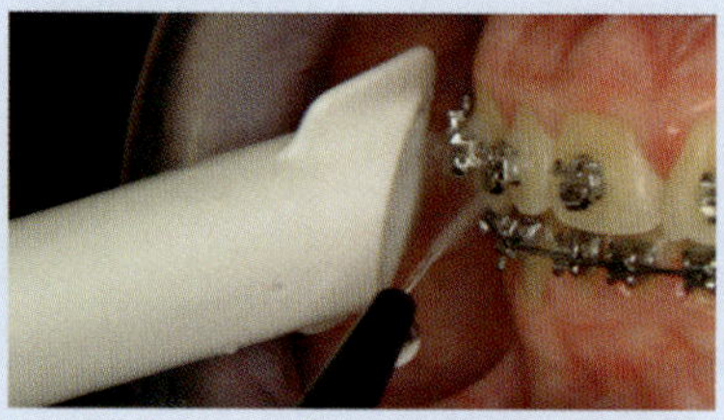

Removal of the archwire. Use of air-water syringe to clean bracket slots

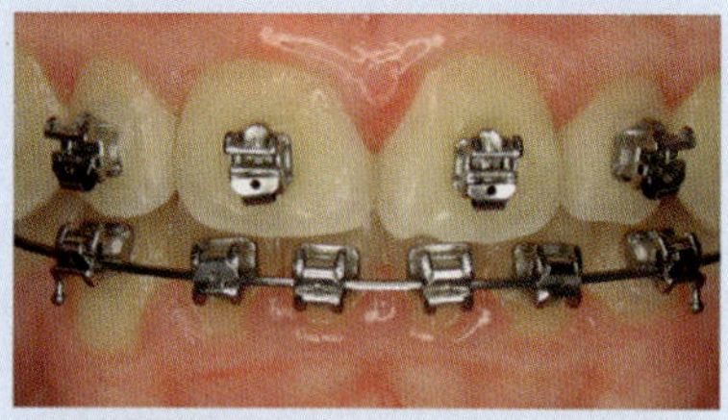

Cleaned slots

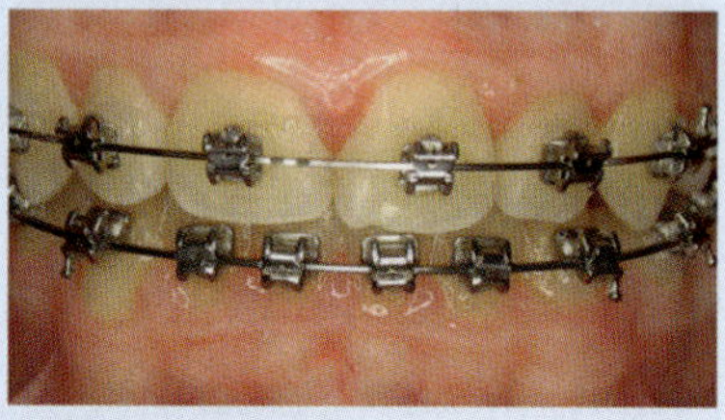

Archwire reinserted

Professional cleaning (when necessary)

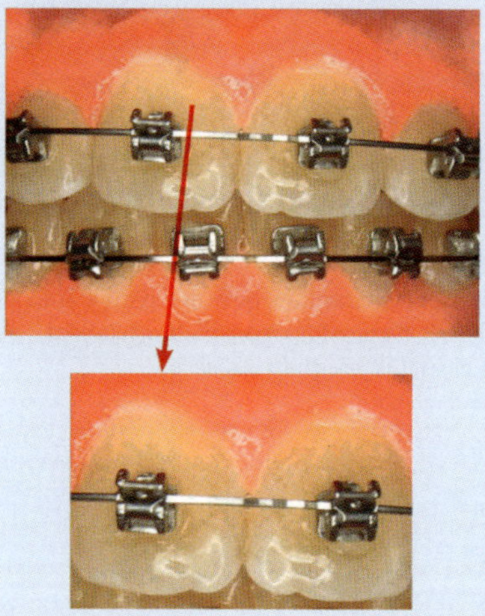

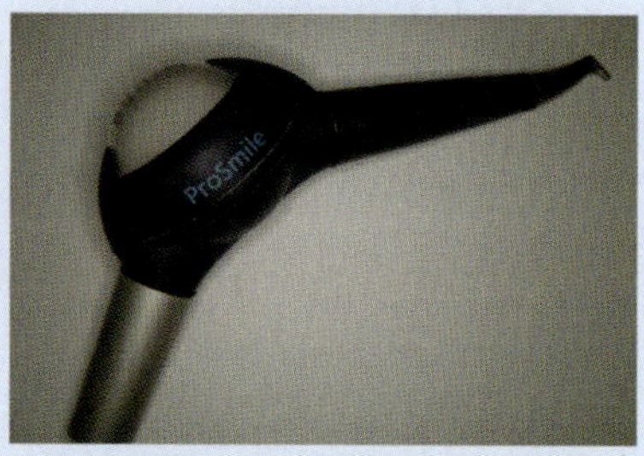

Cleaning tooth surfaces with a Prophy-Jet (Dentsply-Cavitron)

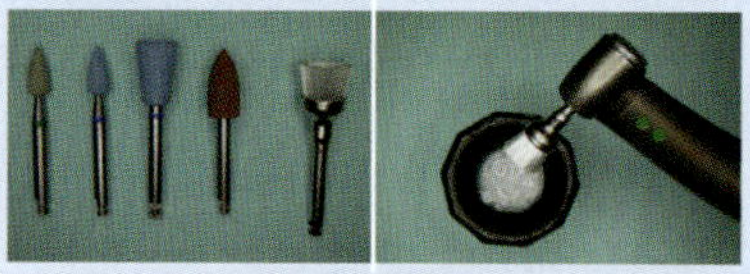

Followed by polishing (hygienist)

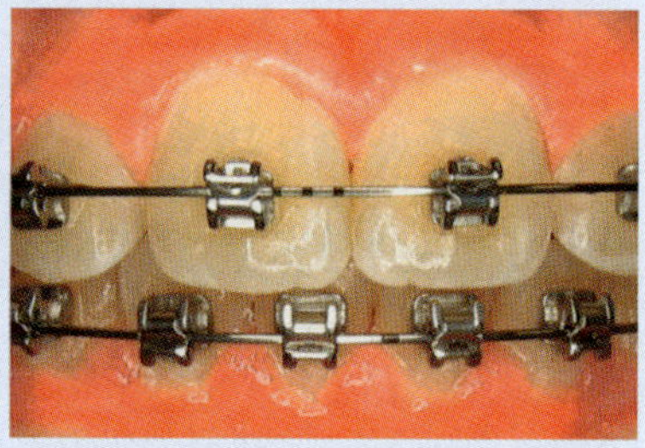

After cleaning

Oral Hygiene after Fixed-Appliance Treatment

The retention phase is important for maintaining orthodontic results and adequate oral hygiene continues to be paramount, and depending on the retainers used, may still involve a number of adjuncts. Removable retainers such as Hawley retainers, vacuum-formed retainers, and positioners allow good cleaning, as they can be removed for brushing. However, patients need to be aware that great care has to be taken when fixed retainers are used. Fixed retention is often used when orthodontic treatment has included extensive tooth movement, in adult patients, and all patients with previous periodontal disease.[2] The advantage of fixed retention is the more or less permanently secured position of the front teeth. However, this has the disadvantage that it can create undercuts in areas that are particularly prone to plaque and calculus accumulation and this may consequently put patients at risk for periodontal problems or tooth decay (**Fig. 5.13**). Appropriate patient information (ideally both written and verbal) and consent to this type of retention is usually advisable. The patient should be instructed to use adjuncts such as interdental brushes (TePe®), Superfloss, and Waterpik water flossers to maintain good oral hygiene around fixed retainers.

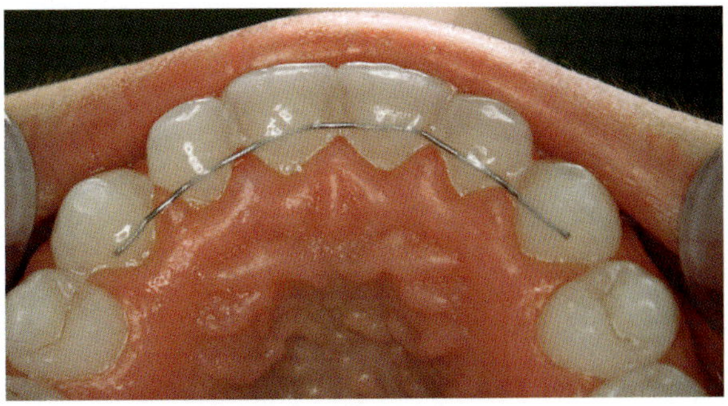

Fig. 5.13 Fixed retainer. This retainer had been fitted several months previously. While oral hygiene appears adequate, there are still signs of gingival inflammation and hyperplasia. The teeth should be professionally cleaned, and the amount of composite around the gingival margin should be reduced to allow for better oral hygiene.

REFERENCES

1. Bishara SE, Oonsombat C, Soliman MM, Warren J. Effects of using a new protective sealant on the bond strength of orthodontic brackets. Angle Orthod 2005;75(2):243–246
2. Bock JJ, Bock J. Grundwissen Kieferorthopädie. Balingen: Spitta Verlag; 2005
3. Chadwick BL, Roy J, Knox J, Treasure ET. The effect of topical fluorides on decalcification in patients with fixed orthodontic appliances: a systematic review. Am J Orthod Dentofacial Orthop 2005;128(5):601–606, quiz 670
4. Derks A, Katsaros C, Frencken JE, van't Hof MA, Kuijpers-Jagtman AM. Caries-inhibiting effect of preventive measures during orthodontic treatment with fixed appliances. A systematic review. Caries Res 2004;38(5):413–420
5. El Bokle D, Munir H. An in vitro study of the effect of Pro Seal varnish on the shear bond strength of orthodontic brackets. World J Orthod 2008;9(2):141–146
6. Hensel E. Langzeitwirkung von Dysgnathien auf den Gesundheitszustand von Zahnhartsubstanzen und Parodontium [postdoctoral dissertation]. Greifswald, Germany: University of Greifswald; 1985
7. Hu W, Featherstone JD. Prevention of enamel demineralization: an in-vitro study using light-cured filled sealant. Am J Orthod Dentofacial Orthop 2005;128(5):592–600, quiz 670
8. Klimek J, Hellwig E. Kariesätiologie und -diagnose. In: Heidemann D, ed. Kariologie und Füllungstherapie. Munich: Urban-Schwarzenberg; 1999:3–42
9. Kneist S, Zingler S, Lux C. Therapiebegleitende Maßnahmen zur Kontrolle des Karies- und Demineralisationsrisikos bei kieferorthopädischer Behandlung. ZWR 2008;117:218–226
10. Micheelis W, Schiffner U, eds. Vierte Deutsche Mundgesundheitsstudie (DMS IV). Neue Ergebnisse zu oralen Erkrankungsprävalenzen, Risikogruppen und zum zahnärztlichen Versorgungsgrad in Deutschland 2005. Cologne: Deutscher Zahnärzte Verlag; 2006
11. Øgaard B, Rølla G, Arends J. Orthodontic appliances and enamel demineralization. Part 1. Lesion development. Am J Orthod Dentofacial Orthop 1988;94(1):68–73
12. Øgaard B, Rølla G, Arends J, ten Cate JM. Orthodontic appliances and enamel demineralization. Part 2. Prevention and treatment of lesions. Am J Orthod Dentofacial Orthop 1988;94(2):123–128
13. Roulet JF, Fath S, Zimmer P. Lehrbuch der Prophylaxeassistentin. Munich: Urban und Fischer; 2006
14. Salar DV, García-Godoy F, Flaitz CM, Hicks MJ. Potential inhibition of demineralization in vitro by fluoride-releasing sealants. J Am Dent Assoc 2007;138(4):502–506

Bonding Techniques

Heiko Goldbecher and Jens Bock

6

The History and Development of Bonding Techniques

When bonding techniques were initially developed, E.W. E. Magill used bands made of precious metals that were cemented directly onto patients' teeth. Some 70 years later, in 1965, G.V. Newman first used direct adhesive bonding techniques. This was an important step in the development from a multiple-band to a multi-bracket appliance. Until then, using fixed appliances required tremendous logistic effort, as it was necessary to have a stock of approximately 30 bands per tooth in order to accommodate the various sizes for each tooth to be banded. Bands are now generally only used for molars; in exceptional circumstances, premolars are banded (for rapid maxillary expansion, for example) (**Fig. 6.1**). The development of bonding thus started with bands cemented, and adhesive techniques were subsequently developed that initially used universal bracket bases. The bracket base was then modified to allow better fitting of individual tooth shapes, and anatomically preformed bracket bases were developed. More recently, individual bracket bases that are custom-made for the patient's individual tooth shape have become commercially available.

The development of self-ligating brackets is not a revolutionary change. The problems generally associated with ligation have not changed. As is described in more detail below, the use of self-ligating brackets requires a certain level of experience which may, at least initially, negatively affect the efficacy of treatment. Successful positioning of a preadjusted bracket in a precise, predetermined location depends on a number of factors, which are generally independent of the ligation mechanism, as the bases of the orthodontic bracket are often identical for each manufacturer, regardless of ligation technique. However, the bracket design itself may have an impact on bracket positioning. Some self-ligating brackets, for example, do not have a vertical slot, and this may make positioning more difficult. The basic principles of ligation are described in detail in Chapter 2; this chapter focuses on the peculiarities of bonding with self-ligating brackets. The following general aspects affect the success of a bonded bracket:

- Congruence of the bracket base with the tooth surface
- Positioning in the vertical and horizontal planes, as well as rotational positioning
- Bond strength (shear, tensile, and torque)
- Debonding characteristics of the bracket

It is only the bracket positioning that is different for self-ligating and conventional brackets.

Positioning of Brackets

Successful treatment with the preadjusted appliance requires precise bracket placement in all three planes of space.

Vertical Positioning

There are numerous suggestions in the literature that can be used as a guide for vertical positioning of brackets on teeth. Most authors use the distance between the incisal edge and the bracket slot as a reference. We recommend the values indicated in **Table 6.1**. There will be a difference between the incisal edge of the central and lateral incisors of approximately 0.5 mm when using these values (**Fig. 6.2**).

In our own studies, we compared the congruence between the bracket base and individual tooth surfaces (**Fig. 6.3**). Scanning the labial surfaces of 500 maxillary central incisors made it possible to develop an average three-dimensional labial tooth surface, which was then compared with bracket bases supplied by various manufacturers in the mesiodistal and occlusogingival directions.

a b

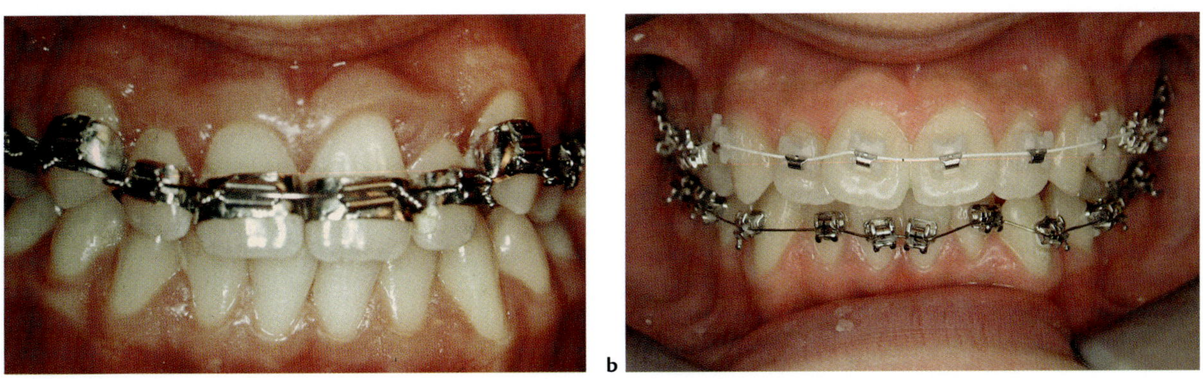

Fig. 6.1 a, b Multiple-band fixed appliances approximately 40 years ago (**a**), and contemporary fixed appliances (**b**).

Table 6.1 Tip and torque values based on McLaughlin, Bennett and Trevisi.[3,4] Depending on the tooth anatomy, bracket positioning can vary by ± 0.5–1.0 mm vertically

	Tooth	1	2	3	4	5	6	7
Distance to the incisal edge in millimeters (standard values) 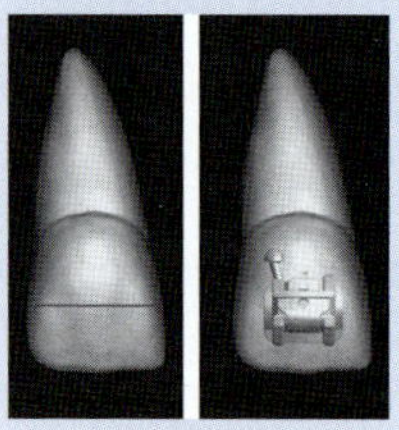	Upper jaw	5	4.5	5	4.5	4	3	2
	Lower jaw	4	4	4.5	4	3.5	2.5	2.5
Open bite tendencies: On anteriors: + 1 mm On posteriors: –0.5 to –1.0 mm 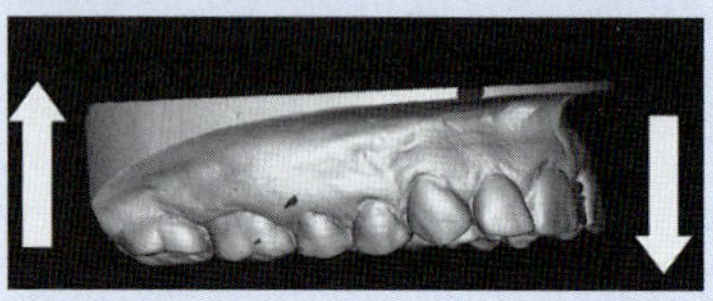	Upper jaw	6	5.5	6	3.5	3	2	2
	Lower jaw	5	5	5.5	3	2.5	2	2
Deep bite tendencies: On anteriors: –1 mm On posteriors: + 0.5–1.0 mm 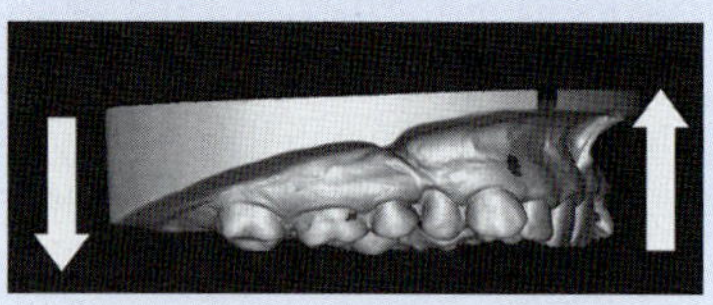	Upper jaw	4	3.5	4	5.5	5	4	3
	Lower jaw	3	3	3.5	5	4.5	3.5	3.5

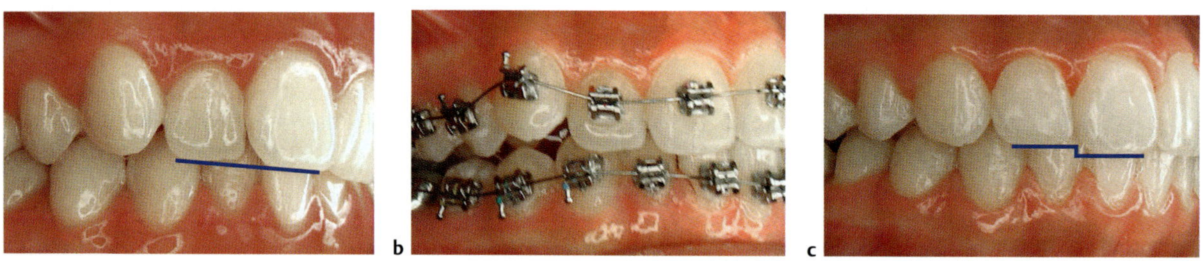

a b c

Fig. 6.2a–c The incisal edge relationship before (**a**), during (**b**), and after orthodontics (**c**).

A good fit of the bracket base is essential, as the bracket slot of a poorly fitting bracket will not be positioned accurately to achieve the desired tooth movement. This is often why teeth sometimes express unwanted movement, which is usually corrected toward the end of the treatment, using artistic bends.

Horizontal Positioning

The positioning of the brackets in the mesiodistal direction is by reference to the height of the tooth contour and contact points to the adjacent tooth (**Fig. 6.4**), while the angulation is determined by the long axis.

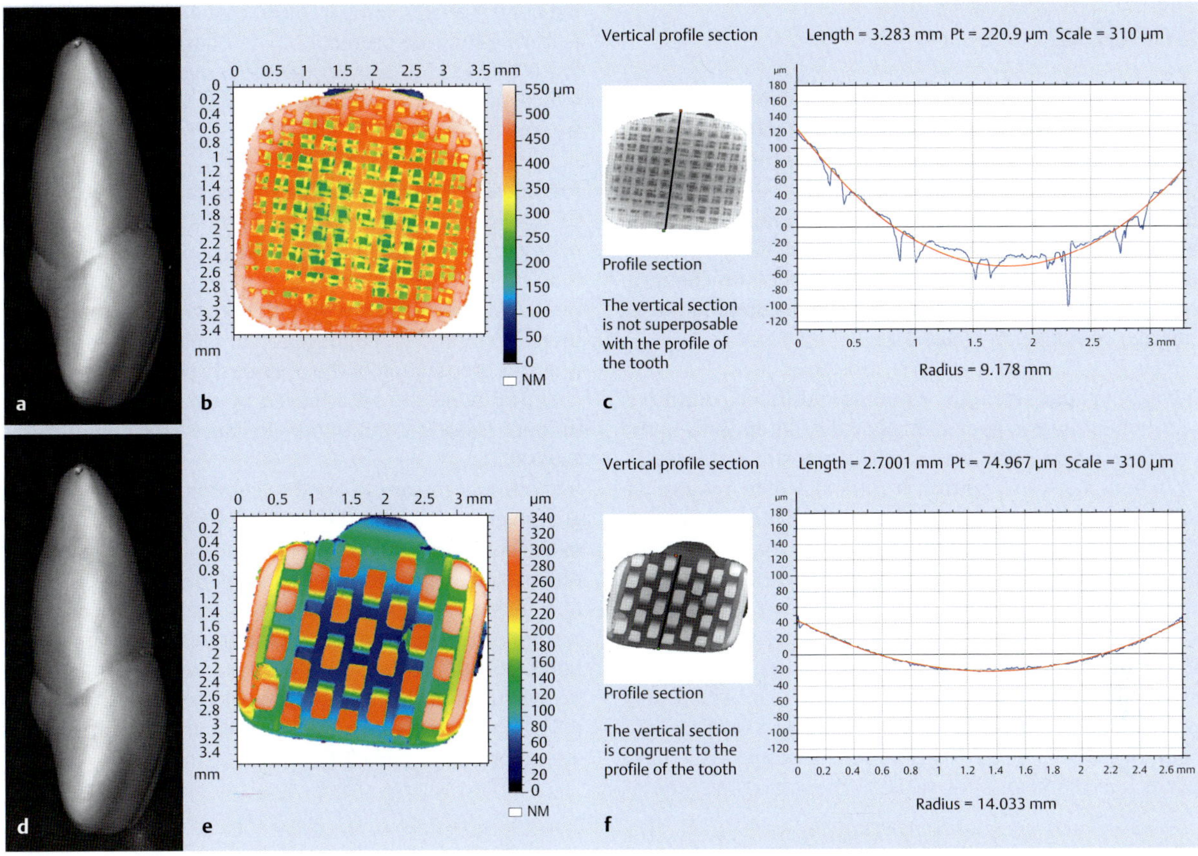

Fig. 6.3 a–f Vertical profile sections of a bracket in a predetermined area.
a–c The radius of the In-Ovation R bracket is narrow. This means that the bracket base has a strong curvature, which does not fit the tooth well.
d–f The radius of the Quick bracket conforms well to the surface of the computer-generated "average" tooth.

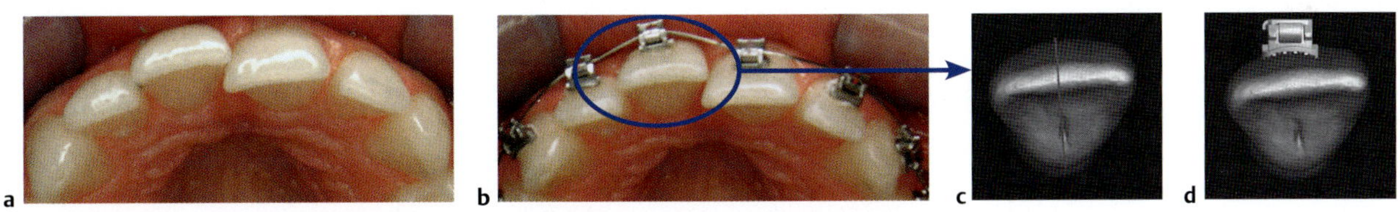

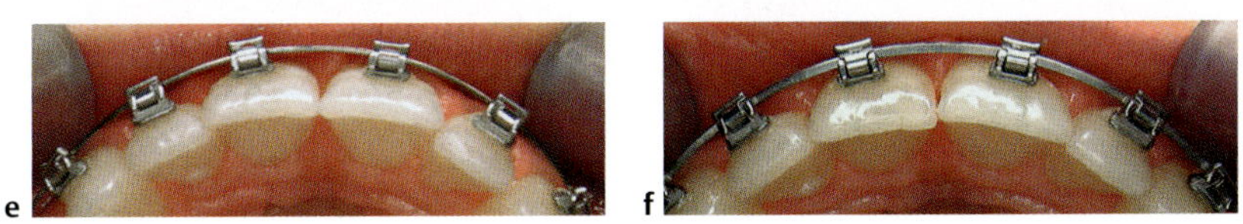

Fig. 6.4 a–f The bracket on tooth 11 was set slightly distal to its ideal position (**a**). The error is not yet fully evident during the initial alignment phase (**b–d**). In the larger rectangular wires, however, the positioning error becomes clear (**e**, **f**).

Bonding

With regard to bonding brackets, there are generally no differences between the various ligation methods, and the same selection criteria for bonding agents therefore apply.

Bonding to the natural tooth surface. Bonding to healthy enamel is a standardized procedure that involves either mechanical bonding (acid-etch technique) or chemical bonding (glass ionomer cements), or a combination of the two components (**Table 6.2**).

Increase in bond strength. Bonding in difficult conditions (e.g., when there is poor enamel quality, alterations in the enamel surface, deciduous teeth, composite restorations, or when moisture control is difficult) may require an adhesion booster such as Enhance (Reliance Orthodontics), which has been on the market for many years and has more recently been replaced by Assure. According to the manufacturer, this product increases the bond strength and has a greater fluoride content. Maximum Cure and Pro Seal (also Reliance Orthodontics), are also sealers but have a higher filler content than Assure and are therefore useful for sealing the tooth surface surrounding the bracket. Both products supposedly have protective characteristics, while at the same time providing bond strength comparable to that of other primers not featuring fluoride protection. The fluoride-releasing sealant is intended to protect the teeth over a 2-year period, which normally covers the duration of fixed appliance treatment.

Priming of previously filled or altered tooth surfaces. Due to the increasing numbers of adults who are seeking orthodontic treatment, orthodontists are more interested than ever to develop bonding strategies for teeth that have previously been filled with either composite, ceramic, or metal restorations. Bonding to composite almost always requires preparation of the previously polished surfaces. A chemical bond can be achieved by using a polymer conditioner (Plastic Conditioner; Reliance Orthodontics, see **Table 6.3**).

It is often necessary to bond to ceramic restorations such as veneers or crowns. The bonding techniques are similar to the bonding protocols for ceramic inlays and prosthetic restorations in restorative dentistry (**Table 6.4**).

It is often necessary to roughen the surface of metal restorations before bonding. Conditioners to increase the bond strength to metal restorations are known as metal primers (Metal Primer; Reliance Orthodontics, see **Table 6.5**). Bonding protocols for the various types of surfaces are described in **Table 6.6**.

Table 6.2

Bonding to enamel	
Mechanical macroretention	Buccal technique: – Lingual technique: microetching
Mechanical microretention	Conditioning of enamel with 30%–40% phosphoric acid
Chemical bonding	Primer—i.e., unfilled monomer or microfilled monomer penetrates into the mechanical microretentions created by enamel etching
Bonding agent	Composite or compomer

Table 6.3

Bonding to existing composite fillings, composite veneers, or acrylic denture teeth	
Mechanical macroretention	Roughening of the surface with a microetcher or with a tungsten carbide burr
Additional bond strength enhancer	Polymer conditioner
Chemical bonding	Primer—i.e., unfilled or microfilled monomer penetrates into the mechanical macroretentions and dissolves the polymer chains of the surrounding acrylic
Bonding agent	Composite

Table 6.4

Bonding to ceramic	
Mechanical macroretention	Roughening of the surface with microetcher or fine diamond burrs
Mechanical microretention	Conditioning of the ceramic with 15%–20% hydrofluoric acid
Additional chemical bonding	Silane agent: porcelain conditioner (Reliance Orthodontics) or silane coupling agent (Espe)
Chemical bonding	Primer—i.e., unfilled or microfilled monomer uses both mechanical macroretention and microretention, and a chemical bond via silane coupling agents
Bonding agent	Composite

Table 6.5

Bonding to metal surfaces (gold, amalgam, and nonprecious metals)	
Mechanical macroretention	Roughening of the surface with microetch or with fine diamonds
Mechanical microretention	Acid-etch conditioning generally not necessary
Additional chemical bonding	Metal primer based on triphosphorus methacrylate
Chemical bonding	Primer: unfilled primer or microfilled, which primarily uses mechanical retention
Bonding agent	Composite

NOTE

Table 6.6 Bonding protocols for various surfaces

	Mechanical macroretention	Mechanical microretention	Additional chemical bond enhancers	Chemical priming agents	Bonding agents
Enamel		30%–40% phosphoric acid		Primer uses mainly mechanical microretention created from enamel conditioning	Composite or compomer
Dentin		Cleaning and "roughening" of surface to reveal dentin channels		Primer, mainly via dentin channels	Compomer or glass ionomer cement
Gold, amalgam, nonprecious metals	Microetch and/or roughening with a fine diamond		Metal primer (triphosphorus methacrylate-based)	Primer uses mainly macroretention	Composite
Composite	Microetch and/or roughening with tungsten carbide burr		Polymer conditioners	Primer uses macroretention and chemical bonding via dissolved polymer chains	Composite
Ceramic	Microetch and/or roughening with a fine diamond	Hydrofluoric acid 15%–20%	Silane agents	Primer uses macroretention and chemical bonding via silane coupling	Composite

Bonding agents with color indicators. Some contemporary bonding agents contain a chemical that changes color either when cured or with a change of temperature (Transbond SB and Blue, 3 M Unitek; and Gréngloo, Ormco). This makes it easier to detect surplus adhesive during bonding or debonding (the latter applies only to temperature-sensitive composites). This can be particularly useful for self-ligating brackets (**Fig. 6.5**), as excess composite may interfere with the self-ligating mechanism. The surplus adhesive is easily seen and can be removed before light-curing of the material.

CLINICAL PEARL

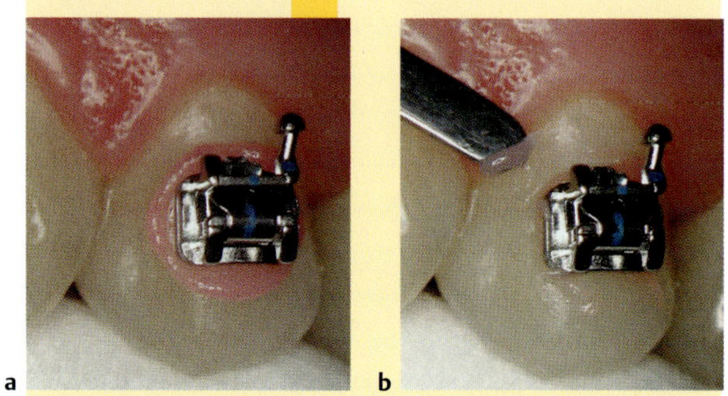

Fig. 6.5 a, b An example of an adhesive with a color indicator, which is useful for visualization and removal of composite remnants. Blugloo and Gréngloo (Ormco), which contain the respective coloring agents, are temperature-sensitive. These bonding agents lose their color when they reach mouth temperature and may need to be cooled down inside the mouth for visualization. Bre.versible (Bredent Medical, Senden, Germany) is yellow in color on delivery but when it is exposed to ultraviolet light it reveals composite remnants by changing its color to blue. Transbond Plus, which is pink (3 M Unitek) is not temperature-sensitive, but becomes transparent once set.

Positioning of Self-Ligating Brackets

Positioning of self-ligating brackets can be facilitated by using special tools such as positioning tweezers and jigs. These can be obtained in a number of designs, depending on the operator's preference. Conventional twin brackets are usually placed using the vertical slot. Apart from the SmartClip, this is not possible with any other self-ligating bracket. The SmartClip bracket has a "classic" bracket design with the traditional twin tie-wings and can therefore be positioned in a similar way to a conventional bracket (**Fig. 6.6**). Self-ligating brackets are delivered open or closed. With closed bracket slots, some inaccuracies in placing the brackets may occur in the hands of an inexperienced operator. Some training (with practice on study models using toffee as an adhesive) may be beneficial before the brackets are directly bonded in patients to avoid inadvertent positioning inaccuracies (**Figs. 6.7** and **6.8**). The vertical positioning of self-ligating brackets is comparable to that of conventional ligation brackets, for both open and closed delivery brackets. However, when a failed self-ligating bracket is being replaced, it should be borne in mind that, if the replacement bracket is delivered closed, it may be difficult to place it in the correct vertical position. The surrounding brackets will be open at this point, as the archwire has been removed for the repair. Conversely, for brackets that are delivered closed, the horizontal pressure used to seat the bracket can lead to positioning inaccuracies due to slippage, which can be avoided if the bracket is opended before placement.

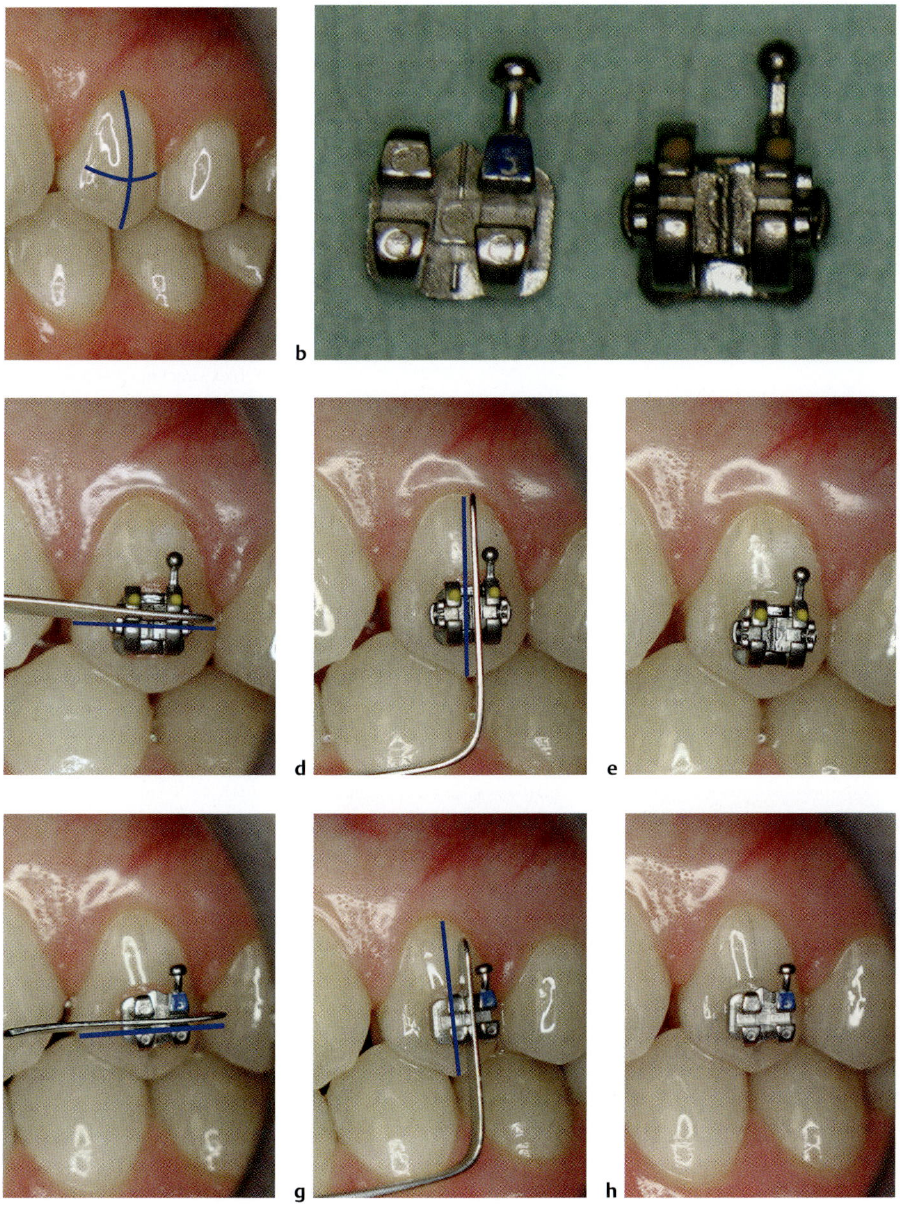

a b c d e f g h

Fig. 6.6a–h Using a small spatula for vertical and horizontal bracket positioning.
a Markings on the enamel surface prior to bonding.
b A conventional bracket (left) and a SmartClip bracket (right) in comparison.
c–e The SmartClip bracket. All the steps for bonding are identical to those for a conventional bracket (**f–h**).

NOTE

The closing mechanisms in self-ligating brackets block the vertical slot. Only the SmartClip (3 M Unitek) bracket can be positioned in the same way as conventional brackets.

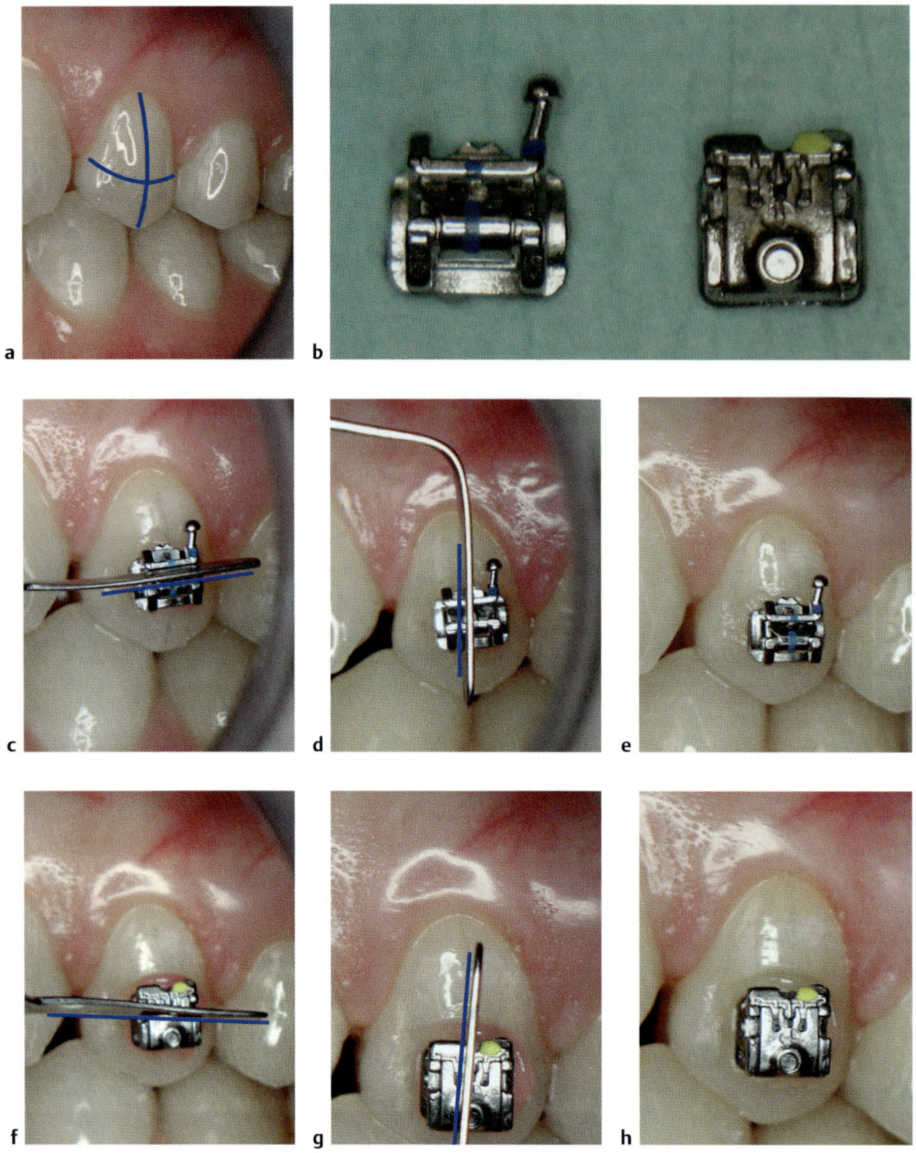

Fig. 6.7 a–h
a Markings on the enamel surface before bonding.
b Quick bracket (left), Carriere LX bracket (right).
c–e Positioning of the Quick bracket.
f–h Positioning of the Carriere LX bracket.
Brackets with closed doors cannot be positioned in the same way as conventional brackets: the Quick and Carriere LX brackets are used here as examples. For the Quick bracket, there are vertical indicators that aid in horizontal positioning of the bracket on the tooth (**c–e**). For the Carriere LX bracket, the vertical markings are not as clear and it is also more difficult to use a probe or spatula as a positioning aid, due to the smooth surface characteristics of the closed bracket. However, in contrast to brackets that are delivered with an open mechanism, the lower border is clearly identifiable and can aid in proper bracket positioning (parallel to the incisal edge).

NOTE

The Quick bracket can be easily positioned horizontally, due to its groove. Accurate vertical positioning is only possible with visual assistance; the vertical slot is occupied by the locking mechanism.
The Carriere bracket is difficult to position, both visually and by touch. Indirect bonding may be helpful for this procedure.

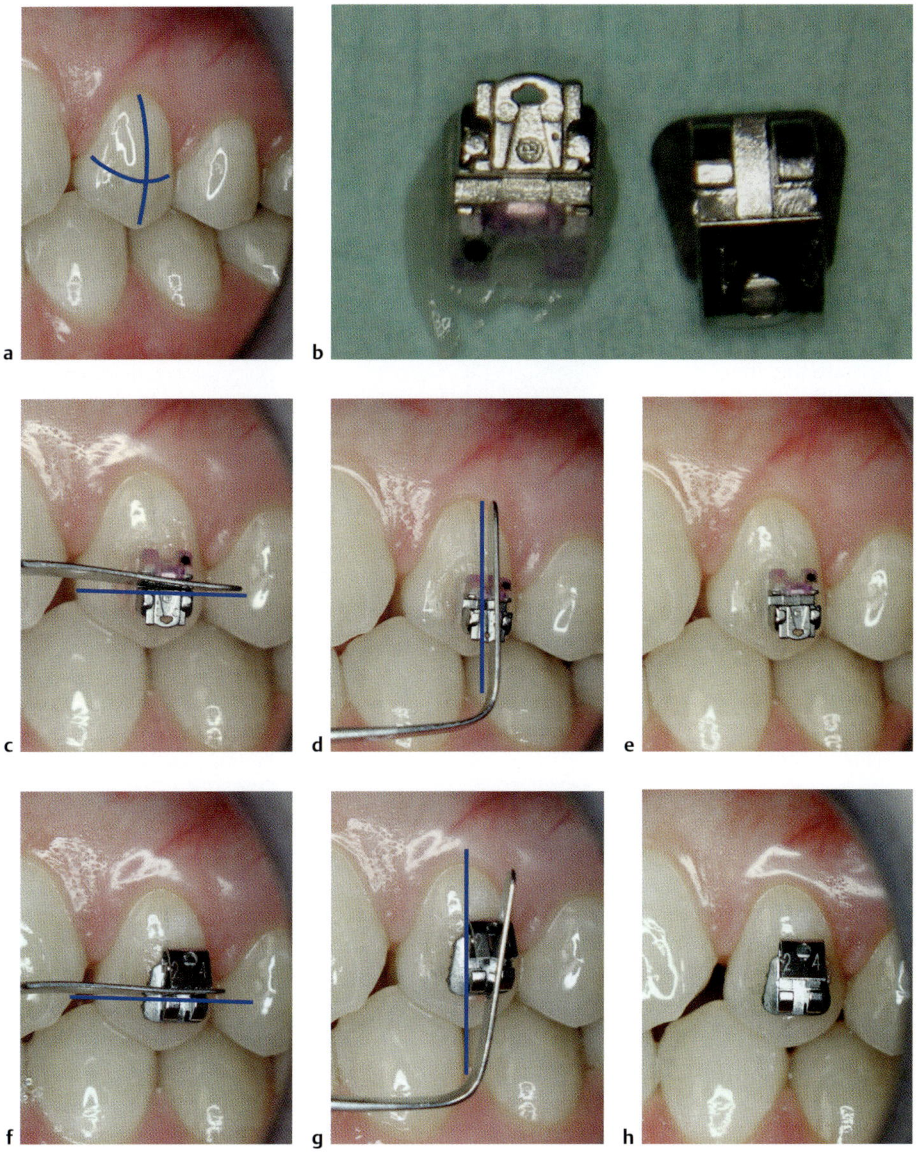

Fig. 6.8a–h Brackets delivered with an opened self-ligating mechanism. An instrument can easily be used for bracket positioning, as with a conventional bracket. However, the open delivery obstructs the view of the bracket base and can interfere with visual positioning. The examples here are Damon 3 and Time 2 brackets.
a Markings on the tooth prior to bonding.
b Damon 3 bracket (left) and Time 2 bracket (right) in comparison.
c–e Positioning of the Damon 3 bracket.
f–h Positioning of the Time 2 bracket.

NOTE

Opened self-ligating mechanisms are a hindrance when the brackets are being positioned vertically, while the open slots aid horizontal positioning.

Direct and Indirect Bonding Techniques

The following sections compare direct and indirect bonding techniques for self-ligating bracket systems. Indirect bonding has a number of distinct advantages for self-ligating systems, due to the demanding mechanical characteristics of the ligation mechanism itself (**Fig. 6.9**).

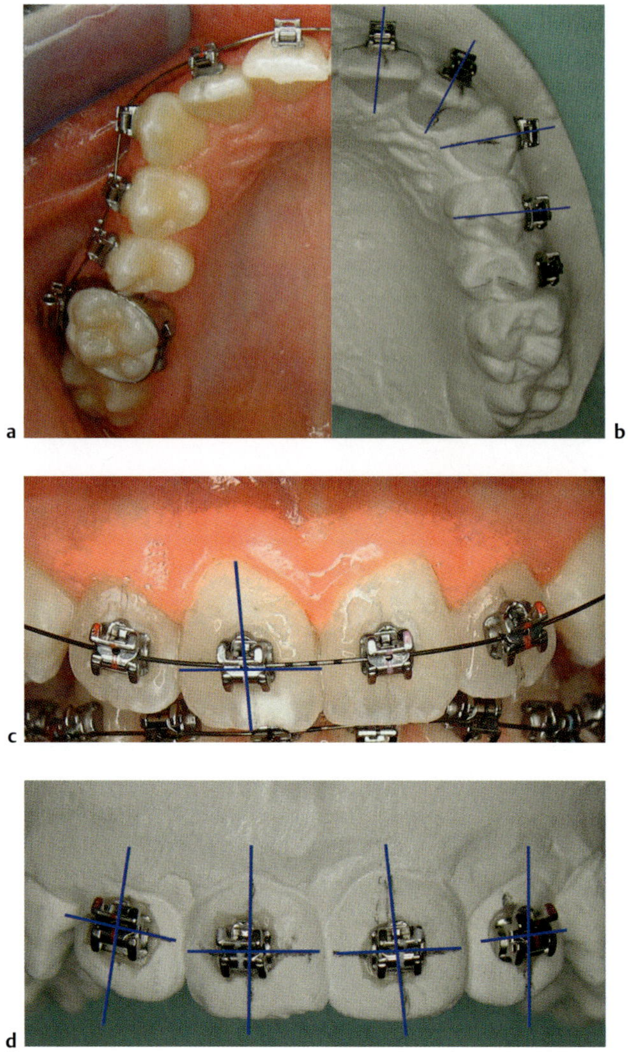

Fig. 6.9a–d Direct and indirect bonding. The advantage of indirect bonding is that brackets are positioned precisely according to vertical and horizontal orientation lines that are directly marked on the plaster cast. Visualization is unobstructed, and the bracket positions can be easily evaluated from all angles. The marks would have to be placed on the conditioned enamel surface, if the tooth surfaces were to be marked for direct bonding.
a, c Direct bonding.
b, d Indirect bonding.

Direct Bonding

The series of images in **Fig. 6.10** illustrate the direct bonding technique in a step-by-step fashion.

CLINICAL PEARL

OptraGate check retractors (Ivoclar, Vivadent, available in several sizes) provide good visibility of the working field.

Advantages

There are no additional laboratory costs associated with this method. The positioning of the bracket is directly visible; residual surface adhesive can be removed immediately.

NOTE

Direct bonding of self-ligating brackets allows visualization and removal of excessive bonding agent, preventing subsequent interference with the ligation mechanism.

Disadvantages

The field of vision may be limited due to access problems, depending on the cheek retractor used, the extent of the patient's mouth opening, and the tightness of the lips. This can be particularly difficult in the premolar and molar areas, and inaccuracies in bracket placement will require either compensatory bending for detailing and finishing, or repositioning of the brackets.

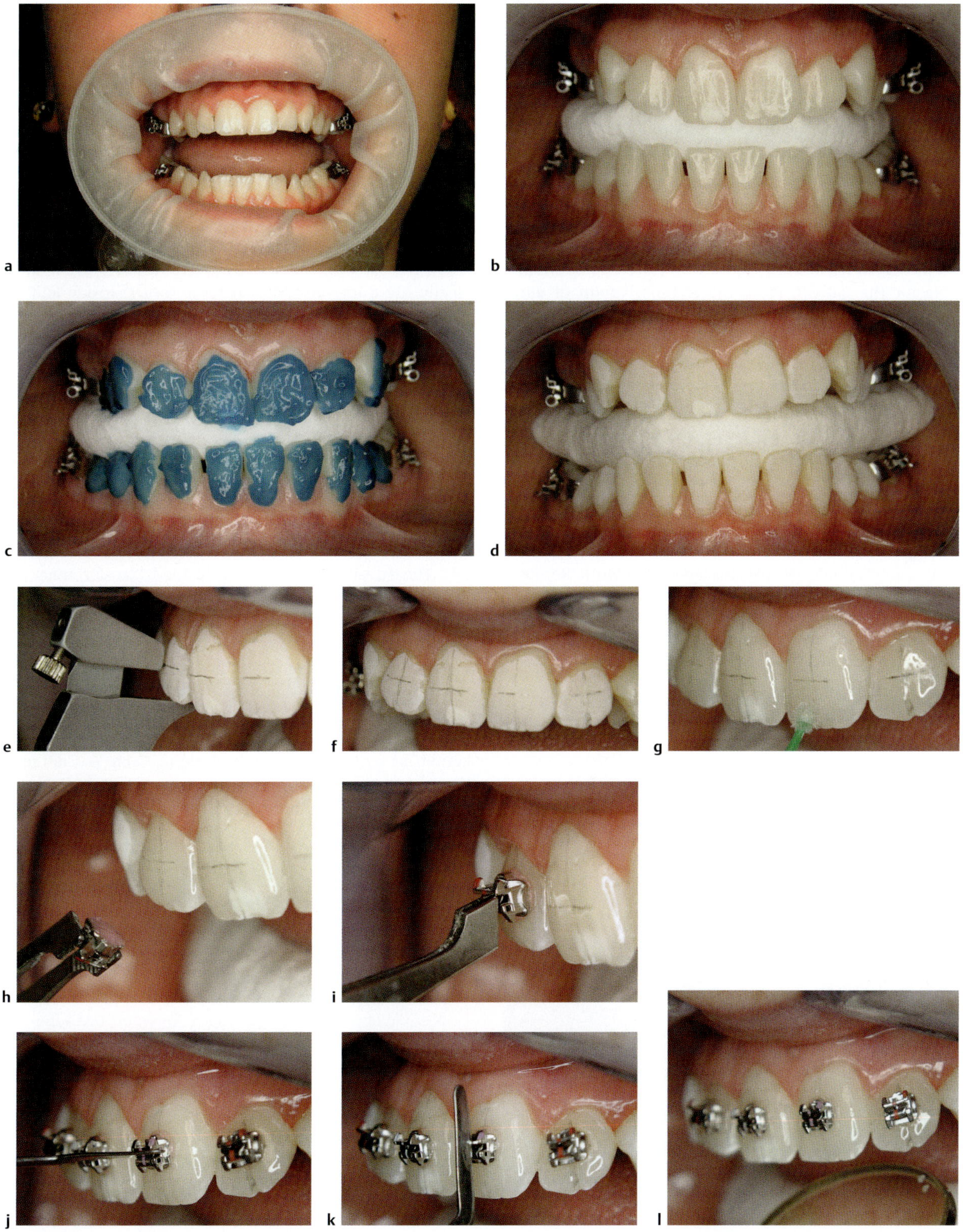

Fig. 6.10 a–l Direct bonding

a, b Use of a cheek retractor to establish a dry field.

c Conditioning of the enamel with phosphoric acid. The whole buccal enamel surface is etched to allow a sealant to be used to protect the enamel surface from decalcification.

d Drying of the field shows the "frosted" appearance of the enamel and thus confirms the etching.

e, f Marking of the reference points for bonding using a Boley gauge with a pencil tip. This can be used for both horizontal and vertical markings.

g Application of the sealant and primer.

h, i Positioning of the bracket at the appropriate site.

j, k Horizontal (**j**) and vertical (**k**) positioning of the bracket.

l Using an intraoral mirror to verify the bracket position before light-curing.

Indirect Bonding

Indirect bonding requires initial positioning of brackets on a working model.[1,2] Following bracket positioning on the model, a transfer tray is fabricated (**Table 6.7**), which is then used to bond the brackets intraorally by transferring the brackets from the model to the patient's teeth (**Table 6.8**).

Advantages

Less chairside time is one of the main advantages claimed for this system, which is more convenient and comfortable for the patient. From the technical point of view, however, it is also significantly easier to bond the brackets on the teeth, as the positioning has already been carried out on the working model. This advantage may be more pronounced if the bonding is being carried out by an inexperienced operator.

Disadvantages

Two appointments are necessary for indirect bonding (one for the study model impression, which allows the laboratory to position the brackets, and one for the bond itself, which is the second stage of the procedure). There will also be additional costs for laboratory work. Removal of excess adhesive may be more labor-intensive, as the surplus composite cannot be removed before it has set. The composite may also inadvertently find its way into the ligation mechanism itself and can interfere with the opening and closing of the mechanism.

Transfer Trays

Silicone Transfer Trays

The brackets are first fixed to the plaster model. The silicone material is subsequently molded to the model with the brackets present. The silicone is adapted to the brackets in a careful fashion that reduces the risk of positioning errors in the transfer tray. The tray can be cut once the silicone has set. Placement of the brackets can be carried out with either a full tray or a partial tray. Very few tools are required for fabricating a silicone positioning tray. The use of a transparent silicone such as Memosil CD (Heraeus Kulzer) improves visibility during the bonding procedure and also allows light-cured composites to be used. One disadvantage of this material is its flexibility even after it has set. Some authors recommend a second layer such as a transparent vacuum-formed tray that sits on top of the silicone tray to increase rigidity (**Fig. 6.11**). If nontransparent silicone trays are used, one should ideally use a low-viscosity material on the inside and a putty (high-viscosity) material on the outside. This increases the precision of the transfer during manufacture as well as bonding. Unfortunately, no visual control is possible when using nontransparent trays, and light-cured adhesives cannot be used.

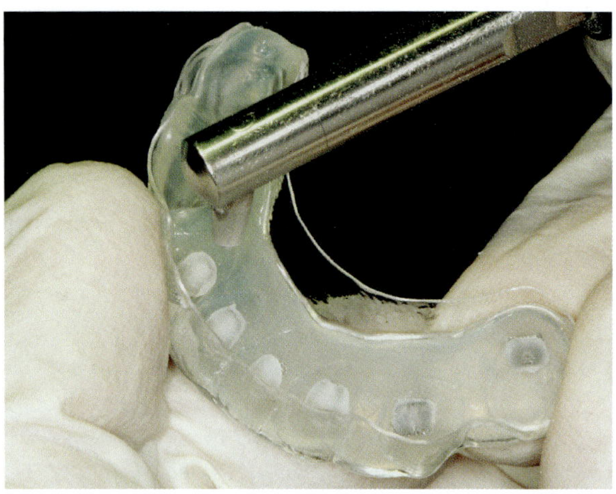

Fig. 6.11 Two-layer transfer with a tray made of a clear silicone putty with an outer shell made of vacuum-formed hard plastic. The latter is used to stabilize the silicone putty.

Vacuum-Formed Trays

Vacuum-formed transfer trays can be made from a variety of materials, which are available in various grades of thickness and hardness. The authors use Erkodent (Scheu Dental). The advantage of vacuum-formed transfer trays is that they are transparent and a light-cured adhesive can be used for bonding of the brackets. The transfer tray is very thin and soft, so that positioning errors sometimes occur during transfer and/or bonding. As with silicone trays, some authors therefore suggest using a second, harder vacuum-formed material to increase the stability and reduce positioning errors. This technique is also known as a "two-foil tray" technique. **Table 6.7** details the exact procedure for this technique, which is the authors' preferred method for indirect bonding.

CLINICAL PEARL

Fixing the Brackets to the Working Model

Two-component composites (e.g., Concise, 3 M Unitek) can be used to seat brackets on the plaster model, but these have the disadvantage that their setting time is very short and no corrections to the bracket position are possible once the material has set. Thermoactive adhesives (e.g., Therma-Cure, Reliance Orthodontics) have no such limitations and are also insensitive to light exposure. Polymerization starts after heating of the model (for 10 minutes at 160°C). Either of these techniques can be used to customize the bracket base to the patient's teeth by filling in the space between the base and the tooth surface with a composite.

Water-soluble adhesives can also be used for bracket positioning on the models, such as "adhesive sticks" or sugar, candy, or toffee. The working time for bracket positioning is considerable when "adhesive sticks" are used. However, water-soluble adhesives do not allow individualization of the bracket base to the patient's teeth because these are too liquid.

Table 6.7 Indirect bonding using a two-layer transfer tray

Impression using alginate material. The impression should be of the highest possible quality and should be cast immediately after the impression is taken, to avoid inaccuracies	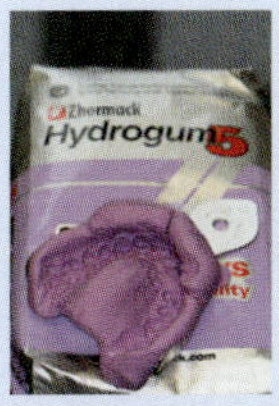
Casting with a hard stone (class III)	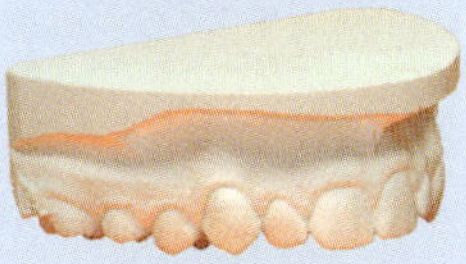
Isolation of the model with an alginate-based material	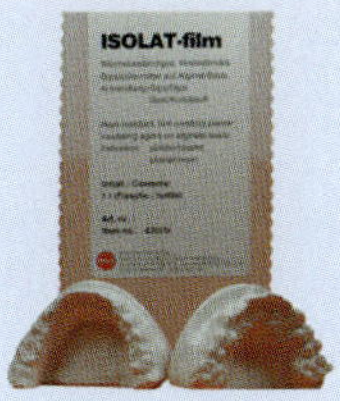
Marking of the bracket position on the plaster model	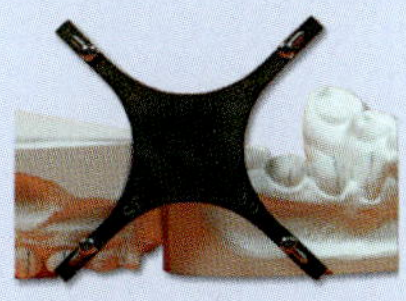
Bonding of the brackets using a light-cure composite or compomer (e.g., Transbond XT, 3 M Unitek or Light Bond, Reliance)	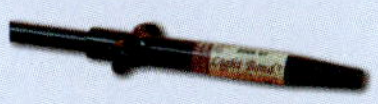
Brackets are positioned on the plaster model	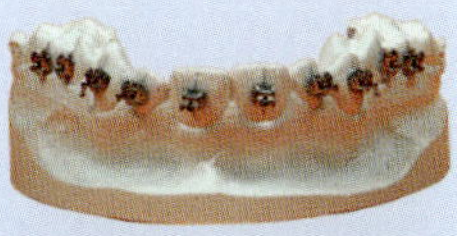
Light-curing after the bracket positions have been verified	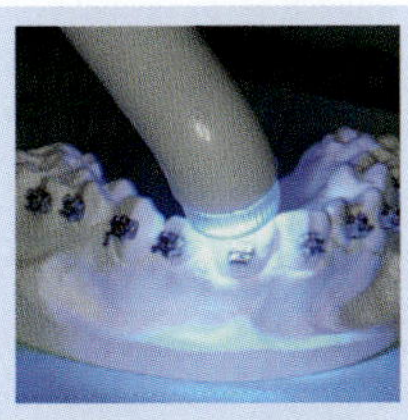
Blocking out the undercuts using thermowax	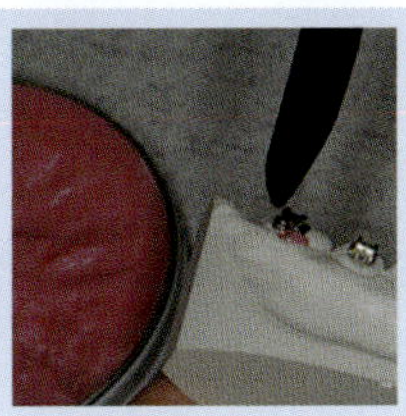
Isolation with silicone spray	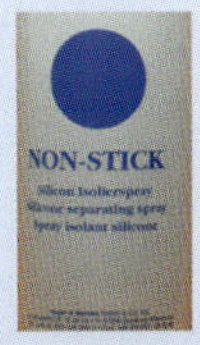
First vacuum-formed tray using a soft silicone material (1.5 mm) Positioning of the model on a Biostar vacuum-forming machine; the model should be placed so that the brackets are free from coverage by the lead balls.	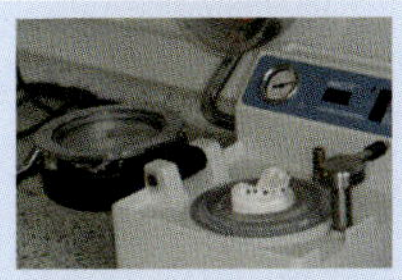
Trimming back the tray and renewed isolation with silicone spray	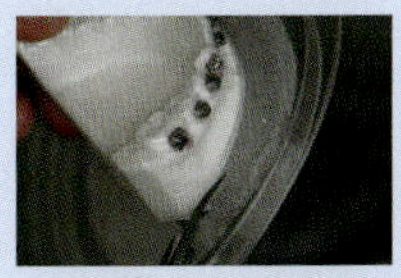
The second tray should be rigid and 1 mm thick	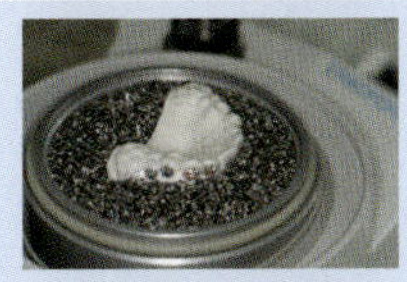
Separation of the outer and inner trays and removal of the isolation residues using a conventional dishwashing agent	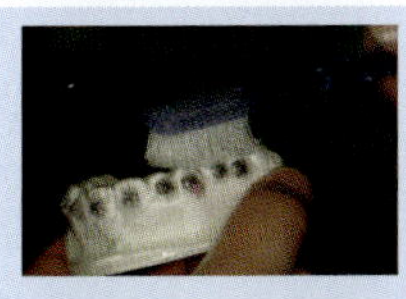
Replace the inner tray and detach the brackets from the plaster model using a wax knife or Buffalo knife. The tray should be protected using a cloth, as shown in this image	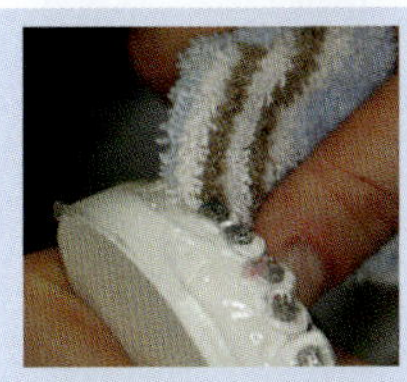
Trimming back of the soft inner positioning tray (approximately 3 mm below the gingival margin). Replacing the tray on the model for verification of bracket position	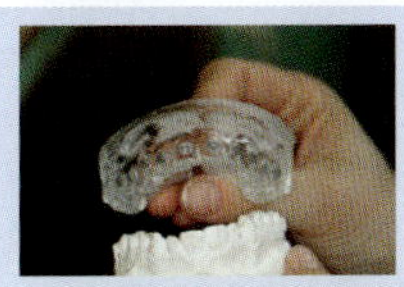
Vertical cuts are placed in the soft tray, using a scalpel, for easier repositioning and removal of the tray	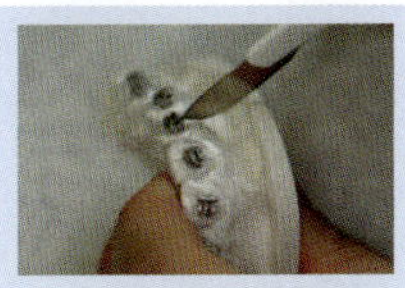
Trimming of the hard tray back to the bracket level and subsequent replacing of the hard tray on top of the soft tray	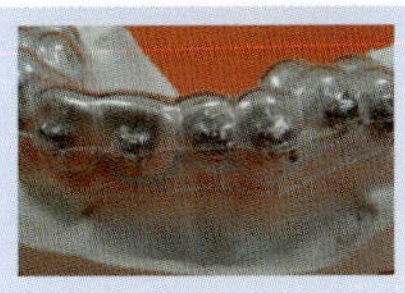

Table 6.8 Indirect bonding in a patient

Removal of any residual plaster	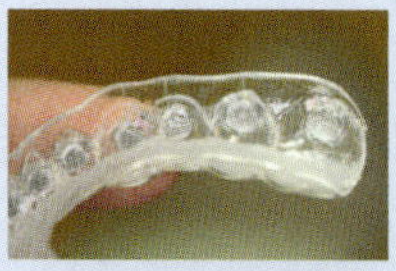
Roughening of the composite surface using a microetcher (e.g., Rondoflex, KaVo)	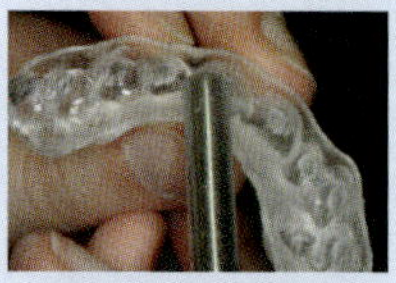
Cleaning of the teeth with fluoride-free paste and drying	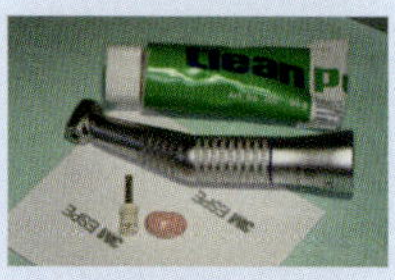
Enamel conditioning	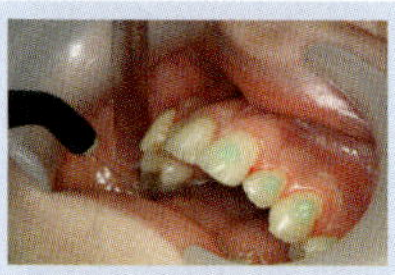
Application of **Resin A** (Sondhi Rapid-Set, 3 M Unitek) on the teeth	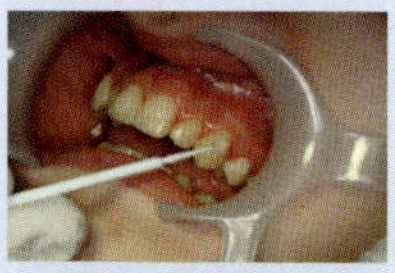
Application of **Resin B** (Sondhi Rapid-Set, 3 M Unitek) on the bracket base	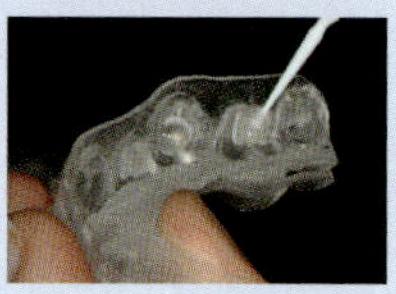
Insertion of the trays	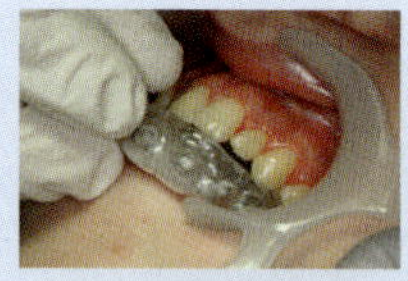
Secure positioning of the tray under pressure for the first 30 s and then maintaining the positioning of the tray for a further 2 min	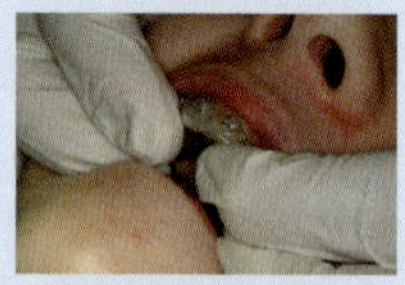
Removal of the outer tray	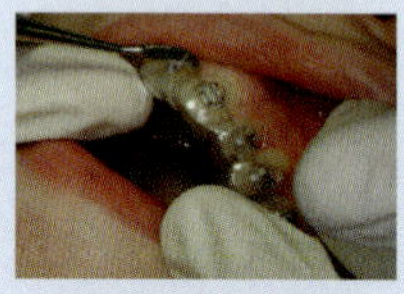
Careful removal of the soft inner tray from the palatal to the vestibular side	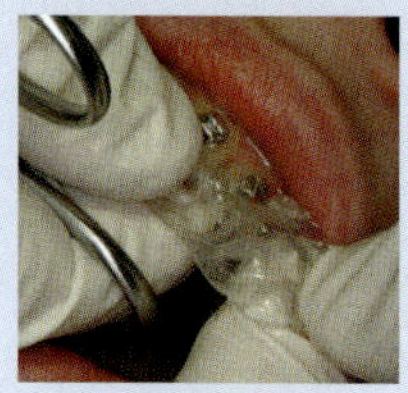
Removal of excess composite using a scaler	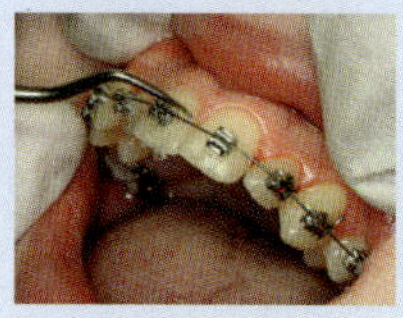

In summary, when direct and indirect bonding techniques are compared, it may be noted that greater precision is likely with the indirect technique, as the bracket positioning procedure is transferred away from the patient's mouth. However, this only provides time savings for the dental practitioner if the positioning is carried out by a dental technician and then checked by the dentist.

REFERENCES

1. Kalange JT. Indirect bonding: a comprehensive review of the advantages. World J Orthod 2004;5(4):301–307
2. Koo BC, Chung CH, Vanarsdall RL. Comparison of the accuracy of bracket placement between direct and indirect bonding techniques. Am J Orthod Dentofacial Orthop 1999;116(3):346–351
3. McLaughlin RP, Bennett JC, Trevisi H. Systemized orthodontic treatment mechanics. Edinburgh: Elsevier Health; 2001
4. Trevisi H. Smart ClipTM Self-ligating appliance system. Edinburgh: Elsevier Health; 2007

Treatment

Bjoern Ludwig and Bettina Glasl

7

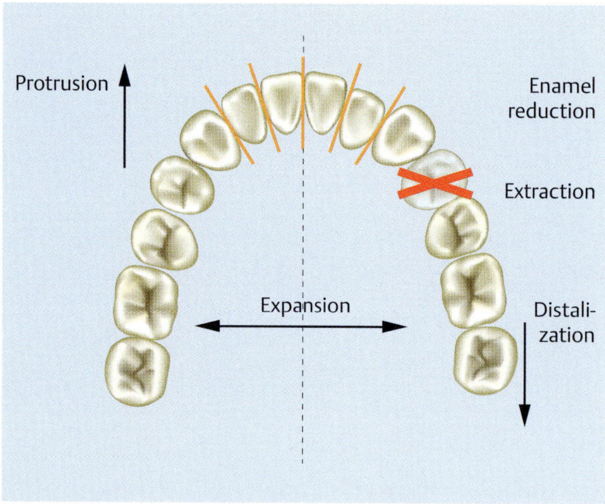

Fig. 7.1 Options for creating space in a dental arch.

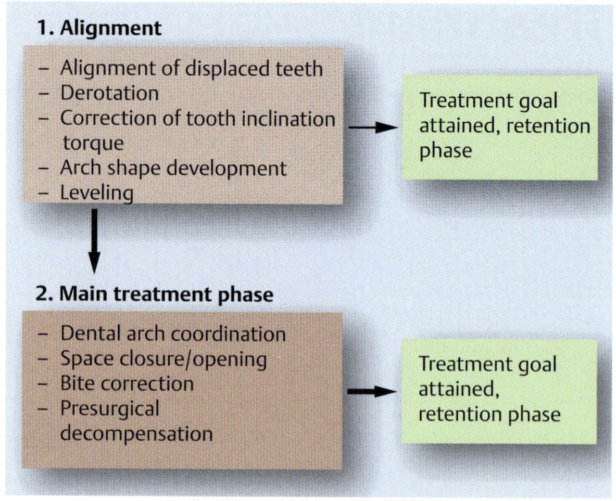

Fig. 7.2 Phases of treatment and treatment goals.

Space Creation

The possibilities for creating space are the same whether self-ligating techniques are employed or conventional ligation is used (**Fig. 7.1**). Space can be created by protrusion of the front teeth, expansion of the posterior dentition, distalization of the posterior dentition, reducing the number of teeth by extraction or by interproximal enamel reduction (stripping)—or a combination of some or all of the above.

Alignment

The first phase of orthodontic treatment immediately after placement of brackets consists of leveling and alignment of the dental arches. This stage of the treatment is usually concerned with derotation and alignment of misplaced teeth into the arch. In a large number of patients, this is the only treatment aim. In others, however, additional treatment aims need to be pursued such as coordination of the dental arches, closure or opening of spaces, correction of the occlusion, or even decompensation of the dental arches before orthognathic surgery (**Fig. 7.2**). One of the major advantages of self-ligation is reduced friction between the archwire and the brackets, which should lead to more rapid alignment during the first phase of orthodontic treatment. It is very useful if this phase of the orthodontic treatment can be shortened to allow the other aims of treatment to be pursued in a more timely fashion.

Biomechanics

In 1932, Schwarz postulated that orthodontic forces applied to a tooth should not be greater than the capillary pressure of its periodontal ligament, which is in the range of 0.22–0.26 N/cm^2 of root surface, to avoid hyalinization and subsequent root resorption. The following criteria determine the level of orthodontic force applied:

- The force required to move a tooth into the desired position (for example, uprighting, physical translation, extrusion, intrusion, or derotation) (**Table 7.1**).
- The effective force that the orthodontic appliances actually exert on the tooth (**Table 7.2**).
- The reactive force, which according to Newton's third law of motion (that action and reaction are equal and opposite) can lead to a reduction in the force acting on the target tooth.

NOTE

Action and reaction are equal and opposite (Newton's third law of motion).

The initial phase of orthodontic tooth movement involves light and flexible archwires that express relatively low and constant force levels. The archwire sizes are subsequently increased gradually until this phase of the treatment has been completed. The amount of force necessary to achieve any particular tooth movement is expressed by the size of the archwires and the material used, as these directly relate to the clinical force levels exerted on the target teeth (**Fig. 7.3**). The resulting forces observed in a clinical scenario often do not correlate directly with those found in experimental situations (**Fig. 7.3** and **Table 7.1**). It is well known that some orthodontic tooth movements take effect more quickly than others: extrusion and elongation of teeth are some of the quickest movements, followed by tipping, which in turn is followed by translation of teeth. Torque expression and intrusion of teeth are the slowest observed movements (**Table 7.3**).

Table 7.1 Recommended force levels by type of tooth movement. The table gives values from the orthodontic literature. Although some of the quoted data are from very old sources that go back more than 50 years, the values are still taught in orthodontic programs today. Agreement on these values is based on the recommendation of different force levels for different types of tooth movement, which are correlated with the root surface areas of different teeth. See **Fig. 7.3**

Type of tooth movement	Incisors, premolars	Canines, molars
Tipping	0.2–0.3 N	0.5–0.75 N
Physical translation	0.4–0.5 N	1.5–2.5 N
Extrusion/ intrusion	0.15–0.3 N The values for intrusion and extrusion are clinically, empirically, and physically suspect; the same value is used for intrusion and extrusion	

NOTE

Orthodontic force levels encountered empirically often do not correlate directly with force levels obtained by experimental studies.

From the biomechanical point of view, self-ligating brackets were developed to reduce the friction of the wire in the bracket slot. Tight ligation of the wires with elastic or wire ligatures actually counteracts the requirements of sliding mechanics. Reports in the literature have shown that frictional resistance reduces the resulting force levels by 50% or more.[2,7,26] For self-ligating brackets, friction can be significantly lower in comparison with normal ligation (between 14% and 40%). However, it is a matter of controversy whether these results derived from ex-vivo situations can be applied to the clinical situation, and it is therefore the individual practitioner who needs to interpret the data available and reach appropriate conclusions for treatment planning of each individual case. A classic example is used here to illustrate the potential physiological benefits of self-ligating brackets (**Fig. 7.4**).

This particular patient presented with a maxillary tooth size–arch length discrepancy (TSALD) and labially crowded canines. Extrusion of the canines requires very little force, while intrusion of the neighboring teeth is very slow and requires greater force levels. The initial archwire was a 0.012 superelastic archwire, which typically creates a force of between 0.2 and 0.5 N; this extrudes the canines but the force levels are well below what is needed for effective intrusion of the neighboring teeth. However, the forces exerted by the archwire are sufficiently large to allow proclination of the incisors. Alignment and space creation result from protrusion of the maxillary anterior segment (**Fig. 7.4c, d**).

Table 7.2 Force levels for various wires with self-ligating brackets. These values are derived from materials-science experiments that allow comparison. There is a lack of standards for material properties, and this table reflects our own measurements

Archwire dimension and type	Force direction: Vertical	Horizontal
0.010 NiTi	0.1 N	0.2 N
0.012 NiTi	0.2–0.4 N	0.2–0.5 N
0.014 NiTi	0.2–0.4 N	0.2–0.7 N

Table 7.3 The time required for various types of tooth movement

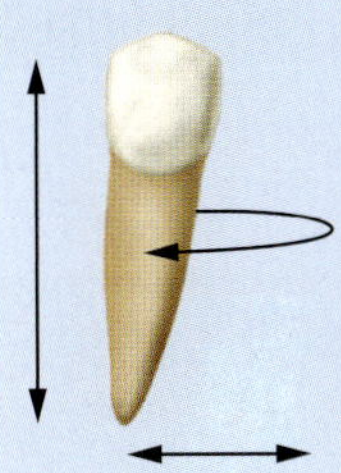

1. Extrusion/ elongation along the long axis
2. Tipping
3. Physical translation
4. Root torque
5. Intrusion along the long axis

Rapid ↕ Slow

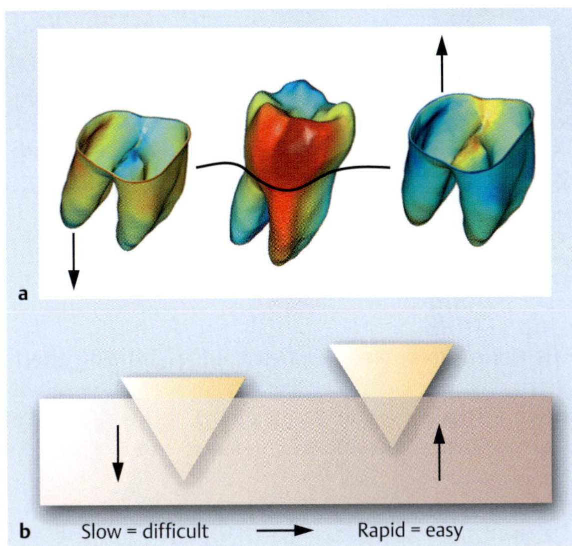

Fig. 7.3a, b Finite-element method (FEM) analysis of root surfaces during intrusion and extrusion. Intrusion of teeth can be compared with forcing a wooden peg into the ground; intrusion requires greater force than pulling the peg out. The amount of force necessary to intrude teeth increases proportionately to their root surface area.

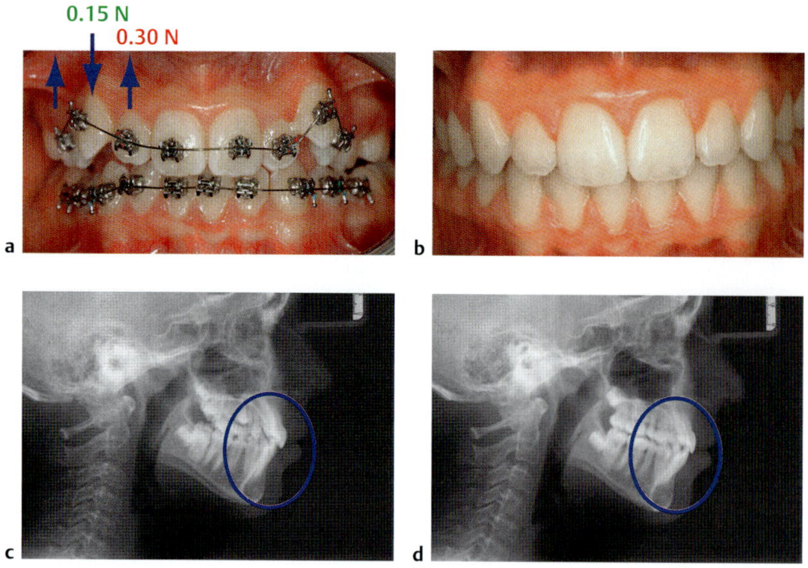

Fig. 7.4a–d Extrusion is possible even with very slight forces of 0.15 N. Reactive intrusion of the surrounding teeth usually starts at force levels of greater than 0.3 N. In order to level teeth by extrusion, only low forces are recommended (0.2 N). See also Chapter 2.

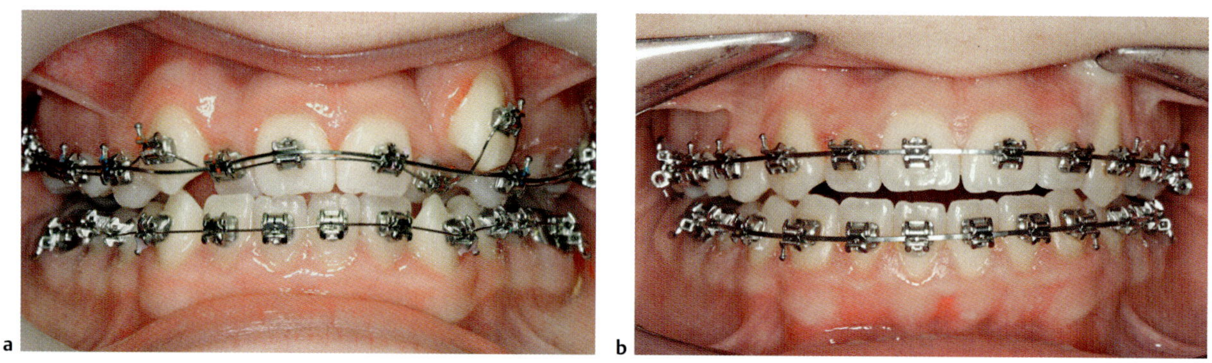

Fig. 7.5a, b An extrusion force of 0.7 N (0.016 superelastic NiTi) can still lead to reciprocal intrusion of the anterior teeth even when a heavy base archwire is used.

This clinical example shows that undesired side effects can largely be avoided by using low force levels in combination with low friction. Using a 0.016 archwire made of the same material would have resulted in force levels of 0.8–1.0 N. This scenario would have created sufficient reciprocal forces for intrusion of the adjacent teeth, which would then cause a biomechanical side effect of additional flaring of the incisors (**Fig. 7.5**).

Expansion of the Arches

Archwire expansion is biomechanically simple and is usually achieved quickly, as the desired tooth position is achieved by tipping of the teeth. However, this can lead to side effects in the vertical dimension that may require additional treatment for correction. Applying force labial to the center of resistance leads to proclination of the incisors during their relative intrusion (**Fig. 7.6**). Transverse expansion of the dental arches can be achieved by dental or skeletal means. In the maxilla, both options can be used on a regular basis due to the presence of the midpalatal suture. In the mandible, the structure equivalent to the maxillary midpalatal suture is the symphysis, which already ossifies before birth and can therefore not be expanded orthodontically. It can only be reopened after surgical intervention and expanded by means of osteogenic distraction.

As transverse dental expansion of the upper jaw usually encompasses buccal tipping of the posterior segments, "hanging palatal cusps" tend to result, which are often responsible for iatrogenic bite-opening (**Fig. 7.7**) and balancing interference.

Dental or skeletal expansion? The treatment strategy should be determined by the primary characteristics of the malocclusion (**Fig. 7.8**). Treatment options for expansion are usually determined by the shape of the lower arch, as good coordination between upper and lower arches is required at the end of the orthodontic treatment. Dentoalveolar expansion is usually achieved by means of the archwire alone. Depending on the amount of expansion necessary, additional auxiliaries can be used, such as quad helices, expansion plates and "jockey wires," to name but a few of the other types of expanders available today (**Fig. 7.9**). Significant transverse discrepancies are

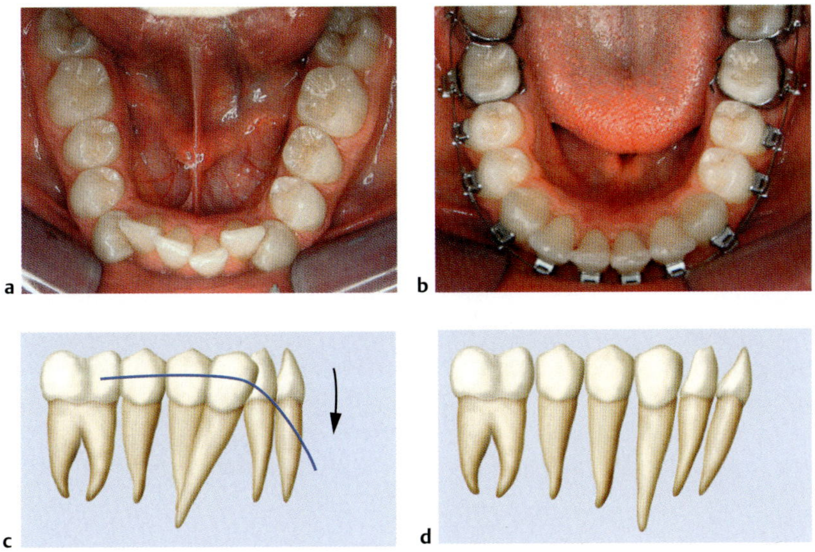

Fig. 7.6a–d The anterior arch segment shows a lack of space, particularly for the canines. The incisors are retroclined and will be proclined during alignment. Due to the inclination of the canines, leveling and alignment using continuous-arch mechanics will lead to proclination and intrusion of the labial segment. Following alignment of the lower front teeth, the canines will eventually upright, but the lower incisors will maintain their proclined position.

Clinical pearl:
"Stripping" from molar to molar and retracting anteriors (**b**)

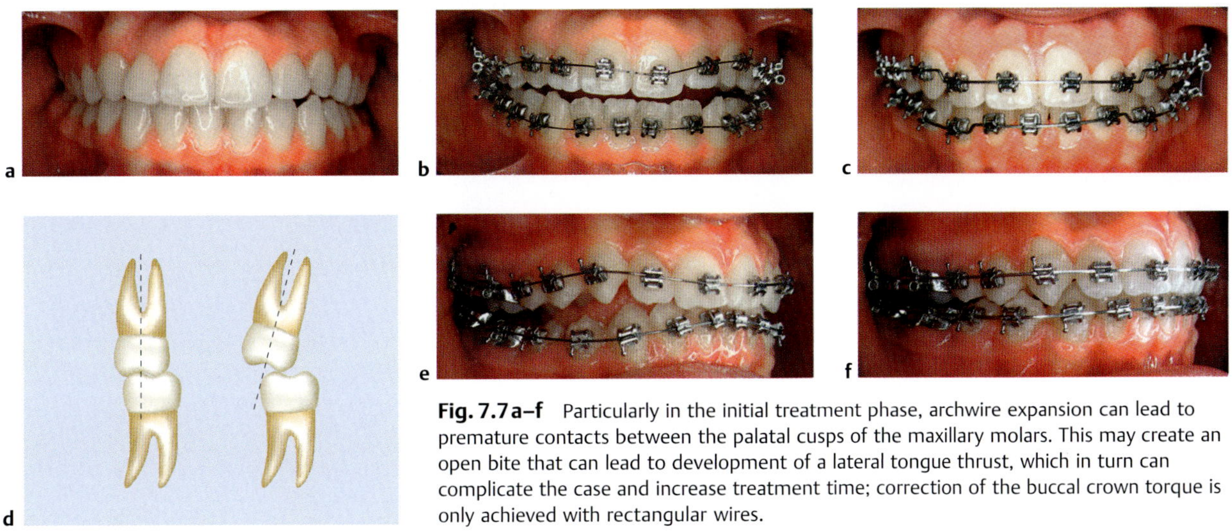

Fig. 7.7a–f Particularly in the initial treatment phase, archwire expansion can lead to premature contacts between the palatal cusps of the maxillary molars. This may create an open bite that can lead to development of a lateral tongue thrust, which in turn can complicate the case and increase treatment time; correction of the buccal crown torque is only achieved with rectangular wires.

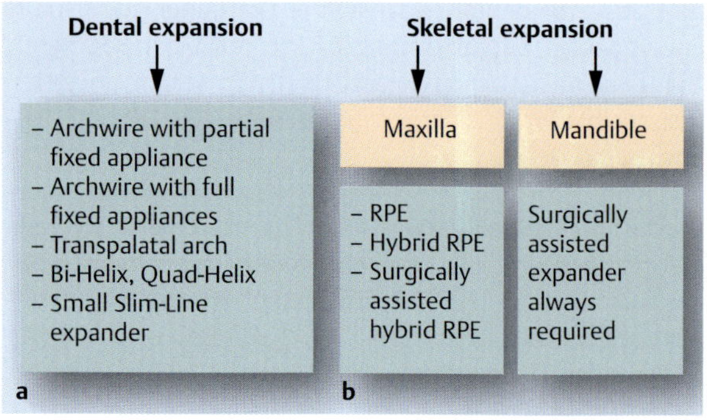

Fig. 7.8 a, b Expansion techniques using (**a**) dental expansion and (**b**) skeletal expansion. RPE, rapid palatal enlargement.

often best addressed by skeletal expansion (i.e., by expansion of the maxillary midpalatal suture; see also the section on "Space Creation by Expansion of Arches" below, p. 135). The presence of the midpalatal suture as well as the thin cortical structure of the maxillary bone are ideal for expansion of the upper jaw. This has to be viewed with the opposite situation in the lower jaw. For the latter, there is an abundance of compact buccal bone, and expansion is consequently more challenging even when surgical assistance is used.

Expansion with archwires. Adequate transverse development of the apical base is a prerequisite of archwire expansion (**Fig. 7.10**). In this particular example, a long-standing thumb-sucking habit had resulted in a V-shaped narrow upper jaw. However, the apical base was sufficiently wide to allow the use of a 2 × 4 appliance during the mixed dentition. The initial archwire was a 0.012 superelastic NiTi, which was followed by a 0.016 wire of the same material. The superelastic archwires were left in situ for 8 weeks each and resulted in a significant development in the arch form, both in the transverse as well as the anterior–posterior dimensions.

For moderate expansion in the permanent dentition, we usually use a 0.012 or 0.016 archwire (for 8 weeks each). We subsequently use a 0.018 × 0.025 superelastic archwire, which fine-tunes the three-dimensional parameters. In cases in which ectopic teeth need to be aligned, this archwire sequence has to be modified; the sequential archwires are 0.010, and 0.012 to 0.016. Further expansion is usually achieved with rectangular archwires such as a 0.018 × 0.025 superelastic archwire. Expansion using an archwire is only of limited value in the lower arch (**Fig. 7.11**), as it really only allows buccal tipping of the posterior segments with correction of the curve of Wilson. The relatively dense bone structure of the mandible prevents skeletal expansion in the absence of surgical assistance—for example, in the form of osteogenic distraction (**Fig. 7.12**).

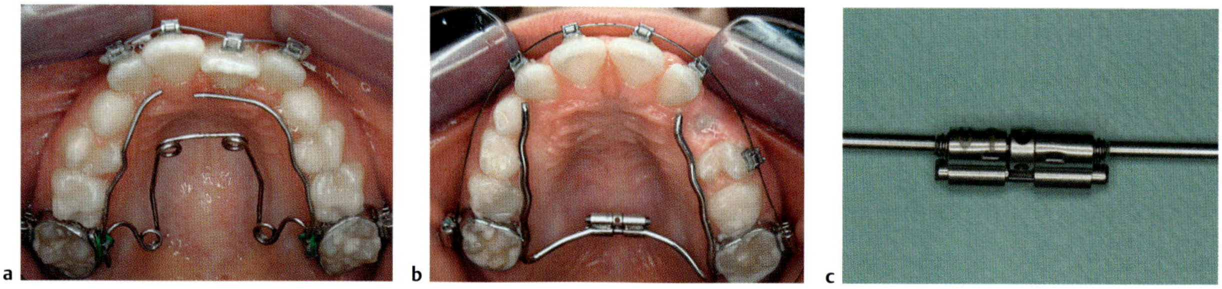

Fig. 7.9 a–c Dental expansion of the upper arch using palatal expansion appliances.
a A quad helix with a 2 × 4 appliance; this method is low-cost and effective, but the actual force levels are difficult to determine. The quad helix is made of stainless-steel wires, which can result in high force levels even after minor activations. It is often difficult to estimate the resulting forces, especially when activating the appliance intraorally.
b, c We have found that the slimline expander (magnified view in **c**) works well, the force levels are more predictable. The patient typically activates the appliance a quarter turn every 3 days.
A full turn of 360° results in 0.8 mm of expansion. This type of expander is better in terms of the applied force levels, although these are high at activation but still intermittent.

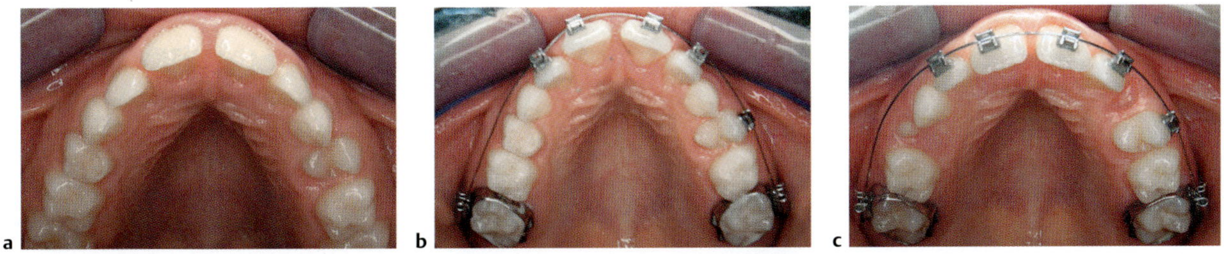

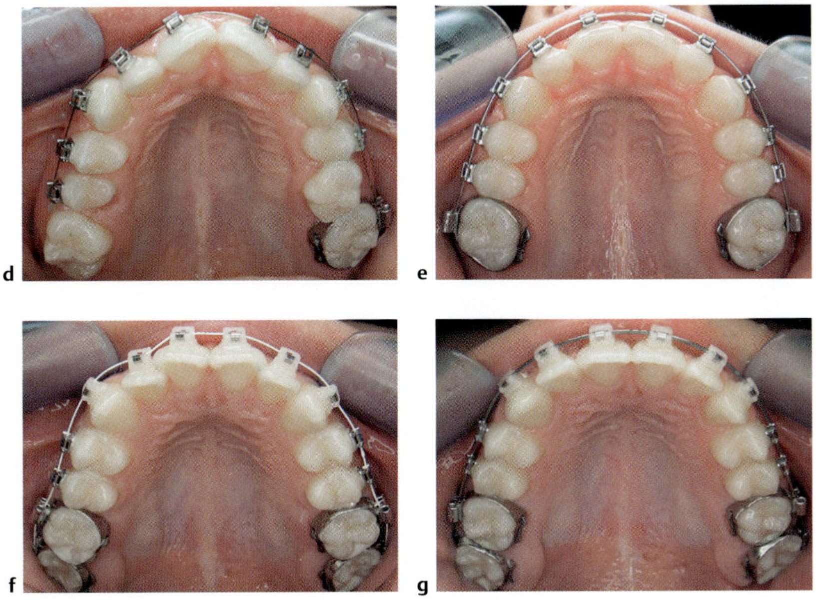

Fig. 7.10 a–g An example of the effects of different archwire shapes on the arch form.

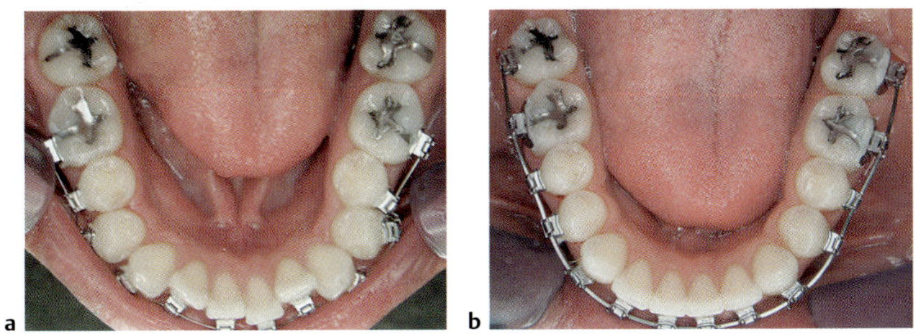

Fig. 7.11 Examples of expansion treatment using an archwire.
a, b Correction of minor irregularities and rotations by protrusion of the lower labial segment. Enamel reduction was performed from bicuspid to bicuspid.

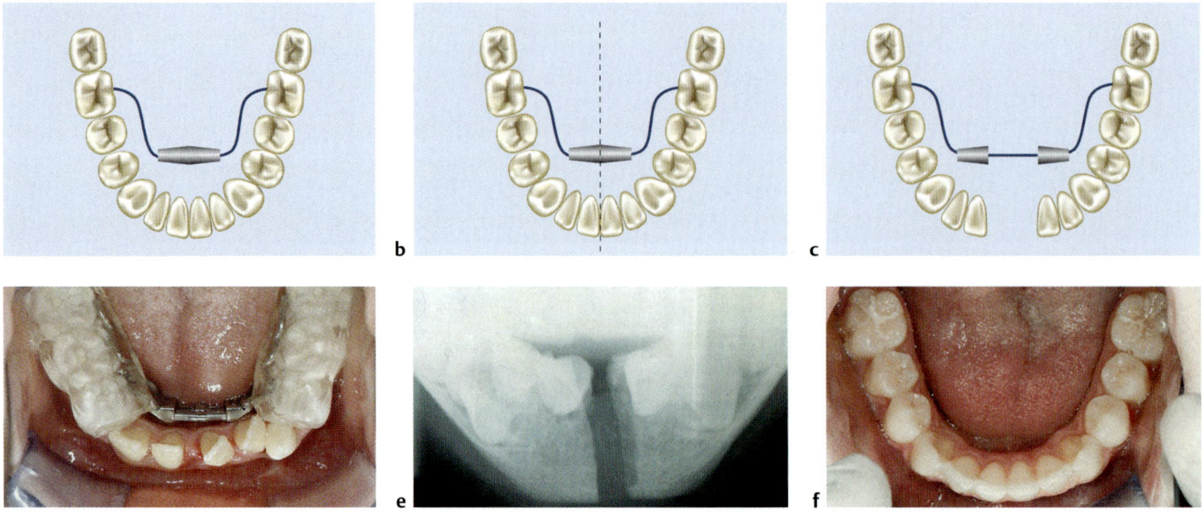
a b c d e f

Fig. 7.12a–f Surgically assisted mandibular expansion (with a slimline screw). (**d–f** courtesy of Dr. Heinz Winsauer, Bregenz, Austria.)

Crowding and Ectopic Canines

The following case studies are examples and illustrate "reduced-friction" full-arch treatments to resolve crowding of the anterior segments. Special emphasis is placed on the alignment of labially positioned maxillary canines. As with all treatment plans, it is important to have well-defined treatment aims before beginning fixed-appliance treatment. This includes the archwire sequence and material, with a view to treating the underlying occlusal discrepancies where present. This should include auxiliaries such as intramaxillary and/or intermaxillary elastics and other adjuncts such as interproximal enamel reduction. An alternative treatment option in cases of severe crowding should encompass the removal of teeth. It is generally thought that dental expansion of the arches is unstable, particularly because most of the alignment is often achieved by tipping movements of the teeth. However, modern retention techniques (see Chapter 9) make it possible to maintain orthodontic results over the longer term. From a scientific point of view, it should also be noted that there appears to be very little difference in the long-term stability of the alignment of the lower labial segment in particular between patients who are treated with an extraction approach or a nonextraction approach.[15]

Case Study 7.1 (Fig. 7.13)

Patient: A.-M.K., female, age 16.
Diagnostic records: models, panoramic radiograph, lateral cephalometric radiograph, intraoral/extraoral photographs, low-dose CT.
Main findings: moderate crowding in both jaws, transverse crowding, class II profile with mild retrognathia.
Treatment aims: protrusion of the front teeth, leveling and expansion of the dental arches and improvement of the patient's profile.
Appliances: self-ligating brackets, molar bands, occlusal stops, and interproximal enamel reduction.
Archwire sequence: 0.012 SE, 0.016 SE, 0.018 × 0.025 SE, 0.019 × 0.025 SS, 0.021 × 0.025 SE.
Alternative treatment strategy: extraction of first premolars.
Active treatment time: 10 months.
Retention: three-dimensional retention with Hawley retainers and bonded retainers.

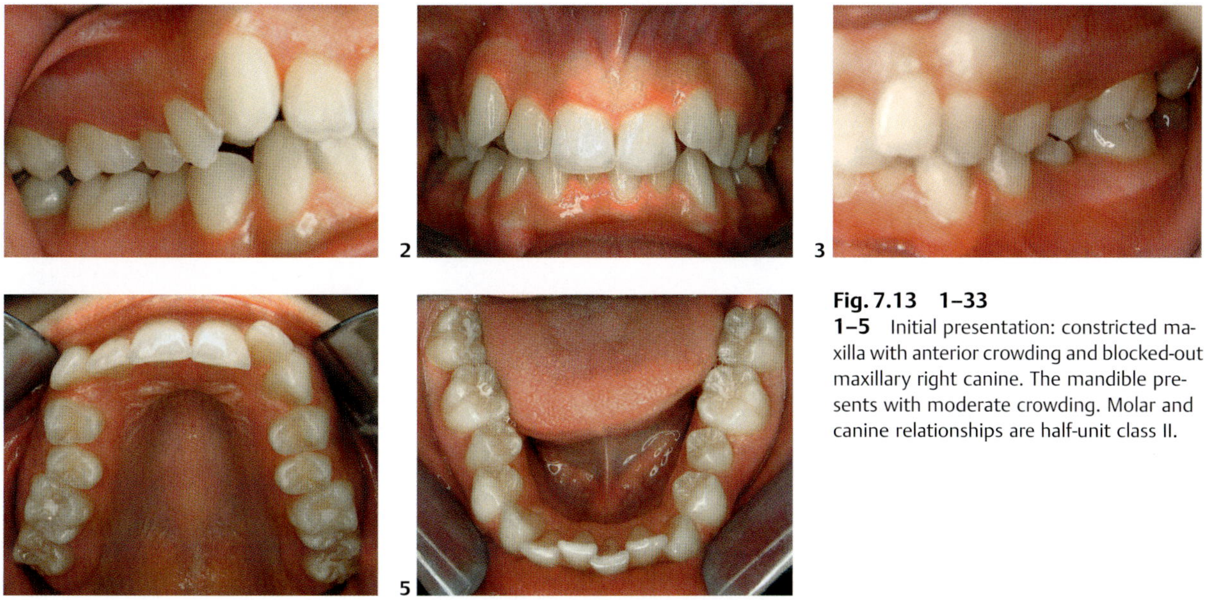

1 2 3 4 5

Fig. 7.13 1–33
1–5 Initial presentation: constricted maxilla with anterior crowding and blocked-out maxillary right canine. The mandible presents with moderate crowding. Molar and canine relationships are half-unit class II.

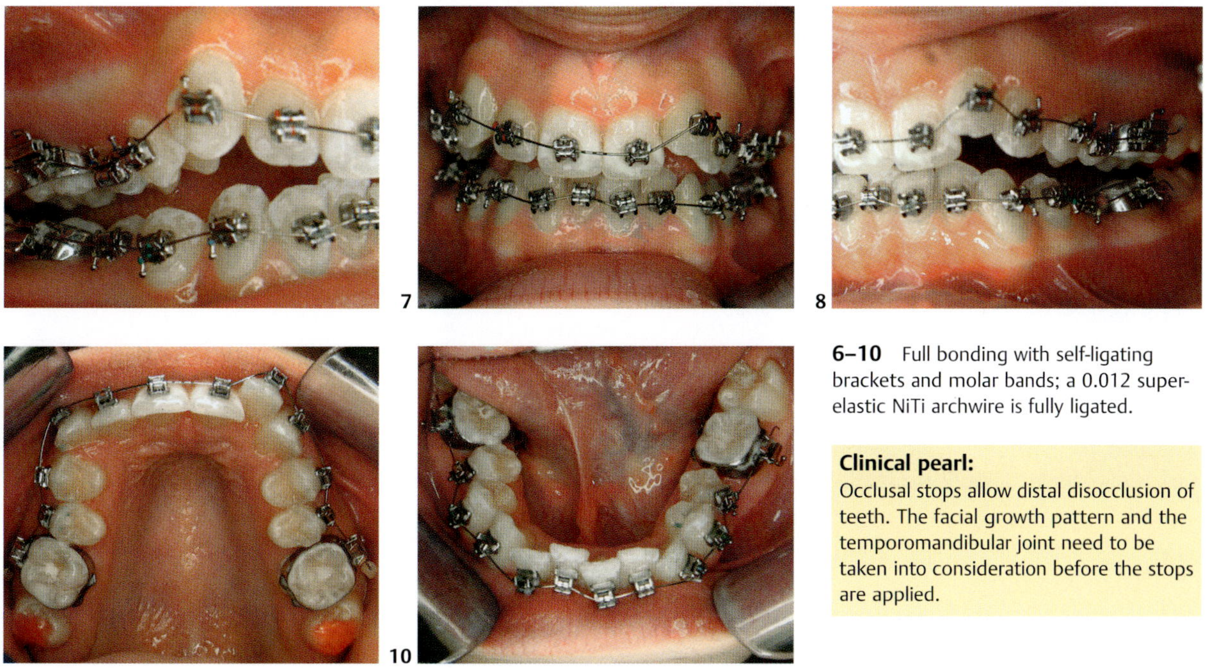

6 7 8 9 10

6–10 Full bonding with self-ligating brackets and molar bands; a 0.012 superelastic NiTi archwire is fully ligated.

Clinical pearl:
Occlusal stops allow distal disocclusion of teeth. The facial growth pattern and the temporomandibular joint need to be taken into consideration before the stops are applied.

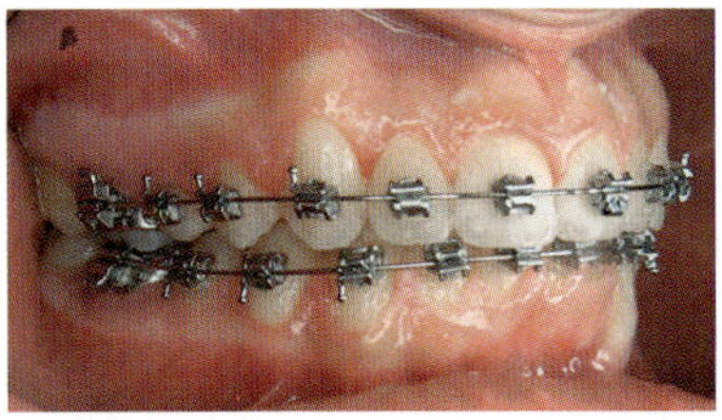
11

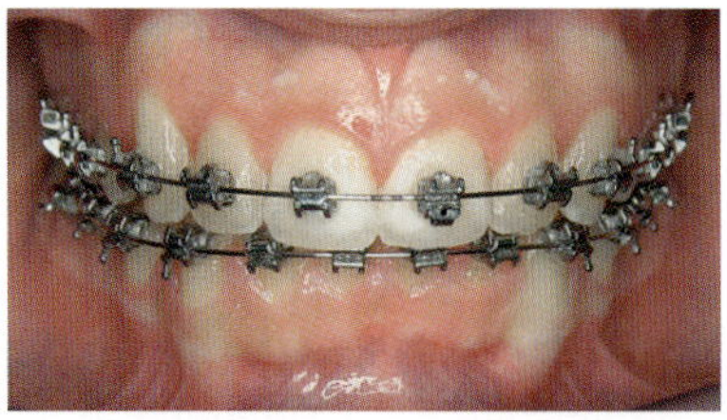
12

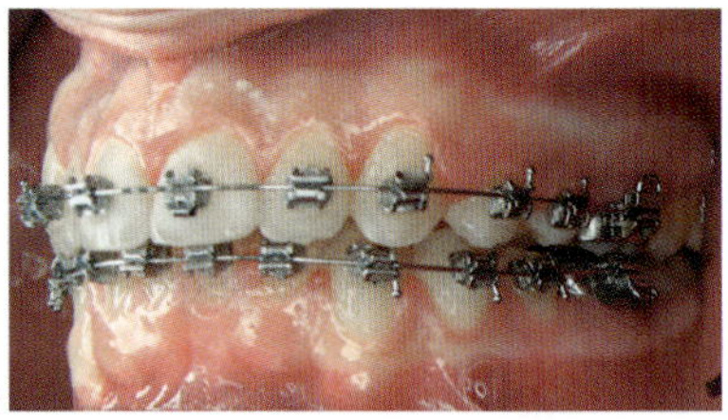
13

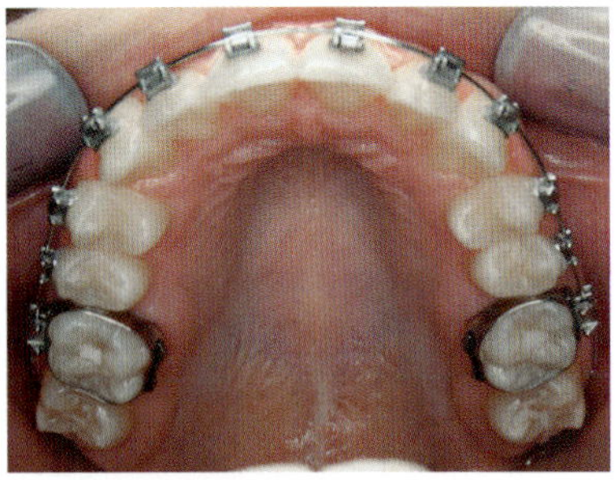
14

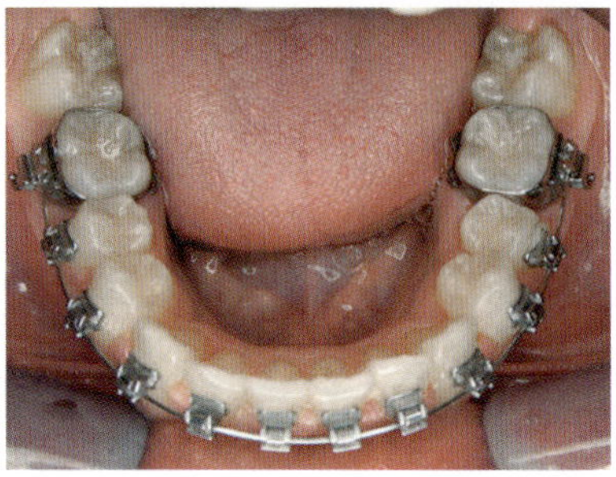
15

11–15 Treatment progress (0.018 × 0.025 superelastic archwires).

Errors and risks:
Space creation in nonextraction treatment may have to include arch expansion as well as interproximal enamel reduction.

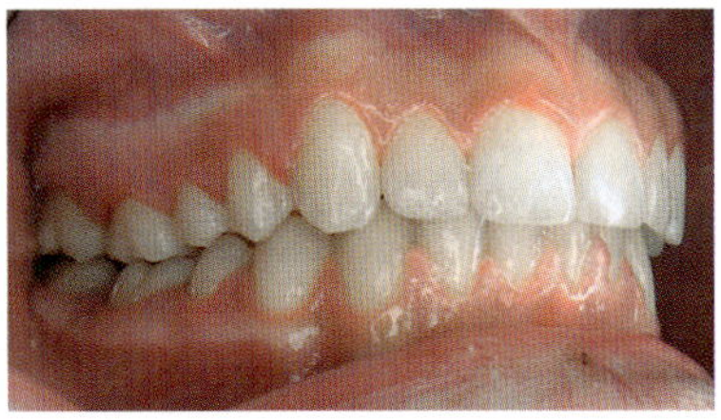
16

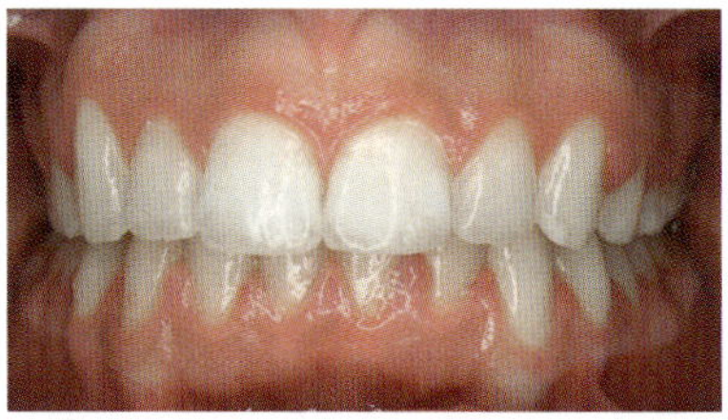
17

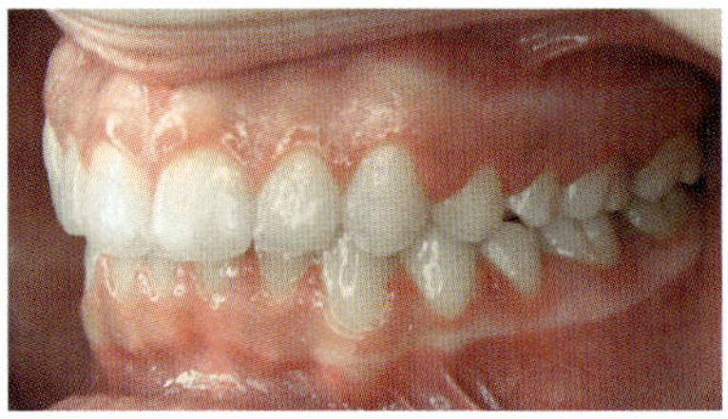
18

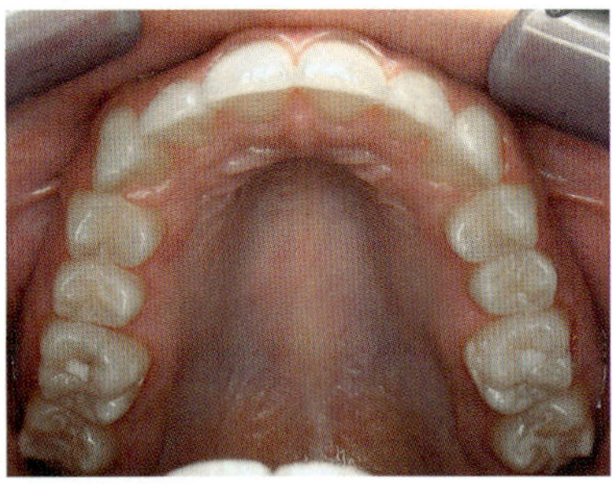
19

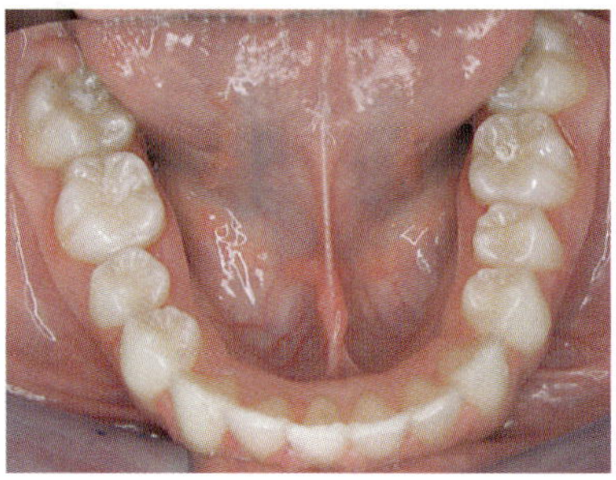
20

16–20 Final result: three-dimensional retention of both maxillary and mandibular teeth is necessary.

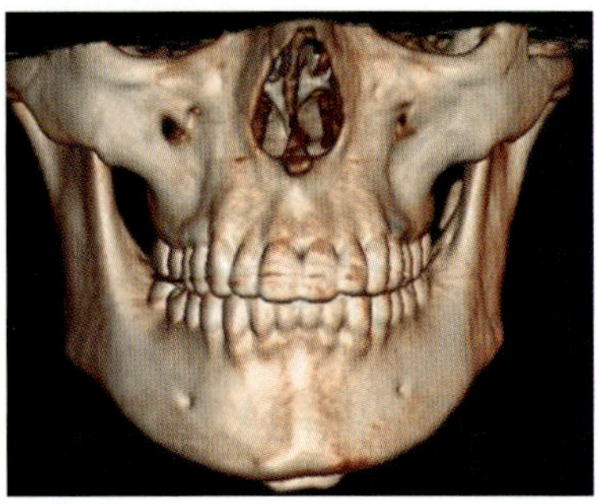
21

21 Low-dose computed tomography shows that none of the teeth have been moved beyond their biological limit; no fenestrations or dehiscences are visible.

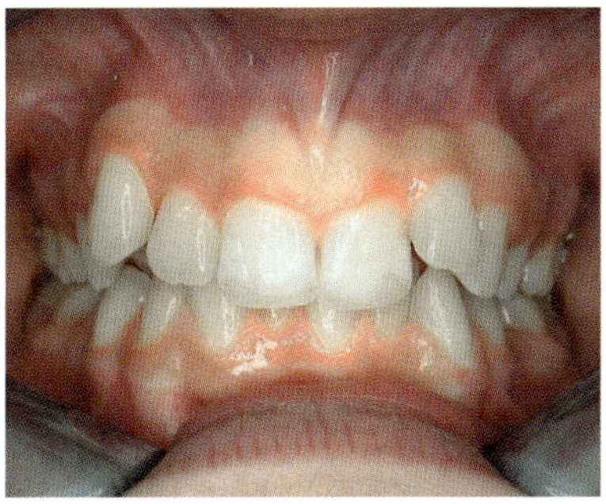
22
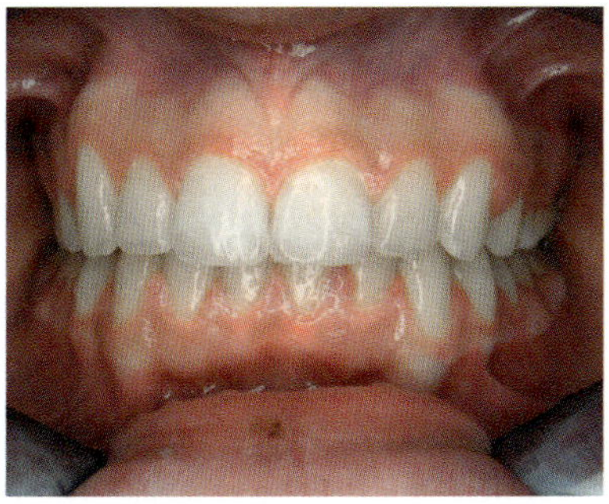
23

22–23 The stability of the sagittal expansion is limited. Approximal enamel reduction will create space for alignment and improved stability.

Errors and risks:
Expansion in the sagittal plane (incisor proclination) is limited by its stability and periodontal concerns. Solution: interproximal enamel reduction (IPR).

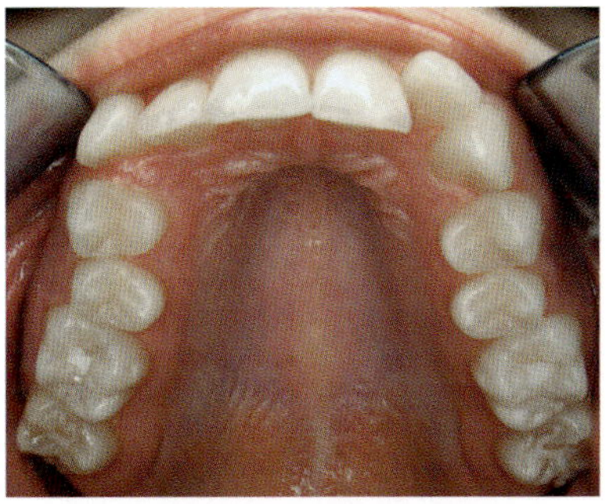
24
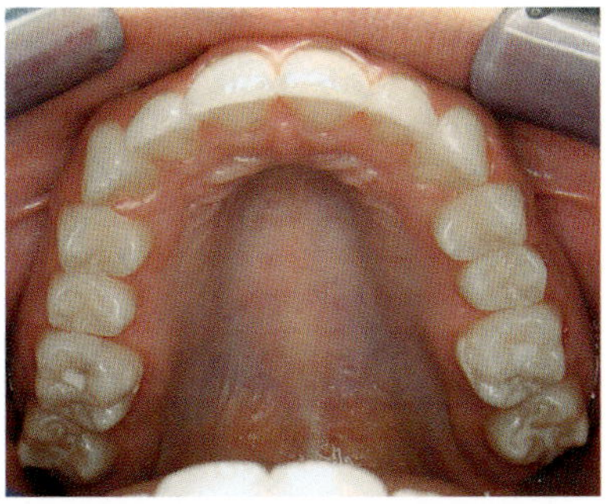
25
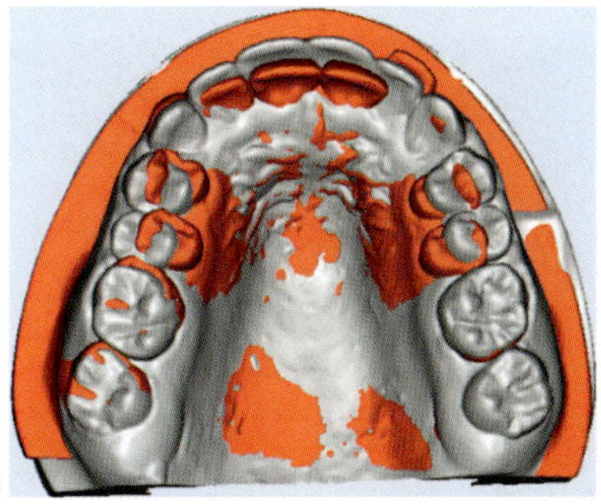
26
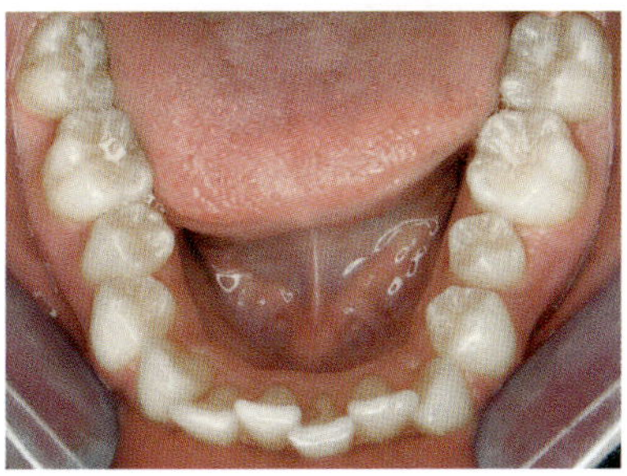
27
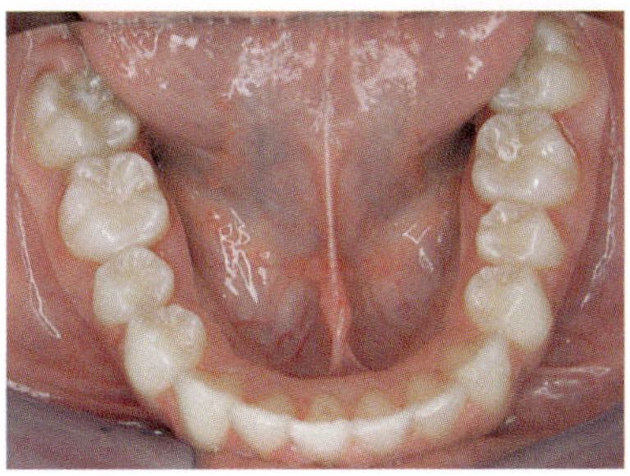
28
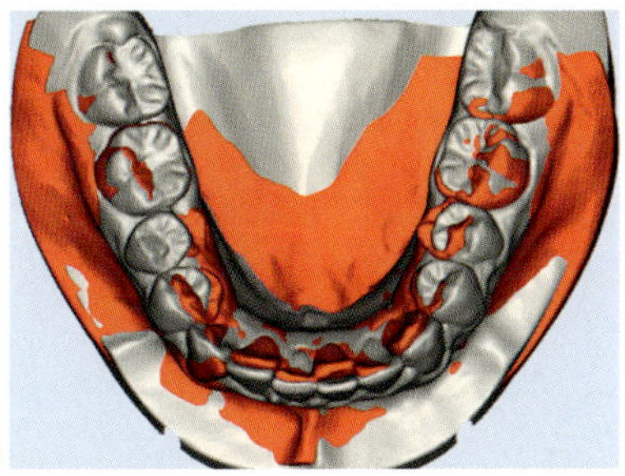
29

24–29 Digital superimposition of the dental arches: initial presentation (images on the left and in red on virtual study models) compared with the result after 1 year in retention. **Caution:** Intercanine width was not changed in lower jaw (**29**)

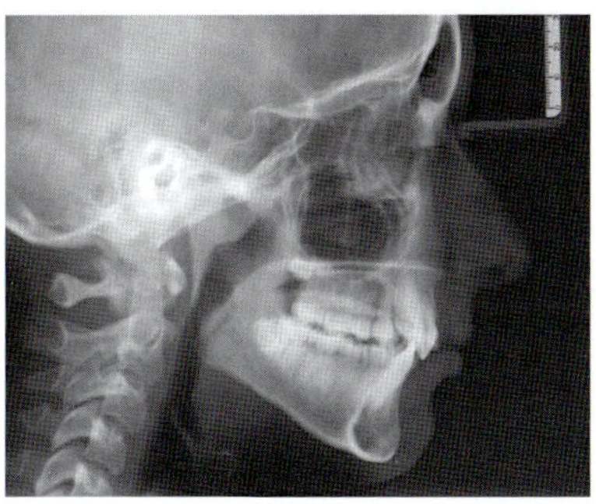
30
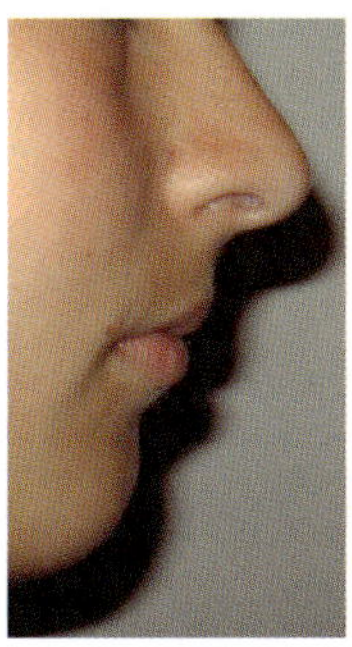
31
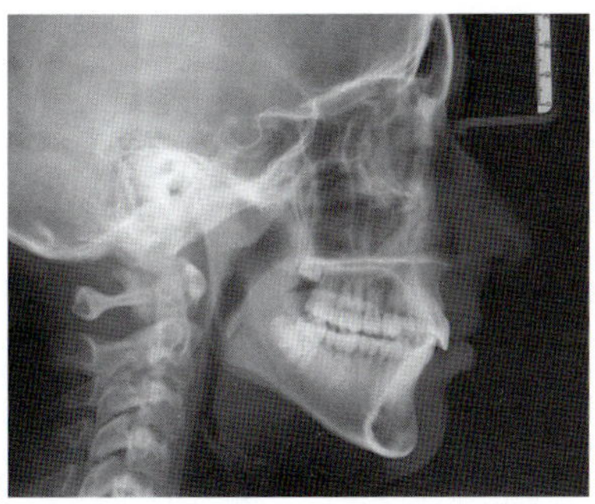
32
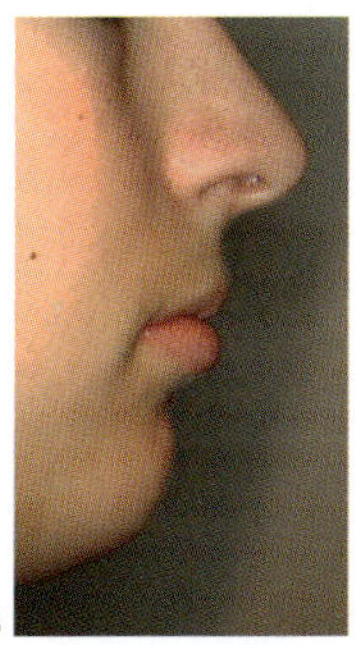
33

30–33 The nasolabial angle improved concomitant with the protrusion of the upper labial segment as it became more acute. Nonextraction treatment improved facial harmony by supporting the position of the upper lip and subsequently reduced the nasal prominence.

Case Study 7.2 (Fig. 7.14)

Patient: M.K., male, age 14.

Diagnostic records: models, panoramic radiograph, lateral cephalometric radiograph, intraoral/extraoral photographs.

Main findings: severe crowding of the upper and lower arches, buccal placement of both upper canines with transverse crowding, and dental alveolar midline discrepancy in the lower jaw to the left.

Treatment aims: alignment of 13 and 33 by expansion, protrusion and interdental stripping, and correction of the midline discrepancy.

Appliances: self-ligating brackets, molar bands, interproximal enamel reduction.

Archwire sequence: 0.010 SE, 0.012 SE, 0.016 SE, 0.018 × 0.025 SE, 0.021 × 0.025 SE.

Alternative treatment strategy: extraction of first premolars.

Active treatment time: 11 months.

Retention: three-dimensional retention with Hawley retainers and bonded retainers.

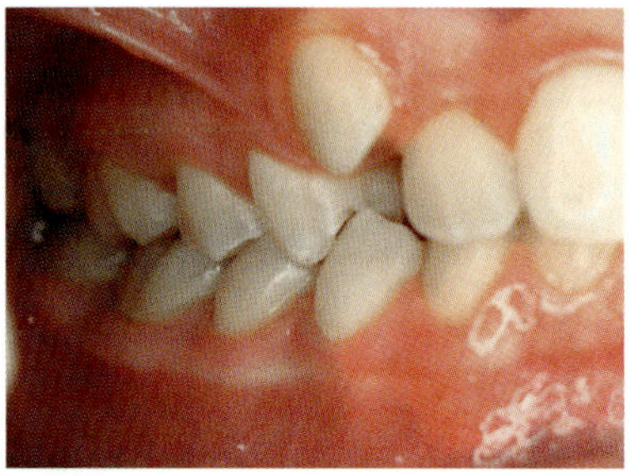
1

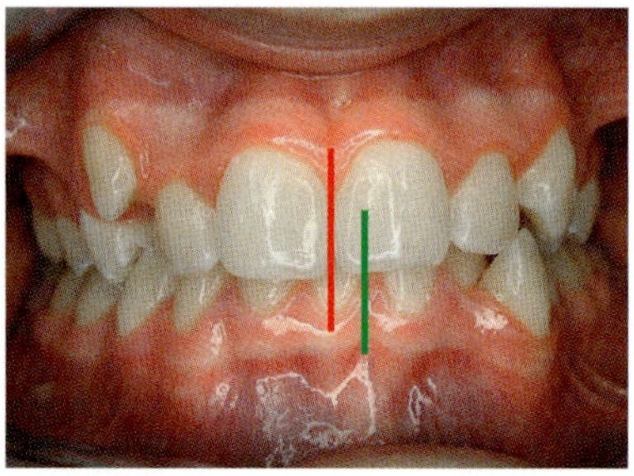
2

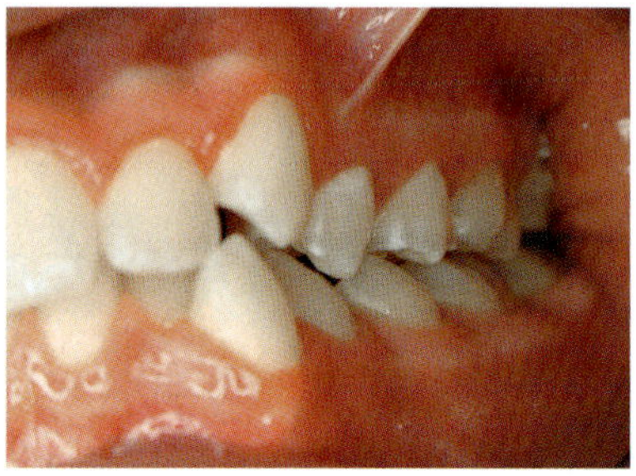
3

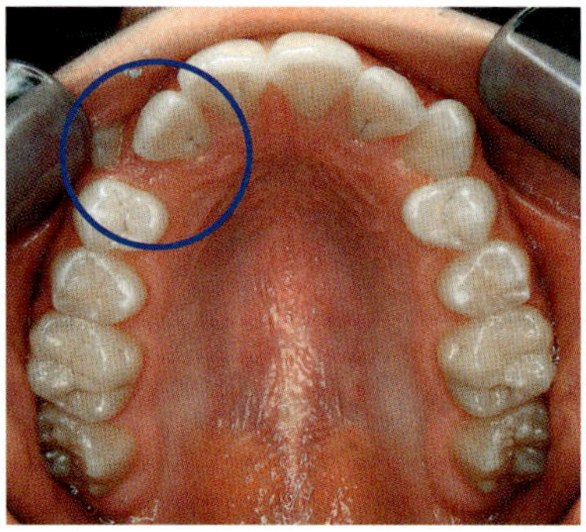
4

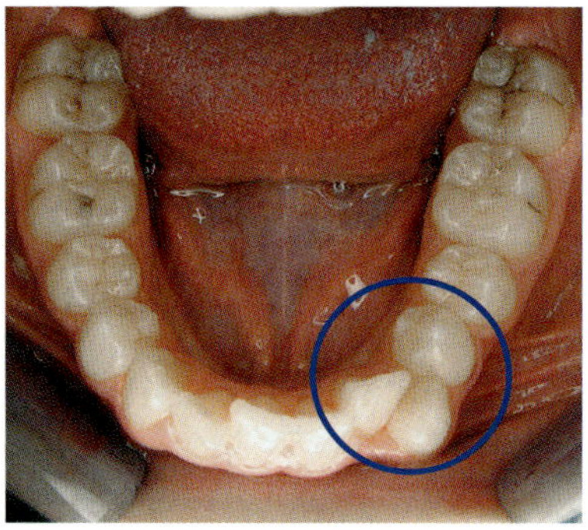
5

Fig. 7.14 1–23
1–5 Initial presentation: constricted maxilla with bucally crowded teeth 13 and 23. The mandible presents with anterior crowding and a buccal 33, with marked deviation of the mandibular dental midline to the left.

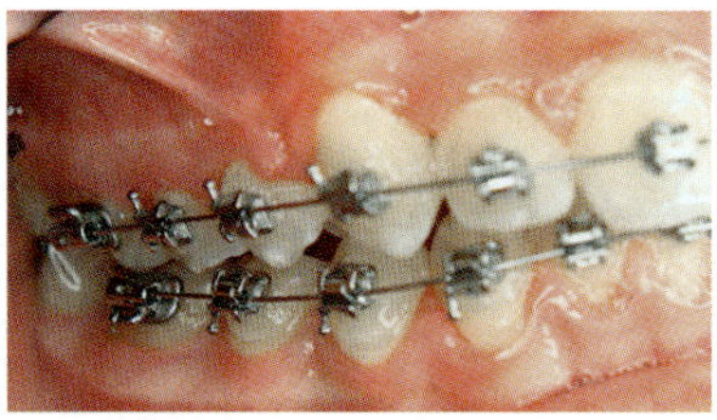
6

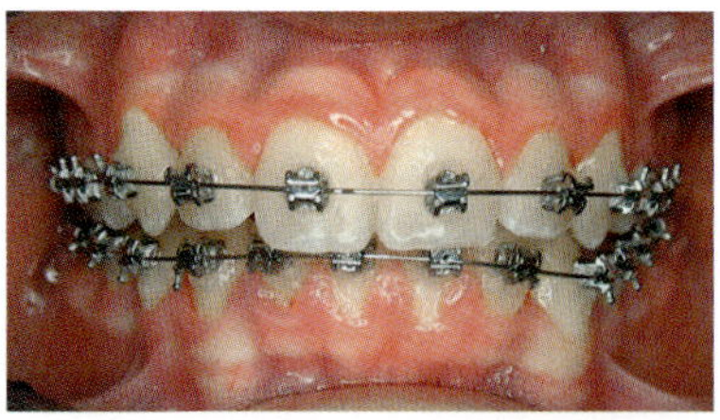
7

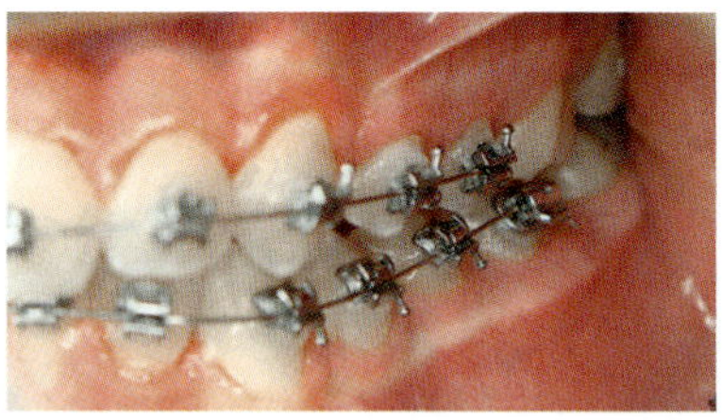
8

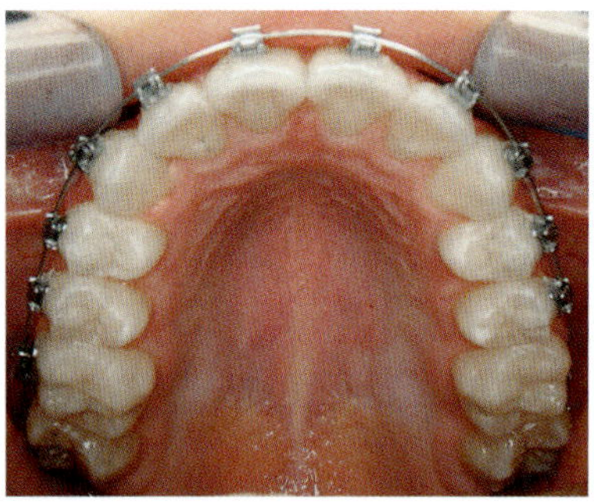
9

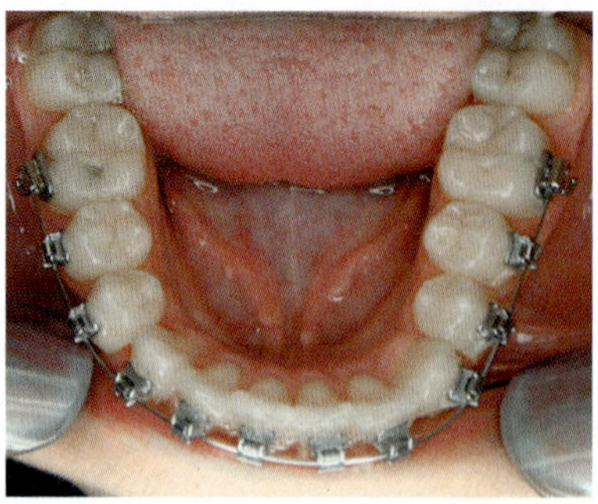
10

6–10 Treatment progress, with fully ligated superelastic 0.016 round archwires.

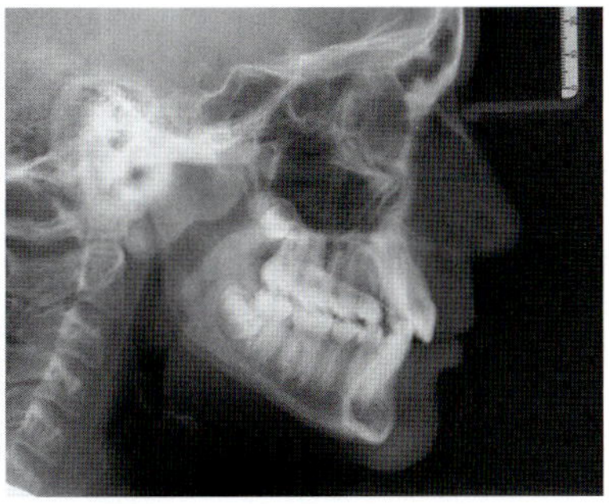
11

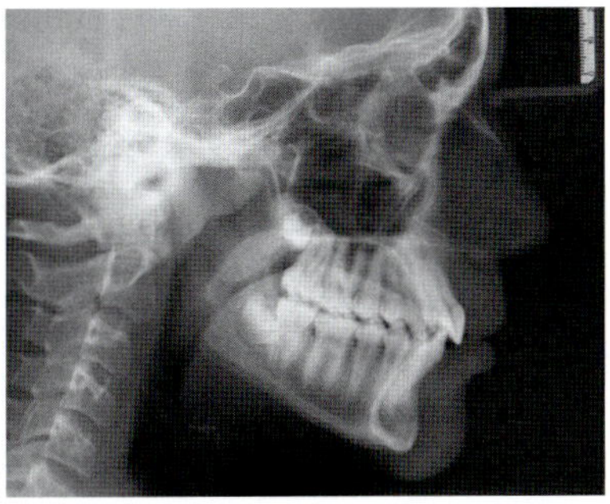
12

11, 12 Caution: unrestricted proclination of the lower labial segment should be avoided. Tip: interproximal enamel reduction can limit the amount of incisor proclination.

CLINICAL PEARL

13–15 Does buccal expansion of the jaws result in fenestration of the buccal cortex?

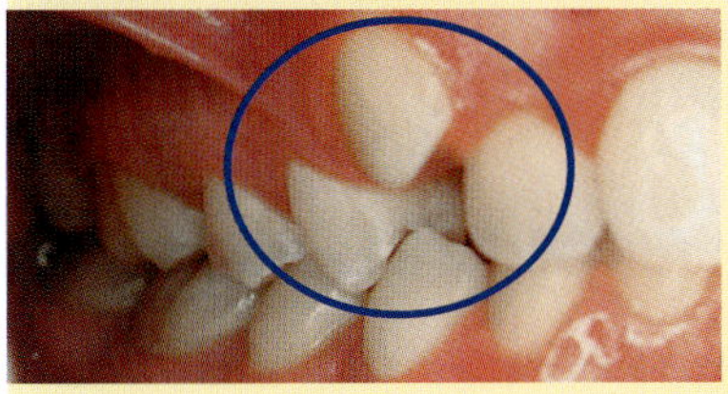
13

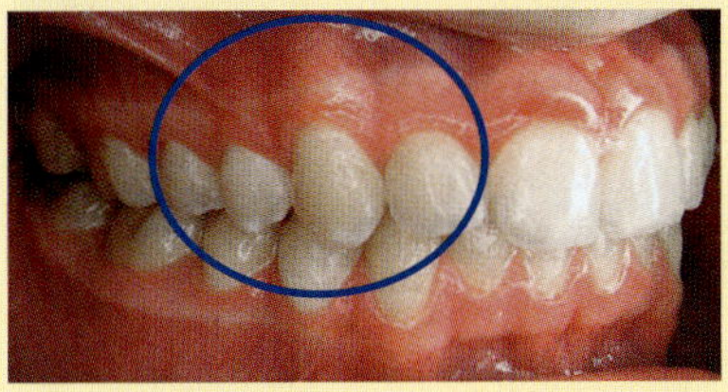
14

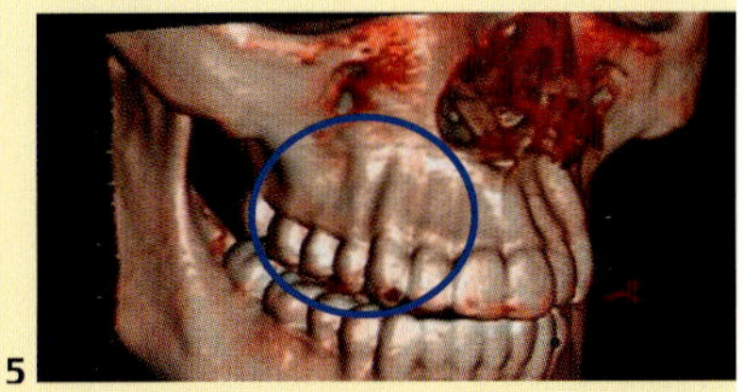
15

Full-sized superelastic archwires such as 0.018 × 0.025 or 0.021 × 0.025 appear, within limits, to be able to transversally expand arches without substantial buccal bone loss. The three-dimensional computed-tomography reconstruction shows good buccal root coverage.

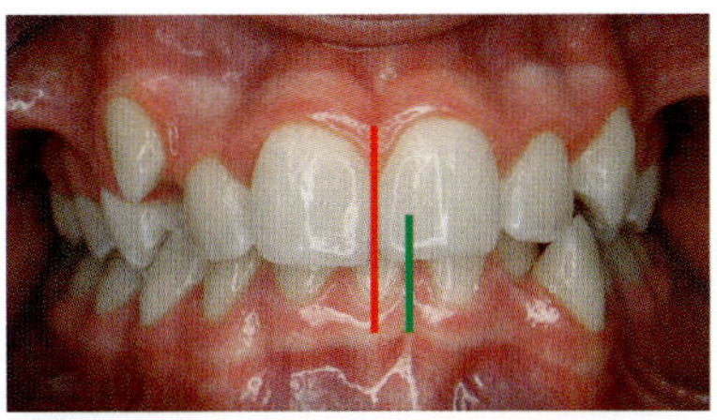
16

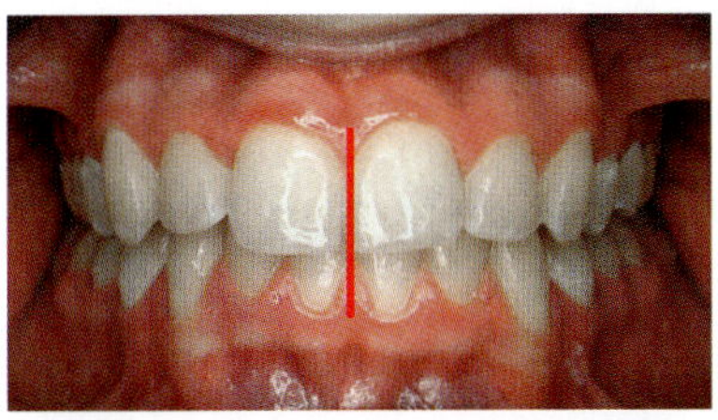
17

16–23 Clinical images and superimposition of the digital study models: initial presentation and final result after 1 year in retention. Retention was with removable appliances, which allowed slight tooth movement during the first year.
Caution: Intercanine width was not changed (**23**)

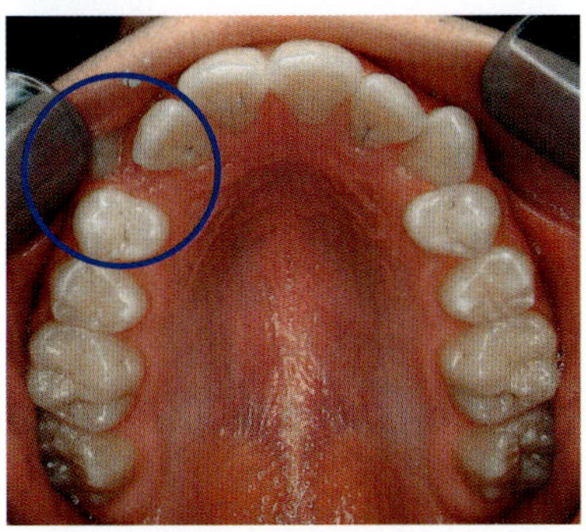
18

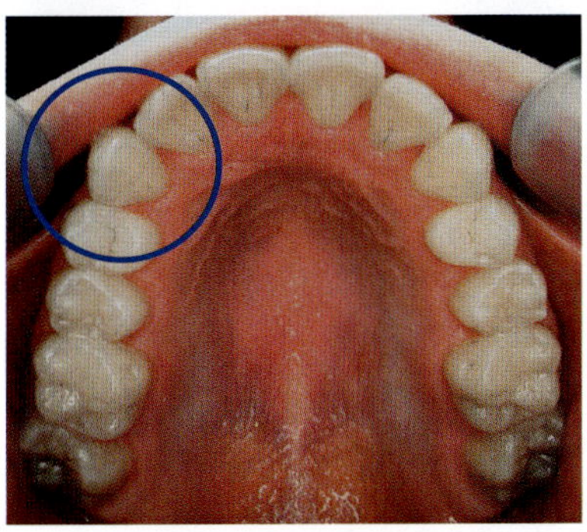
19

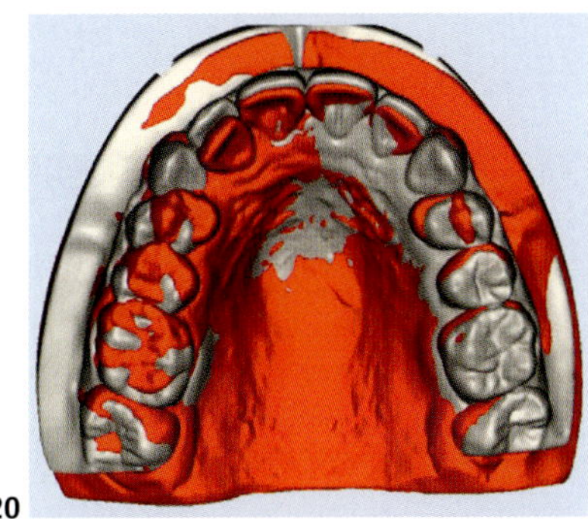
20

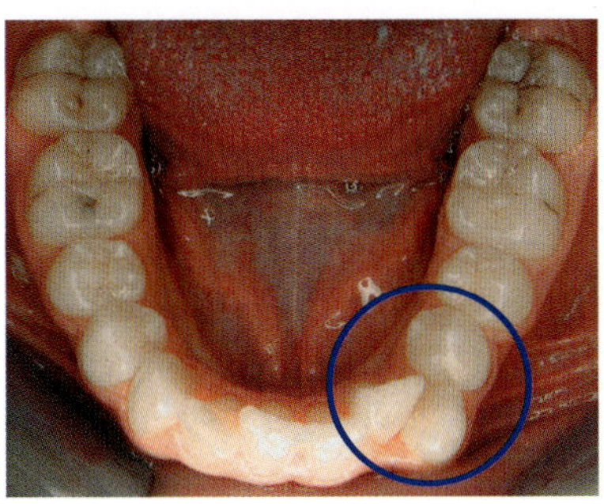
21

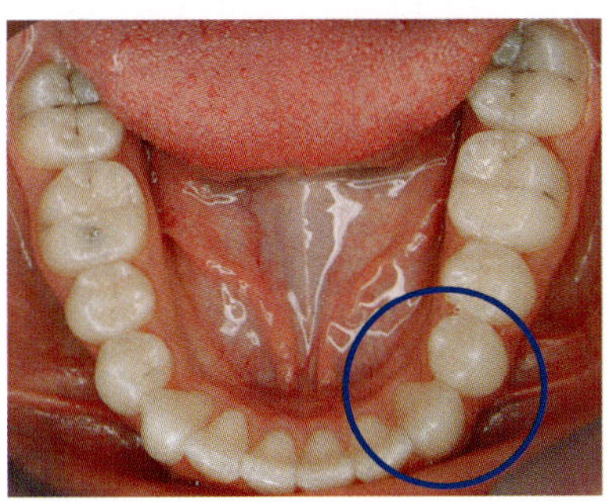
22

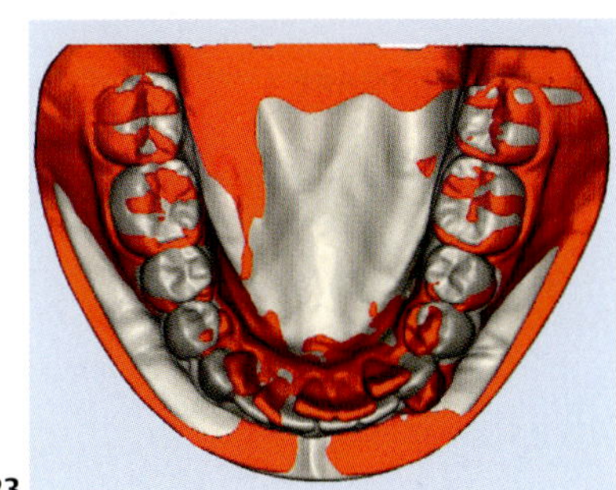
23

Case Study 7.3 (Fig. 7.15)

Patient: B.C., male, age 15.
Diagnostic records: models, panoramic radiograph, lateral cephalometric radiograph, intraoral/extraoral photographs.
Main findings: transverse deficiency of maxilla, tendency to prognathia, buccal positioning of 13 and 23.
Treatment aims: expansion of the upper jaw, alignment of 13 and 23, reduction of the slightly increased overjet and overbite.
Appliances: self-ligating brackets and molar bands.
Archwire sequence: 0.012 SE, 0.016 SE, 0.016 × 0.022 SE, 0.018 × 0.025 SE, 0.019 × 0.025 SS.
Active treatment time: 9 months.
Retention: bonded retainers and three-dimensional retention in the upper jaw with a Hawley retainer.

1 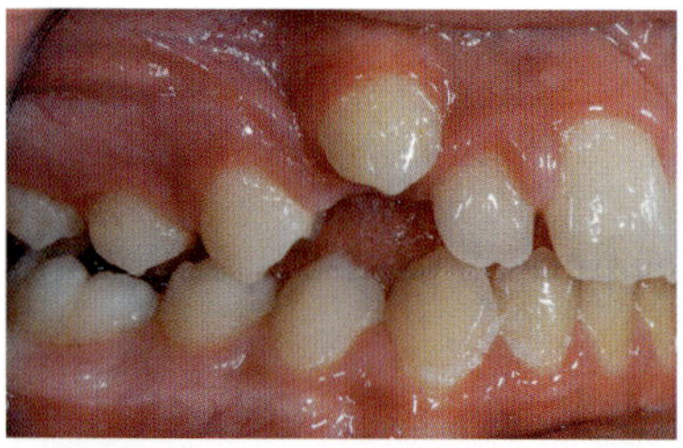
2 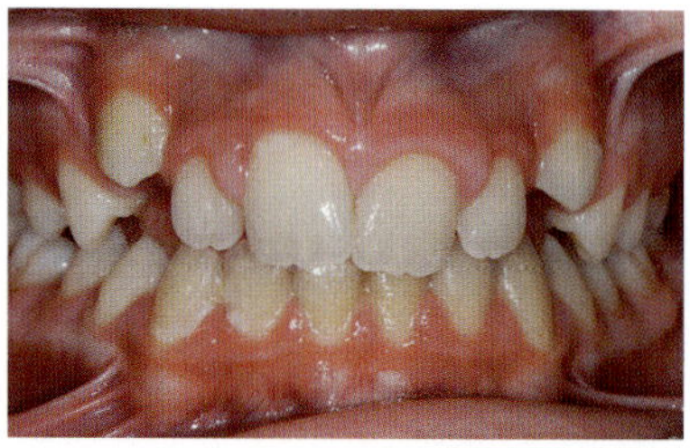
3 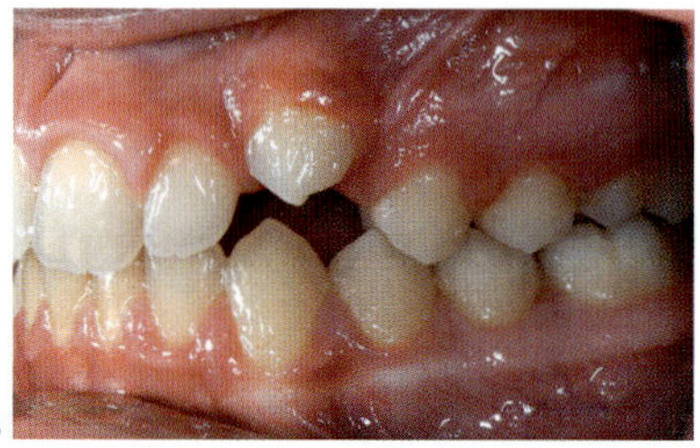
4 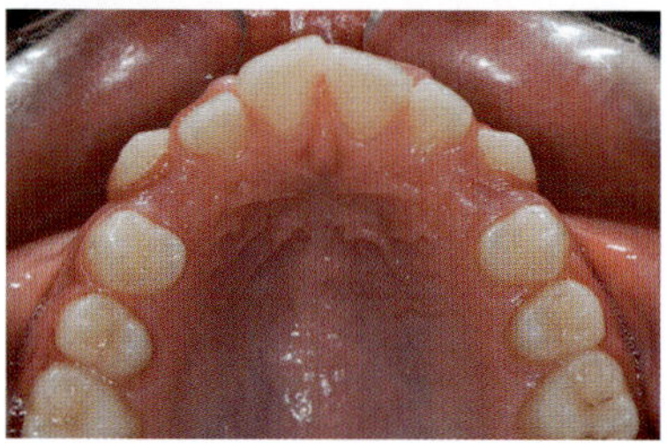
5 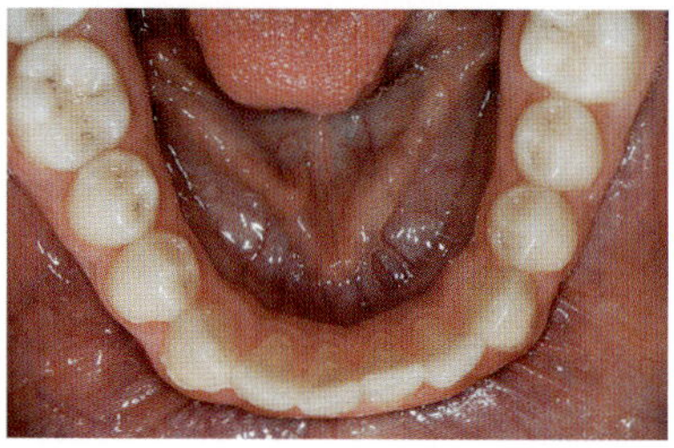

Fig. 7.15 1–21
1–5 Initial presentation; buccally displaced teeth 13 and 23 and a class III tendency in the buccal segments.

6 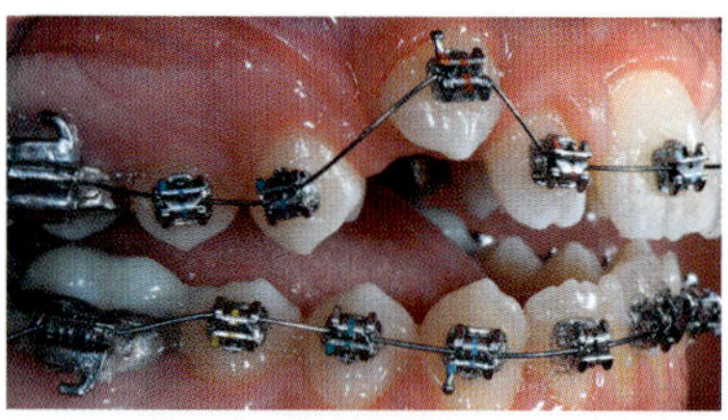
7 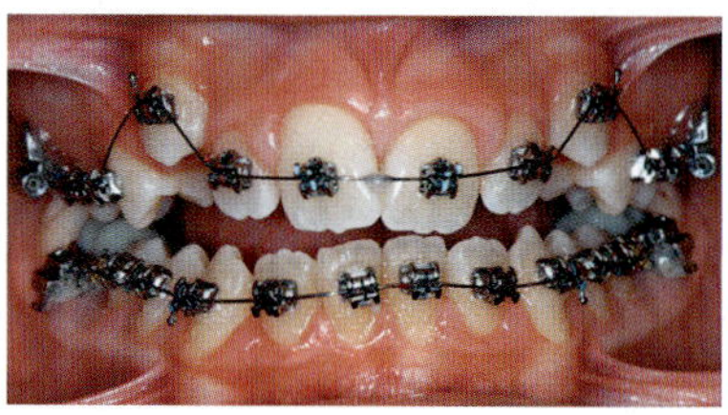
8 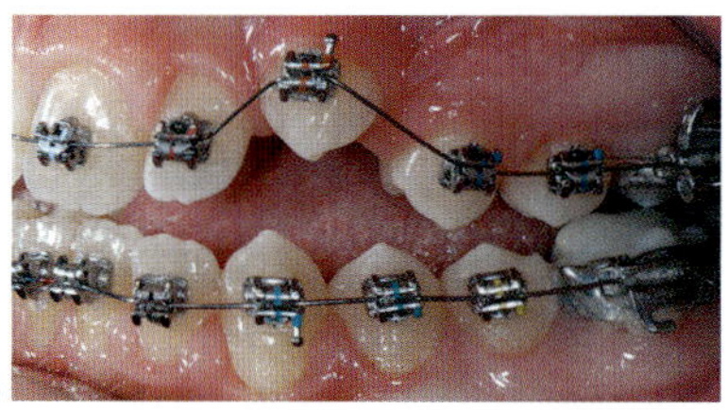
9 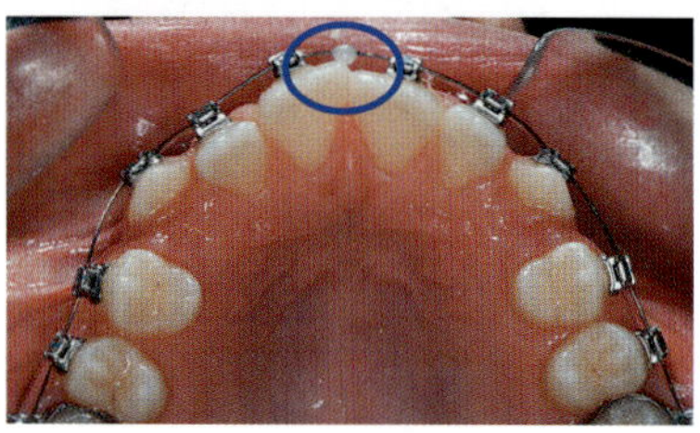

6–9 Initial alignment with a superelastic NiTi archwire 0.012, which was fully ligated.

CLINICAL PEARL

A "stop" made of light-cured composite material can be used to avoid shifting of the archwires, which may cause patient discomfort.

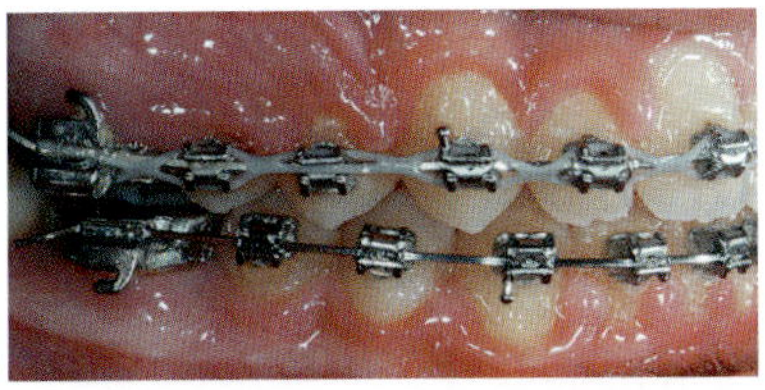
10

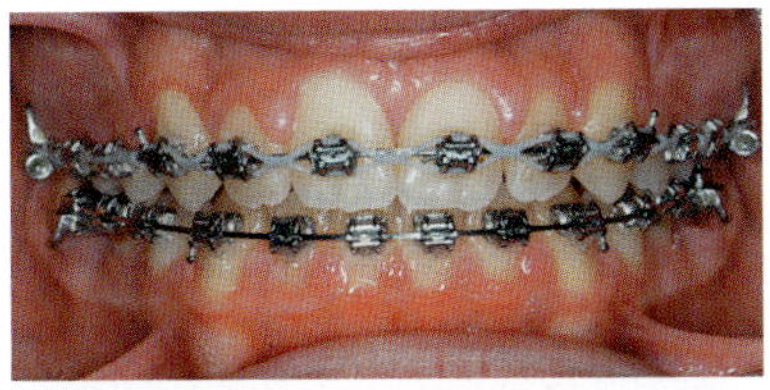
11

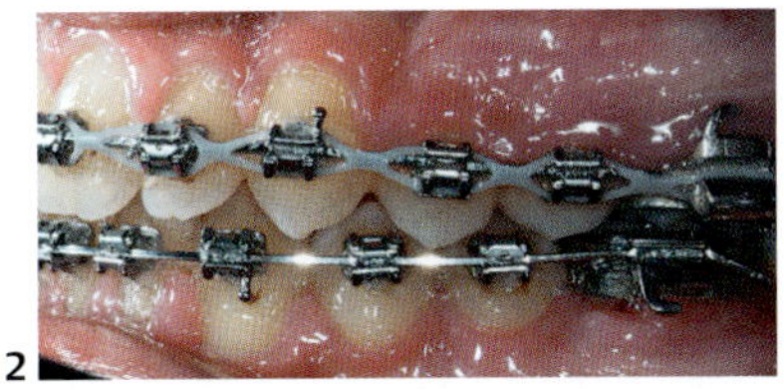
12

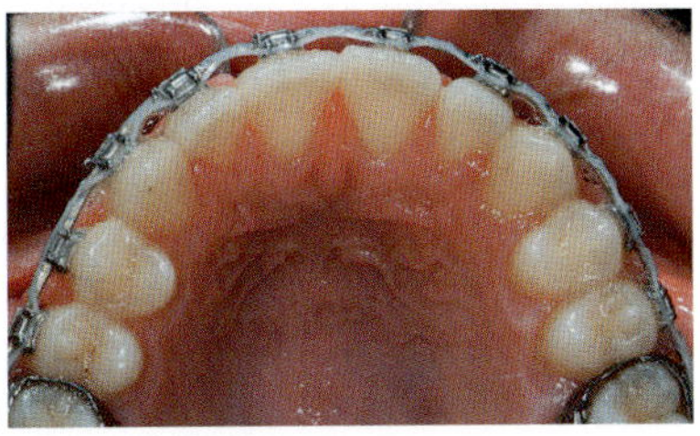
13

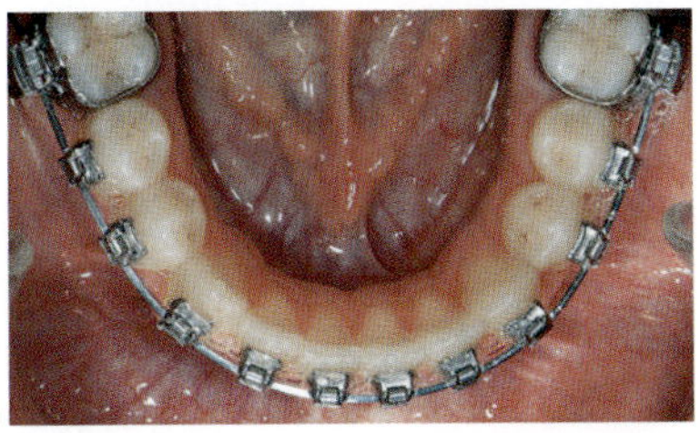
14

10–14 0.019 × 0.022 stainless-steel archwires with an elastomeric chain in the upper jaw.

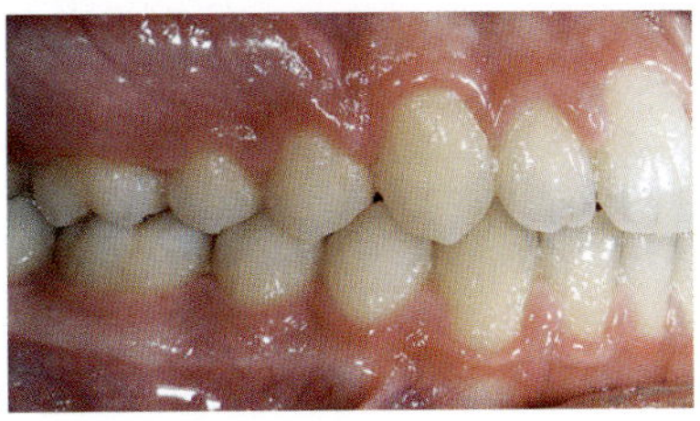
15

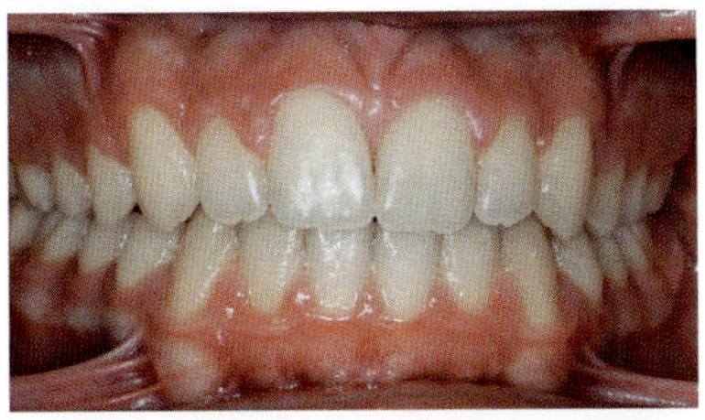
16

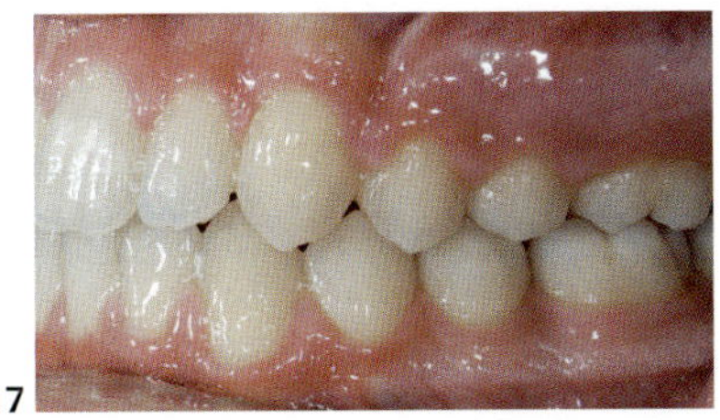
17

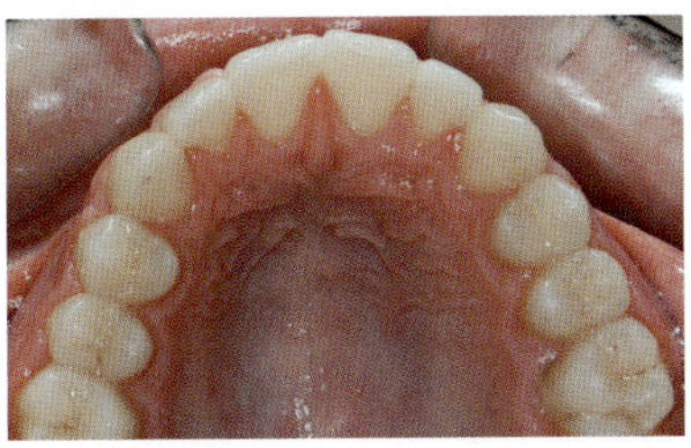
18

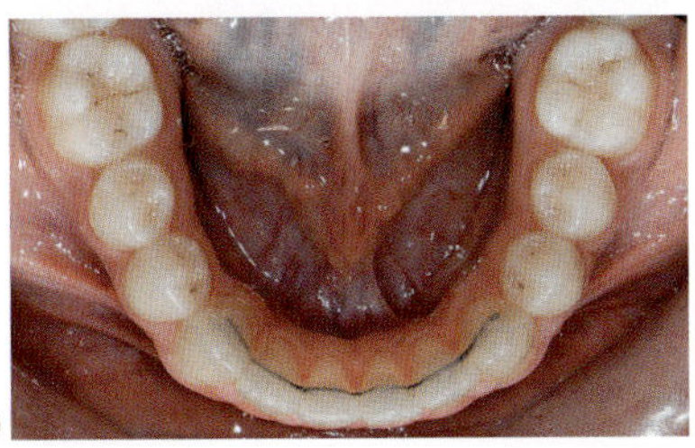
19

15–19 One year in retention using a fixed retainer in the mandible and a removable retainer in the maxilla.

Errors and risks:
Rapid, short treatments require careful retention.

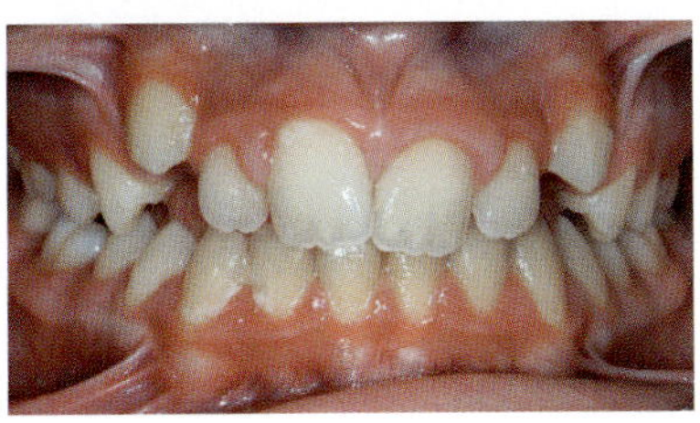
20

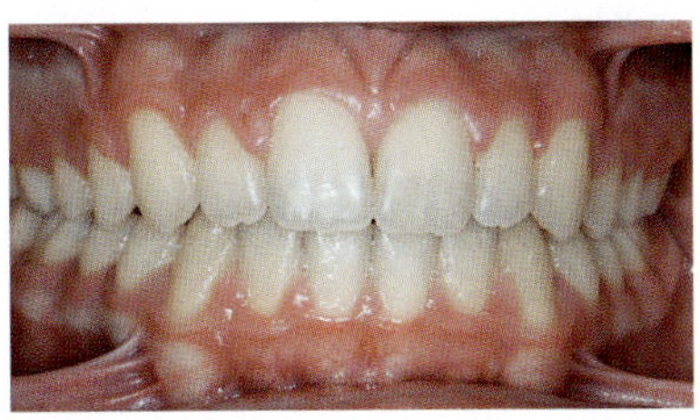
21

20–21 The initial presentation and final result after approximately 9 months of active treatment. (Images courtesy of Vittorio Cacciafesta, Milan, Italy.)

Case Study 7.4 (Fig. 7.16)

Patient: M.Y., female, age 15.

Diagnostic records: models, panoramic radiograph, lateral cephalometric radiograph, intraoral/extraoral photographs.

Main findings: anterior crowding, tipping of the occlusal plane.

Treatment aims: resolution of crowding and correction of the occlusal plane.

Appliances: self-ligating brackets, molar bands and interproximal enamel reduction.

Archwire sequence: 0.012 SE, 0.016 SE, 0.016 × 0.022 SE, 0.018 × 0.025 SE, 0.021 × 0.025 SE.

Active treatment time: 8 months.

Retention: fixed retention to the labial segments and further retention with vacuum-formed retainers.

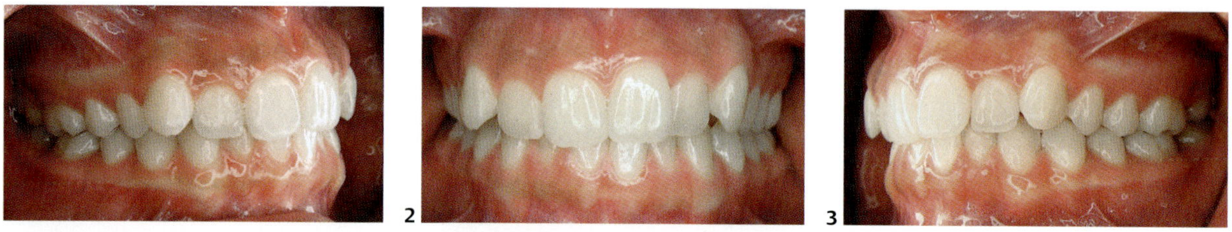

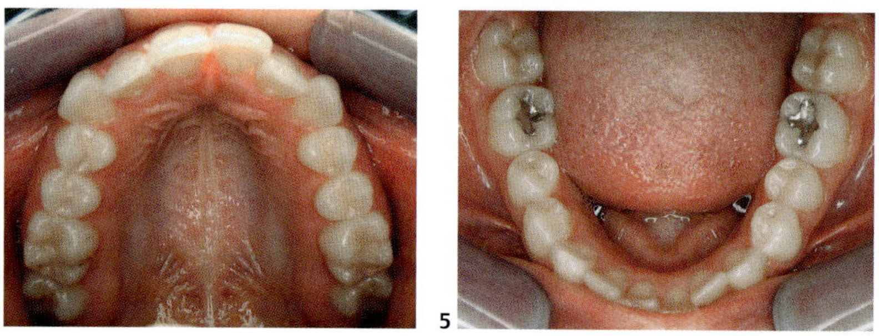

Fig. 7.16 1–22
1–5 Initial presentation: class I with maxillary and mandibular anterior crowding.

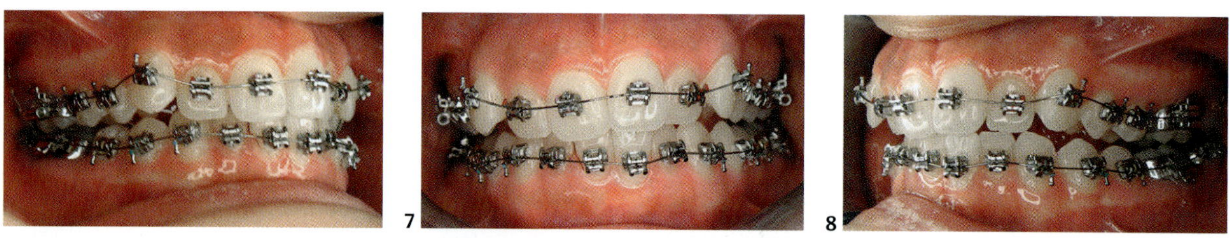

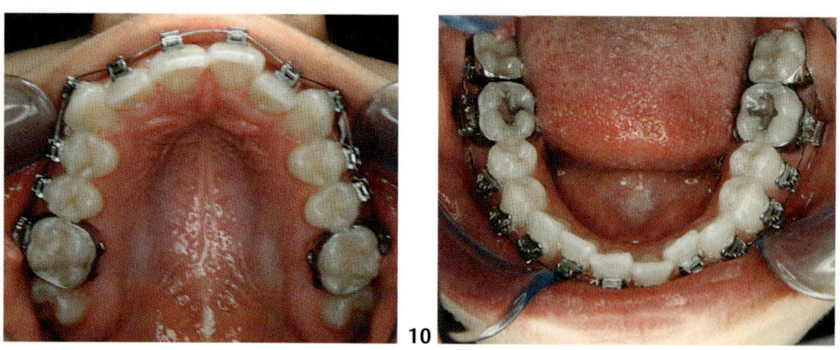

6–10 Self-ligating brackets with superelastic 0.012 NiTi wires in both arches.

Errors and risks:
Limitation of incisor proclination by interproximal enamel reduction before placement of orthodontic appliances.

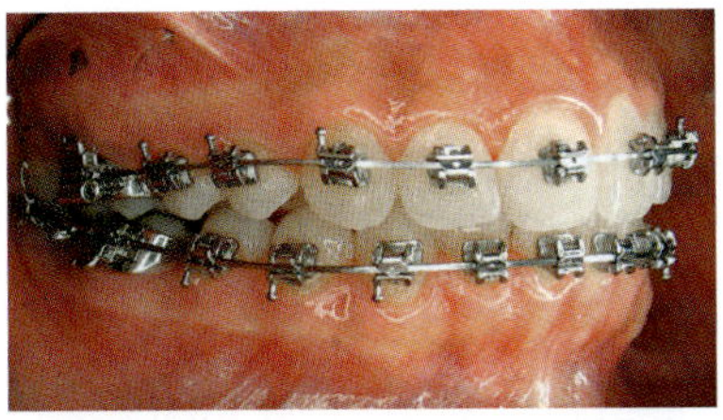
11

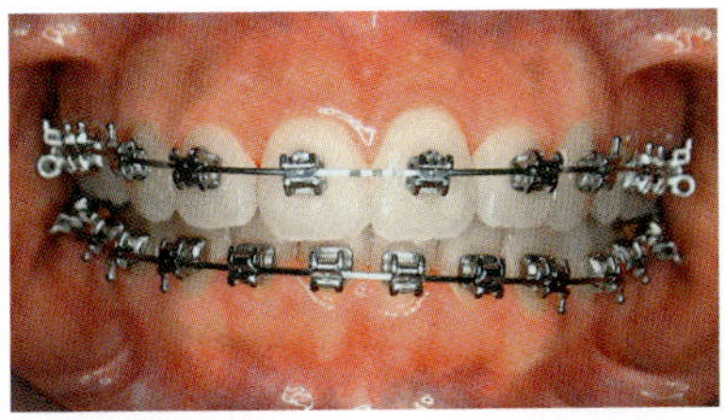
12

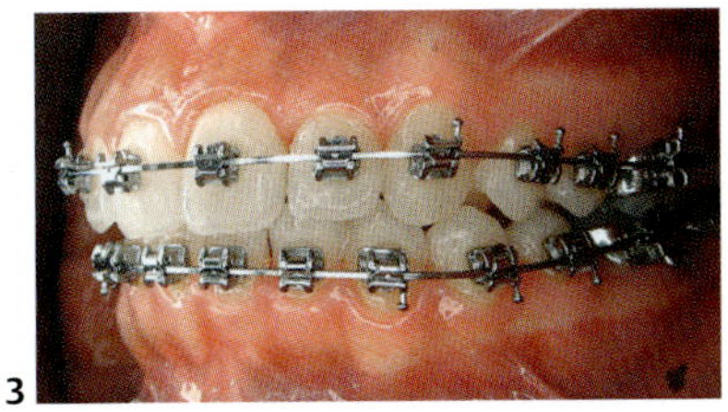
13

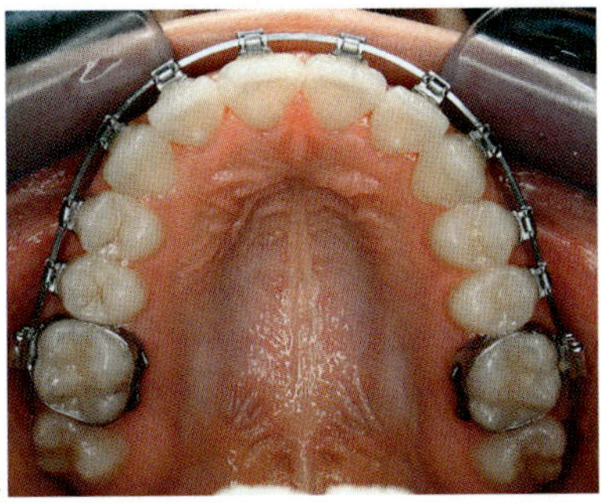
14

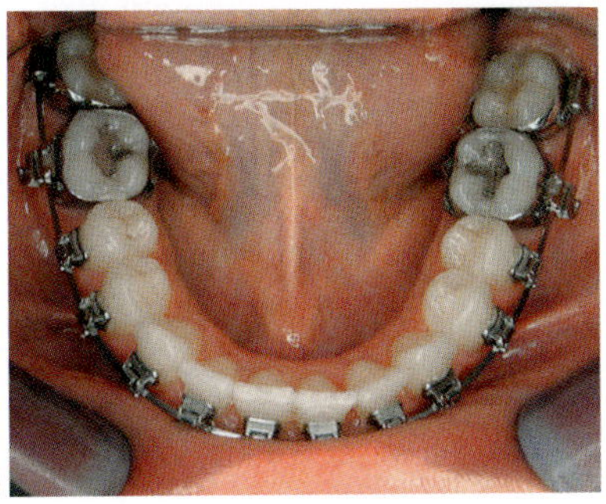
15

11–15 Leveling and alignment of the occlusal plane with square BioFinisher archwires.

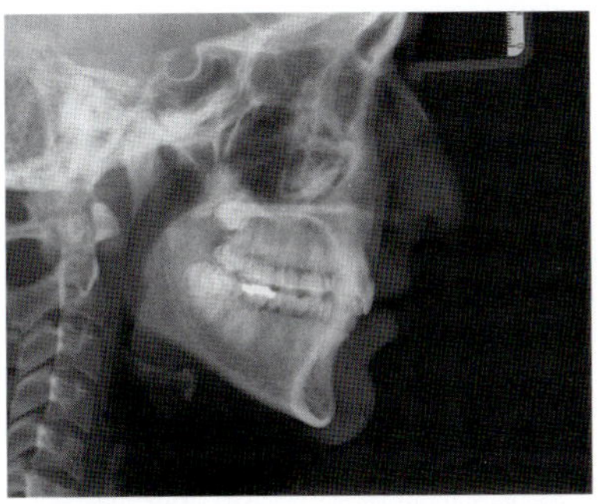
16

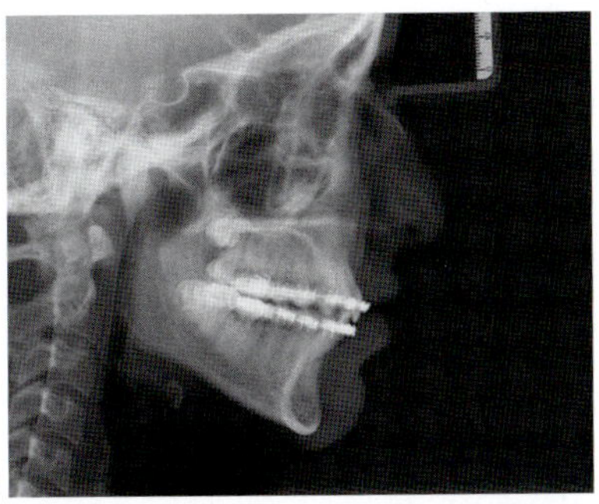
17

16, 17

Clinical pearl:
Taking the lateral cephalogram before the debonding appointment allows analysis of enamel to incisor inclination with the appliances still in place. It is still possible to improve it by means of interproximal enamel reduction or even dental extractions at this point.

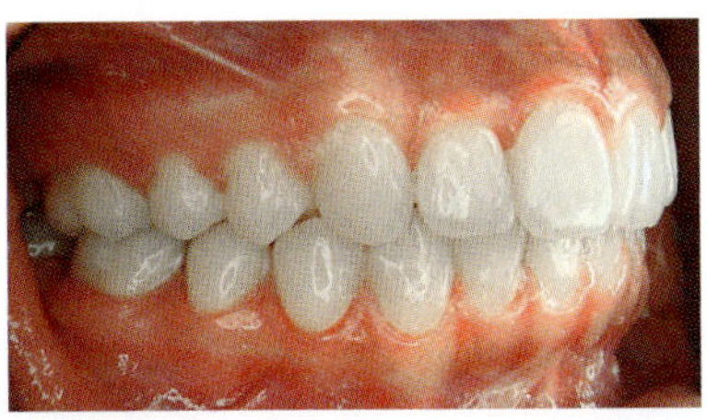
18

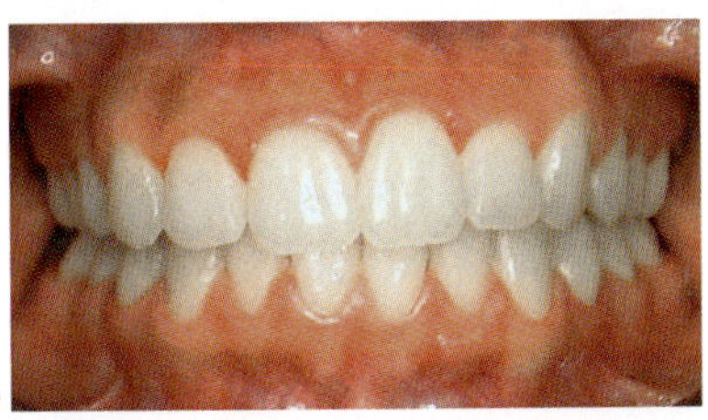
19

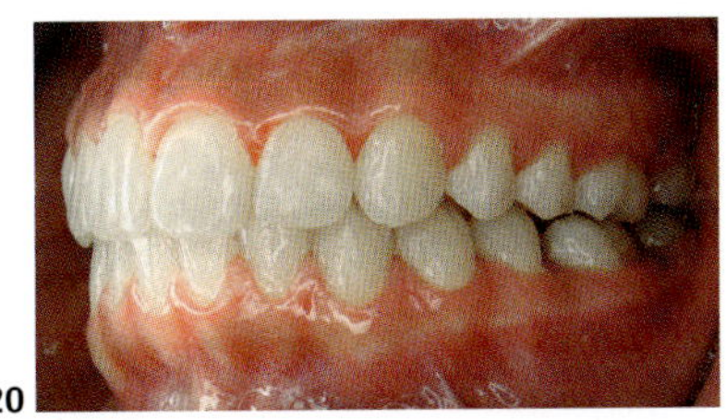
20

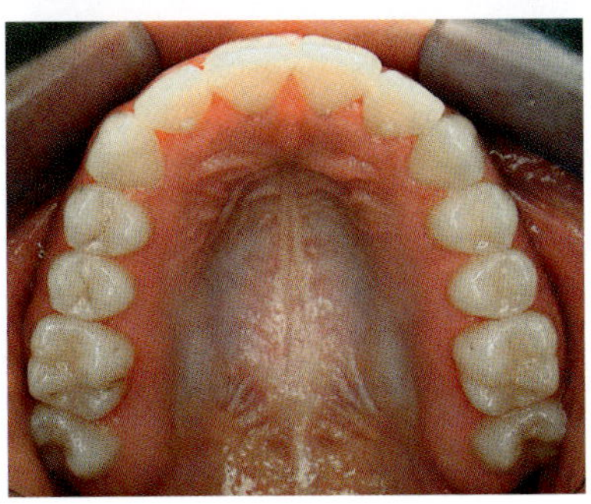
21

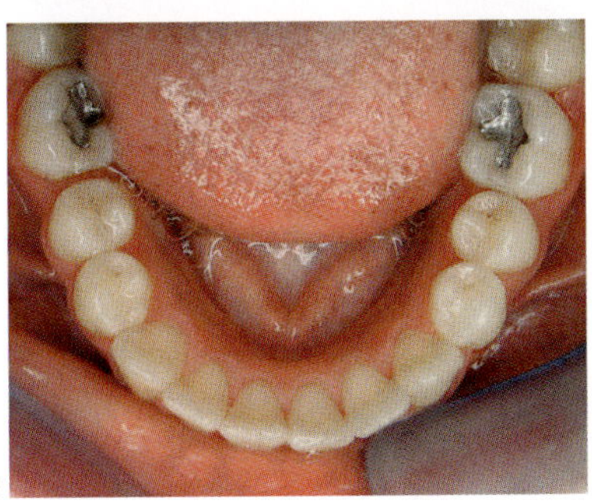
22

18–22 One year after retention with vacuum-formed retainers.

Errors and risks:
Stability: fixed retention should be considered if the patient's compliance with retainer wear is expected to be poor.

Case Study 7.5 (Fig. 7.17)

Patient: A.B., male, age 17.

Diagnostic records: models, panoramic radiograph, lateral cephalometric radiograph, intraoral/extraoral photographs.

Main findings: asymmetric buccal segment relationship, crowding of the upper front teeth.

Treatment aims: alignment of the upper front teeth only (the patient requested limited treatment), including interproximal size reduction (stripping).

Appliances: self-ligating brackets, approximal enamel reduction.

Archwire sequence: 0.012 SE, 0.016 SE, 0.016 × 0.022 SE, 0.018 × 0.025 SE 0.021 × 0.025 SE.

Alternative treatment strategy: lingual fixed appliance.

Retention: fixed retainer to the upper front teeth.

1
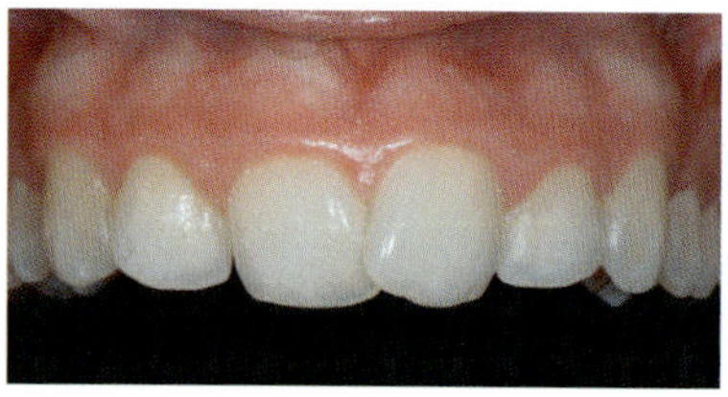

Fig. 7.17 1–17

1 Crowding of the anterior teeth, particularly of the central incisors, was the patient's chief complaint.

2 3 4
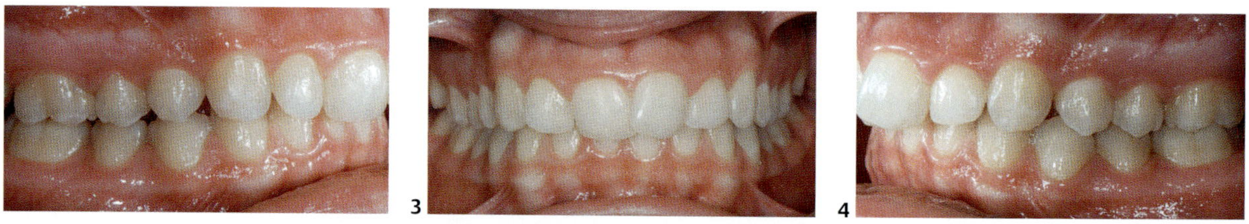

5 6
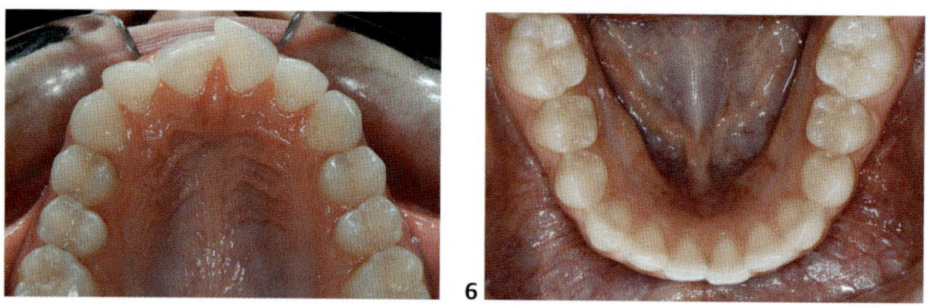

2–6

Caution:
Retroclination of 11 (upper right central incisor) limits extrusion and proclination of the lower labial segment and it may potentially restrict mandibular excursions, also holding the mandible in a class II situation.

7 8 9
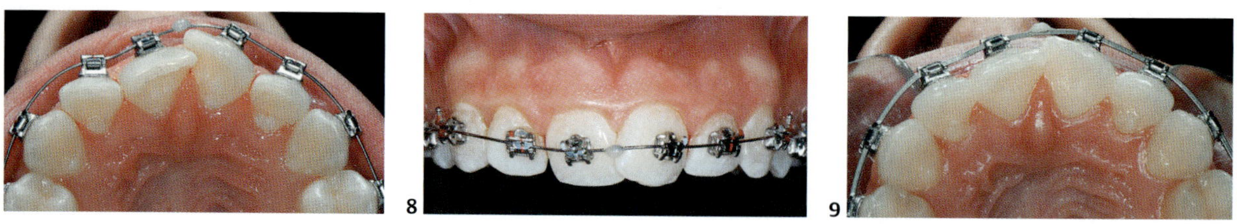

7–9 Following placement of 0.012 and 0.016 superelastic NiTi archwires, torque values are improved by using square superelastic wires.

CLINICAL PEARLS

- Composite stops palatal to the upper central incisors.
- Interproximal enamel reduction before archwire placement.

CLINICAL PEARL

The fixed retainer is only fitted to the upper incisors. The canines have not been bonded, in order to avoid occlusal contact between the retainer and the lower teeth, which could lead to higher failure rates.

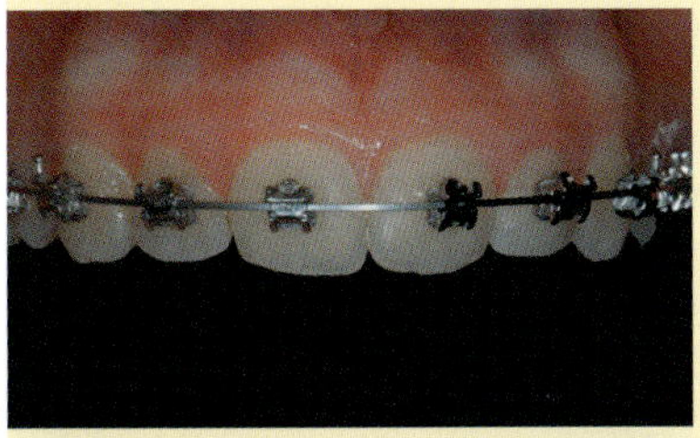
10
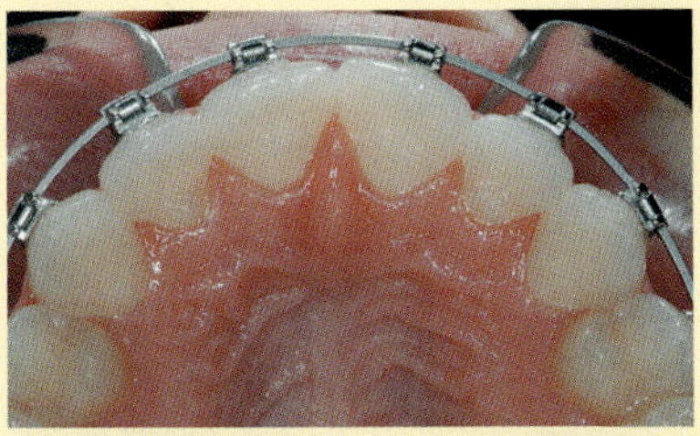
11
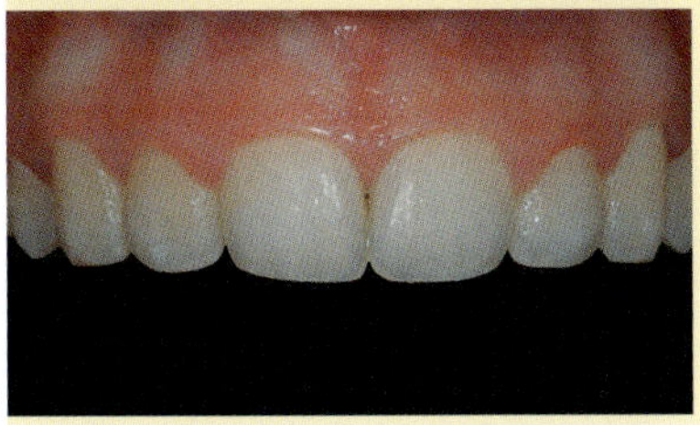
12
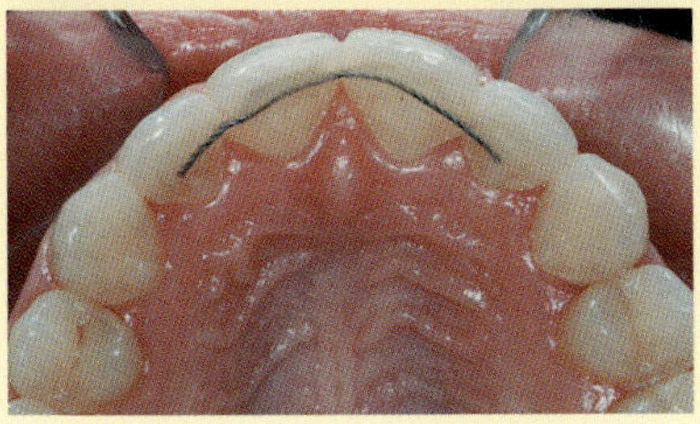
13

10–13 0.021 × 0.025 superelastic NiTi archwire and subsequent retention.

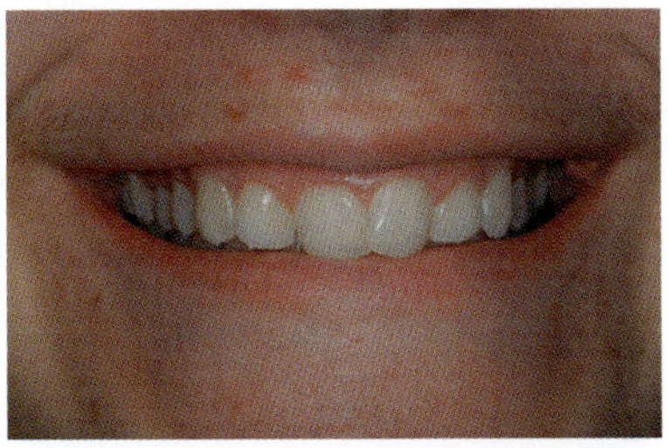
14
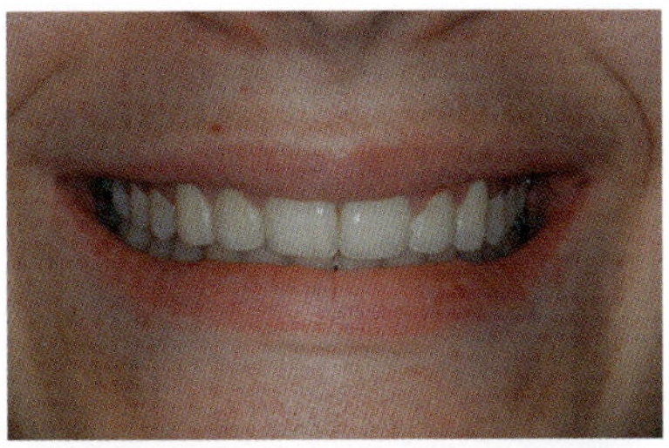
15
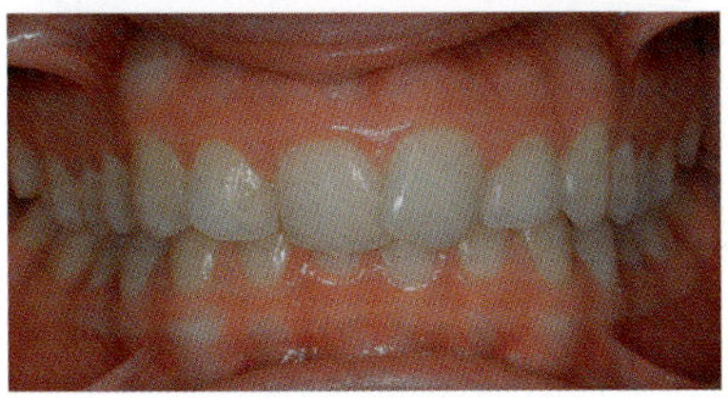
16
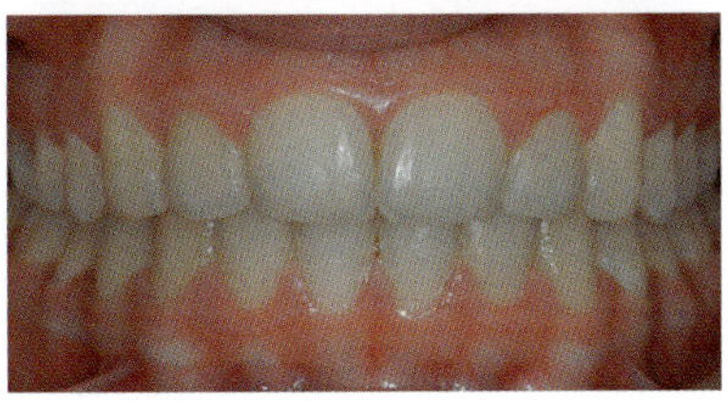
17

14–17 The initial presentation and the treatment result after 1 year in retention (right-hand side). (Treatment and images courtesy of Vittorio Cacciafesta, Milan, Italy.)

Case Study 7.6 (Fig. 7.18)

Patient: J.J., male, age 9.
Diagnostic records: models, panoramic radiograph, lateral cephalometric radiograph, intraoral/extraoral photographs.
Main findings: distal displacement of the lower jaw due to excessive retroclination of the upper labial segment (Class II/2 occlusion), deep traumatic overbite, and anterior crowding.
Treatment aims: resolve posterior displacement by protrusion and expansion of the upper jaw.
Appliances: self-ligating brackets, molar bands (2 × 4 appliance).
Archwire sequence: 0.012 SE, 0.016 SE, 0.016 × 0.022 SE, 0.019 × 0.025 SS.
Alternative treatment strategy: removal of appliances with expansion plate to the upper jaw and protrusion springs for the upper labial segment.
Active treatment time: 7 months.
Retention: three-dimensional retention using an upper removable appliance or functional appliance to potentially avoid more complex treatment in the teenage years.

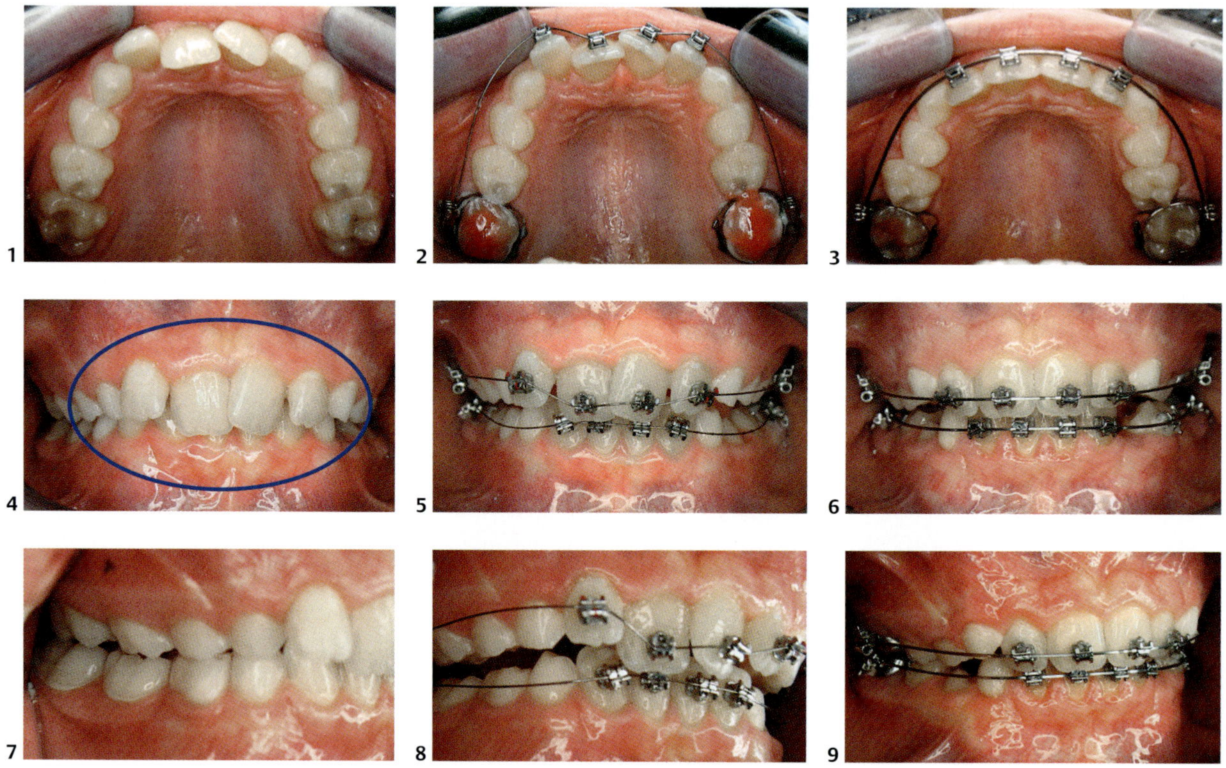

Fig. 7.18 1–9
1–9 Class II/2 occlusion, with severely retroclined and overerupted central incisors.
Left column: before treatment.
Middle column: 0.012 superelastic NiTi archwires ligated.
Right column: after correction of the maxillary incisor angulation, the mandible is free to develop in a forward direction.

CLINICAL PEARL

The 2 × 4 fixed appliance is often a good alternative to removable appliances, as it is not dependent on patient compliance. Early alignment, particularly of the upper front teeth, can lead to spontaneous correction of a class II molar relationship, as seen in **Fig. 7.18**.

Treatment of Occlusion after Leveling and Alignment

It is often noticed that occlusal interference persists after the leveling and alignment stage. It can be eliminated by using harmonized arch shapes. After good coordination between the dental arches has been established, spontaneous improvement of the occlusion often occurs without any need for extensive intermaxillary elastic wear (see Case Studies 7.7–7.9).

Case Study 7.7 (Fig. 7.19)

Patient: M.K., female, age 15.
Diagnostic records: models, panoramic radiograph, lateral cephalometric radiograph, intraoral/extraoral photographs.
Main findings: crowding of 13 and 43, open bite tendency with tongue interposition in the area of 13, 43 and 23, 33.
Treatment aims: align 13 and 43 and secure the reduced overbite.
Appliances: self-ligating brackets, molar bands, approximal enamel reduction, intermaxillary elastics.
Archwire sequence: 0.012 SE, 0.16 SS, 0.016 × 0.022 TMA, 0.018 × 0.025 SE, 0.019 × 0.025 SS.
Alternative treatment strategy: extraction of premolars.
Active treatment time: 12 months.
Retention: bonded retainers to upper and lower front teeth and follow-up of the overbite situation with monitoring of growth.

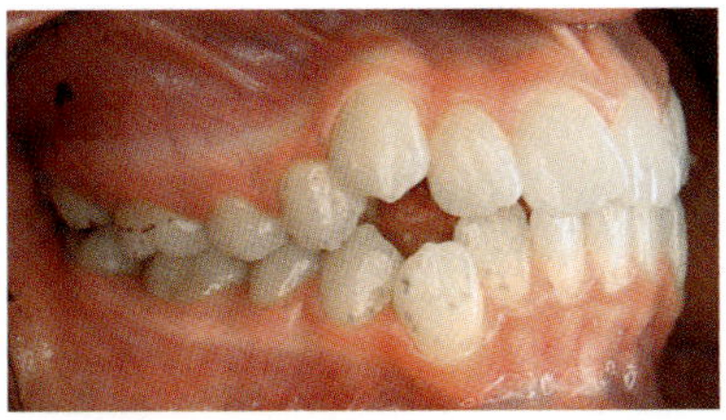
1

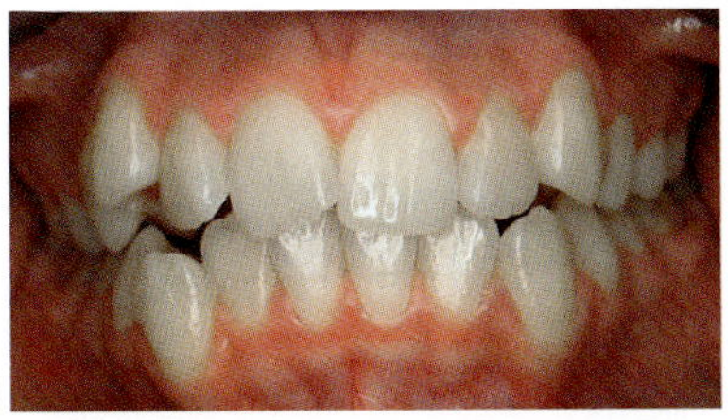
2

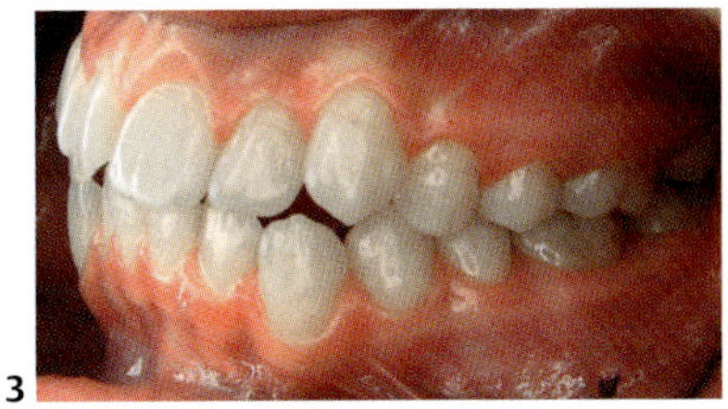
3

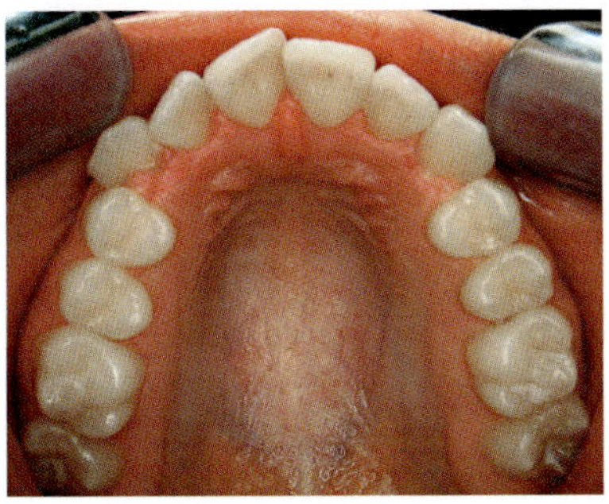
4

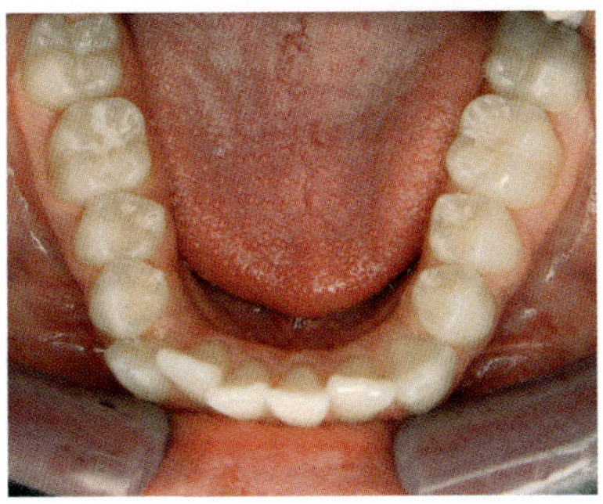
5

Fig. 7.19 1–28
1–5 Initial presentation: there is crowding in both arches but a normal buccal segment relationship, with reduced overbite and overjet.

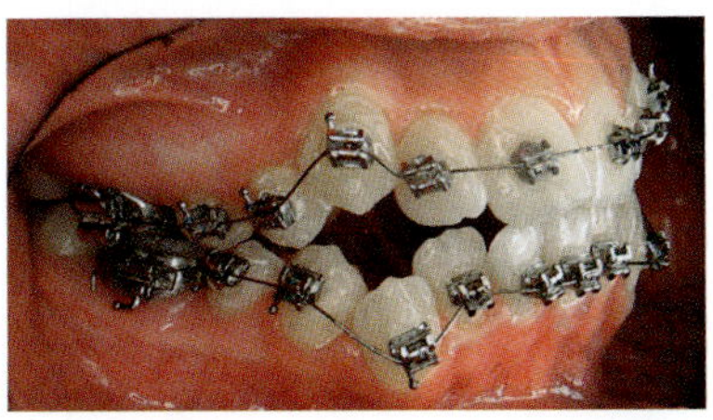
6

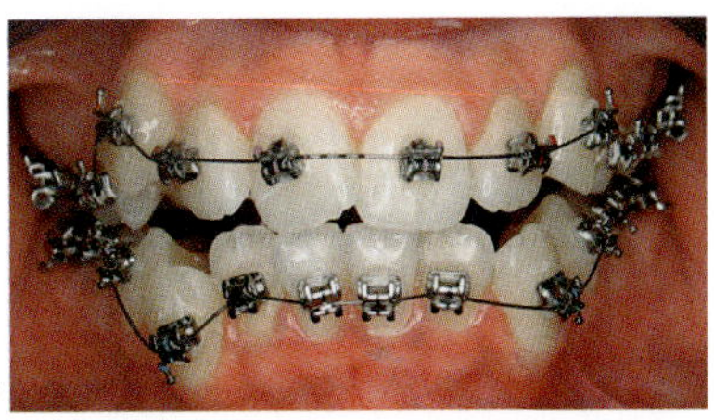
7

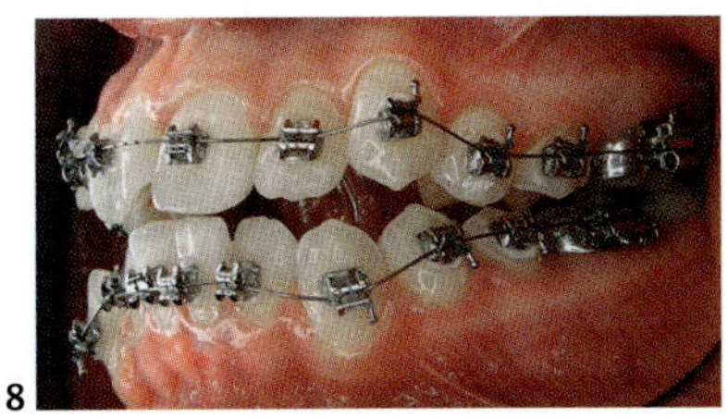
8

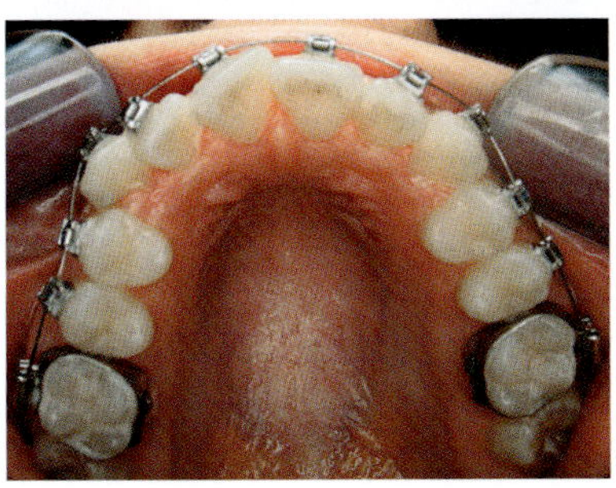
9

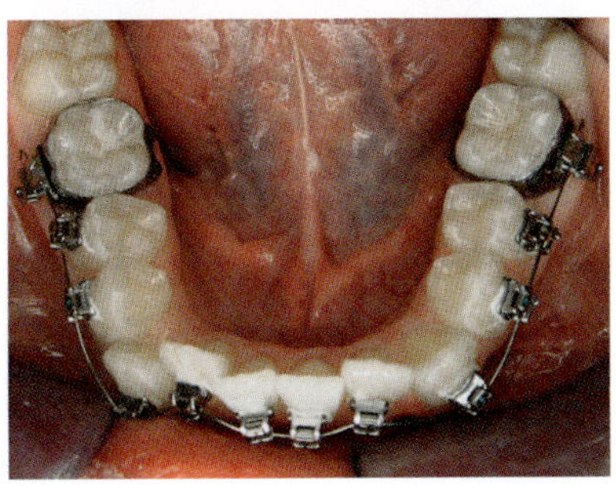
10

6–10 0.012 superelastic NiTi archwires fully ligated to all brackets.

Note:
Full ligation into all teeth can cause an anterior open bite, and subsequent interposition of the tongue between the teeth should be monitored carefully. IPR should be considered at the start of treatment.

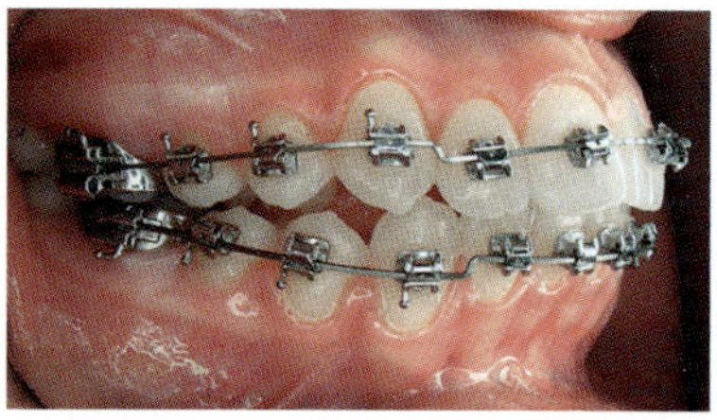
11

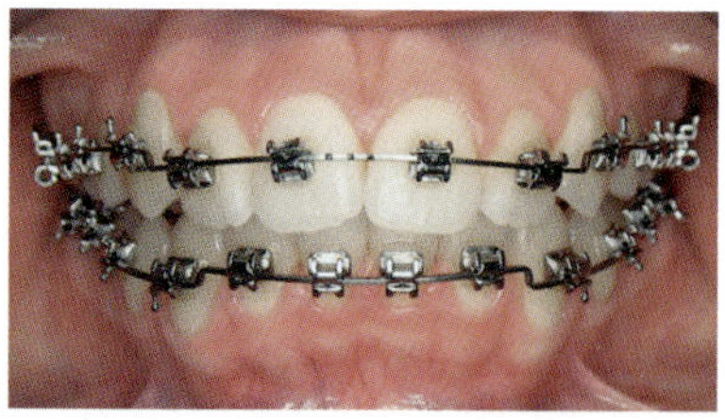
12

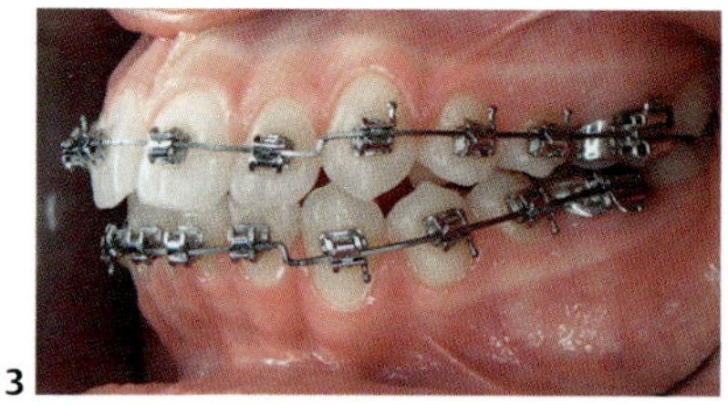
13

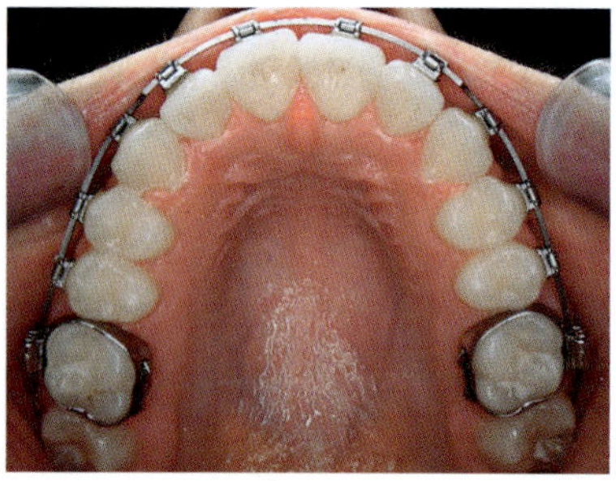
14

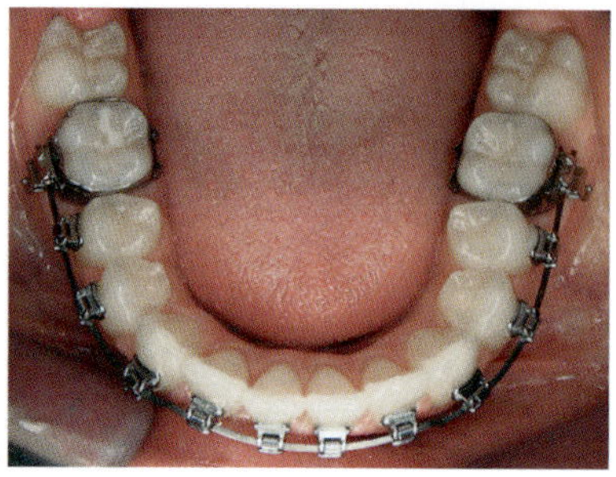
15

11–15 A 0.016 × 0.022 titanium–molybdenum alloy (TMA) archwire with extrusion bends for the anterior segments.

Caution:
Inclination problem! Enamel reduction in the lower jaw from 5–5 and in the upper premolars must be performed.

CLINICAL PEARL

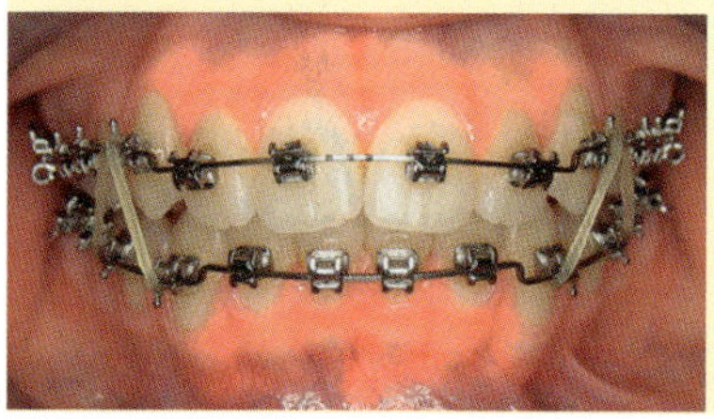
16

Question: How should the overbite be preserved?
Answer:
- Apply vertical elastics to the maxillary canines.
- Do not bond the second molars.
- Interproximal enamel reduction and retroclination of the incisors.

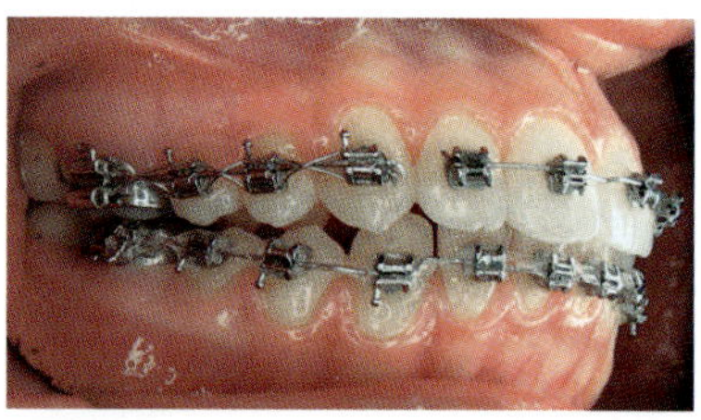
17

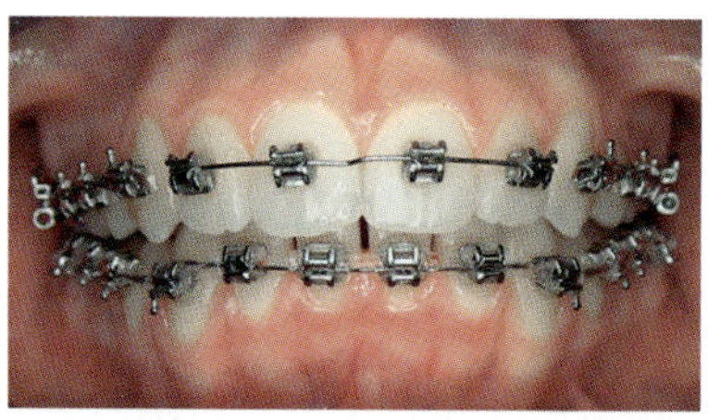
18

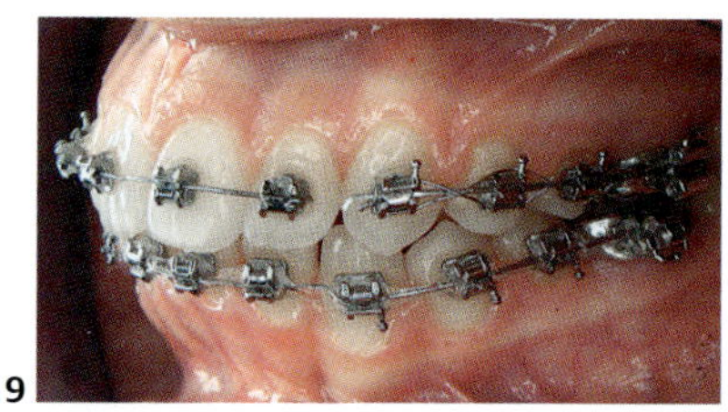
19

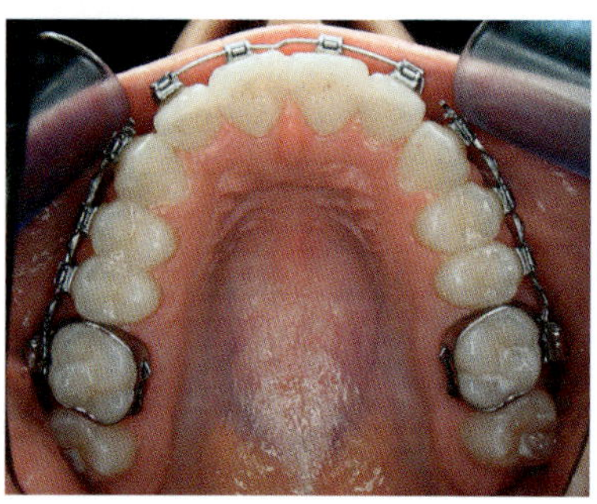
20

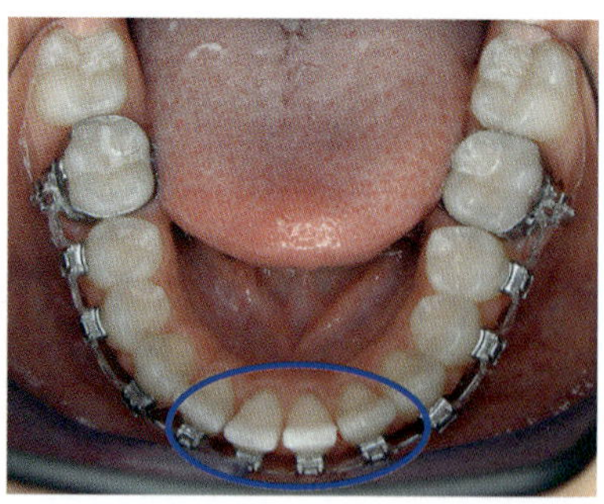
21

17–21 Interproximal enamel reduction of the maxillary incisors was carried out; there is significant stripping of the lower labial segment, with subsequent retroclination of the teeth. Segmental archwires can be used to improve settling.

CLINICAL PEARL

Space for retroclination of the anterior segment is created by interproximal reduction, and the labial segments are retroclined by subsequent use of a continuous elastic chain.

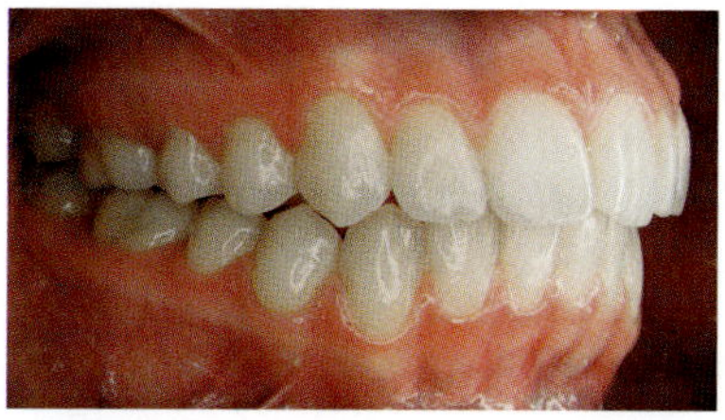
22
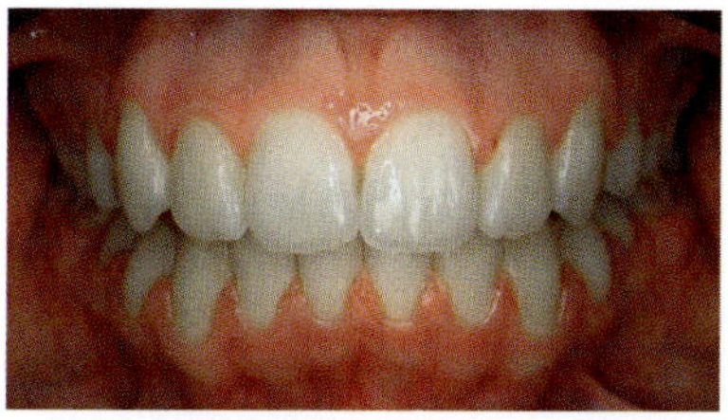
23
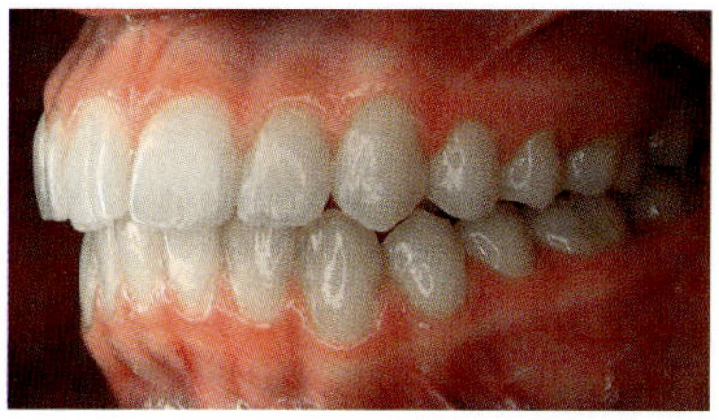
24
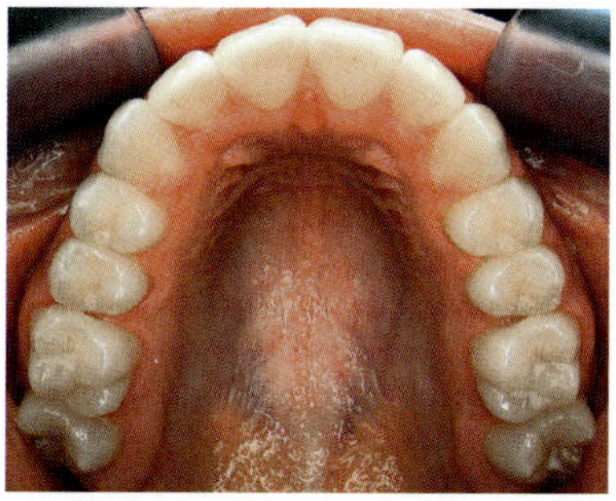
25
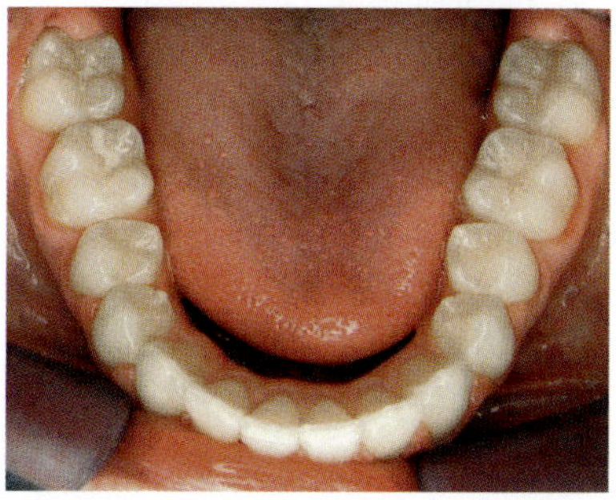
26

22–26 Result after 1 year in retention.

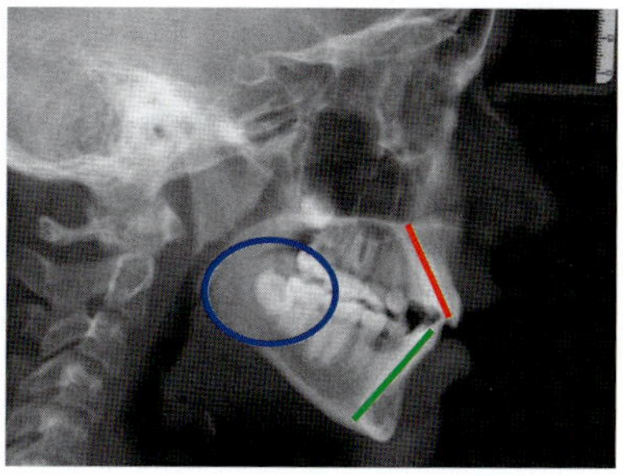
27
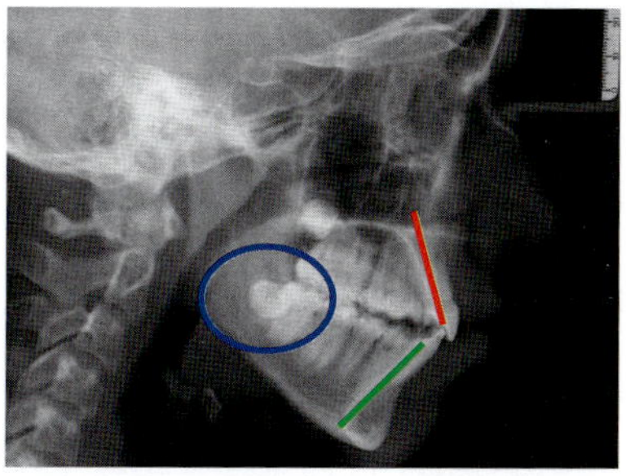
28

27, 28 Lower incisor inclination at the start of treatment and following orthodontic treatment; lip competence at end of treatment.

Errors and risks:
Incisor inclination was preserved despite the initial crowding. However, fixed retention should be considered in borderline nonextraction cases. The development of the third molar should be monitored during the follow-up.

CLINICAL PEARL

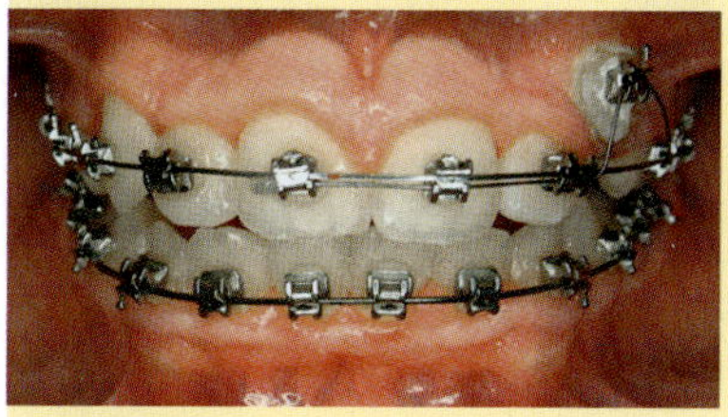
1
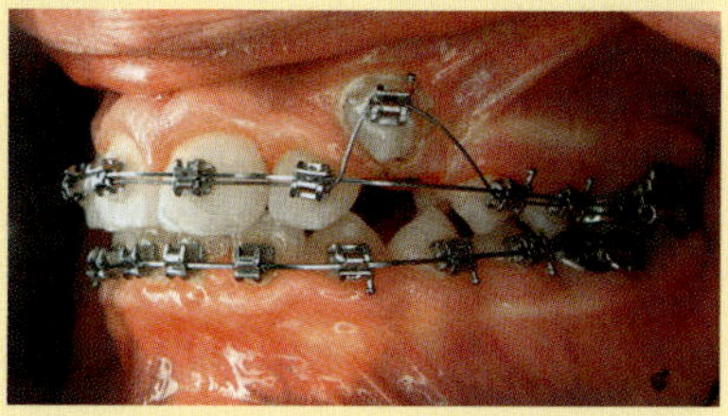
2

Fig. 7.20

1, 2 Delayed or ectopically erupting canines can be corrected using a superelastic overlay wire (piggyback technique). Other teeth can still be moved on the rigid base arch. Using self-ligating brackets with an auxiliary slot can be beneficial, as shown here.

Case Study 7.8 (Fig. 7.21)

Patient: A.N., female, age 15.

Diagnostic records: models, panoramic radiograph, lateral cephalometric radiograph, intraoral/extraoral photographs.

Main findings: increased overjet, anterior crowding, and rotations.

Treatment aims: coordination of the arches, alignment of the upper and lower labial segments, and reduction of the overjet.

Appliances: self-ligating brackets, molar bands, approximal enamel reduction.

Archwire sequence: 0.012 SE, 0.016 SE, 0.016 × 0.022 SE, 0.018 × 0.025 SE, 0.021 × 0.025 SE.

Alternative treatment strategy: n/a.

Active treatment time: 12 months.

Retention: three-dimensional retention, including bonded retainers.

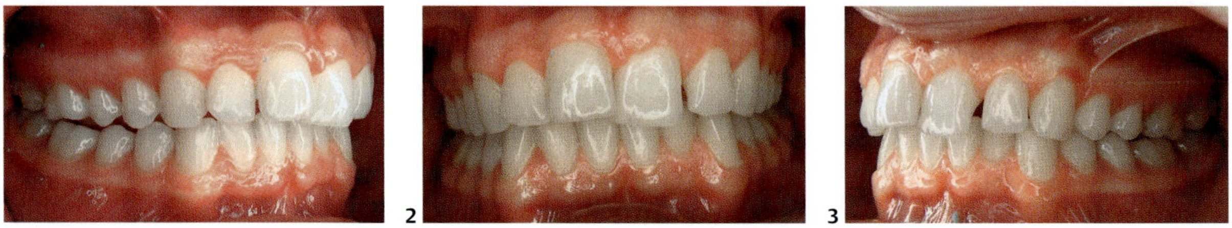

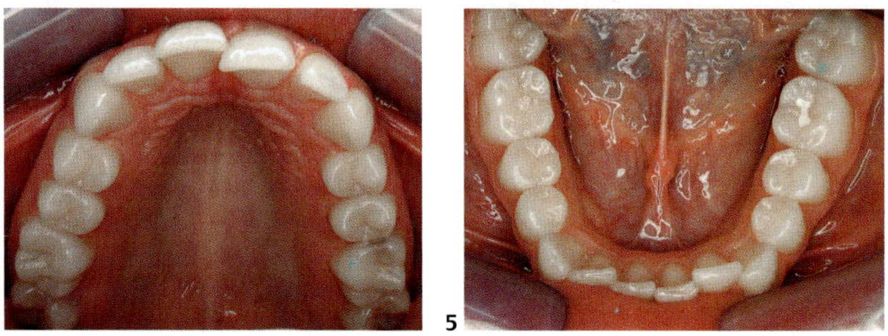

Fig. 7.21 1–22

1–5 Initial presentation: maxillary and mandibular crowding combined with a constricted maxillary arch. Class II tendency.

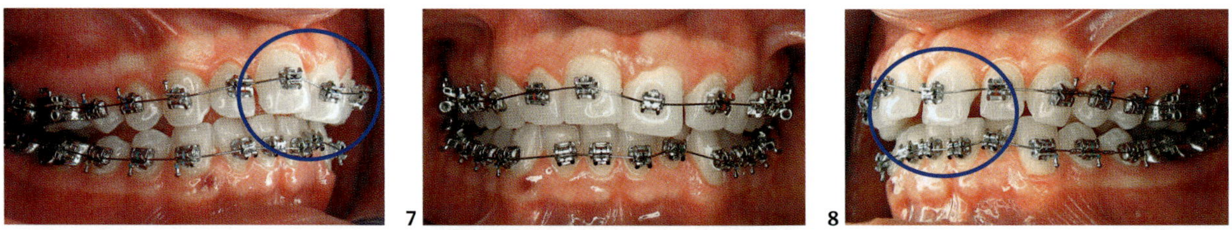

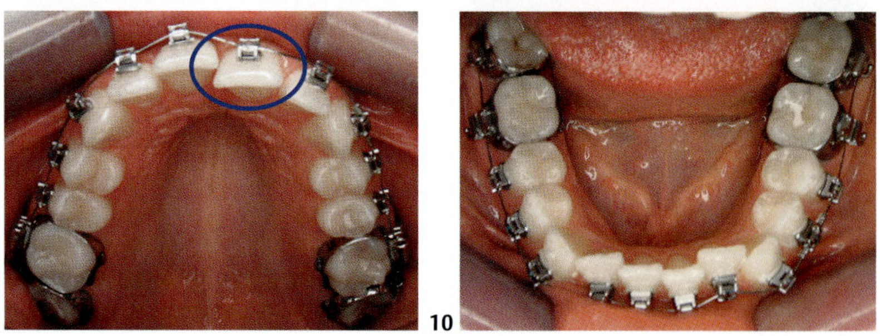

6–10

Clinical pearl:
The retroclined maxillary left incisor is restricting mandibular excursions.

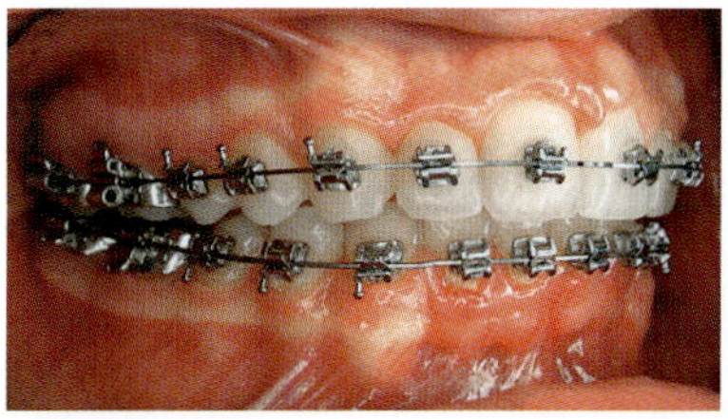
11

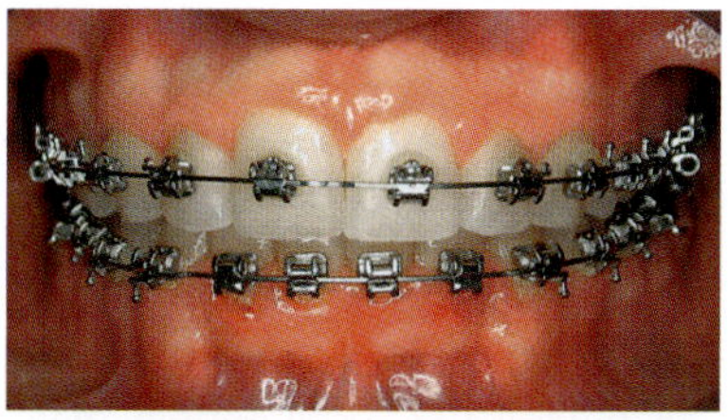
12

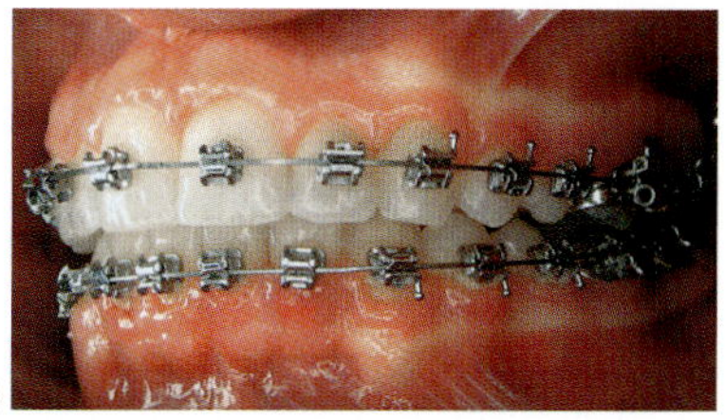
13

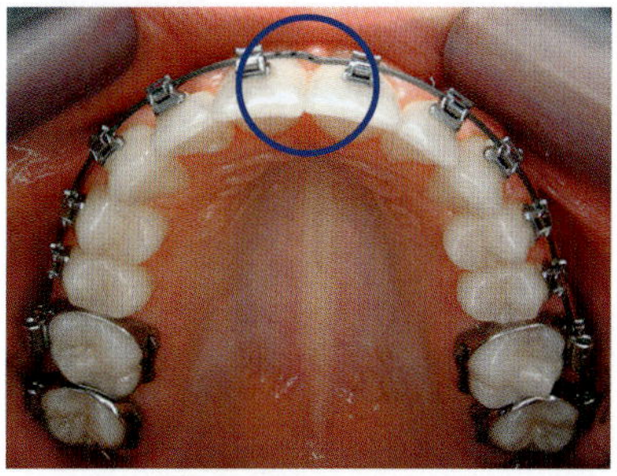
14

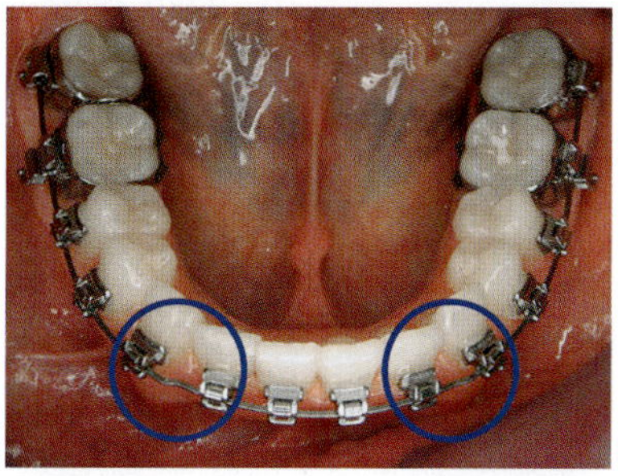
15

11–15 Alignment of the upper and lower arches leads to spontaneous correction of the initial class II discrepancy.

Errors and risks:
Self-ligating brackets may also require individual finishing bends in the later stages of treatment.

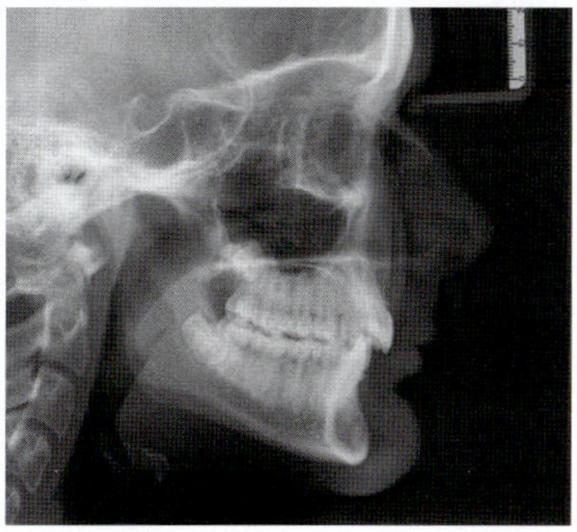
16

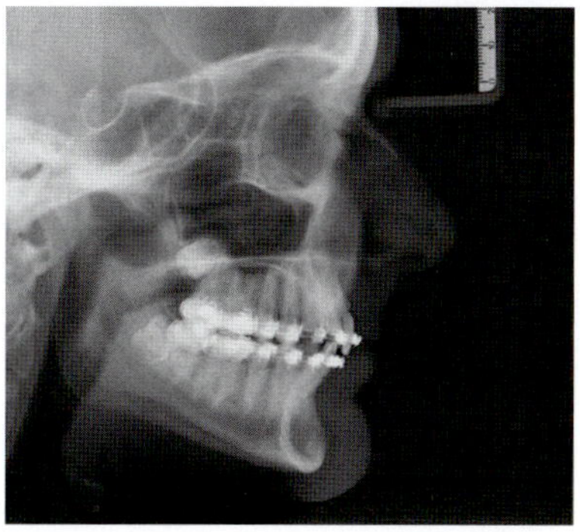
17

16, 17

Clinical pearl:
Comparison of lateral cephalograms before treatment and before appliance removal makes it possible to assess the incisor angulation. Adjustments of incisor inclinations are still possible using interproximal reduction and continuous elastic chains, as the appliances are still in place. Uppers need additional torque in this case to allow a mandible class I.

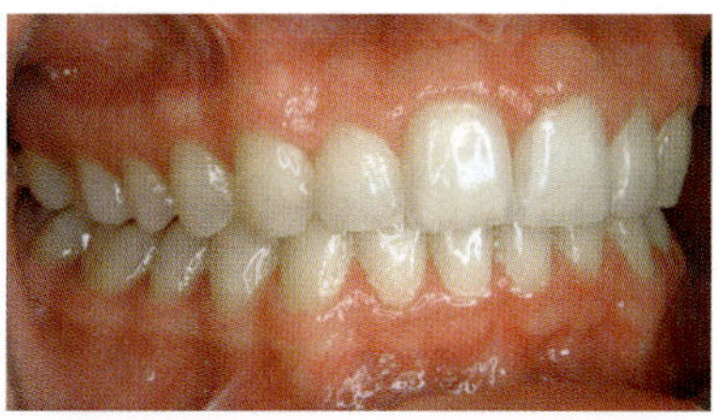
18

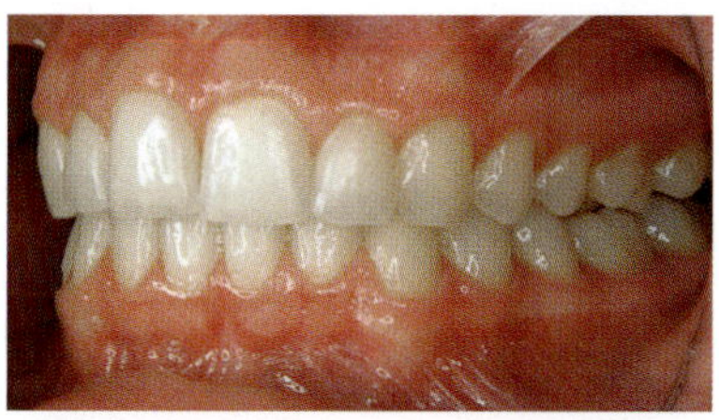
19

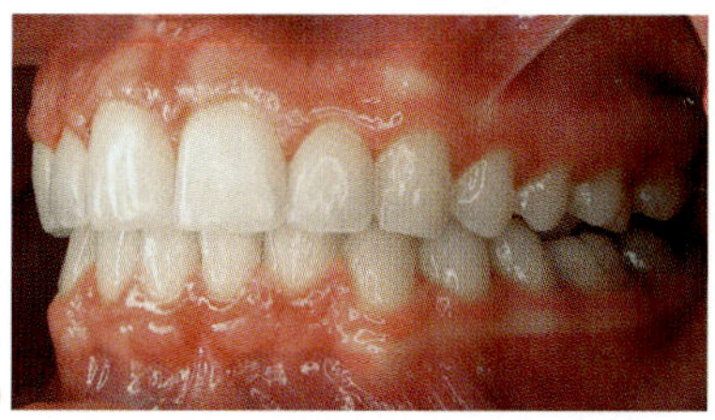
20

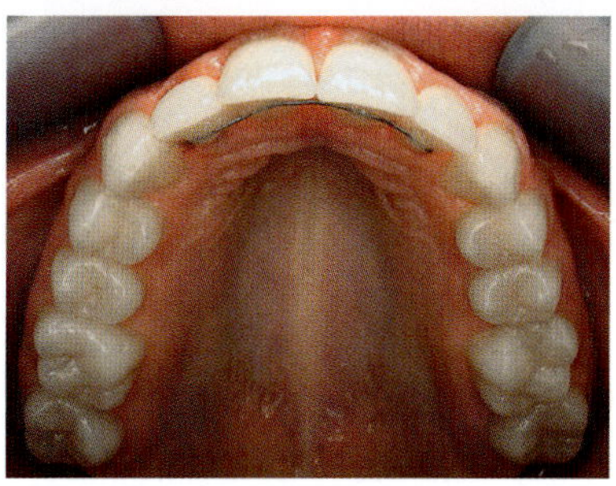
21

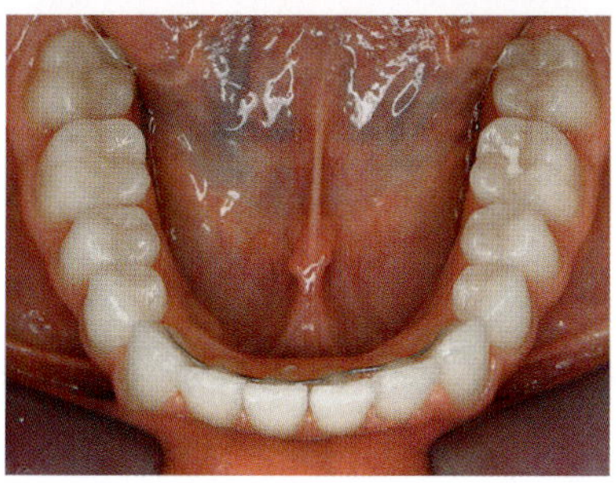
22

18–22 The final result after 1 year of retention using fixed retainers combined with Hawley retainers.

Case Study 7.9 (Fig. 7.22)

Patient: K.H., female, age 15.
Diagnostic records: models, panoramic radiograph, lateral cephalometric radiograph, intraoral/extraoral photographs.
Main findings: bilateral crossbite, open bite in the premolar areas affecting the left more than the right, tendency to mandibular prognathism.
Treatment aims: expansion in the upper jaw and establishment of good intercuspation.
Appliances: self-ligating bracket, molar bands, approximal enamel reduction in the lower jaw.
Archwire sequence: 0.012 SE, 0.016 SE, 0.016 × 0.022 SE, 0.018 × 0.025 SE, 0.019 × 0.025 SS.
Alternative treatment strategy: rapid maxillary expansion.
Active treatment time: 11 months.
Retention: maintenance of the alignment with bonded retainers with additional three-dimensional retention in the upper jaw.

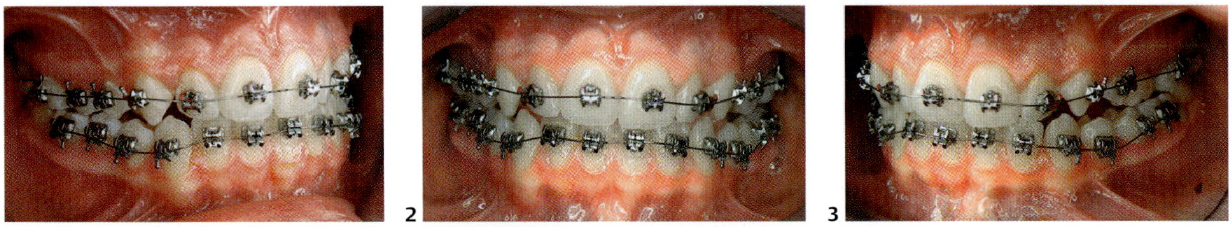
1 2 3

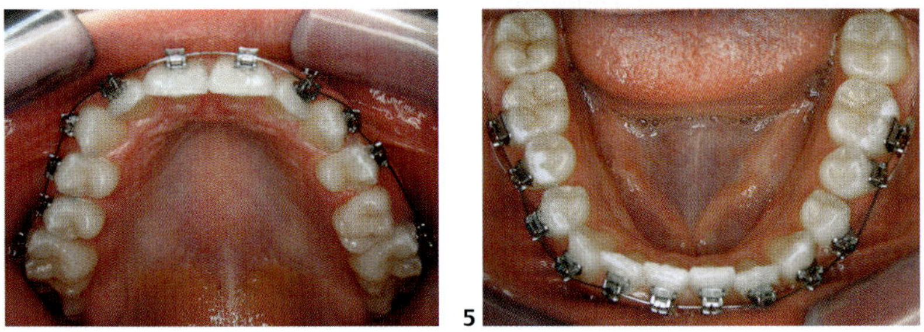
4 5

Fig. 7.22
1–5 Initial presentation: anterior crowding with a constricted maxilla and bilateral crossbite.

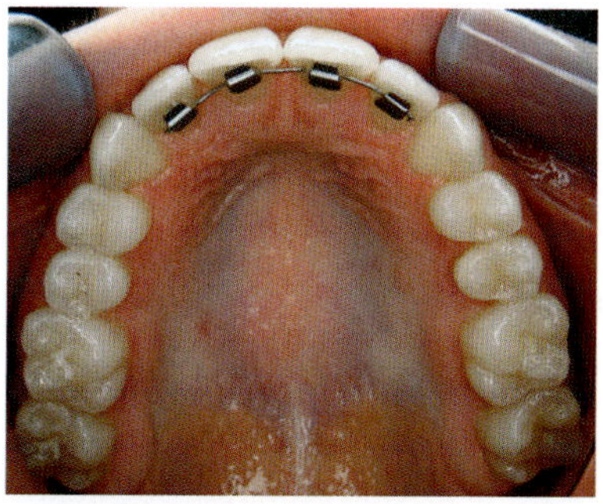
7

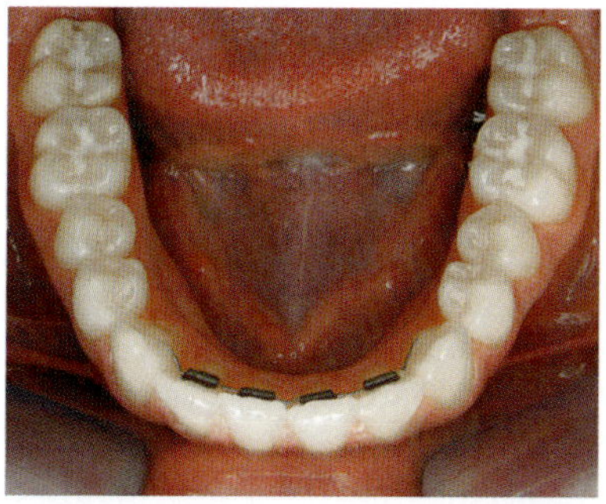
8

7–11 The final result after 1 year of retention with anterior fixed retainers combined with Hawley retainers.

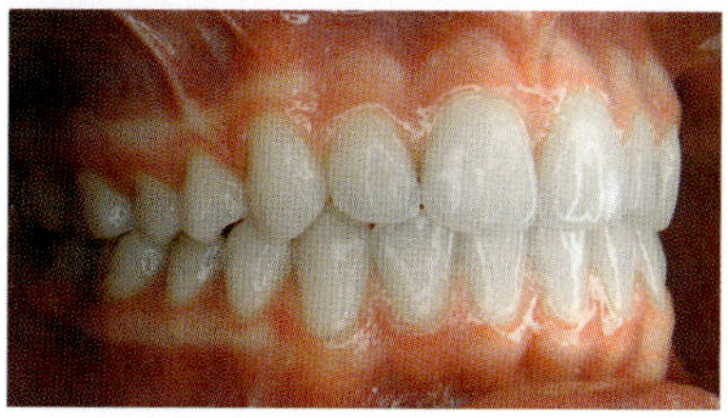
9

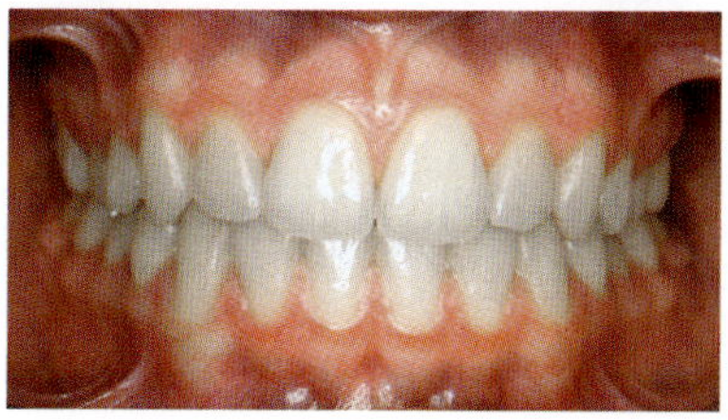
10

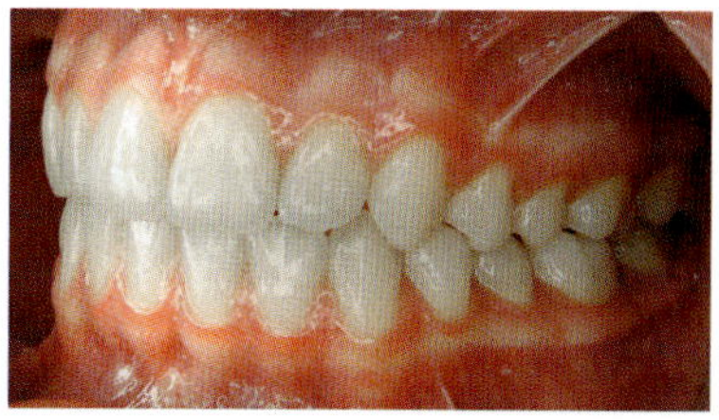
11

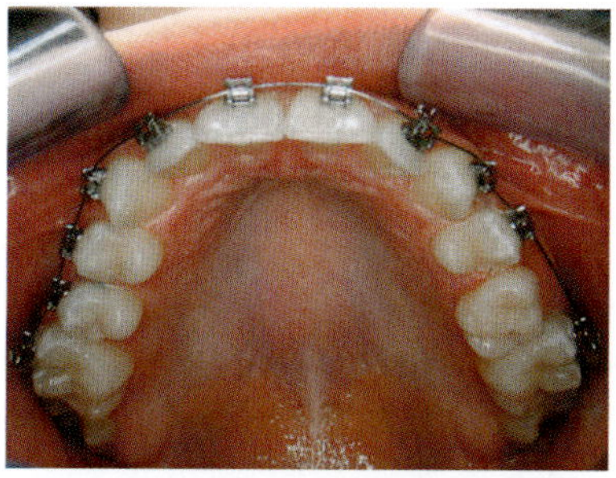
12

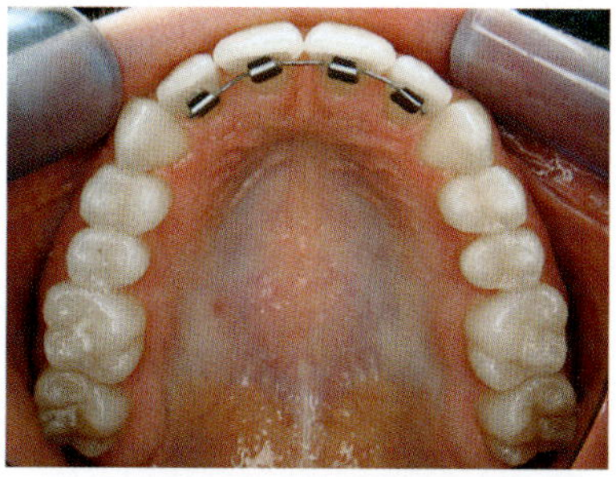
13

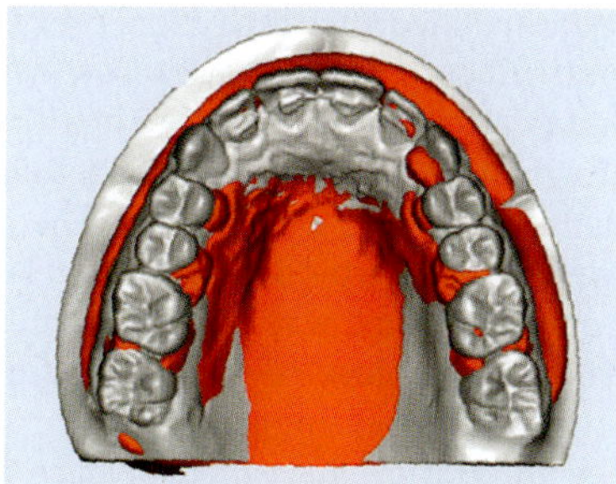
14

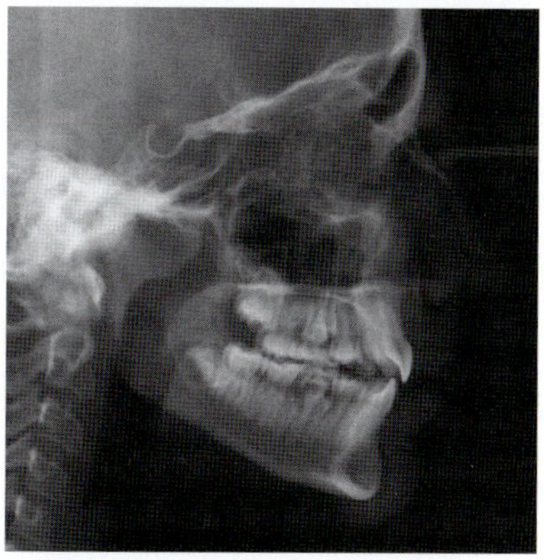
15

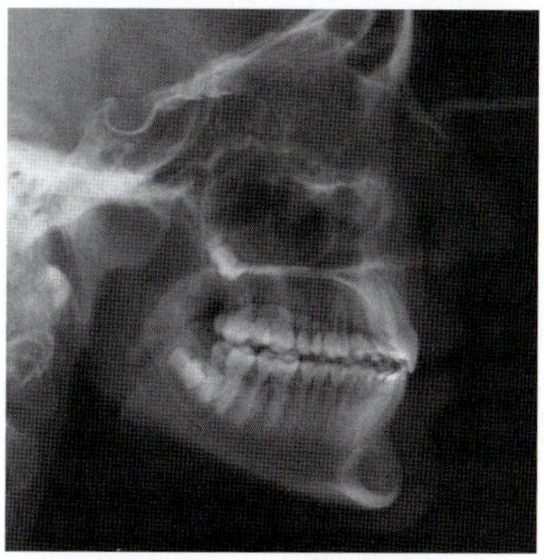
16

12–18 Comparison of the pretreatment and post-treatment situation intraorally, cephalometrically, and by superimposition of the digital study models of the maxilla. Superimposition of the study models shows that very little actual expansion was necessary to correct the bilateral crossbite.

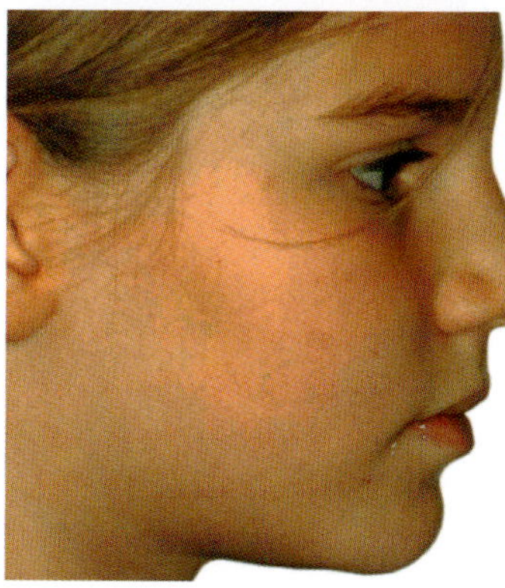
17

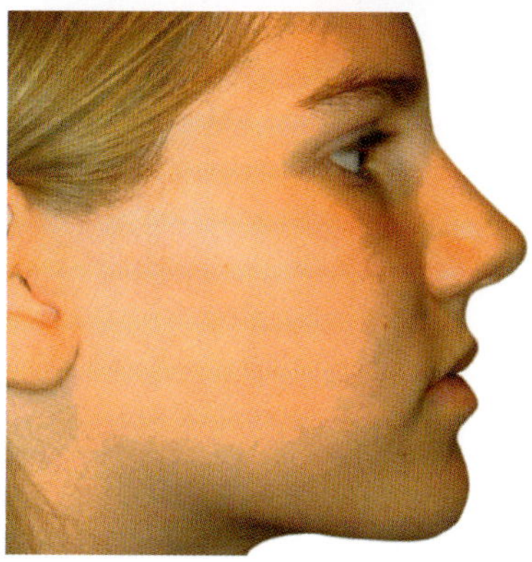
18

Errors and risks:
The mandibular prominence increased within 2 years.

Space Creation by Distalization

Most conventional distalizers use the anterior dentition and the palate as the retentive element for distalizing the posterior teeth. This was first described by Hilgers in 1992.[13,14] The pendulum appliance showed a distalization of 63.5%–73.5% and reciprocal mesial protrusion of the anchorage teeth in the anterior segment between 26.5% and 36.5%.[4,9,18] In addition, there was distal tipping of the molars between 10.6° and 18.5°.[4,9]

A simplified distalizer known as a Frog appliance was first described by Walde. It is also known as a "simplified molar distalizer" (**Fig. 7.23**).[32]

The basic design features (**Fig. 7.24**) consist of a custom screw, which is connected to the first molars via a transpalatal arch. This element is anchored by an acrylic (Nance-type) button, which itself is cemented to the first and second premolars via wire extensions. The transpalatal arch is designed in such a way that it can be removed, modified, and activated. It can also be left in place once the distalization components have been removed. Walde recommended one activation every 4–5 weeks, with a total of approximately five turns, which results in molar distalization of 1–2 mm every month. The screw has been designed in such a way that a full turn distalizes the elements by half a millimeter. The authors recommend one turn (a quarter of 360°) every 3 days.

A more efficient way of using the Frog device relies on skeletal anchorage of the mesial aspect, by measures of orthodontic mini-implants.

The anterior palate is an ideal place for secure placement of mini-implants. The ideal insertion point is mesial to the connecting point between the two upper first premolars (this point has been chosen as it is often easily identifiable due to the nonerupted canines at the start of treatment), 4.5 mm behind the distal aspect of the incisal papilla (**Figs. 7.25** and **7.26**).[10,11,35] The ideal transverse distance to the midpalatal suture is approximately 3 mm on either side, as this has the best bone tissue available for secure placement.[35]

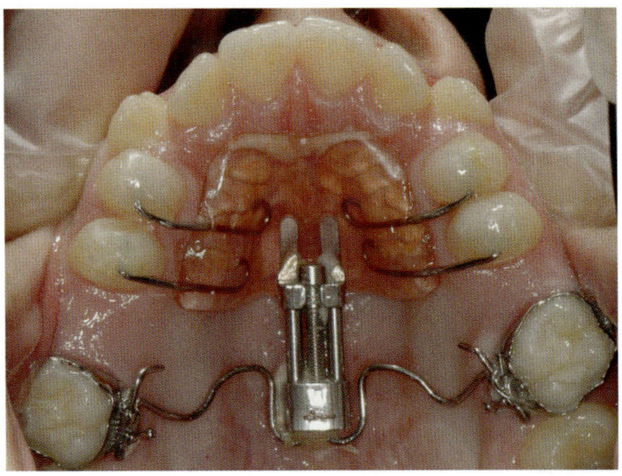

Fig. 7.23 The Frog appliance (Forestadent), with a combination of tooth-borne and tissue-borne anchorage.

The skeletal anchorage and sectional wire approach allows orthodontic treatment mesially to the second premolars during distalization of the posterior segments, which can decrease the overall treatment time—particularly in comparison with the original design of this distalization device, which required orthodontic treatment in several stages.

The first-generation skeletal Frog still used an acrylic button in which the mini-implants were anchored. Although it was effective, it had the familiar disadvantage of restricted oral hygiene, with subsequent irritation and inflammation of the gingiva. This led to the development of the skeletal Frog without the acrylic button, in which an abutment directly connects the mini-implants to the distalizing screw. Further refinements of the design led to an abutment that is compatible with the Ortho-Easy system, which doubles as a transfer aid and coupling unit (**Fig. 7.27**). The steps required to fabricate the appliance are as follows: after insertion of the implants, the abutments are mounted on the heads of the mini-implants and an impression is taken. "Transfer implants" are then attached to the abutments before pouring of the impression. This creates a model containing two implant heads that correspond to the situation in the patient. The abutments are then replaced on the implants and are integrated into the final appliance by soldering or laser-welding them to the screw–transpalatal arch complex (**Fig. 7.28**). The abutment is first tried-in to make sure that the fit is adequate. A diverging insertion in the direction of the abutments may become necessary in case the mini-implants are not completely parallel. The abutments may then need modification so that they can be inserted without interference. Once the abutments have been tested and found to give a satisfactory fit, glass ionomer cement can be used to securely fasten the distal component of the Frog appliance, while the abutments are secured with a flowable composite (**Fig. 7.28**). The small size of the abutments allows good cleaning of the palatal mucosa, as well as reduced interference of the Frog appliance with the tongue, particularly compared to the traditional design using an acrylic button.

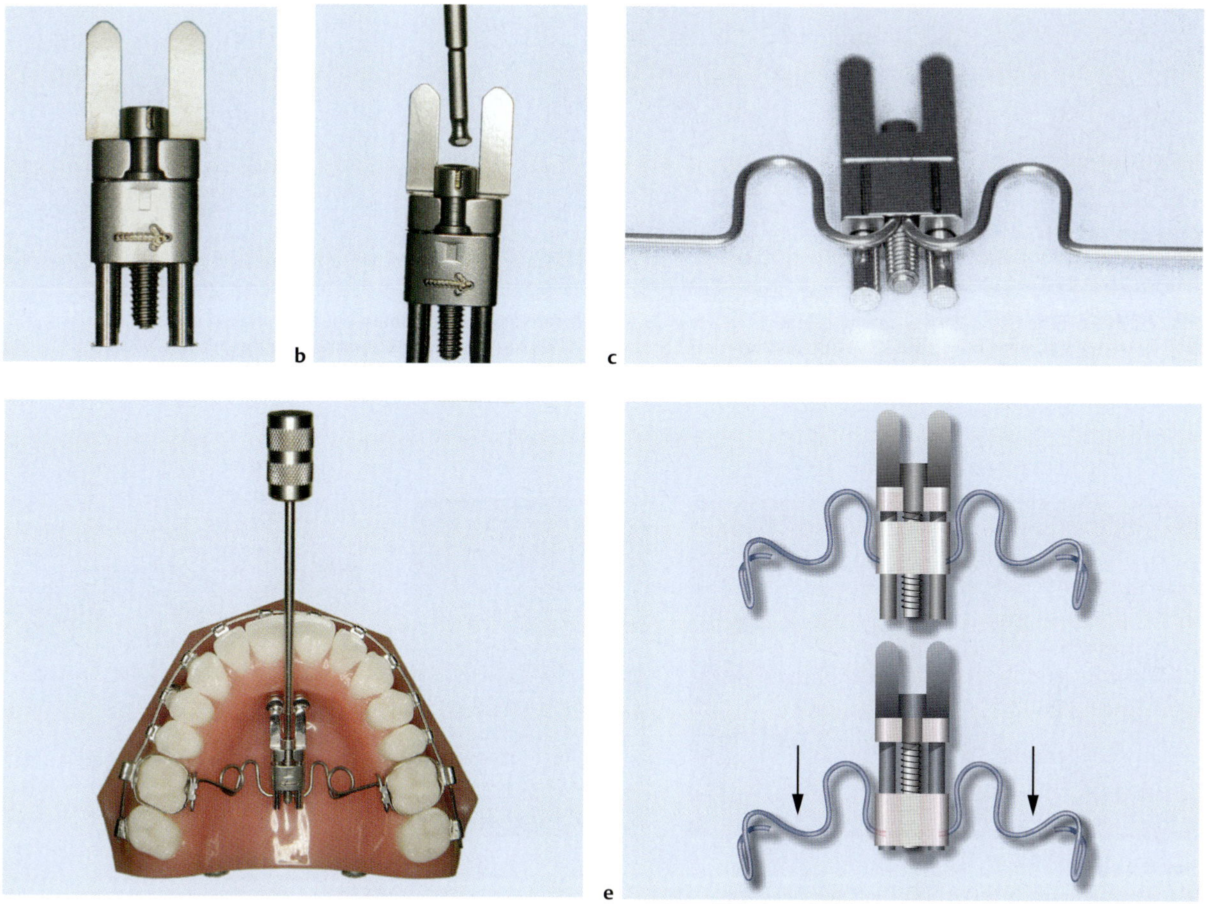

Fig. 7.24a–e The Frog appliance (Forestadent) consists of several prefabricated parts, which are assembled in a laboratory. The parts include a distalization screw, a prefabricated transpalatal arch made of 0.032 stainless steel, and a key for activating the distalizing screw. The connection between the transpalatal arch and the distalizing screw is removable (**a–c**). Activation occurs at the anterior part of the screw, so the key can be inserted sagittally. The easy access makes activation simple and helps ensure good patient compliance (**d, e**).

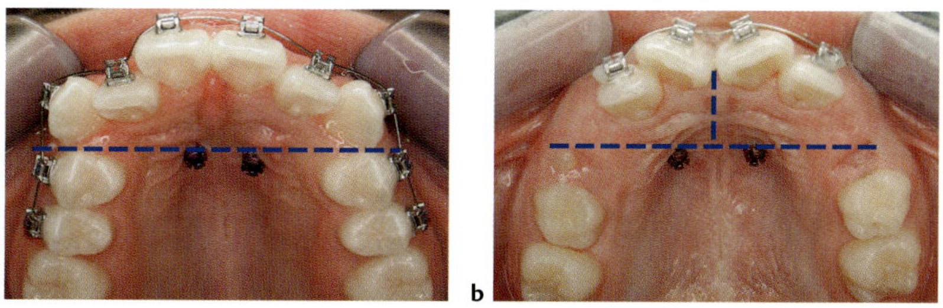

Fig. 7.25a, b Mini-implants should be inserted mesial to the line connecting the two upper first premolars. This appears to be a stable position with sufficient bone for secure retention of the Frog appliance (Forestadent). It can sometimes be difficult to locate this point due to mesially migrated premolars or previous extractions. Another anatomical landmark that can be used to position the mini-implants is a point 4–5 mm distal to the posterior end of the incisal foramen.

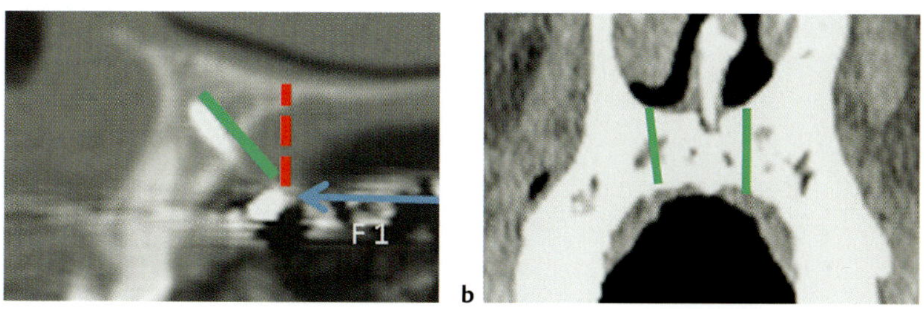

Fig. 7.26a, b
a Computed tomography of positioned mini-implants that have been inserted perpendicular to the palatal surface.
b The frontal view shows the amount of bone available for anchorage.

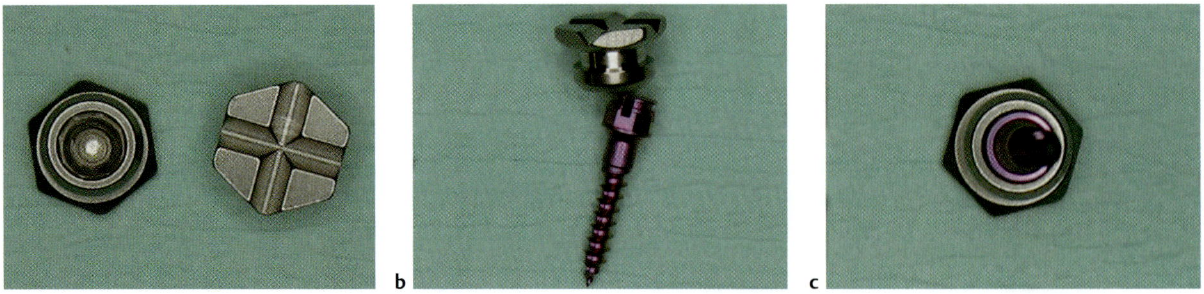

Fig. 7.27 a–c The Ortho Easy system (Forestadent).
a View of the abutment from both sides (top and bottom).
b Lateral view. The abutment has a built-in undercut.
c Precise fitting of the abutment to the mini-implant head.

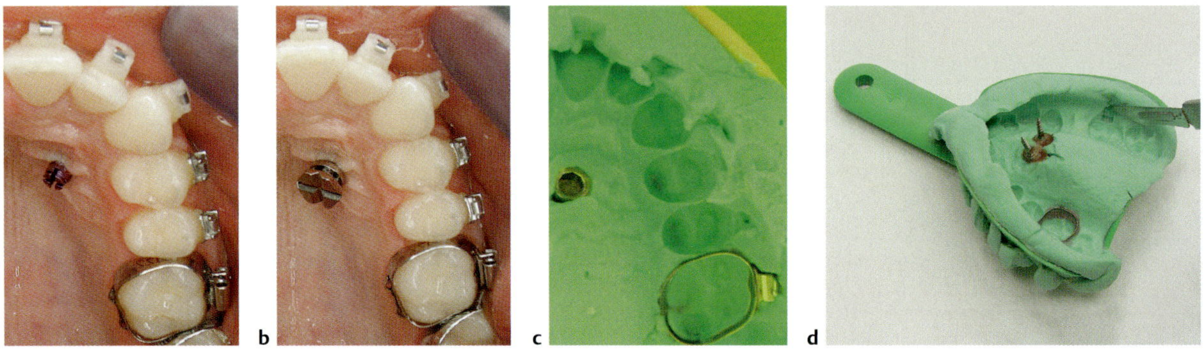

Fig. 7.28 a–j
a The mini-implant has been placed in the patient's mouth.
b The circular undercut ensures good retention in the impression material (**c**) and secure repositioning of the transfer screws (**d**). Now the impression can be cast in high-strength (type 4) dental stone.
e–j See p. 127.

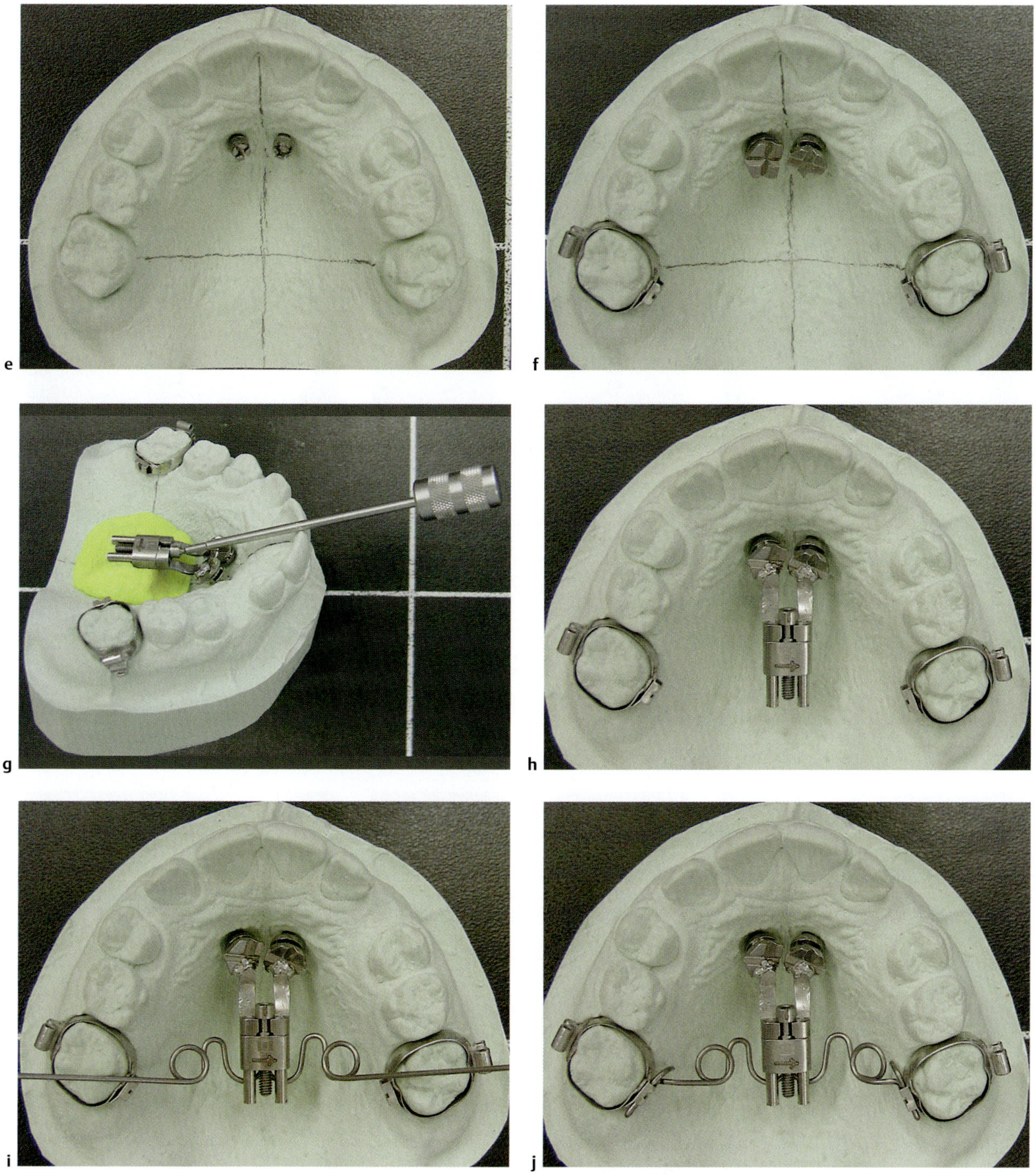

Fig. 7.28 a–j (continued)
e, f The manufacturing process for the skeletal K-pendulum.
e The working model made of high-strength (type 4) dental stone, with the transfer screws.
f Abutments on the transfer screws and molar bands are in place.
g Positioning of the Frog screw with correct angulation, which allows the activation key to fit.
h Completed laboratory work after soldering of the abutments to the distalizing screw.
i Fitting of the titanium–molybdenum alloy (TMA) transpalatal arch.
j The all-metal framework of the K-pendulum allows good oral hygiene.

Case Study 7.10 (Fig. 7.29)

Patient: S.W., female, age 11.
Diagnostic records: models, panoramic radiograph, lateral cephalometric radiograph, intraoral/extraoral photographs.
Main findings: crowding of 13 and 23 buccally.
Treatment aims: distalizing the upper molars to create space for alignment of 13 and 23.
Appliances: self-ligating brackets, molar bands, mini-implants, Frog appliance.
Archwire sequence: 0.012 SE, 0.016 SE, 0.016 × 0.022 SE, 0.018 × 0.025 SE, 0.019 × 0.025 SS.
Alternative treatment strategy: removal of premolars in the upper jaw.
Active treatment time: 12 months.
Retention: three-dimensional retention with Hawley retainers.

1 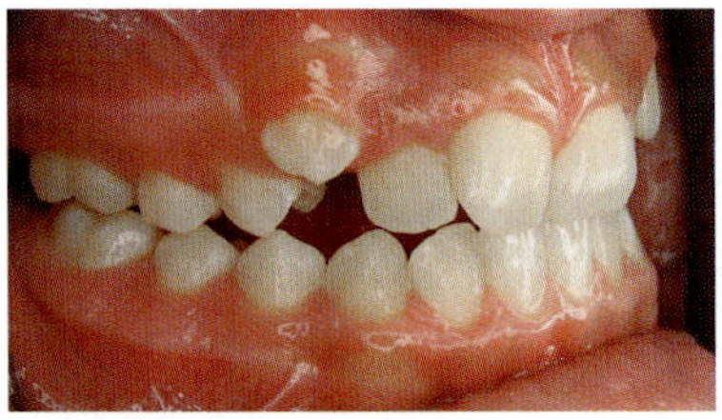
2 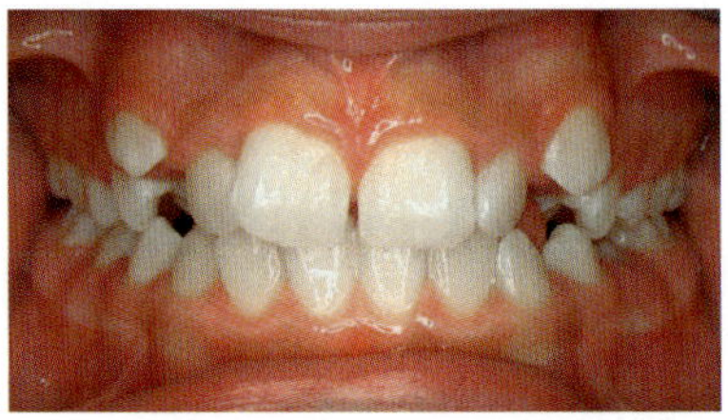
3 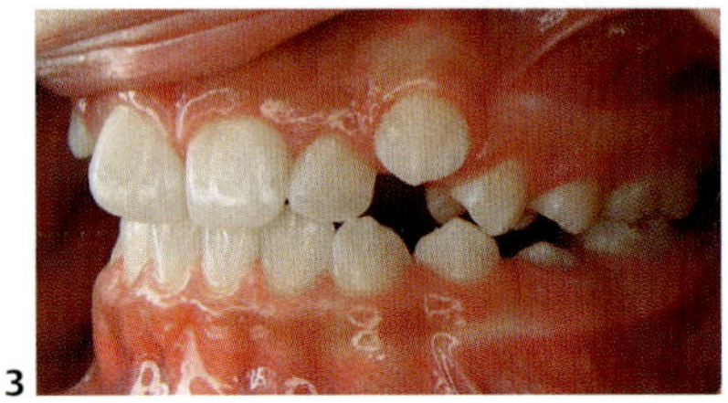
4 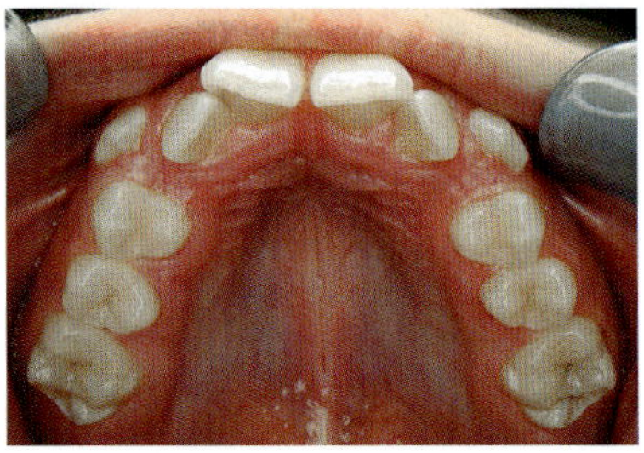
5 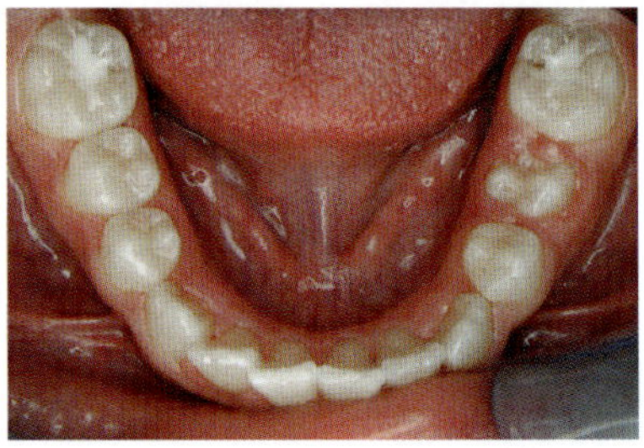

Fig. 7.29 1–31
1–5 Initial presentation: blocked-out maxillary canines and mild anterior mandibular crowding.

6 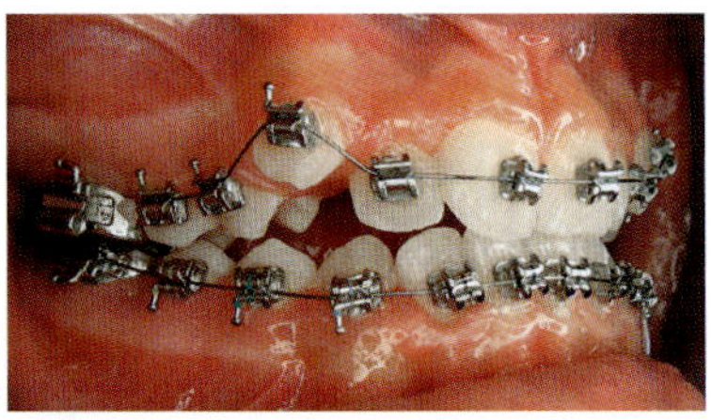
7 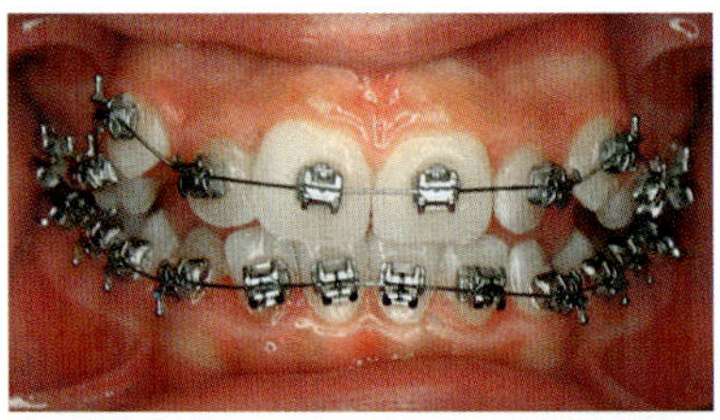
8 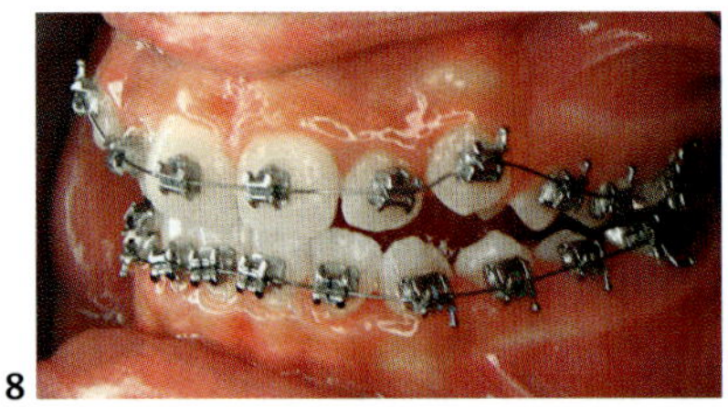
9 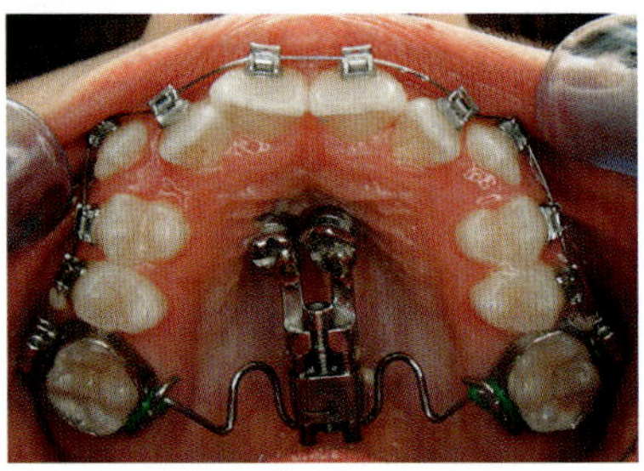
10 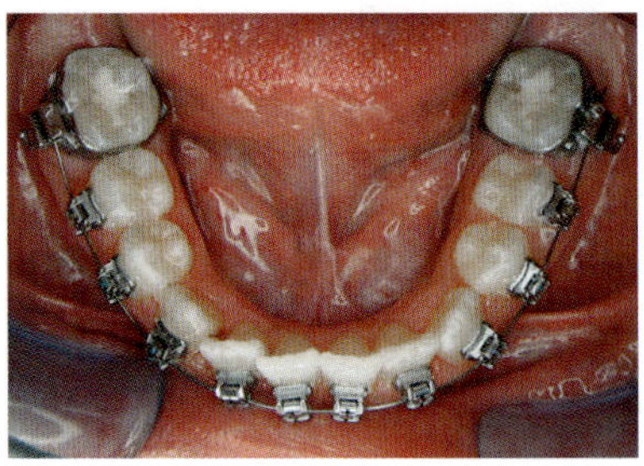

6–10

Clinical pearl:
The Frog appliance is activated immediately after insertion by four to five turns.

ERRORS AND RISKS

The maxillary archwire extends only to the second bicuspids.

Caution:
If the first molars are included in the continuous archwire, the distally directed force can lead to undesired retroclination of the incisors.

11

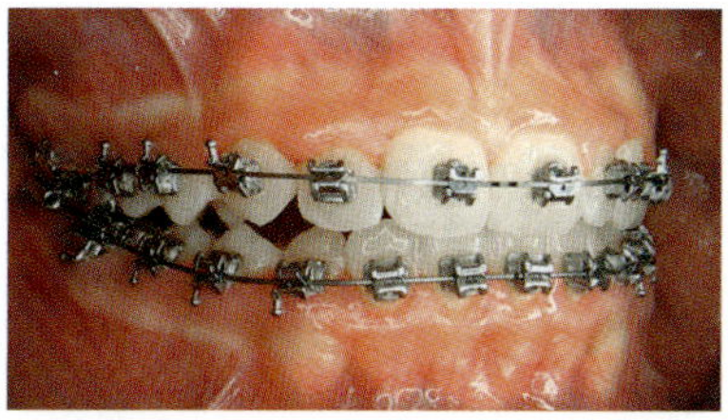

12

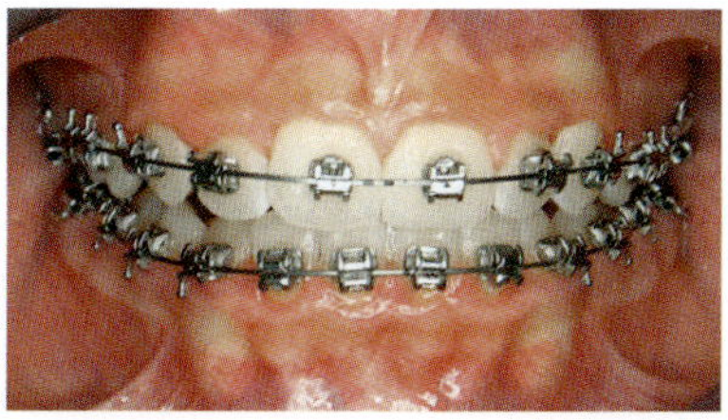

13

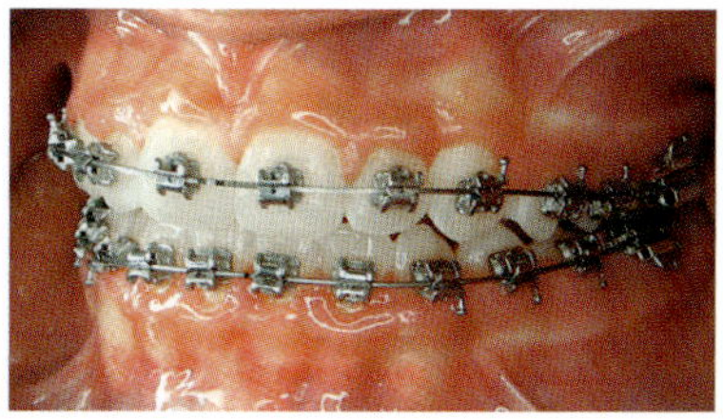

14

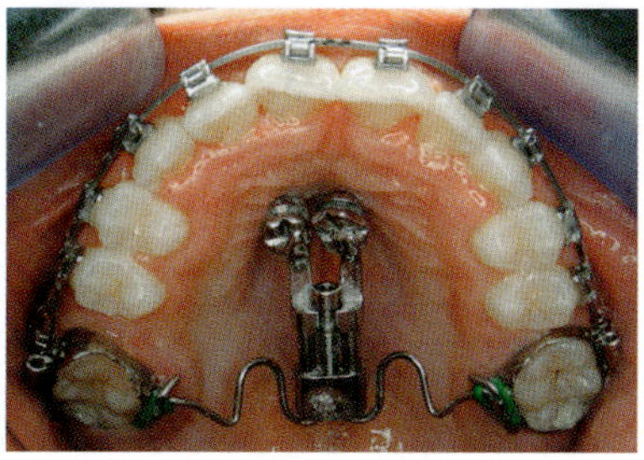

15

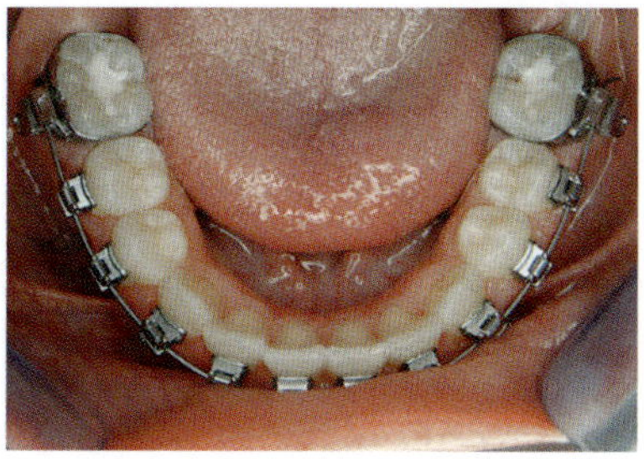

11–15 The results of distalization 5 months into treatment, with overcorrection of the maxillary molars.

16

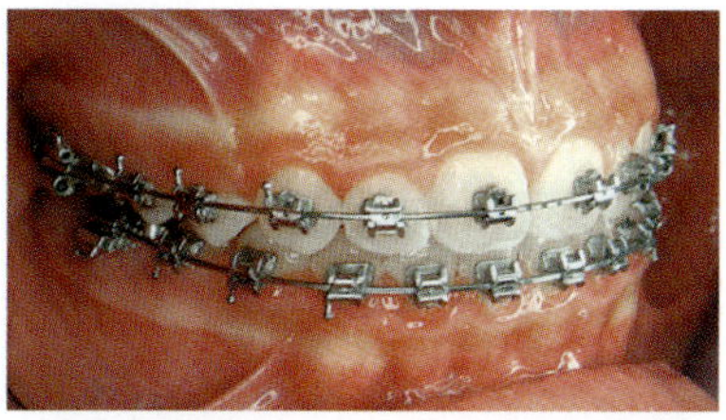

17

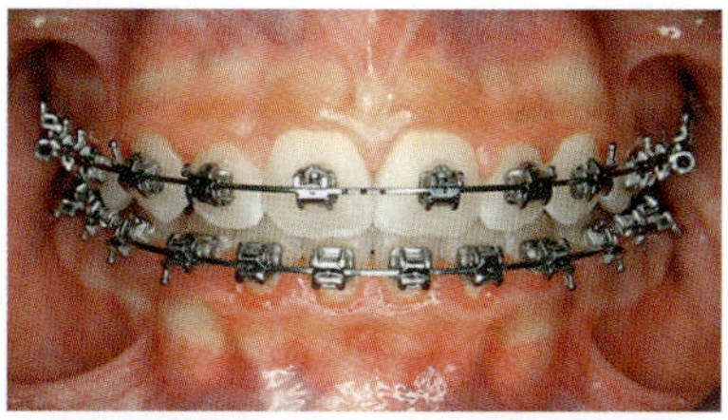

18

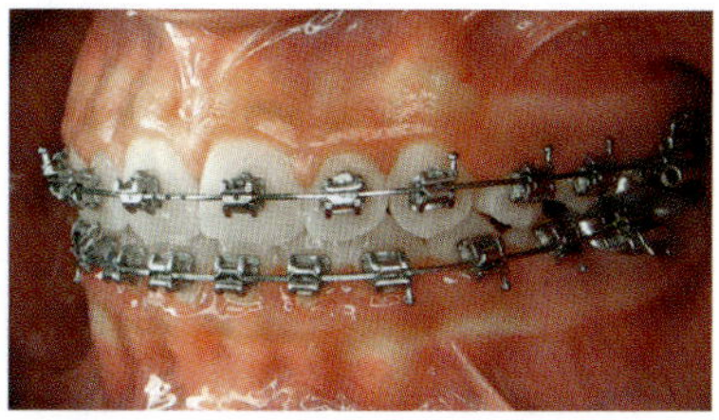

19

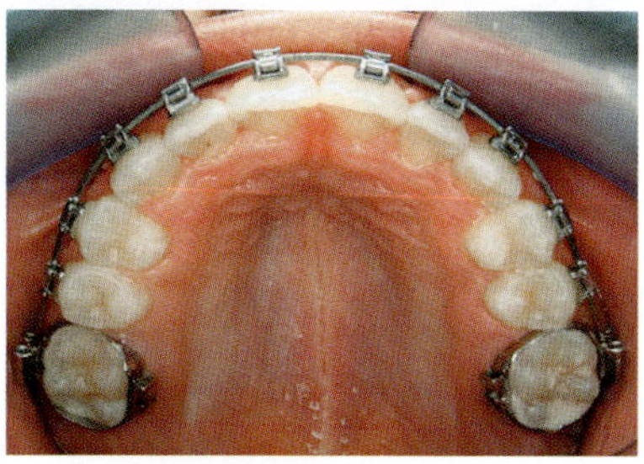

20

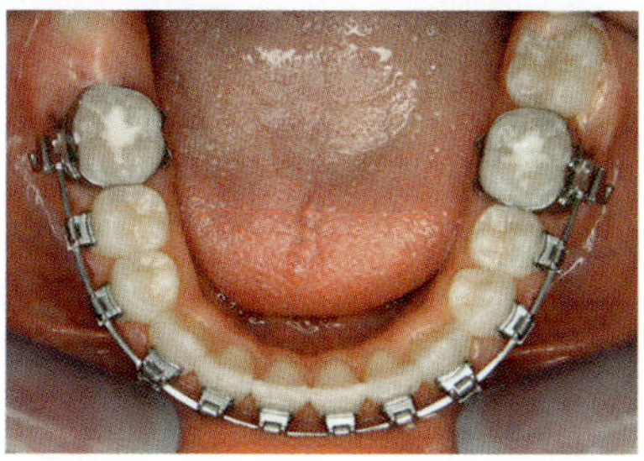

16–20 Ten months into treatment, the occlusion has been corrected.

21 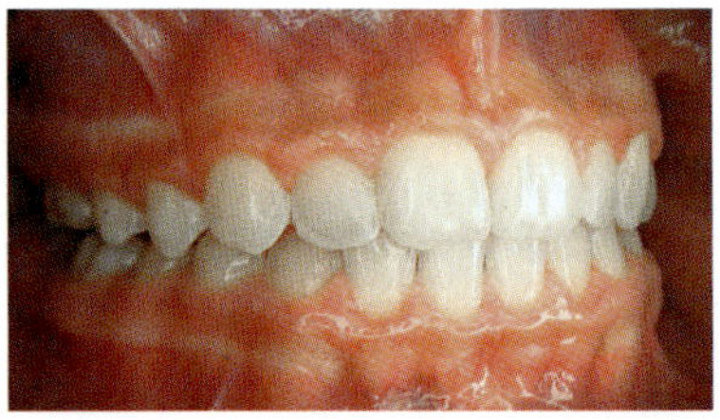 22 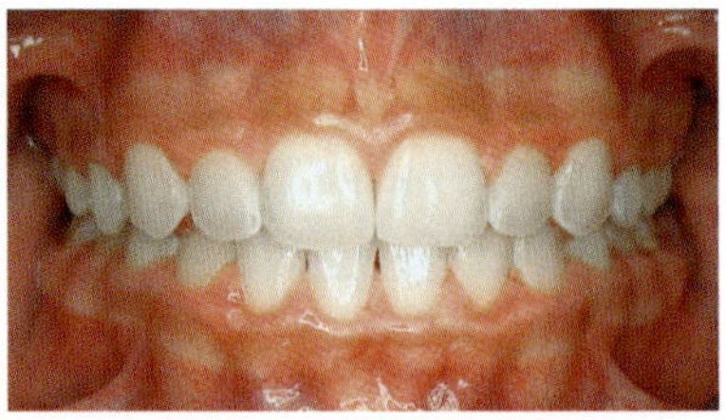 23 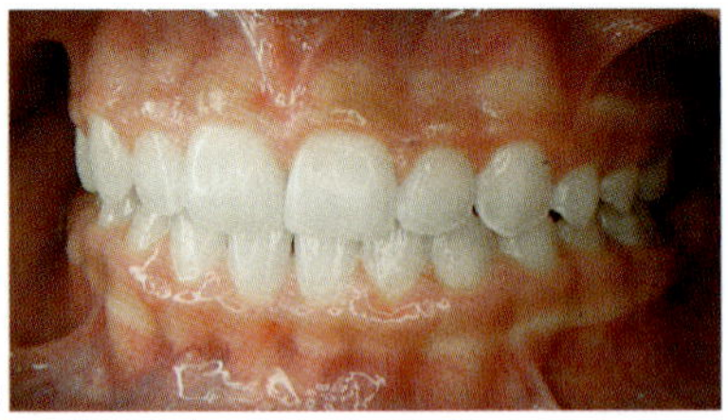

24 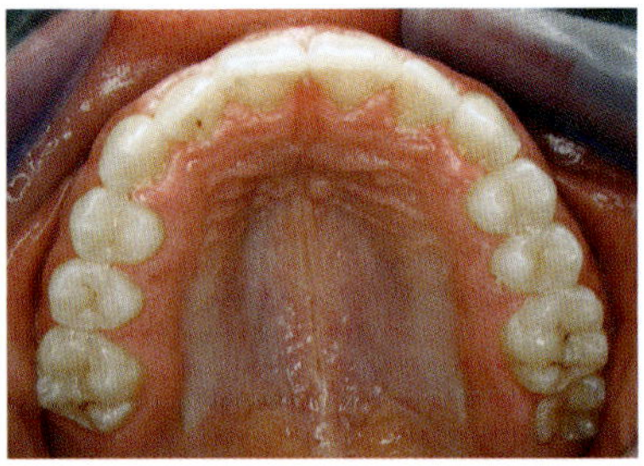 25 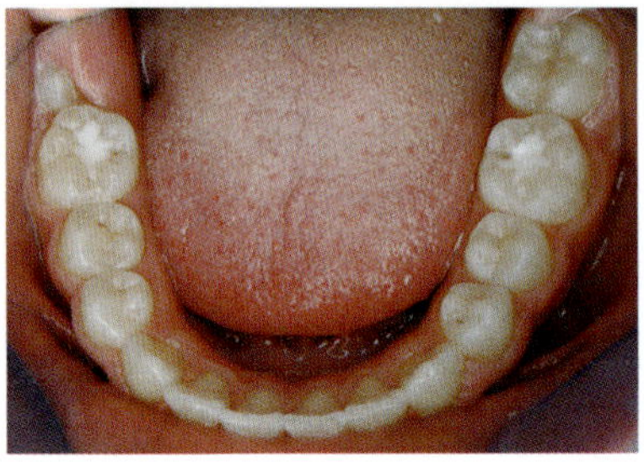

21–25 The start of the retention phase, with removable retainers.

26 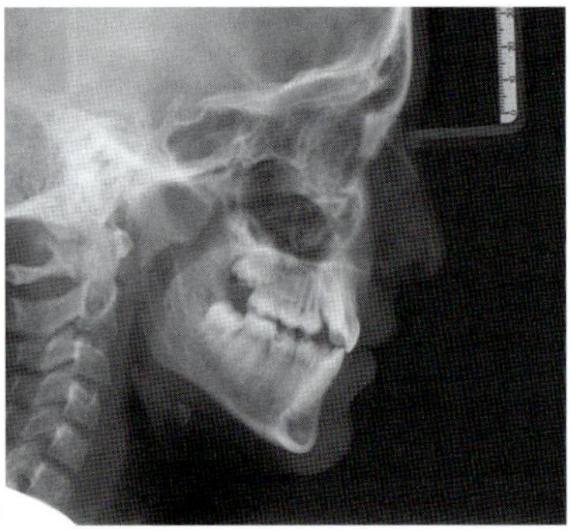 27 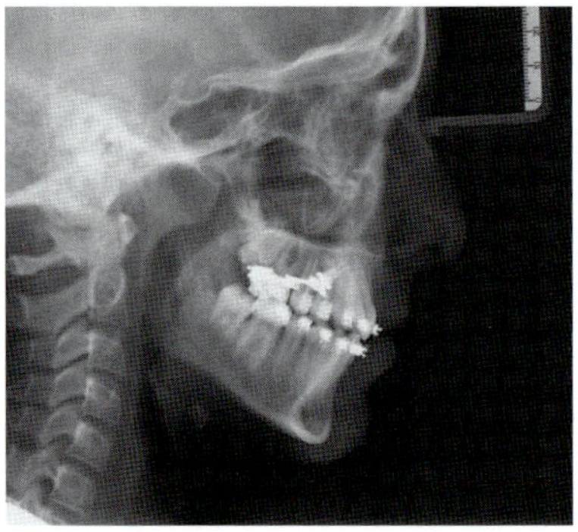 28 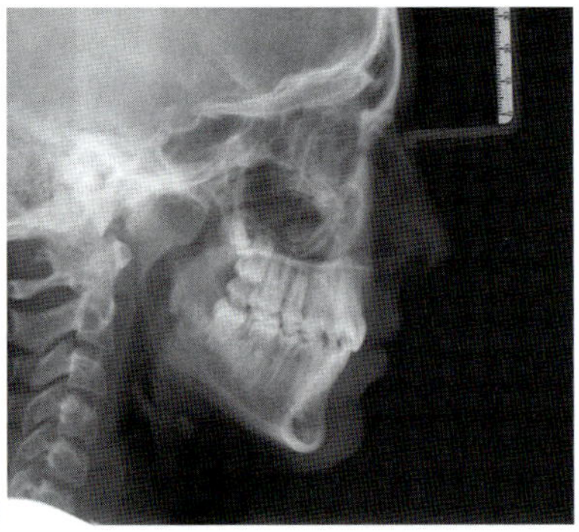

26–28 Lateral cephalometric radiographs before treatment, after distalization, and post-treatment.

29 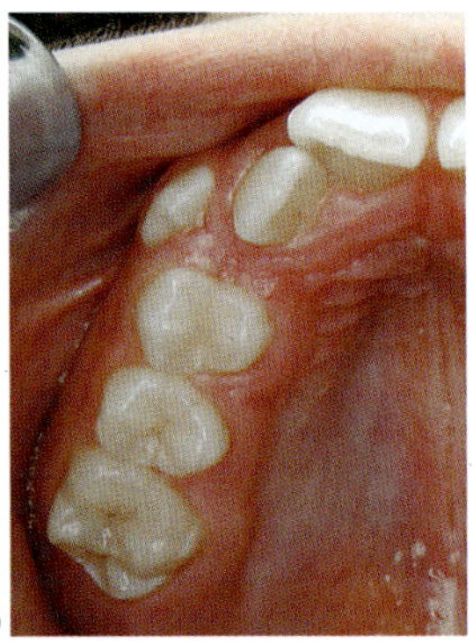 30 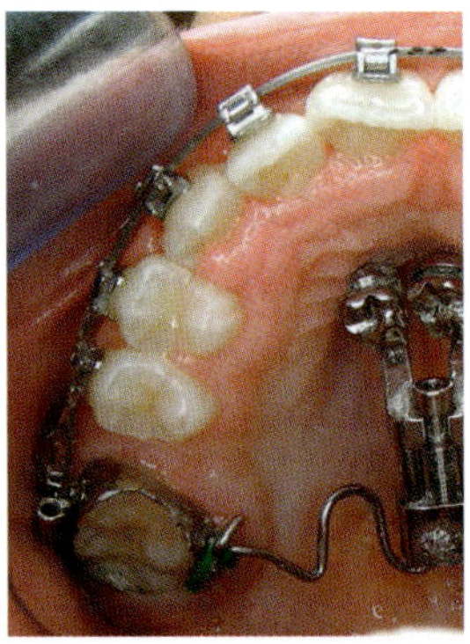 31 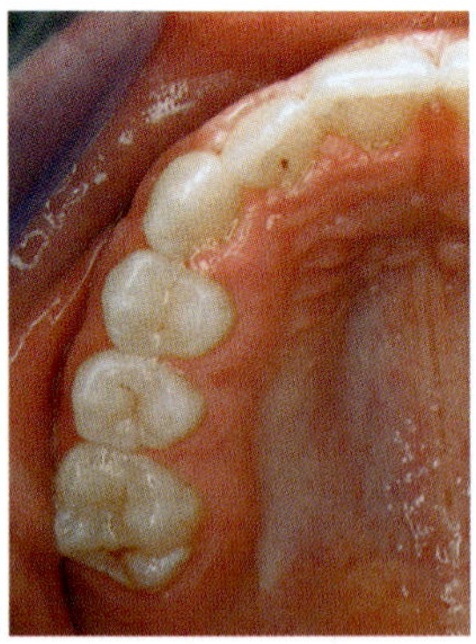 32 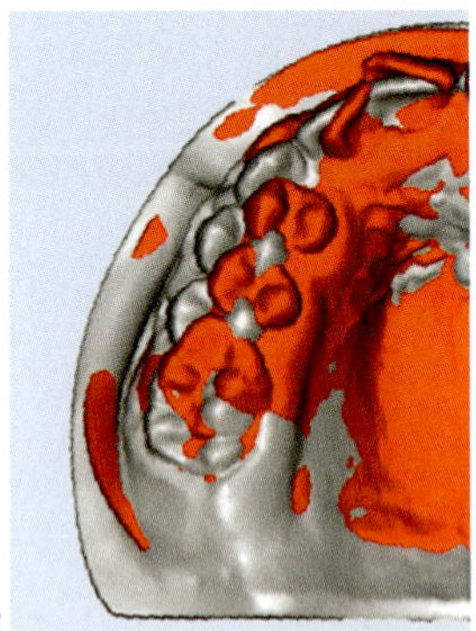

29–32 Distalization of the first molars: comparison of the situation before treatment and after 1 year of retention: superimposition of the digital study models.

ERRORS AND RISKS

Does the skeletal Frog appliance prevent protrusion of the labial segments?

This case report suggests that incisor angulation remains largely unchanged (see **Fig. 7.29**, **26–28** and **29–32**).

Case Study 7.11 (Fig. 7.30)

Patient: A.P., female, age 11.
Diagnostic records: models, panoramic radiograph, lateral cephalometric radiograph, intraoral/extraoral photographs.
Main findings: crowding of 13 and 23.
Treatment aims: distalizing of the molars to create space in the maxillary canine area.
Appliances: self-ligating brackets, molar bands, mini-implant, Frog appliance.
Archwire sequence: 0.012 SE, 0.016 SE, 0.016 × 0.022 SE, 0.018 × 0.025 SE, 0.019 × 0.022 SS.
Alternative treatment strategy: extraction of the first premolars in the upper jaw.
Active treatment time: 10 months.
Retention: three-dimensional retention with Hawley retainers.

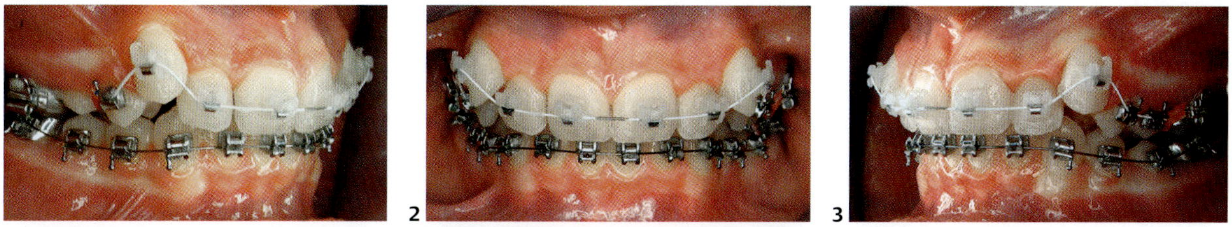

1 2 3

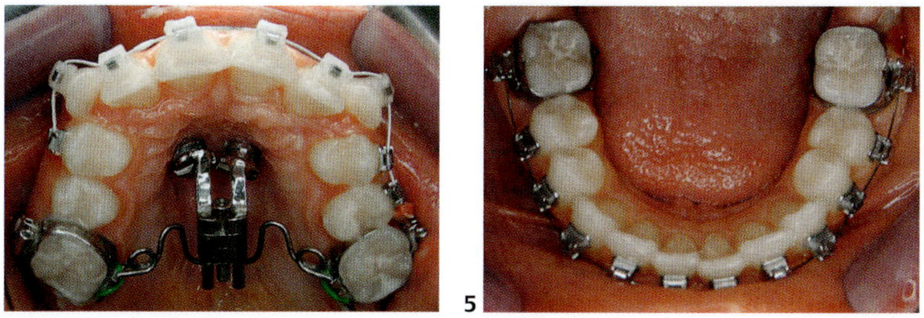

4 5

Fig. 7.30 1–24
1–5 Initial presentation: buccally crowded maxillary canines and mild anterior mandibular crowding.

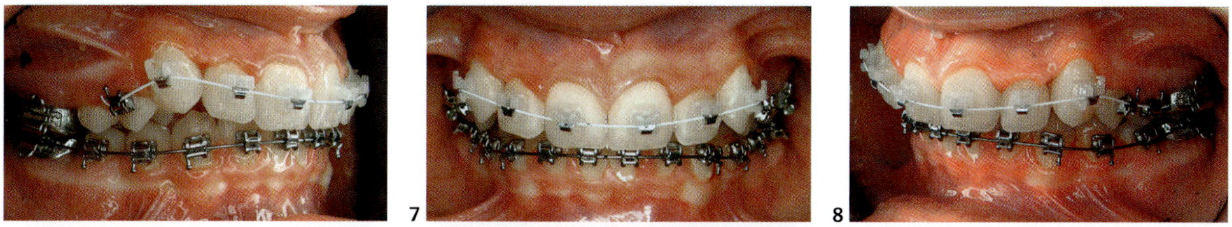

6 7 8

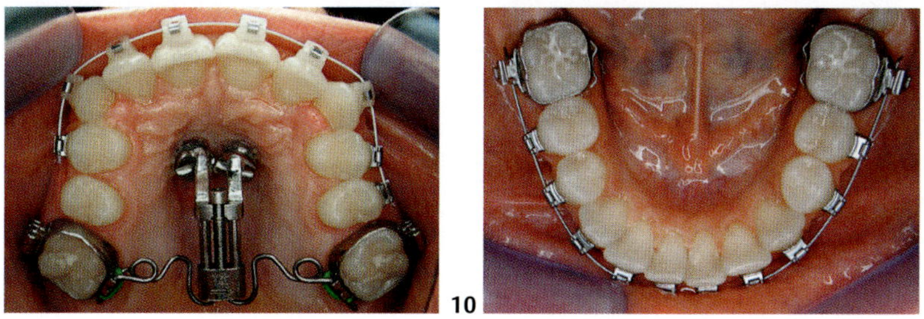

9 10

6–10 Treatment progress: alignment and distalization.

Errors and risks:
The maxillary archwire extends only to the second bicuspids. If the first molars are included, retroclination of the upper front tooth may result.

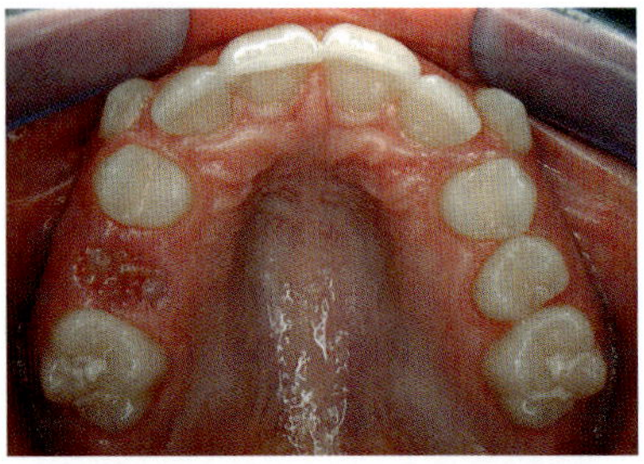
11

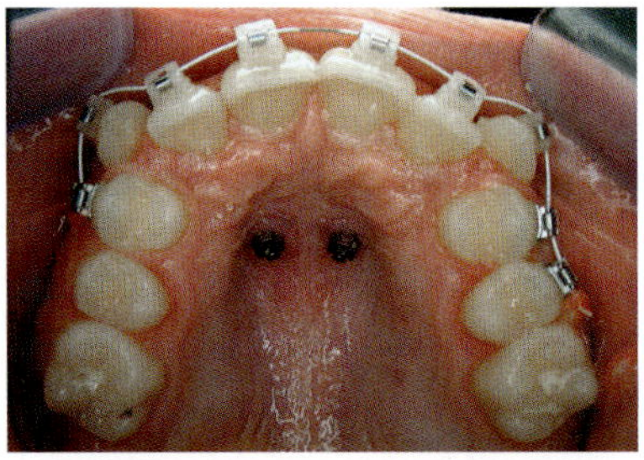
12

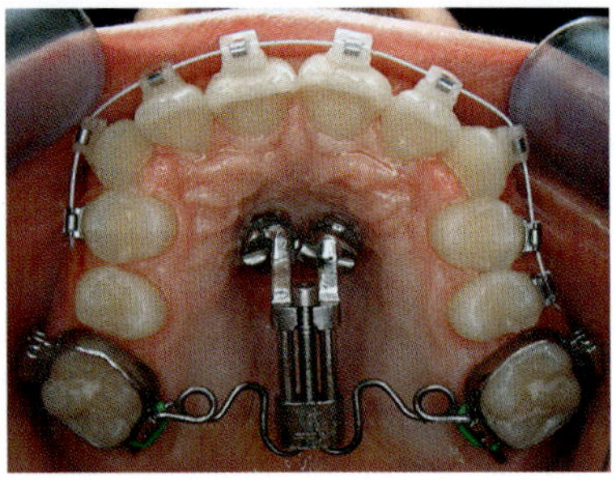
13

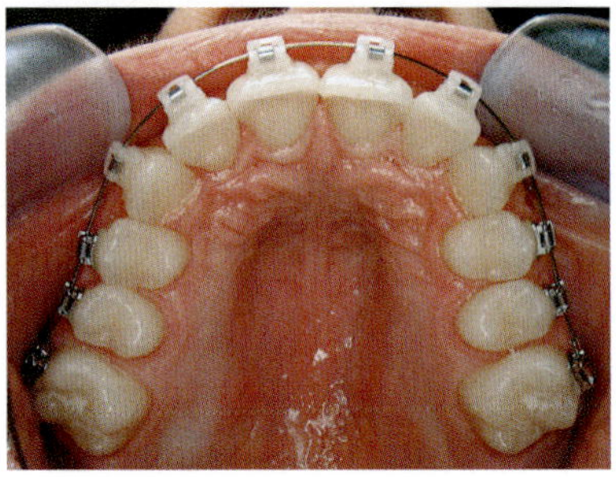
14

11 Before treatment.
12 Placement of mini-screws and self-ligating brackets.
13 The Frog appliance has been active for 5 months.
14 End of distalization.

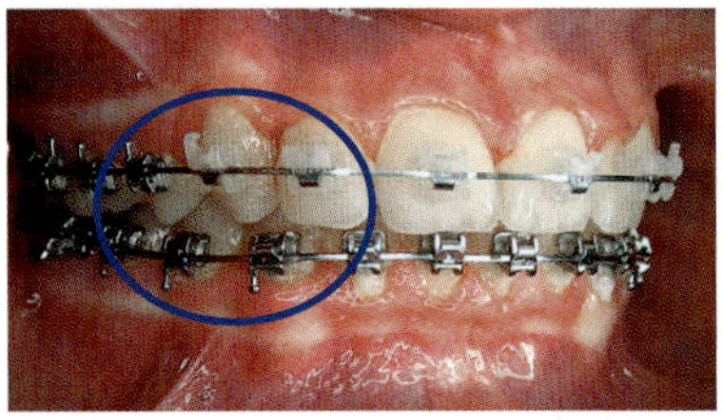
15

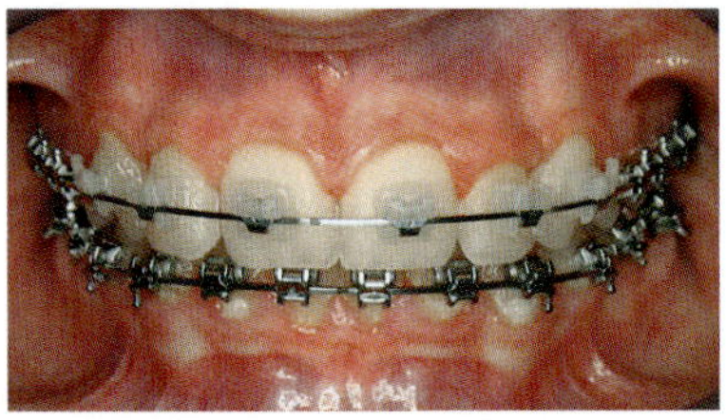
16

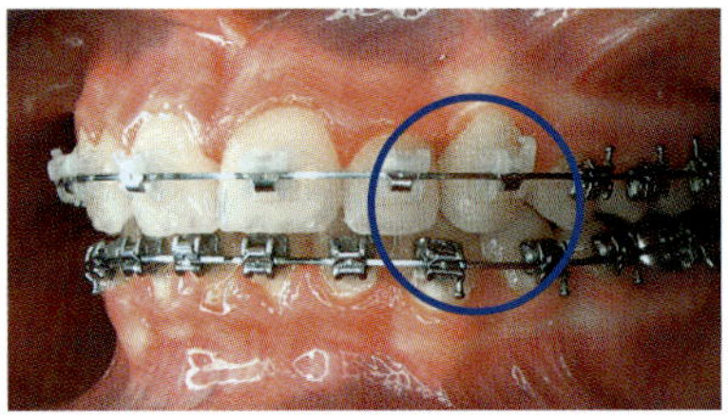
17

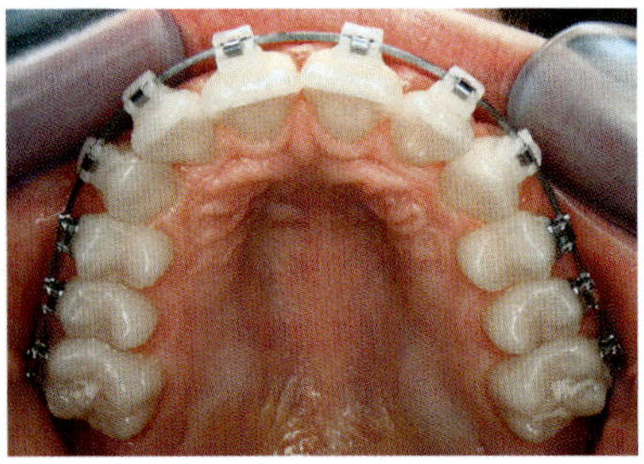
18

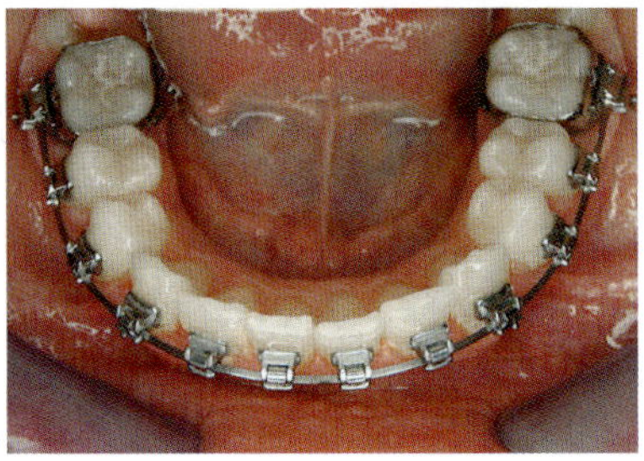
19

15–19 After approximately 10 months, good alignment, molar and canine relationship has been achieved.

CLINICAL PEARL

Ectopically positioned teeth, particularly canines, may show an esthetically compromised gingival margin after alignment (circled in 15). Using an electric toothbrush with a soft head may be advisable, as it can help protect the gingival tissues. A gingival graft can be considered for correction.

20 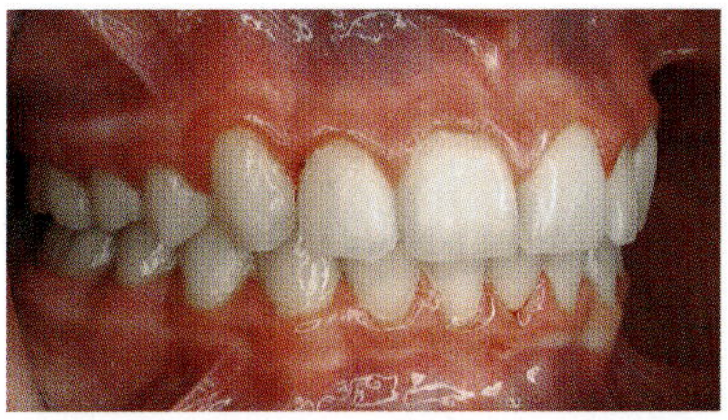 21 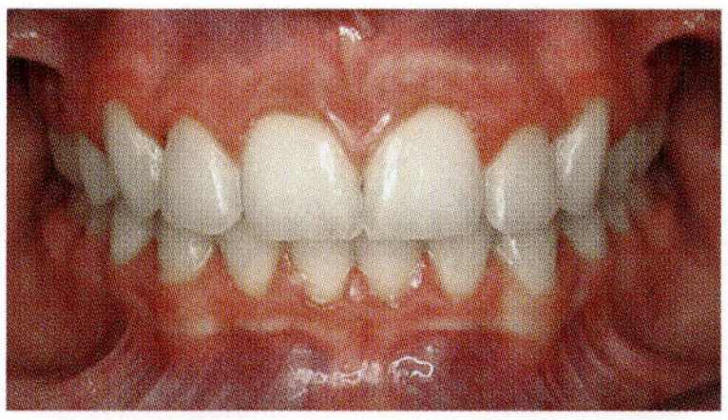 22 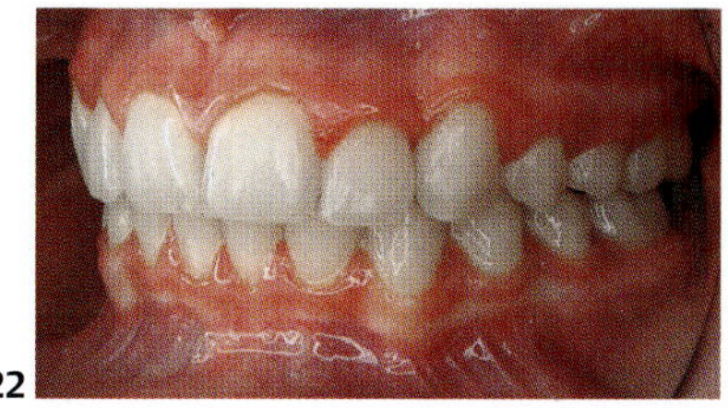

23 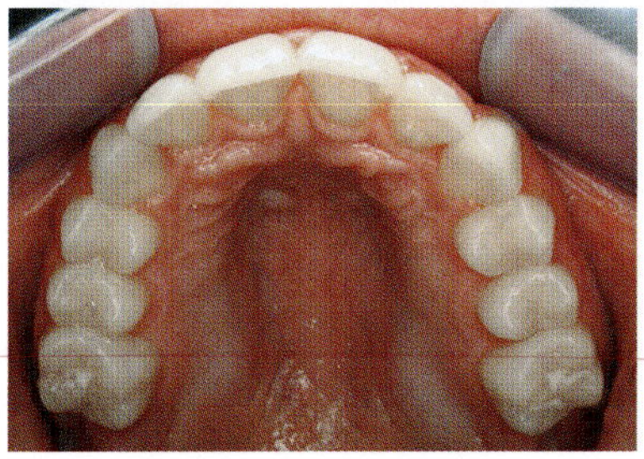 24 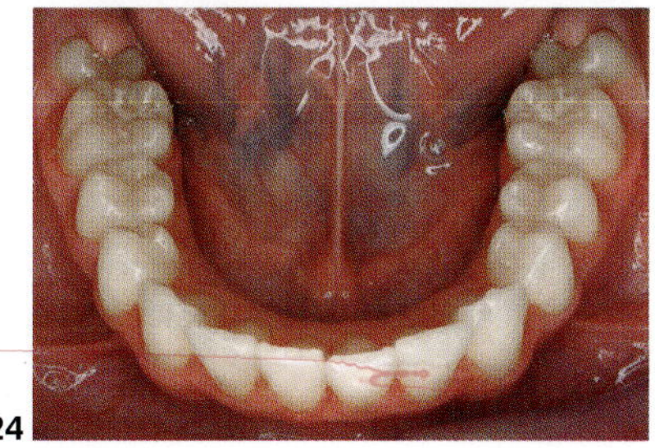

20–24 Start of retention with removable retainers.

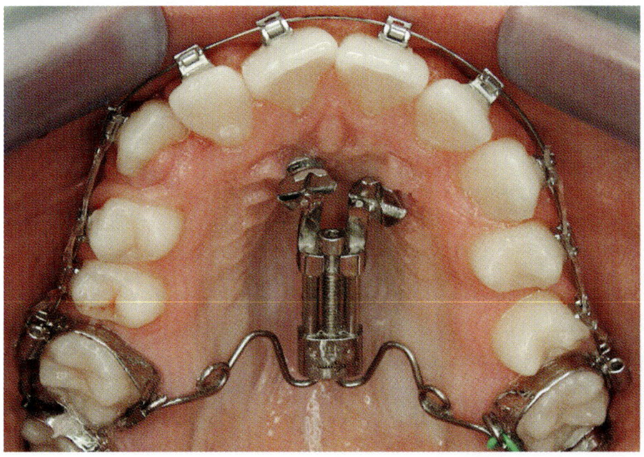

Fig. 7.31 The skeletally supported Frog appliance at the end of the distalization phase. The molars have tipped distally and are rotated due to biomechanical side effects. This can be corrected after distalization.

The design of the original Frog appliance used a transpalatal arch made of stainless steel. The design did not allow correction of previously rotated molars or iatrogenic distal tipping (**Fig. 7.31**), and it was therefore replaced in second-generation appliances with a round 0.032 titanium–molybdenum alloy (TMA). This is similar to the approach used in the K-pendulum (Kinzinger). This transpalatal arch is designed with loops that can be adjusted to derotate teeth, expand the archwire, or counteract the distal tipping movement that normally occurs during distalization (**Fig. 7.32**). Several investigations of the force levels provided by the TMA transpalatal arch have shown that its initial activation and periodic reactivation can lead to effective control of the side effects occurring during molar distalization. The tendency for maxillary constriction that results from activation of the screw can also be counteracted by expansion of the transpalatal arch. In other words, the reactivation of the modified Frog appliance is similar to that of the K-pendulum, the effects of which have been well investigated. The Frog appliance is therefore also known as a skeletal K-pendulum.[18] **Figure 7.33** illustrates the position of the pendulum springs resulting from bending and activation.

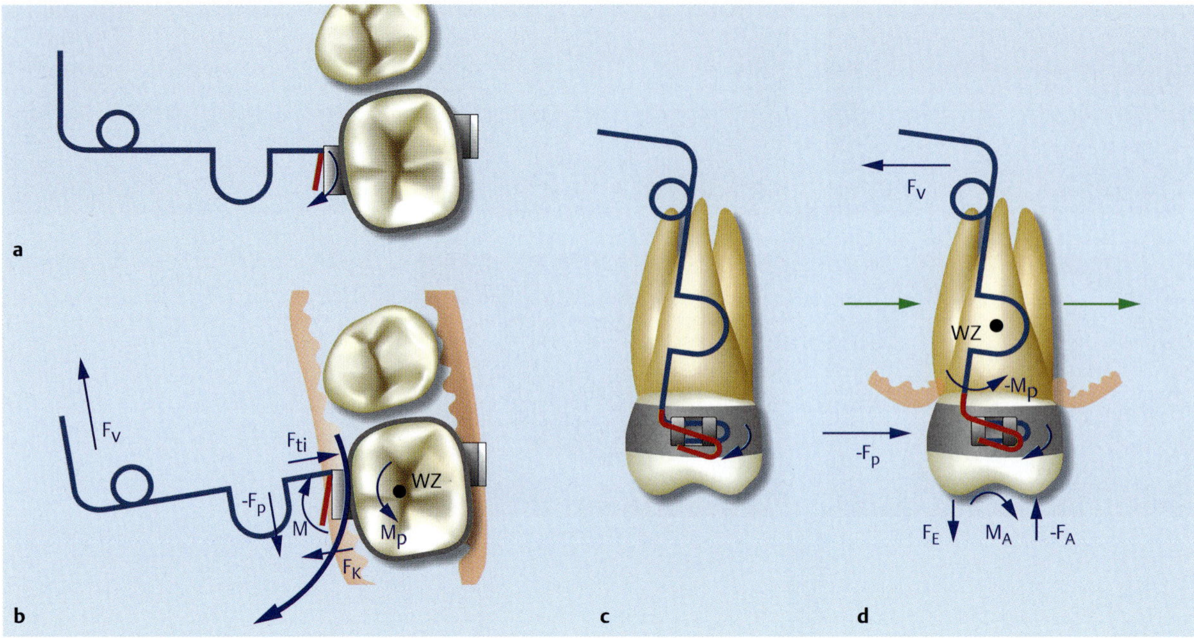

Fig. 7.32a–d Activating the components of the pendulum appliance.
a, b Toe-in bend of the transpalatal arch for derotation.
c, d Uprighting activation to counteract the distal crown tip on the molars.

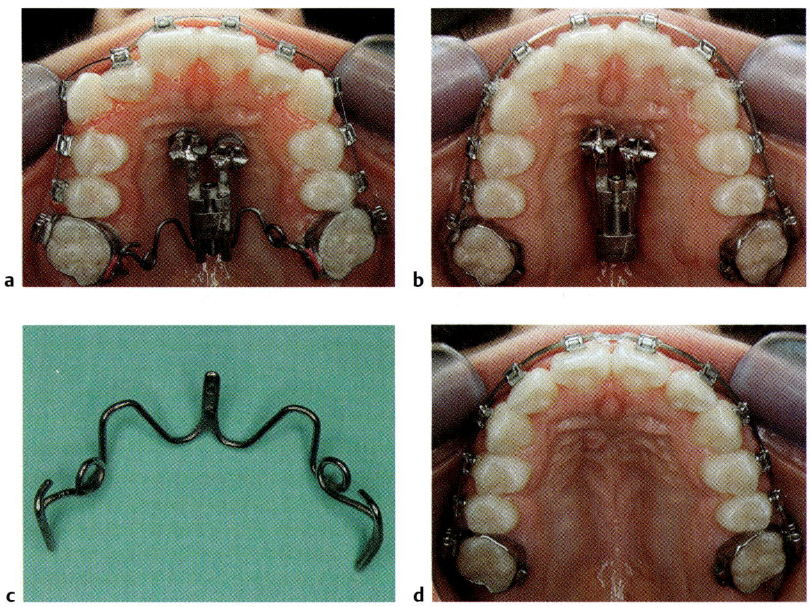

Fig. 7.33a–d
a At the start of distalization.
b After 3 months, with significant rotation of the molars (too little “toe-in” of the transpalatal arch).
c Extraoral reactivation to increase the “toe-in.”
d At follow-up examination 8 weeks later shows an improved molar position.

Space Creation by Expansion of Arches

Skeletal expansion of the upper jaw by expanding the midpalatal suture was first described by Angelle in 1860, but this form of treatment only gained wider acceptance after 1953, mainly inspired by the work of Derichsweiler and Korkhaus. Conventional rapid maxillary expansion uses forced expansion of the midpalatal suture by four-point retention, usually on the first molars and the first premolars. Modifications of this device involving a bonded expander design rely on acrylic capping of the posterior segments. The present authors prefer a combined tooth-borne/bone-borne anchorage solution. This hybrid maxillary expander replaces the premolar bands with mini-implants.[34] Insertion of the mini-implants is similar to the method described in section on "Space Creation through Distalization" above (**Fig. 7.34**). The screws are inserted roughly 2 mm paramedian to the suture and on a line connecting the mesial aspects of the first premolars. It is important that the implants should not be inserted too close to the median suture, otherwise the stability of the implants may be compromised during expansion (**Fig. 7.34**). We recommend activating the expansion screw three times a day (**Figs. 7.34** and **7.35**).

The fabrication of the expansion device is similar to that described for the Frog appliance. The abutments are filled with Vaseline and placed over the mini-implant heads, and an alginate impression is taken. The rapid maxillary expansion device is subsequently fixed to the mini-implants in the anterior palate and to the first molars in the posterior palate via the abutments, which also double as coupling devices (**Fig. 7.36**).

The advantage of the bone-borne expansion approach in the anterior maxilla lies in the application of forces directly onto the skeletal structures in that area; the dentition is not affected. This allows more efficient expansion of the midpalatal suture, with potentially fewer dental

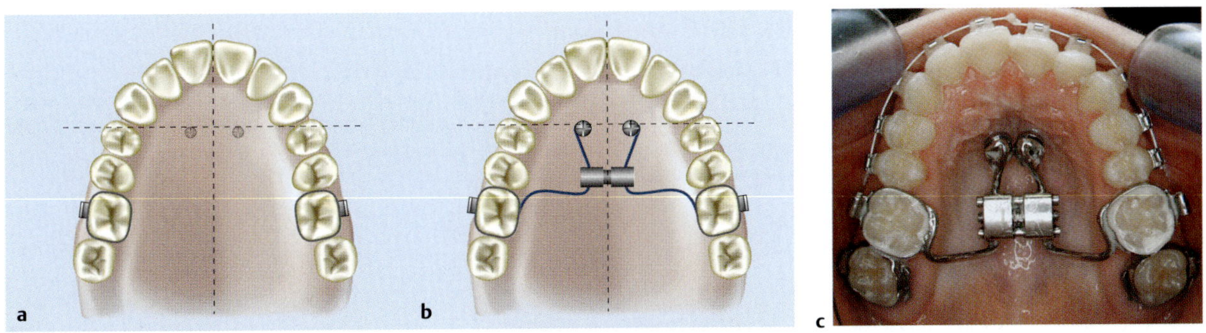

Fig. 7.34a–c The mini-implants are placed on a line mesial to the two upper first premolars, 4 mm distal to the incisive papilla. The implants should be inserted approximately 2 mm lateral to the maxillary suture.

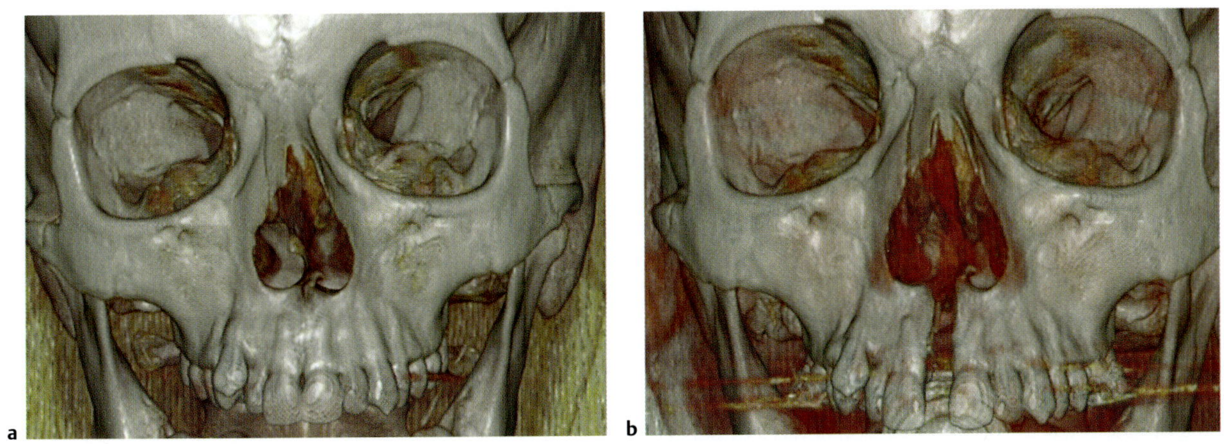

Fig. 7.35a, b Three-dimensional computed-tomography images. Immediately after expansion of the maxilla, the midline suture opens.

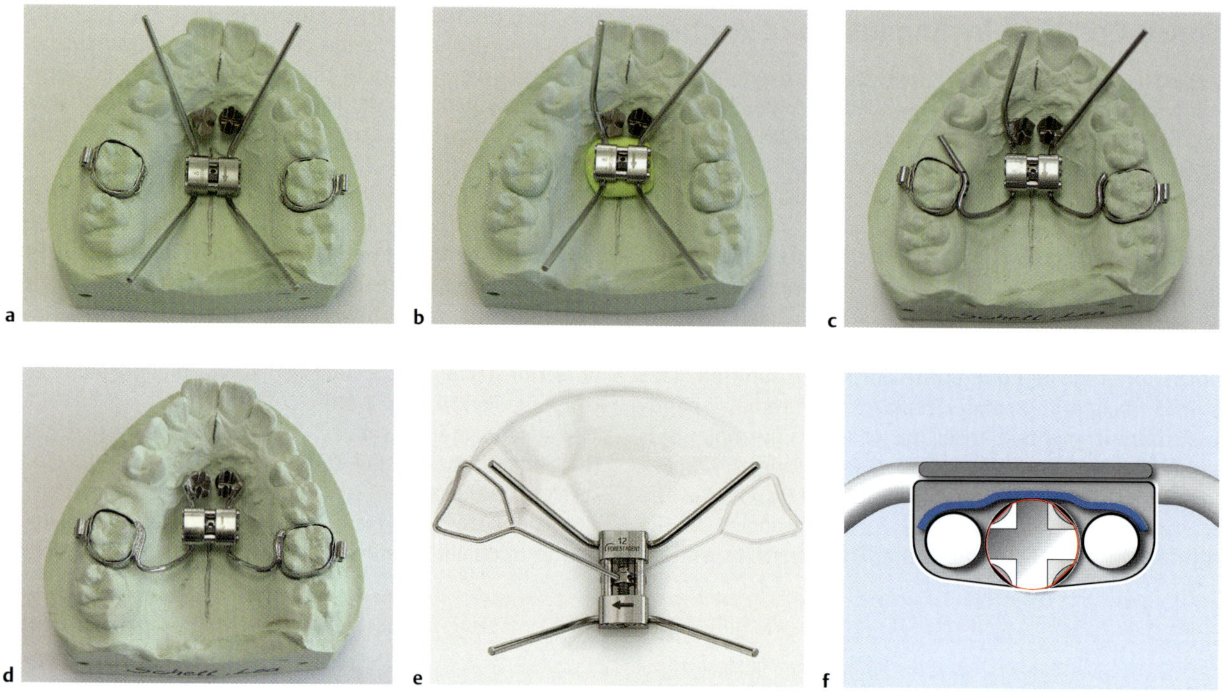

Fig. 7.36 a–f The laboratory procedure for hybrid rapid palatal expansion (RPE).
a Fixation of the abutments.
b, c Seating of the expansion screw. The frontal arms are shortened and welded to the abutments. The posterior arms are adapted to fit the molar bands and are also welded.
d The completed hybrid RPE.
e, f An example of a safety screw (Snap Lock, Forestadent). After each activation, a leaf spring engages the screw and prevents it from inadvertently turning backward.

side effects. An additional advantage is that orthodontic treatment mesial to the upper first molars can be carried out simultaneously (such as leveling and alignment) and archwire progression is possible during the retention period. The final 0.019 × 0.025 stainless-steel archwires can then be used to maintain the transverse changes without the need to keep the expansion device in place for long periods of time (**Fig. 7.37**). This approach allows more efficient overall treatment (one phase instead of two phases). This hybrid maxillary expansion device is suitable for patients in the mixed permanent dentition period, as well as adults. It is now widely known that the midpalatal suture does not completely fuse, so even adults can be treated in this way. The increased difficulty of maxillary expansion in the upper jaw in adults is mainly thought to be due to solidification of the lateral skeletal structures of the skull, such as the maxillary abutment of the zygoma, rather than to solidification of the midmaxillary suture.[20,31,38] In patients over the age of 25, we recommend a cut in the zygomatic structures of the lateral maxilla (rather than a complete osteotomy) to aid maxillary expansion.

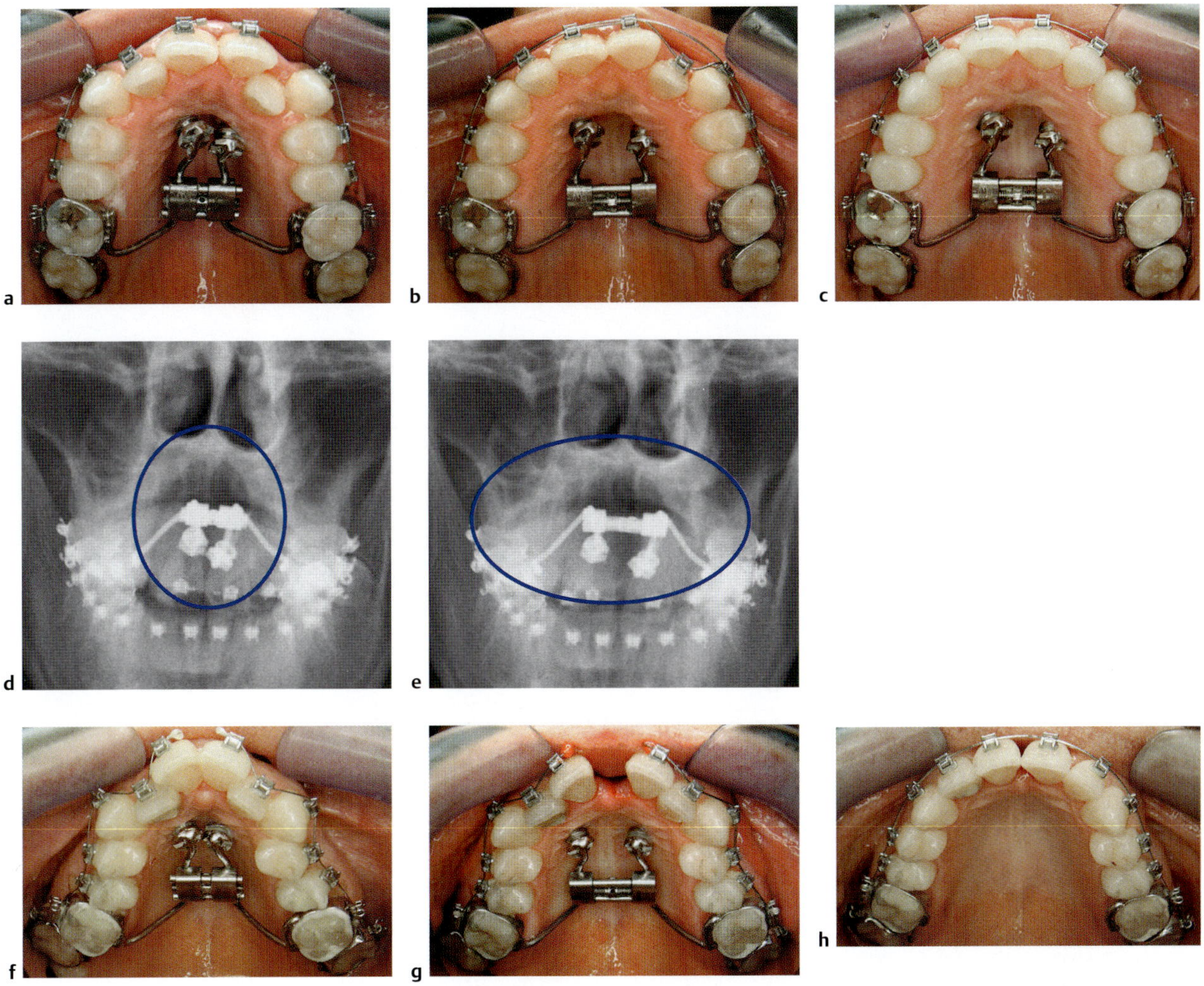

Fig. 7.37 a–h A clinical example of maxillary expansion using hybrid rapid palatal expansion (RPE) (**a–e**). The skeletal effect is clearly visible on the intraoral photographs; the abutments are spread apart (**a–c**). Radiographs confirm this (**d, e**). **f–h** Surgically assisted hybrid RPE in a 45-year-old man.

Case Study 7.12 (Fig. 7.38)

Patient: N.H., male, age 8.

Diagnostic records: models, panoramic radiograph, lateral cephalometric radiograph, intraoral/extraoral photographs.

Main findings: bilateral crossbite, reduced overjet, and overbite.

Treatment aims: forced expansion of the upper jaw, alignment of both upper and lower front teeth.

Appliances: self-ligating brackets, molar bands, mini-implants, hybrid rapid maxillary expander.

Archwire sequence: 0.012 SE, 0.016 SE, 0.016 × 0.022 SS: after eruption of 22 0.012 SE, 0.016 SE, 0.017 × 0.025 SE.

Alternative treatment strategy: conventional rapid maxillary expansion.

Active treatment time: 10 months (including waiting for eruption of 22).

Retention: upper and lower retainers, with a midline screw to allow for expansion if necessary.

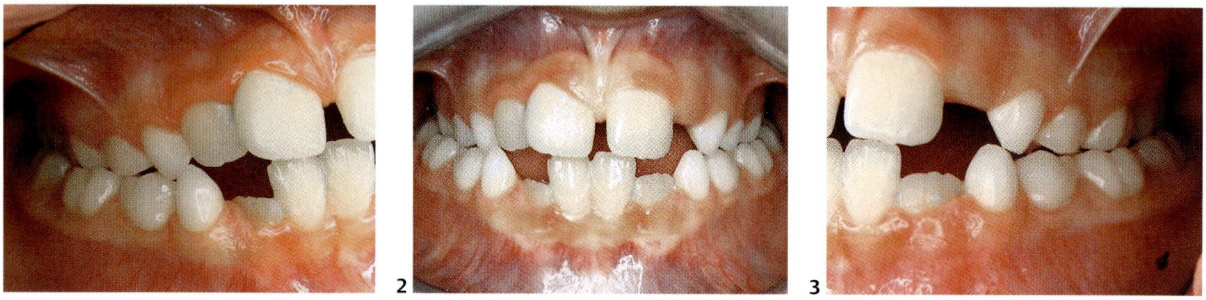

1 2 3

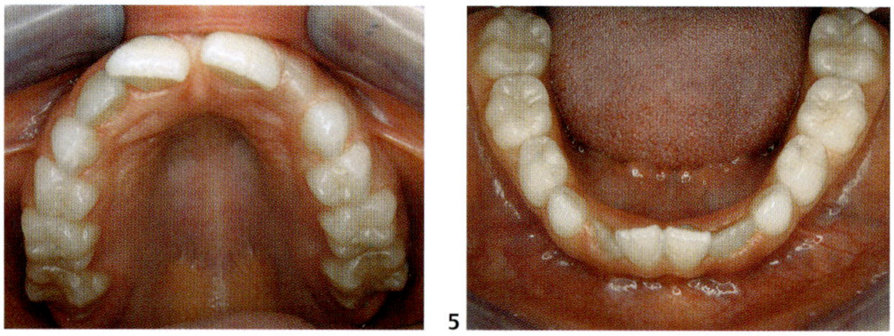

4 5

Fig. 7.38 1–18

1–5 Initial presentation: bilateral crossbite with a constricted maxilla in the mixed dentition.

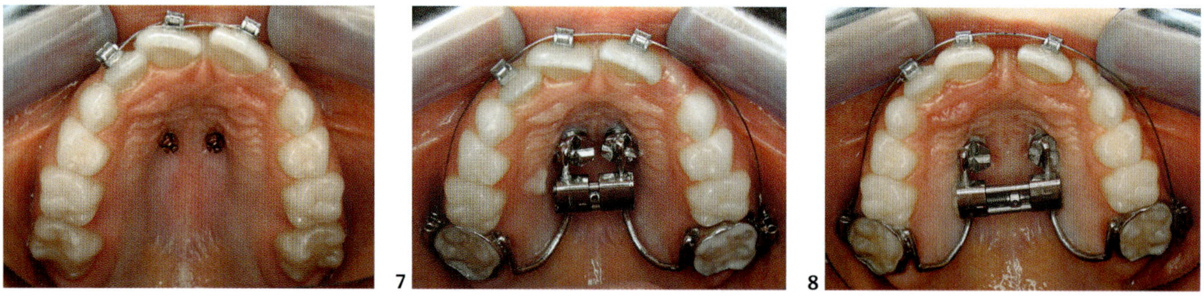

6 7 8

6–8 Mini-implants placed and self-ligating brackets in place (**6**), hybrid rapid maxillary expander inserted (**7**), and the appliance after 2 weeks of expansion (**8**).

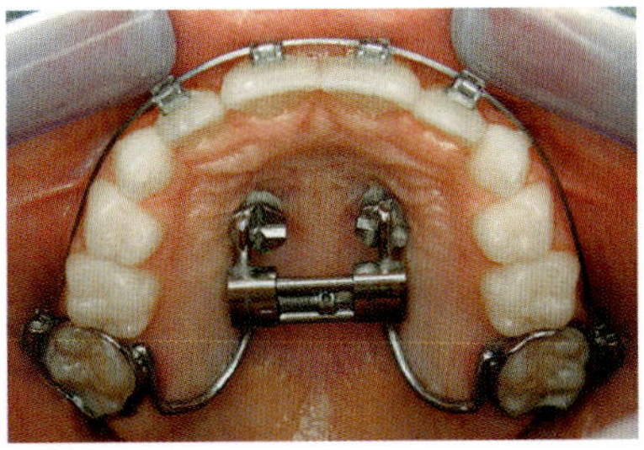
9
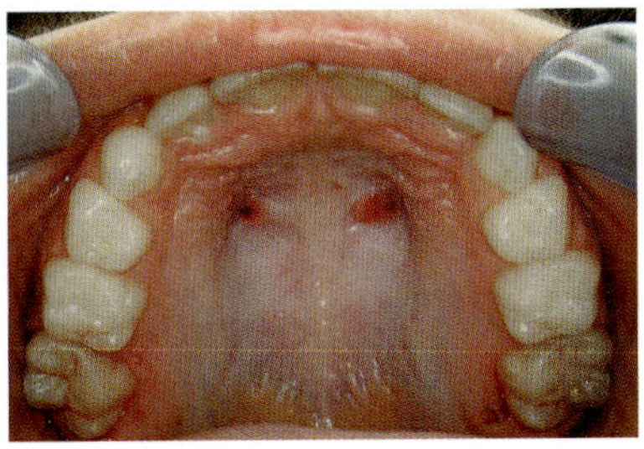
10
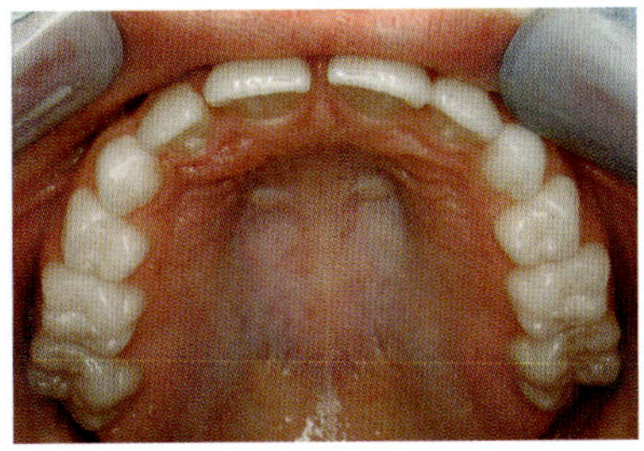
11

9–11 The site of the hybrid expander immediately after removal and 1 year after retention.

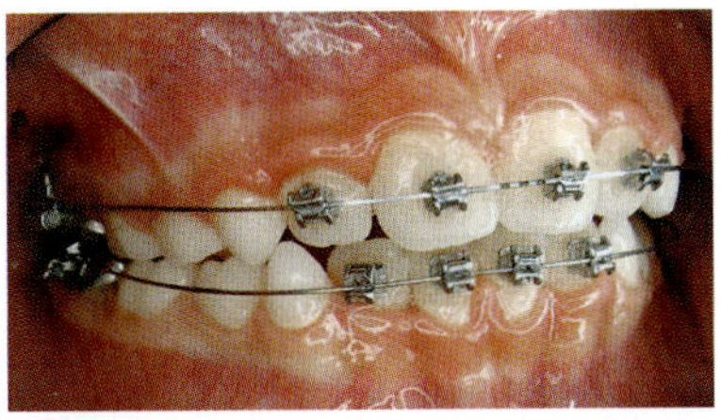
12
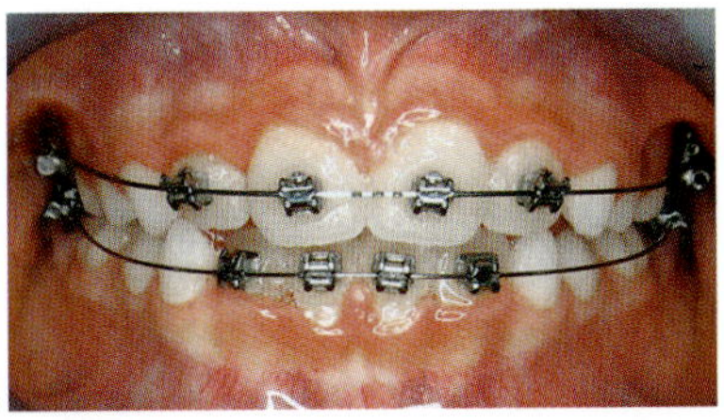
13
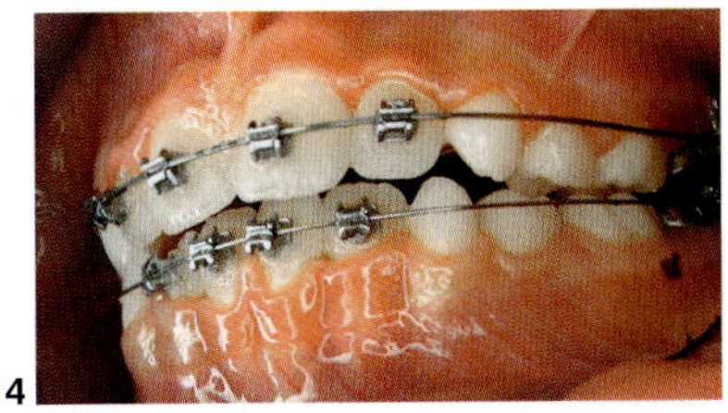
14

12–14 After 10 months of interceptive treatment.

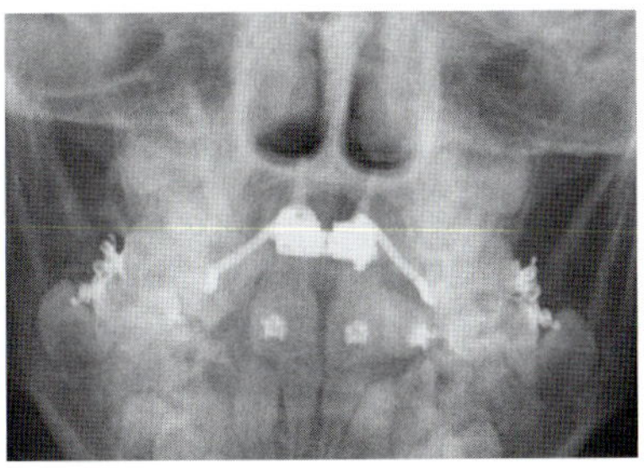
15
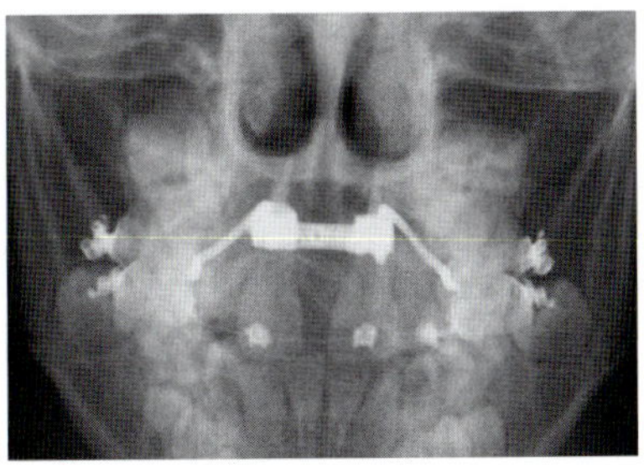
16

15, 16 Posteroanterior cephalograms before expansion and immediately after expansion.

CLINICAL PEARL

Question: Does the skeletal anchorage of the hybrid rapid maxillary expander prevent buccal tipping of the molars used for retention?

Answer: In addition to confirming the sutural effects, analysis of the frontal cephalogram shows that the position of the anchoring molars is largely stable.

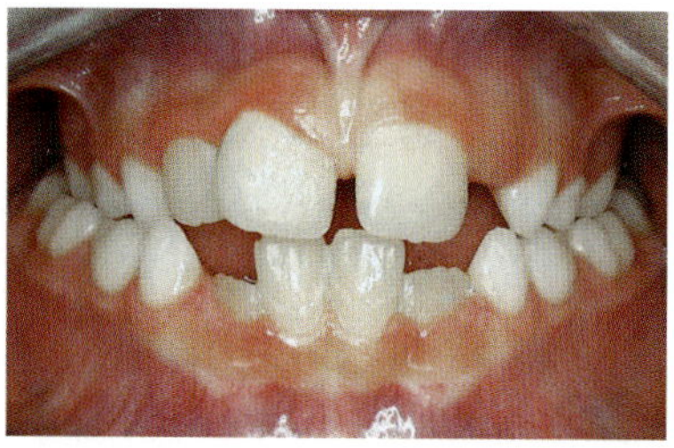

17

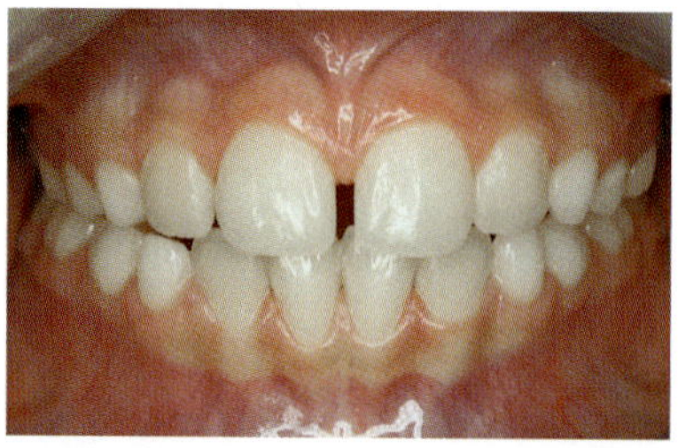

18

17, 18 Before treatment and 1 year after completion of interceptive treatment, with occlusal relationships appropriate for the patient's age.

ERRORS AND RISKS

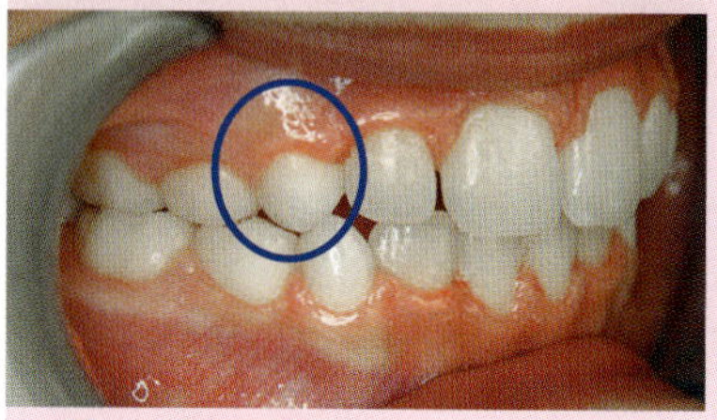

1

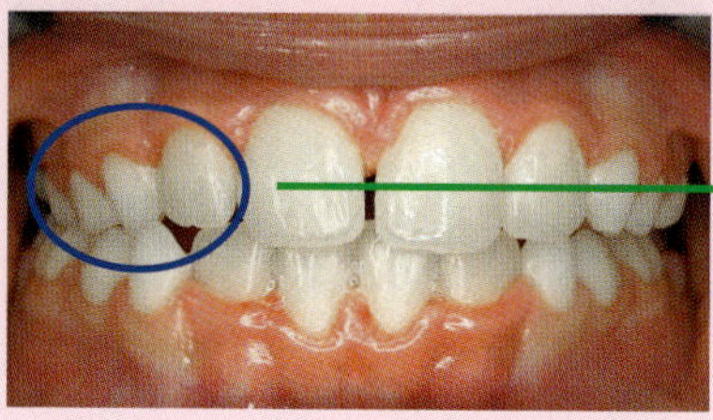

2

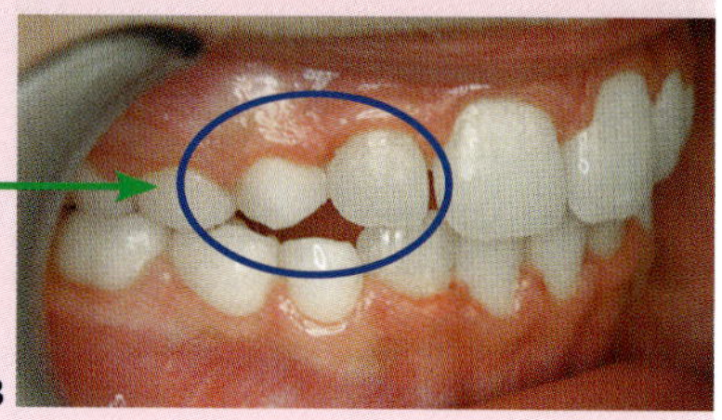

3

Fig. 7.39 1–3

1–3 In the mixed-dentition phase, premature occlusal contacts between the deciduous teeth may lead to a functional shift in the mandible. These contacts should be eliminated at an early stage by simple occlusal adjustment.

Case Study 7.13 (Fig. 7.40)

Patient: J.L., female, age 13.
Diagnostic records: models, panoramic radiograph, lateral cephalometric radiograph, intraoral/extraoral photographs.
Main findings: skeletal class III with maxillary hyperplasia and blocked out of 13, reduced overjet, and open bite tendency.
Treatment aims: skeletal expansion of the upper jaw, space creation in the area of 13, and improvement of the overjet and overbite.
Appliances: self-ligating brackets, molar bands, mini-implants, hybrid rapid maxillary expansion.
Archwire sequence: 0.012 SE, 0.016 SS, 0.016 × 0.022 SE, 0.018 × 0.025 SE, 0.019 × 0.025 SS.
Alternative treatment strategy: conventional rapid maxillary expansion.
Active treatment time: 13 months.
Retention: three-dimensional retention encompassing a removable retainer with the potential for further expansion (midline screw).

1
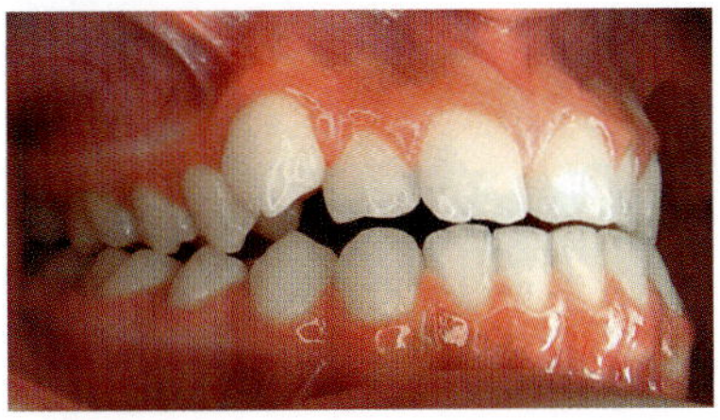
2
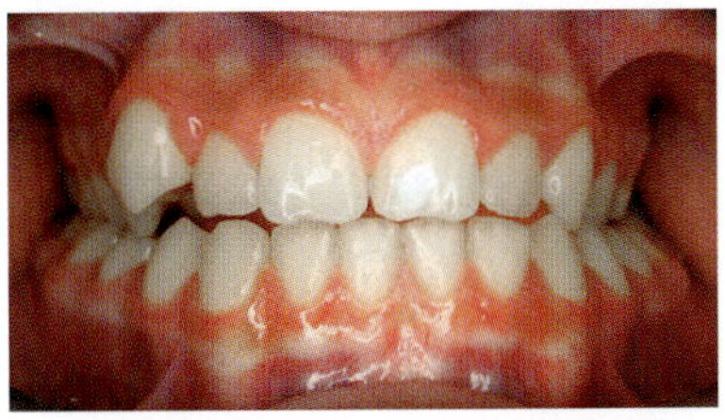
3
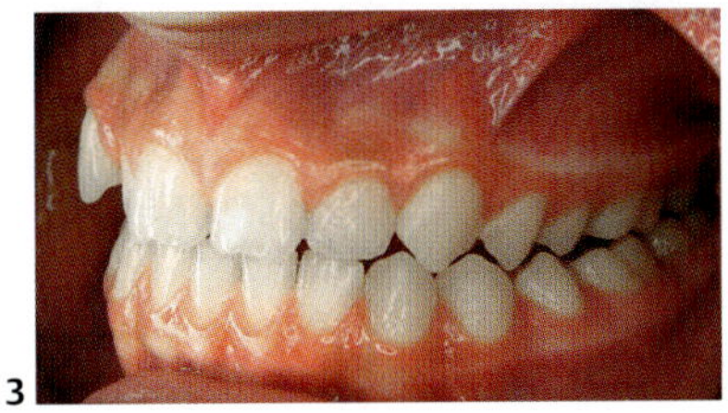
4
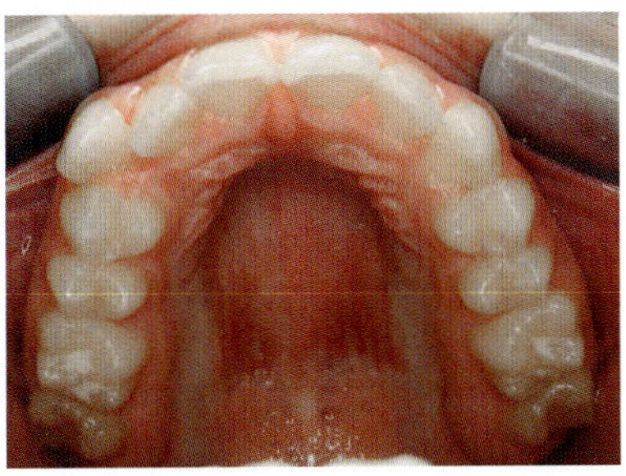
5
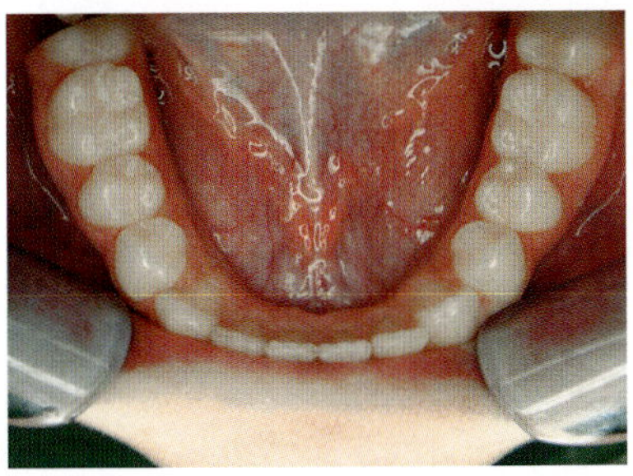

Fig. 7.40 1–21
1–5 The initial presentation: constricted maxilla, unilateral crossbite (left); tooth 13 is blocked out buccally.

Errors and risks:
Maxillary constriction causing a functional shift to the left creating a unilateral crossbite.

6
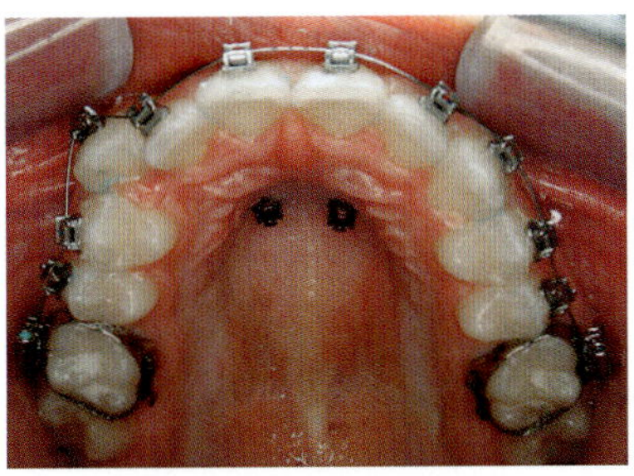
7
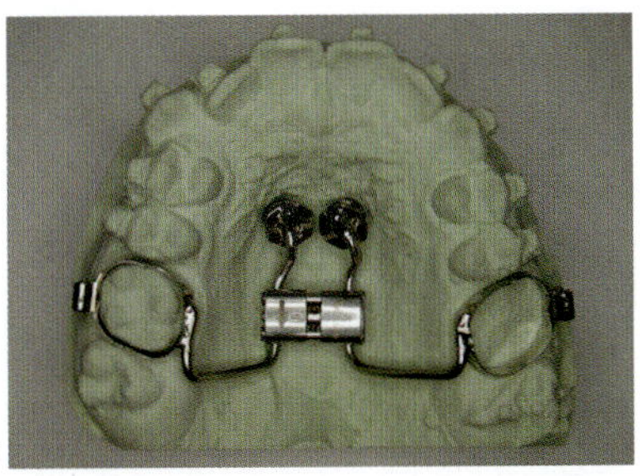
8
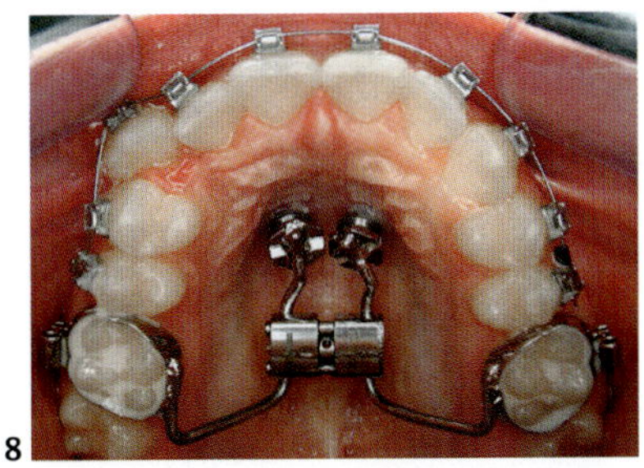

6–8 Simultaneous use of a hybrid rapid palatal expander and self-ligating brackets for transverse expansion in the upper jaw.

9
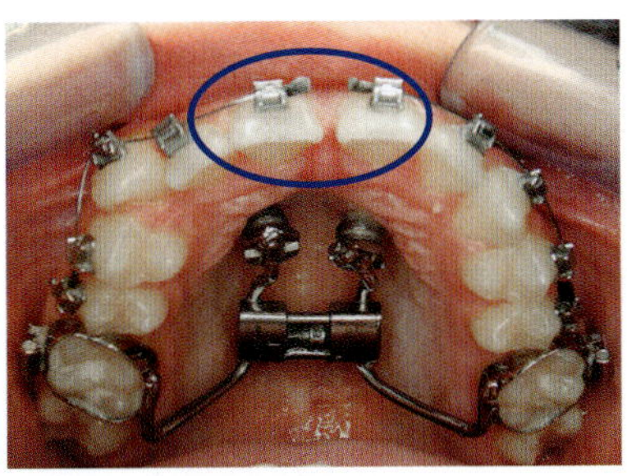
10
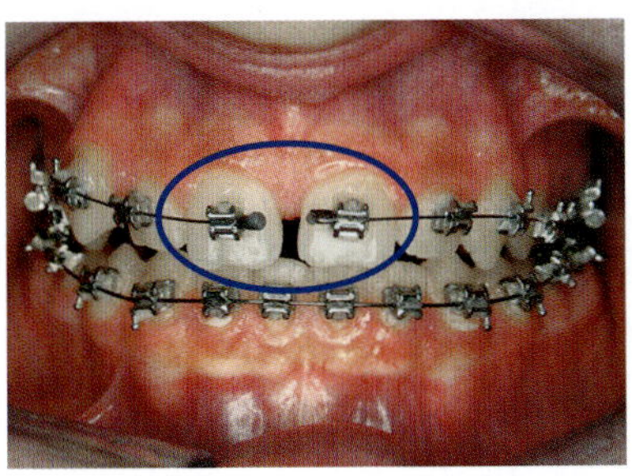
11
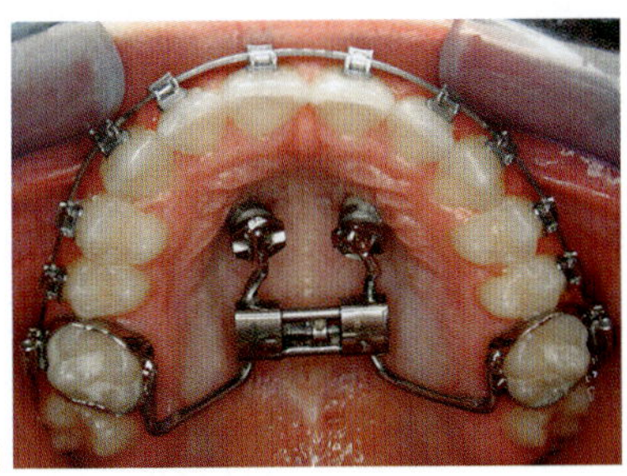

9, 10 After 10 days of activation of the hybrid rapid palatal expander (the archwire has been cut in the midline).

11 3.5 months into treatment.

ERRORS AND RISKS

The maxillary archwire should be sectioned between the maxillary central incisors before expansion.

CLINICAL PEARL

Settling of the occlusion using vertical elastics to the canines.

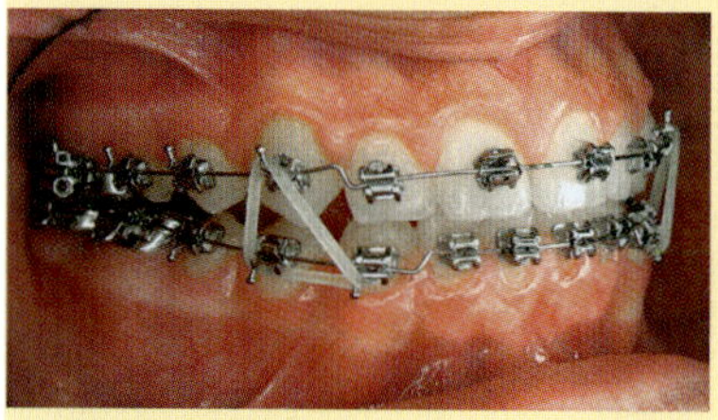
12
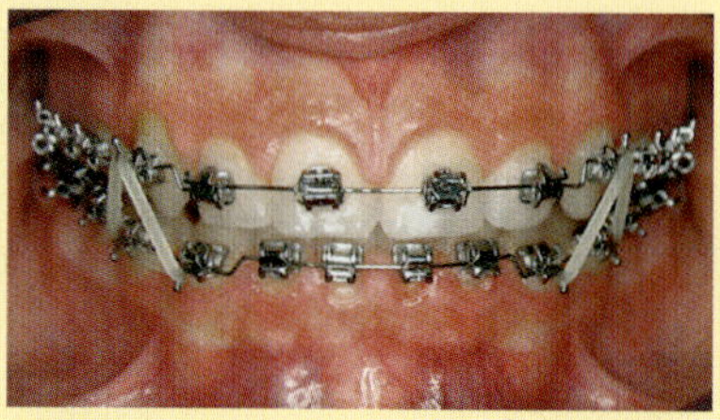
13
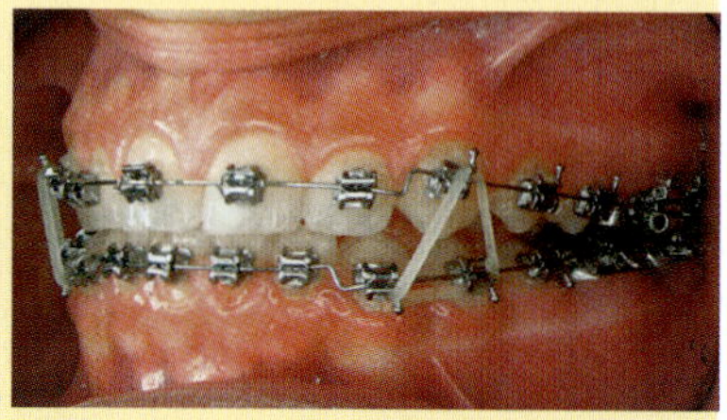
14

12–14 The maxillary anterior segment is stepped down and the mandibular anterior segment is stepped to increase the overbite. Vertical triangular elastics are worn for further support.

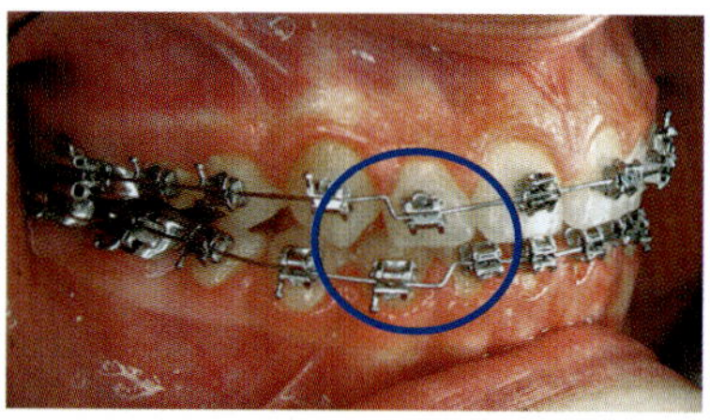
15
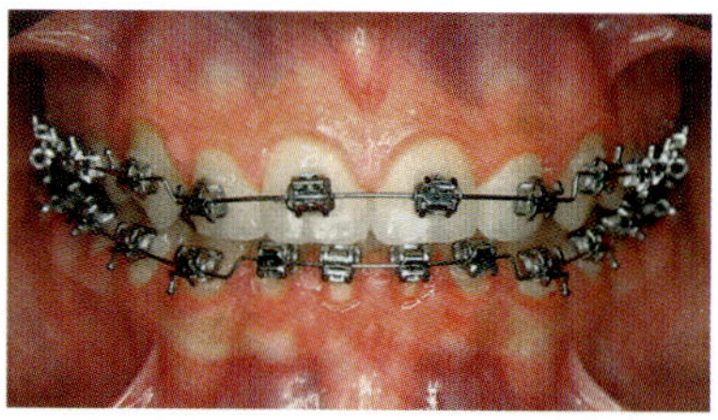
16
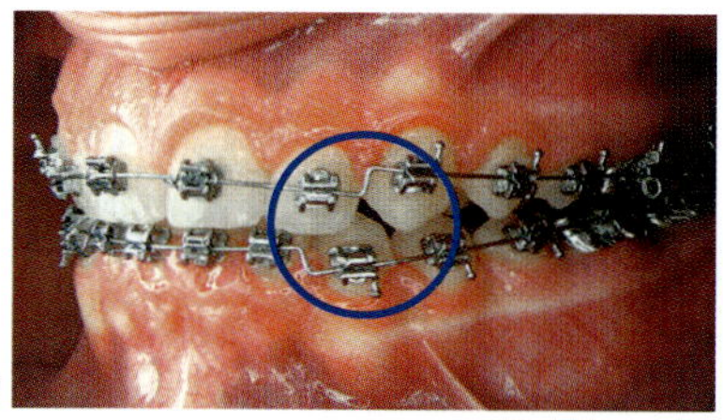
17
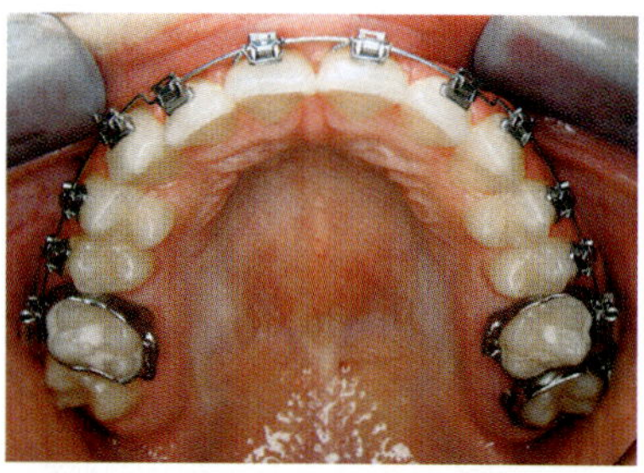
18
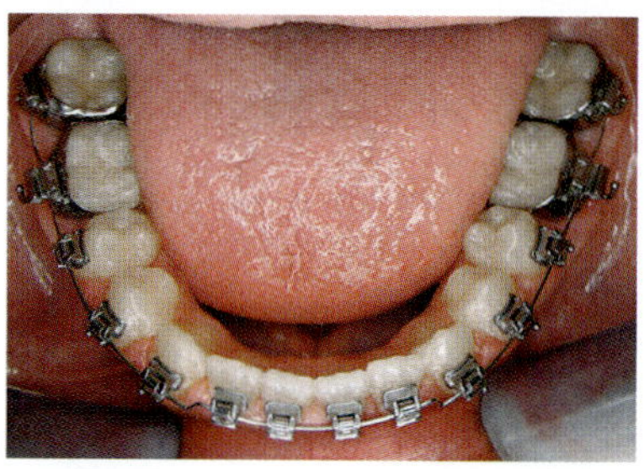
19

15–19 The situation before debonding.

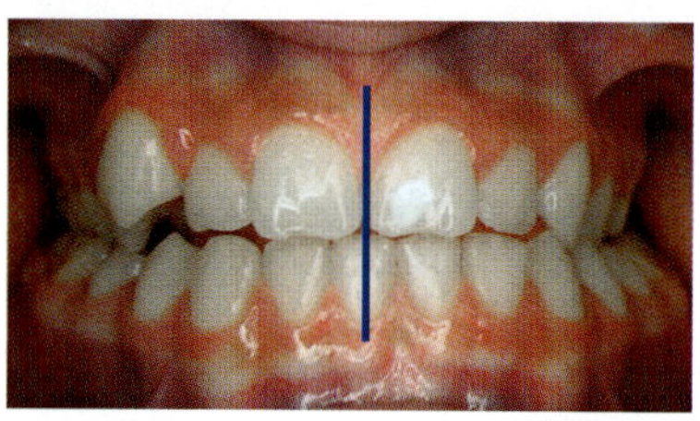
20
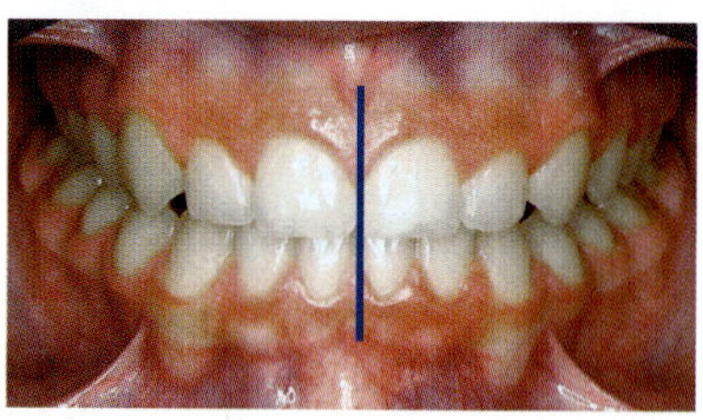
21

20, 21 The midline discrepancy was resolved by expansion of the upper jaw and correction of the crossbite.

Space Creation by Extracting Teeth

Extraction in the permanent dentition is one of the oldest, quickest, easiest, and most predictable ways of creating space. Holinder and also Herbst recommended extracting premolars routinely to create space in orthodontics as early as 1882. Removing a single premolar creates about 7–8 mm of space, and symmetrical extraction of two premolars will create approximately 16 mm of space. In a large number of patients, this is more space than is actually required to align the teeth. In select cases, however, extractions are beneficial and necessary. The most common reason for removing premolars in our practice is to correct primary or secondary crowding and for camouflage treatment of underlying skeletal base discrepancies that do not warrant a surgical approach.

Case Study 7.14 (Fig. 7.41)

Patient: J.F., female, age 14.
Diagnostic records: models, panoramic radiograph, lateral cephalometric radiograph, intraoral/extraoral photographs.
Main findings: crowding, with all four canines blocked out labially.
Treatment aims: Extraction of all four first premolars, alignment of all teeth.
Appliances: Self-ligating brackets, molar bands.
Archwire sequence: 0.012 SE, 0.016 SE, 0.016 × 0.022 SE, 0.021 × 0.025 SE, 0.019 × 0.025 SS for sliding mechanics.
Alternative treatment strategy: skeletally anchored Frog appliance, interproximal reduction for mandibular space creation.
Active treatment time: 13 months.
Retention: three-dimensional retention.

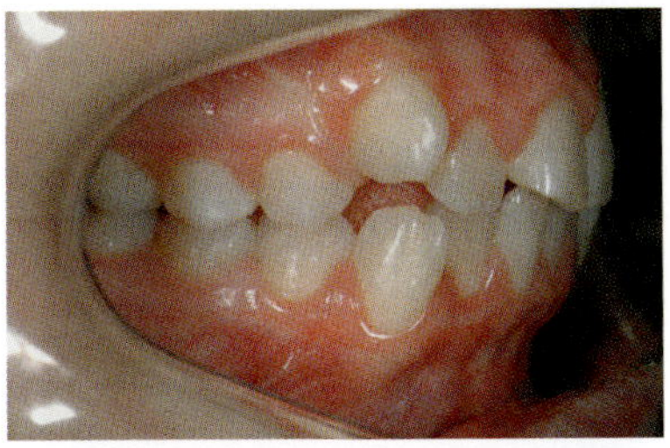
1
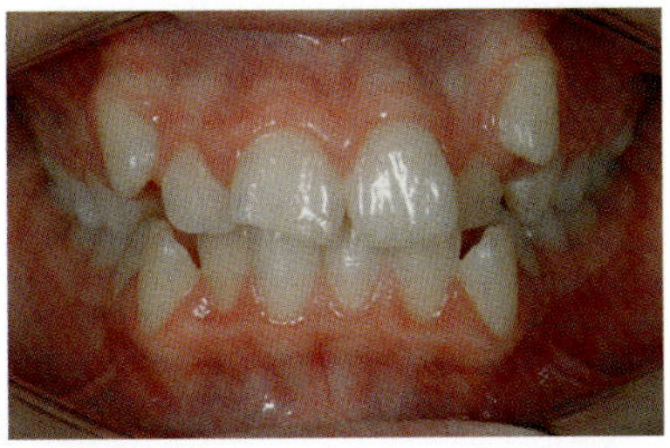
2
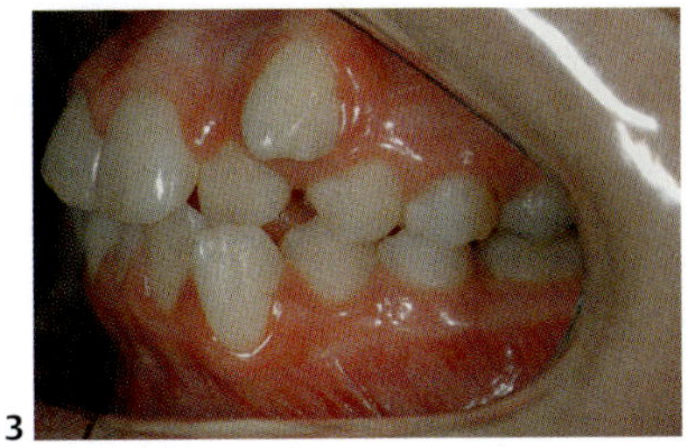
3
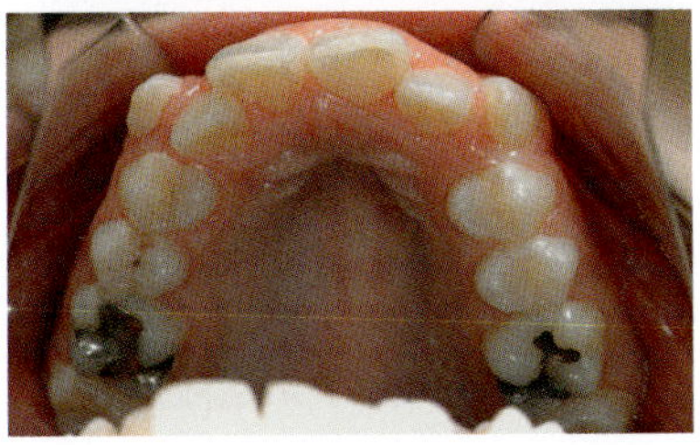
4
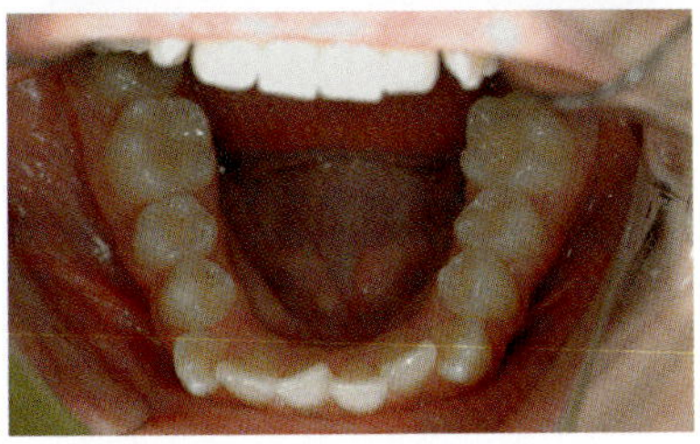
5

Fig. 7.41 1–18
1–5 The findings before treatment: significant crowding in both dental arches.

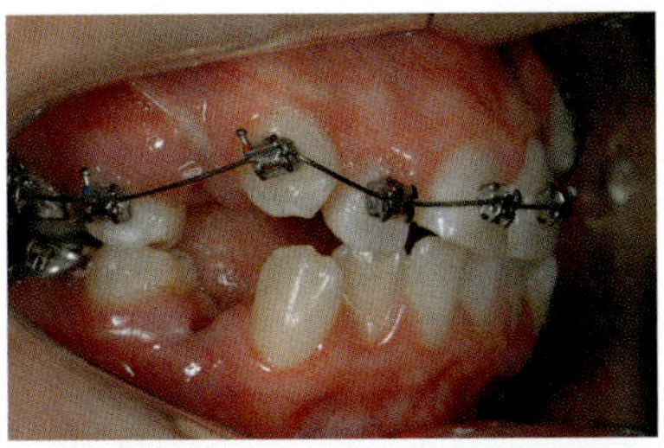
6
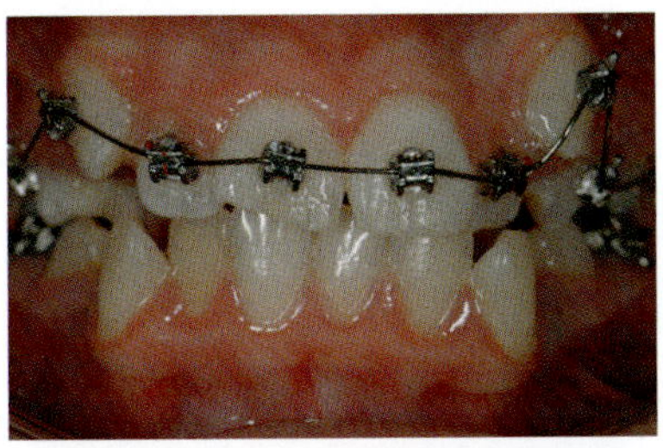
7
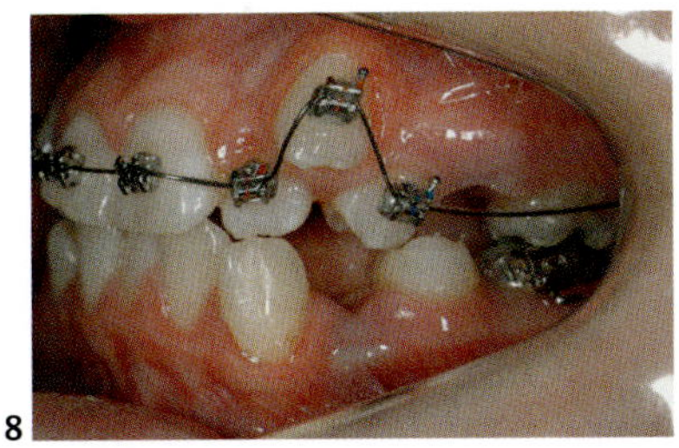
8
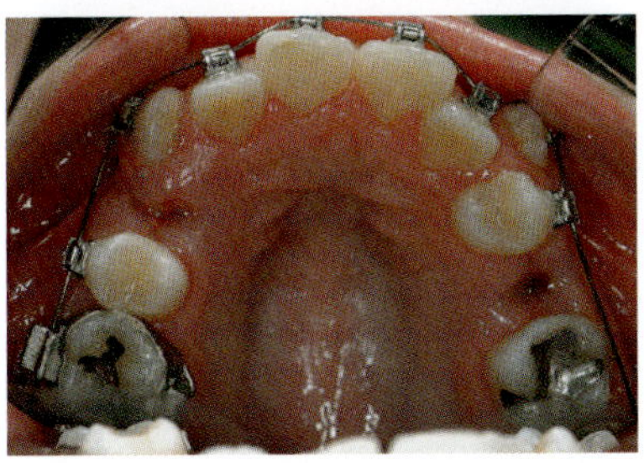
9
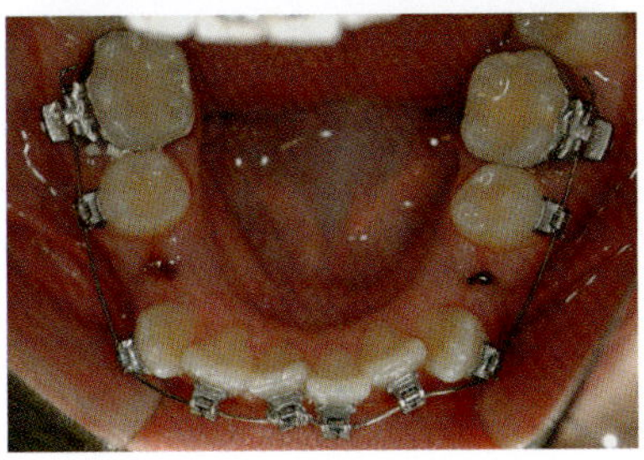
10

6–10 0.012 SE archwires and self-ligating brackets placed in the maxillary arch.

Clinical pearl:
There is immediate tooth movement into a fresh extraction socket. The dental surgeon should be asked not to compress the alveolus after the extraction, to avoid constriction of the site.

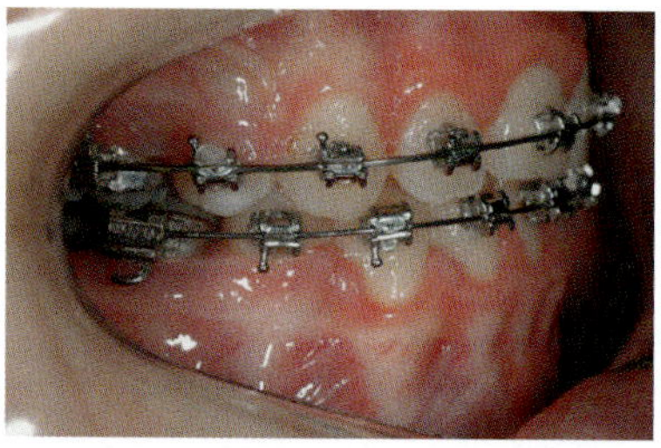
11

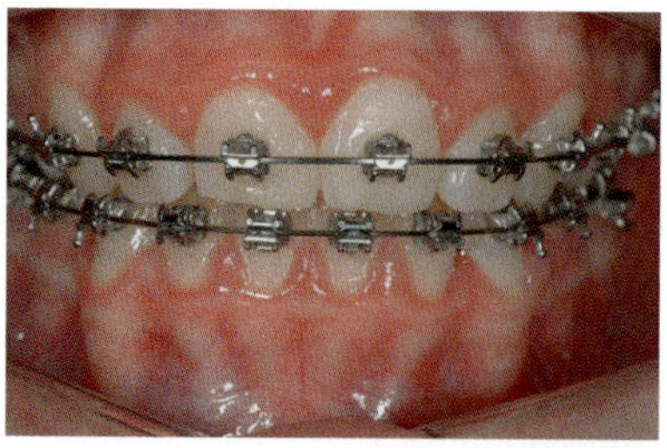
12

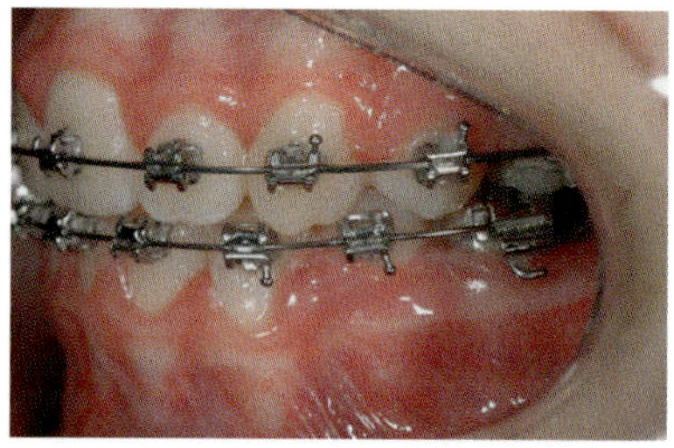
13

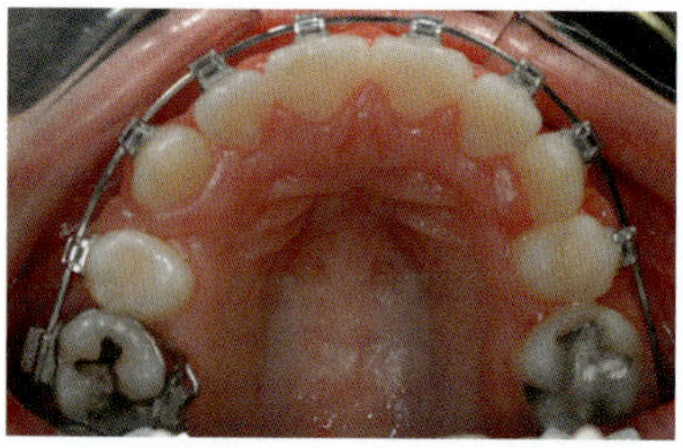
14

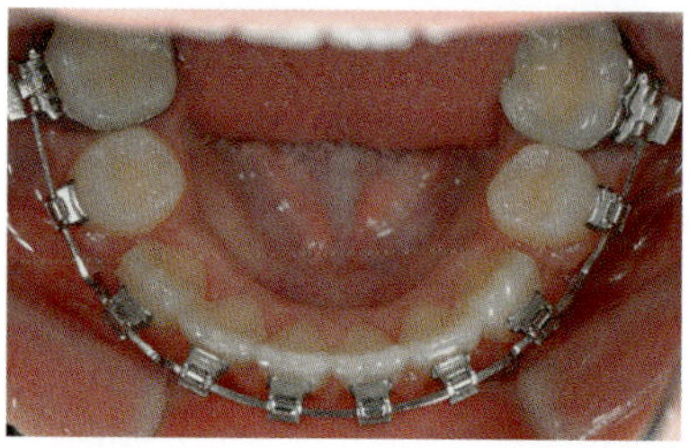
15

11–15 0.021 × 0.025 SE archwires.

Clinical pearl:
In patients with crowding, the combination of square superelastic wires and a low-friction environment allows teeth adjacent to an extraction site to gently migrate into the site, often without the use of space-closing adjuncts such as elastics.

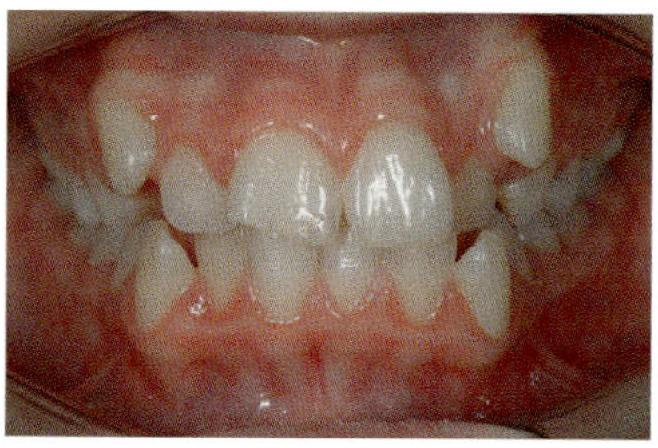
16

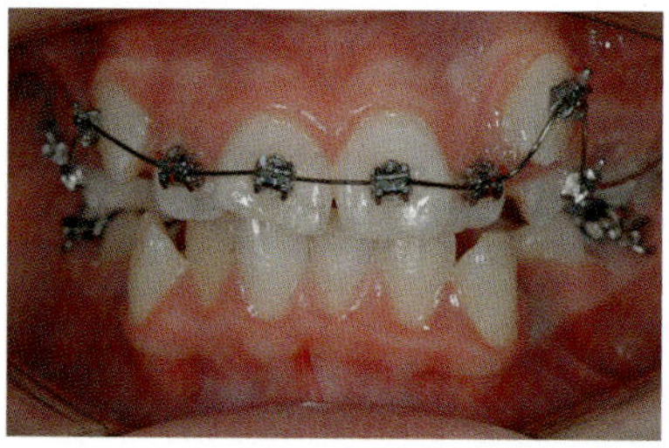
17

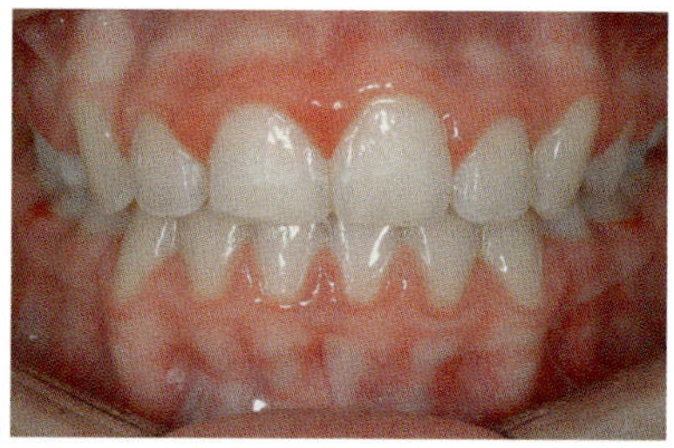
18

16–18 Before treatment, maxillary appliances, final result. (Images courtesy of Dr. Javier Frenck, Cordoba, Argentina.)

Case Study 7.15 (Fig. 7.42)

Patient: A.H., female, age 12.
Diagnostic records: Models, panoramic radiograph, lateral cephalometric radiograph, intraoral/extraoral photographs.
Main findings: maxillary prognathism with proclined maxillary incisors; moderately retrognathic mandible on cephalometry.
Treatment aims: extraction of maxillary first premolars, anterior retraction (camouflage treatment).
Appliances: self-ligating brackets, molar bands.
Archwire sequence: 0.012 SE, 0.016 SE, 0.016 SS, 0.016 × 0.022 SE, 0.018 × 0.025 SE, 0.019 × 0.025 SS.
Alternative treatment strategy: distalization, Herbst appliance, orthognathic surgery after completion of growth.
Active retention time: 14 months.
Retention: three-dimensional retention with a Hawley retainer.

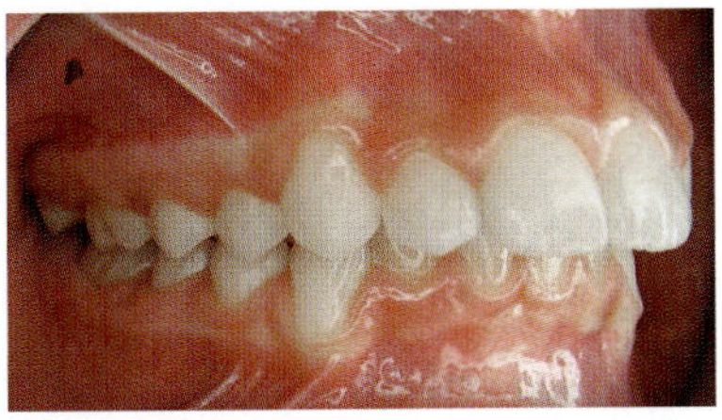
1

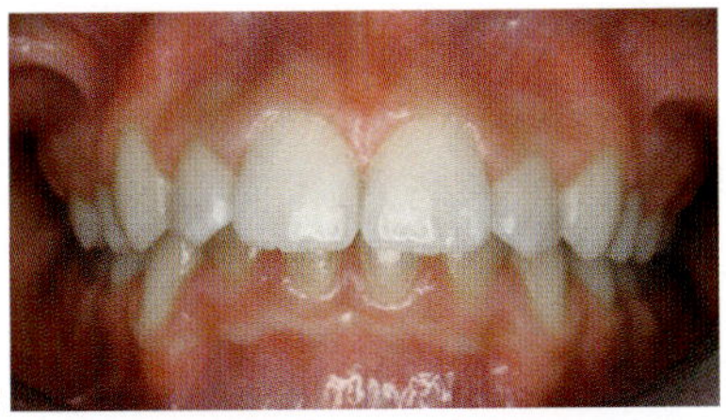
2

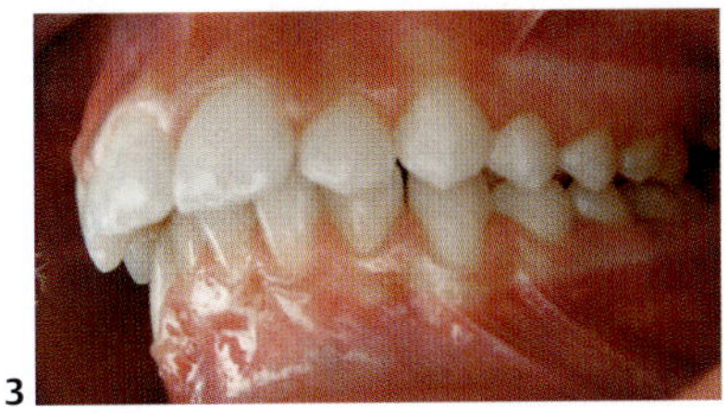
3

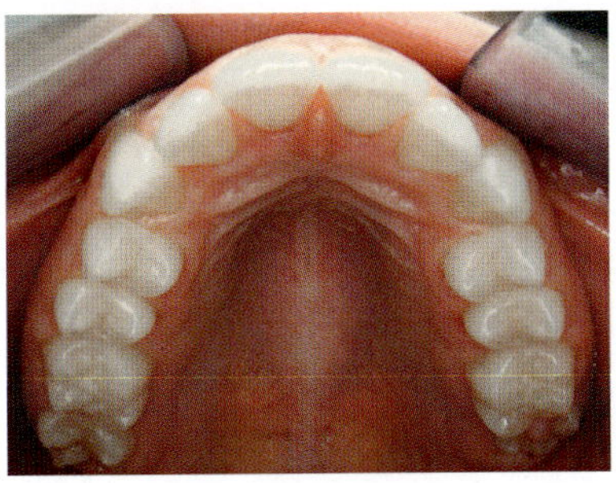
4

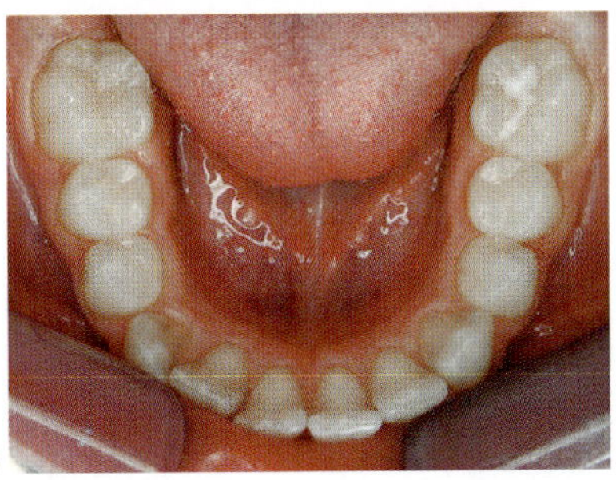
5

Fig. 7.42 1–30
1–5 The situation before treatment, with increased overjet (12 mm) due to maxillary prognathism and only moderate mandibular retrognathism.

CLINICAL PEARL

- Attention should be paid to the patient's habits and habitual positioning of the lower lip.
- Orthodontic camouflage should be considered as a valid alternative.
- The advantages and disadvantages of the different treatment options need to be explained to the patient.

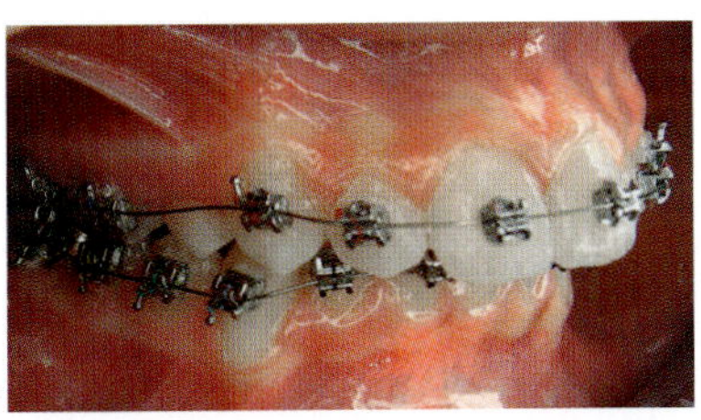
6

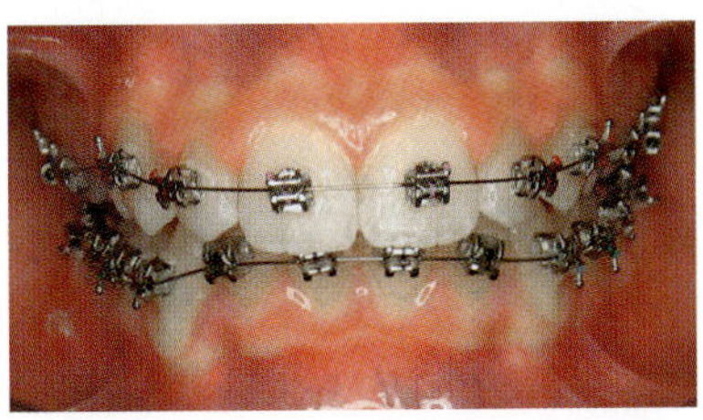
7

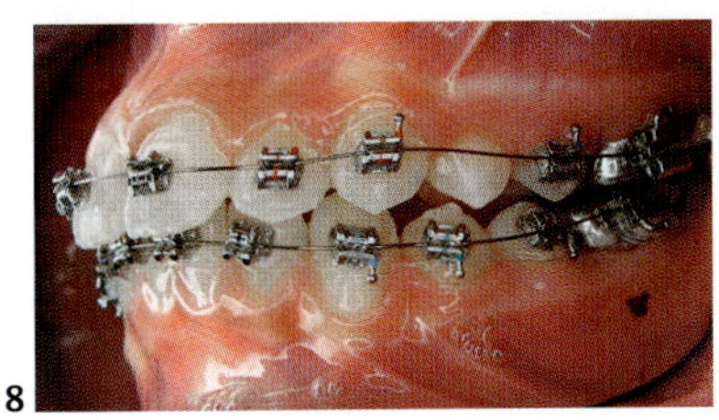
8

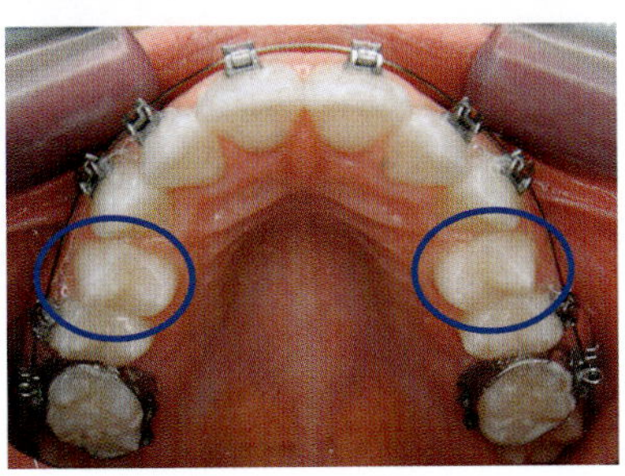
9

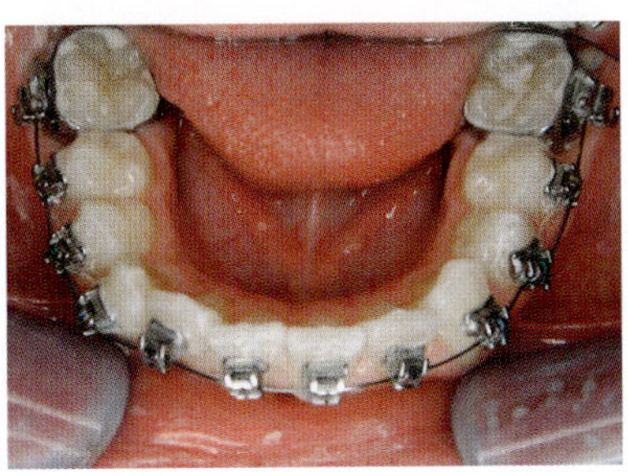
10

6–10 0.012 SE archwires with self-ligating brackets.

Clinical pearl:
The premolars that will be extracted are not bonded, so space closure can occur immediately after extraction.

ERRORS AND RISKS

Action is equal and opposite to reaction, so that anchorage loss may occur.
Mesialization of the posterior segments needs to be avoided to allow for en-masse retraction of the anterior teeth.
Strategies:

11
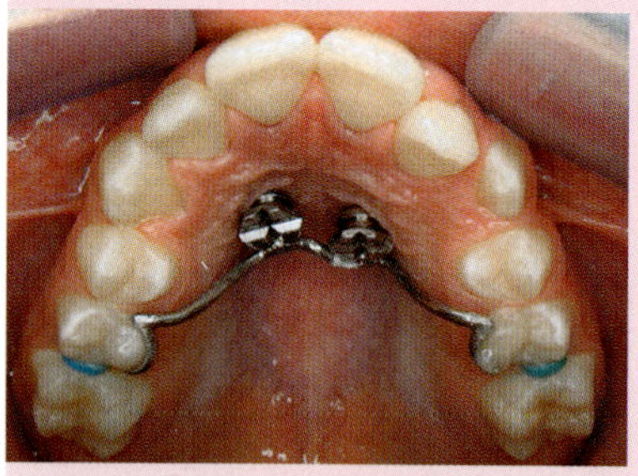

12
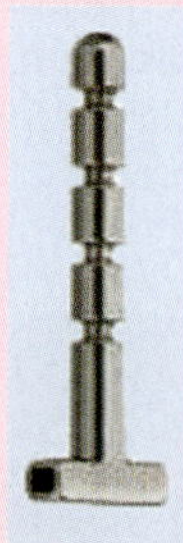

13
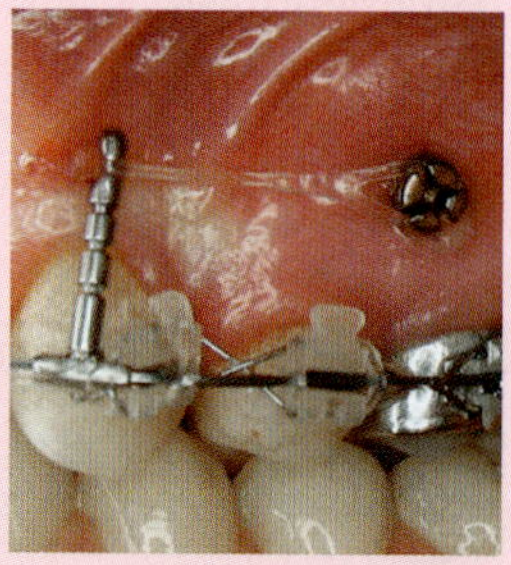

14
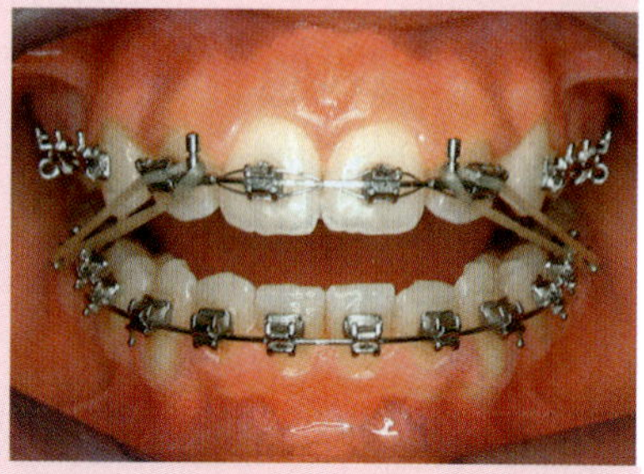

11 Skeletally anchored transpalatal arch.

12, 13 Buccal mini-implant with a power arm.

14 Class II elastics (¼ 6 oz) for sliding mechanics.

Predictable ⟶ **Unpredictable**

15
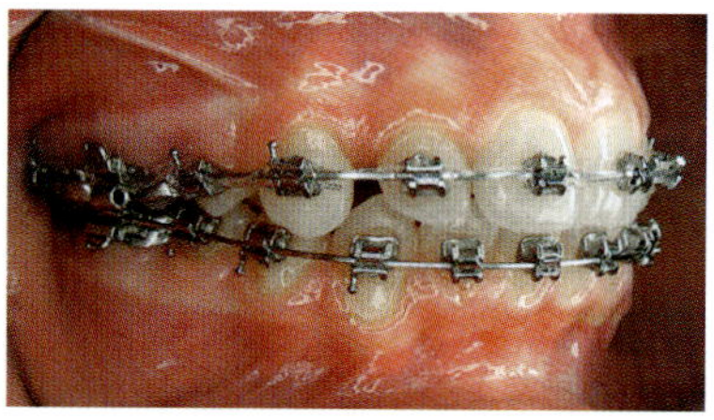

16
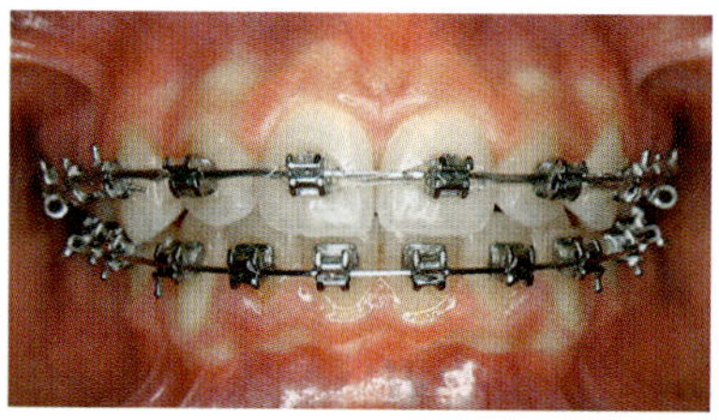

17
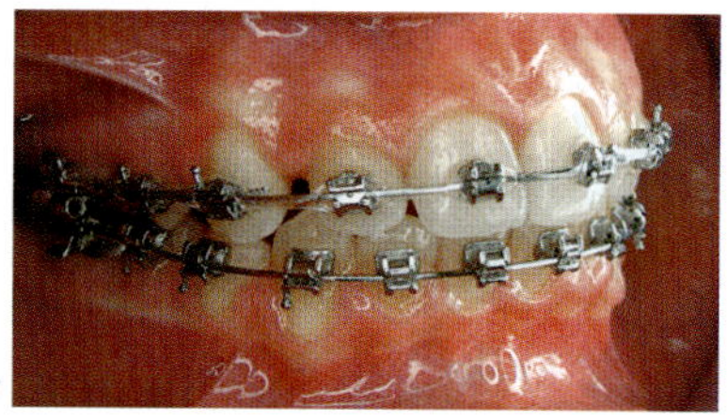

18
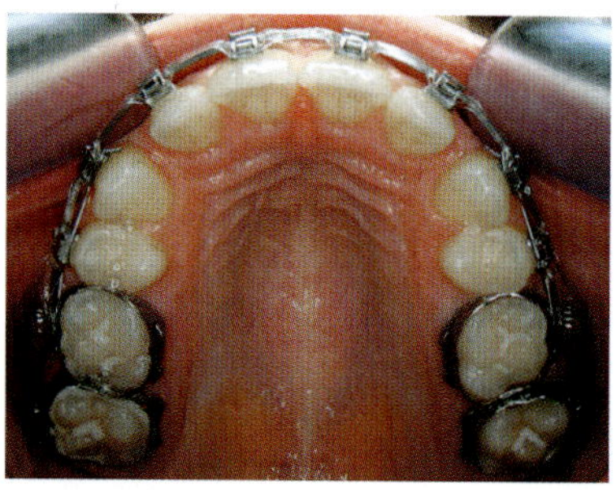

19
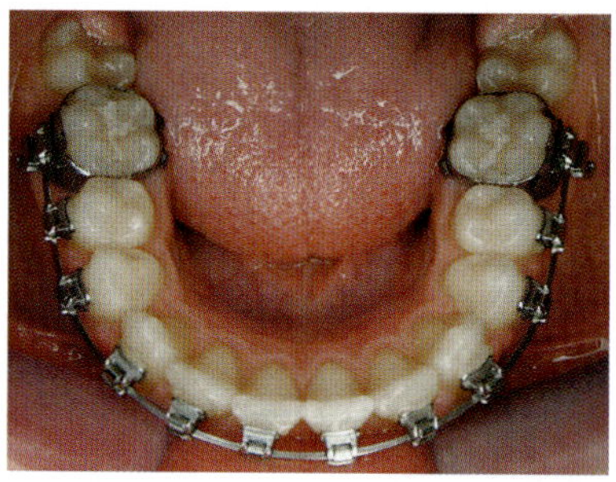

15–19 A mild class III canine relationship, with residual space closure still to follow.

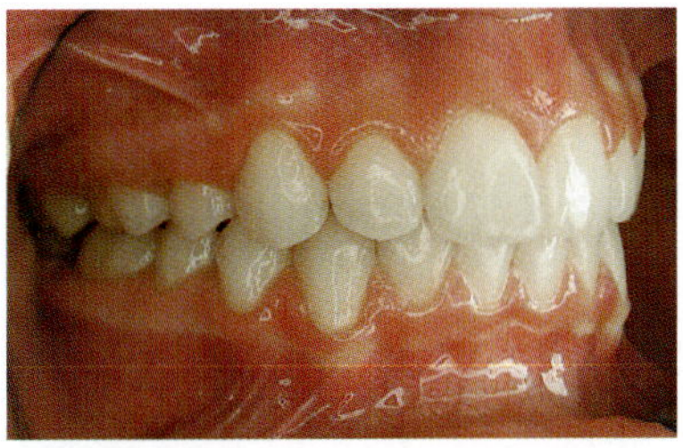
20

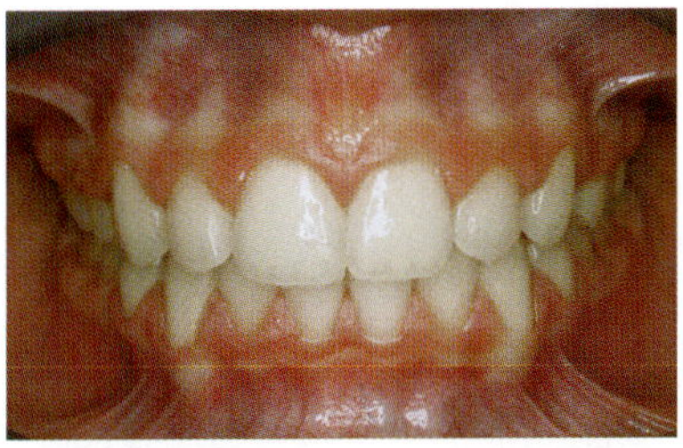
21

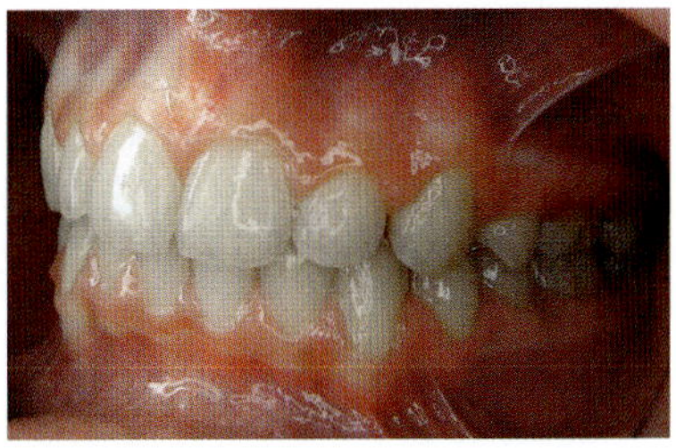
22

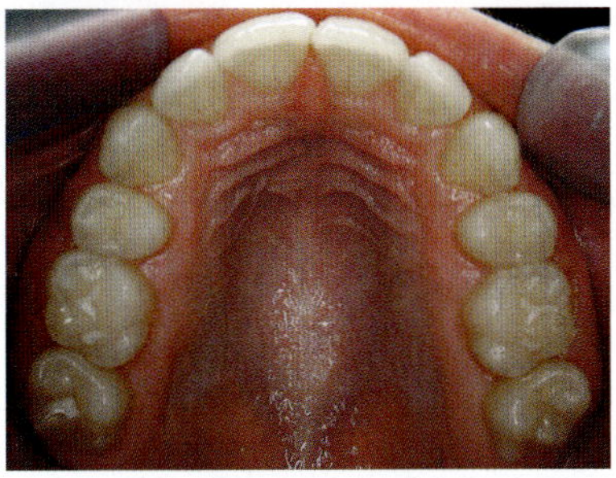
23

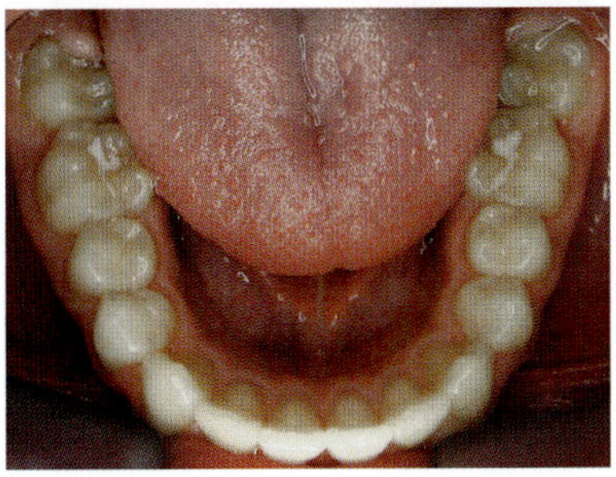
24

20–24 After 1 year of retention with a removable mandibular advancement appliance.

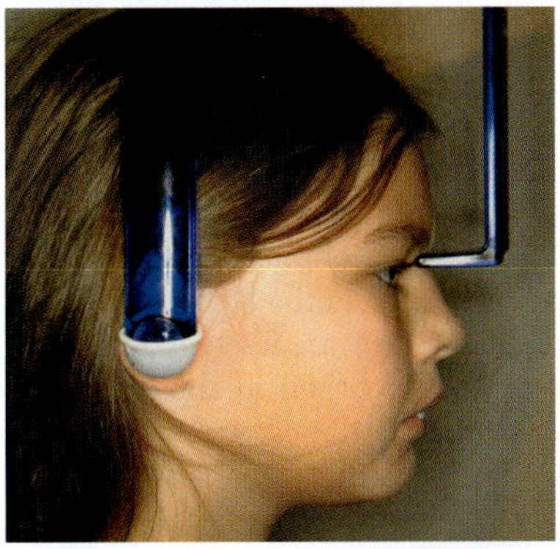
25

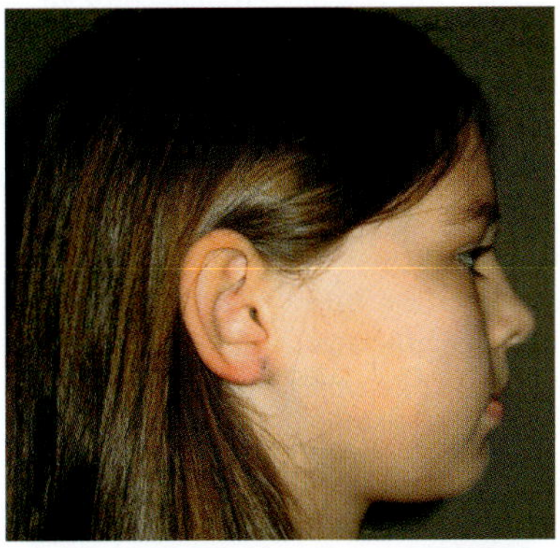
26

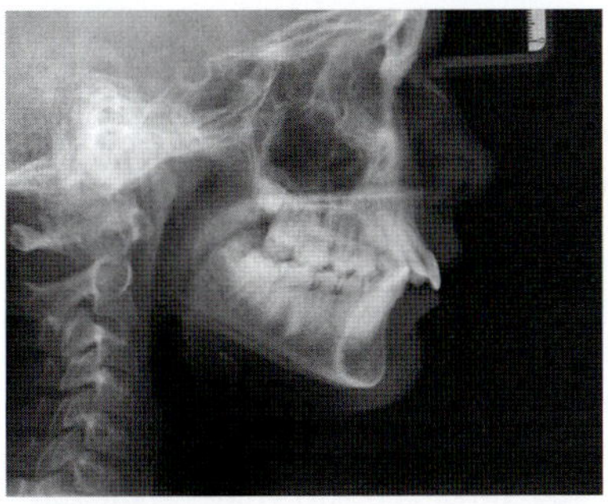
27

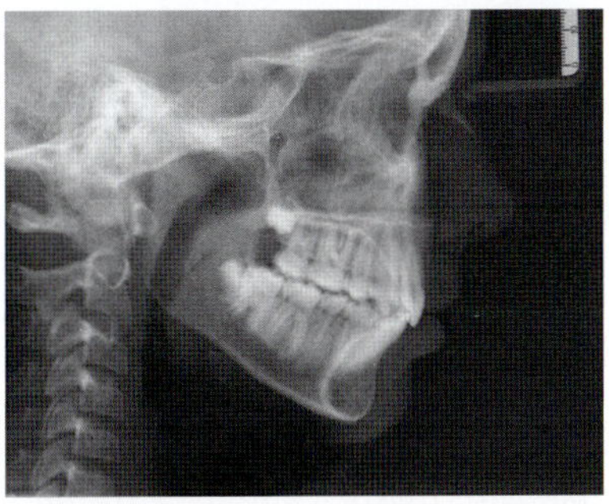
28

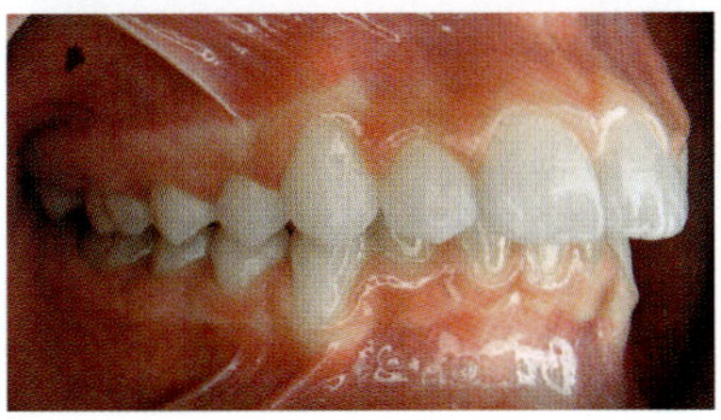
29

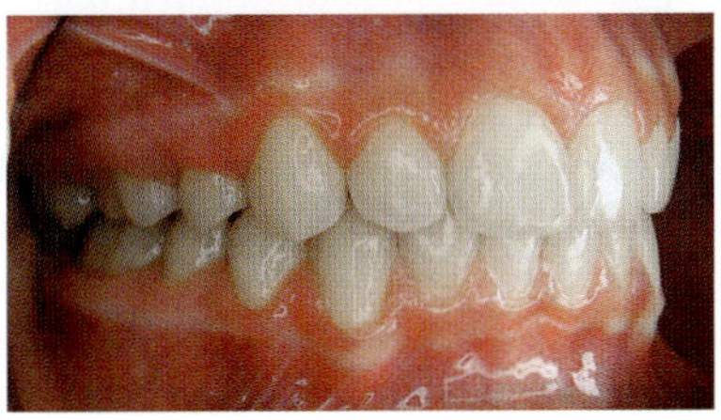
30

25–30 Comparison of the situation before and after treatment: extraoral photographs, cephalometric radiographs, and intraoral photographs.

NOTE

The decision on whether to carry out camouflage treatment for an underlying skeletal base discrepancy (such as the removal of the upper first premolars to compensate for a class II skeletal base) depends on cephalometric analysis including soft and hard tissues, patient preferences and medical history.
In Case Study 7.15, maxillary prognathism rather than mandibular deficiency was diagnosed. We felt that surgical correction by bringing the lower jaw forward was not indicated.
The soft-tissue profile before treatment shows incompetent lips. Before treatment the patient was unable to close her mouth even with pronounced lip straining. The retrusion of the maxillary anterior segment and simultaneous proclination of the mandibular anterior segment led to a very favorable soft-tissue response, with an improvement in the facial profile and competent lips as the final result.

In cases in which premolars have been extracted and space closure follows, a low friction bracket system can be extremely useful. It allows more efficient space closure and retraction of the anterior segment via sliding mechanics. Another option in these cases is to combine active self-ligating brackets in the anterior segment (for improved torque control) and passive self-ligating brackets in the posterior segments for reduced friction. While this will maintain or improve incisor torque, it allows controlled sliding mechanics at reduced force levels, which prevents side effects such as bowing of the archwire.

Space Creation by Interproximal Enamel Reduction (IPR)

Interproximal enamel reduction (IPR or stripping) is a recognized alternative to extraction of teeth in selected cases. The space created for the anterior segments can be between 4 mm and 9 mm per arch.[12,37] According to Fillion, maxillary incisors can be reduced by approximately 0.3 mm for each contact and mandibular incisors by approximately 0.2 mm. Buccal teeth can generally be reduced by 0.6 mm.[8] Sheridan showed that an overall space gain of nearly 6.5 mm can be achieved on a regular basis.[28,29] Reduction of the enamel by about 50% of its original thickness is considered acceptable and does not create long-term problems. This would theoretically allow for more than 9 mm of space to be created in each arch.[30] Neither increased sensitivity of the teeth nor greater susceptibility to developing dental caries has been demonstrated in long-term follow-up studies of patients who underwent this form of treatment. In fact, some authors reported that 10 years after orthodontic treatment with IPR, the irregularity index compared favorably with patients who had undergone orthodontic treatment without IPR.[36] The clinical procedure is described in the section on "Interproximal Enamel Reduction (Stripping)" in Chapter 8.

Correction of Skeletal Discrepancies

Correction of a Class II Buccal Segment Relationship

Based on the findings by Roux that functional occlusal stimuli affect the growth of the maxilla and mandible, Andreesen and Häupl introduced the now-classical concept of functional orthodontics in 1935. Most of the functional appliances were originally removable, and patient compliance was an issue. Adequate wearing time is of paramount importance for achieving the treatment aims, and this issue led to the development of the noncompliance myofunctional systems that are now routinely used in many orthodontic practices. It was the rediscovery of the "Herbst appliance" (originally dating from 1904) by Pancherz in the 1970s that led the way to noncompliance class II correctors during the past 20 years. Other examples of noncompliance functional appliances are the Mandibular Anterior Repositioning Appliance (MARA), the Functional Mandibular Advancer (FMA), and other successors to the Herbst appliance such as the Sabbagh Universal Spring (SUS) and the Forsus spring.
All of these appliances have been used successfully, and they have been extensively described in the literature. Apart from the very effective therapeutic principles, all noncompliance functional appliances can also demonstrate unwanted side effects such as significant proclination of the lower incisors. This is a well-known unwanted side effect that is particularly prevalent with use of Herbst appliances.

Functional Mandibular Advancer

The Functional Mandibular Advancer (FMA) was developed by Kinzinger in 2002 (**Fig. 7.43**).[16,17,19] The concept is similar to the twin-block concept in that it has guide planes that train the mandible forward on final closure, achieving the desired myofunctional effect (see Case Study 7.16). In the FMA, however, the guide planes are positioned buccally and are usually part of a cast framework.

Modification of FMA. During function, the molars that retain the appliance undergo intrusive forces and tipping moments. The mandibular molars, for example, tend to tip mesially, which can lead to proclination of the anterior segment. These effects can be prevented by using skeletal anchorage to maintain the position of the lower molars. A modified cast FMA is currently being developed to allow skeletal anchorage.

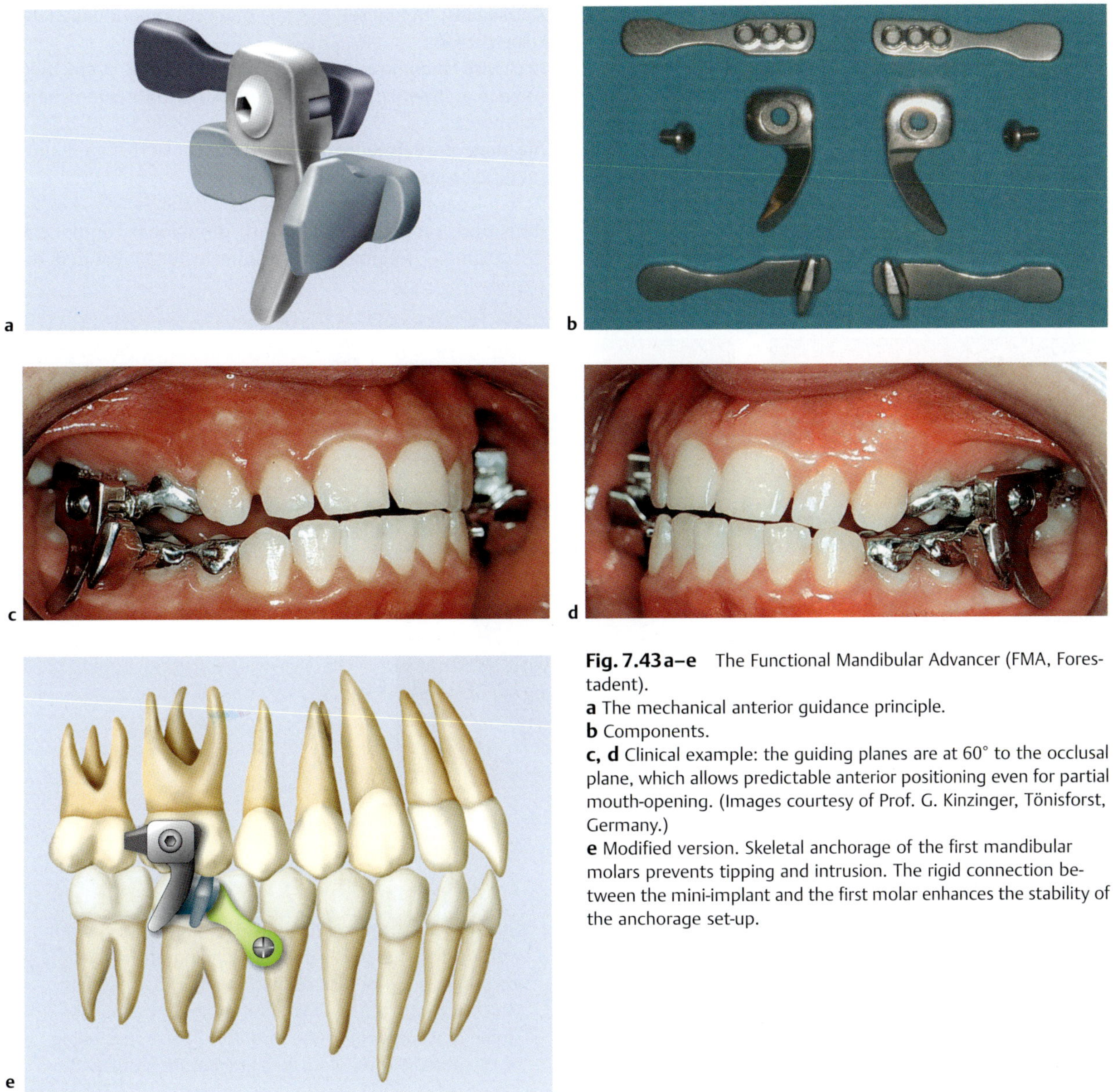

Fig. 7.43 a–e The Functional Mandibular Advancer (FMA, Forestadent).
a The mechanical anterior guidance principle.
b Components.
c, d Clinical example: the guiding planes are at 60° to the occlusal plane, which allows predictable anterior positioning even for partial mouth-opening. (Images courtesy of Prof. G. Kinzinger, Tönisforst, Germany.)
e Modified version. Skeletal anchorage of the first mandibular molars prevents tipping and intrusion. The rigid connection between the mini-implant and the first molar enhances the stability of the anchorage set-up.

Orthodontic mini-implants are inserted distal to the mandibular second premolars to reinforce anchorage of the lower molars. The mini-implants are placed before the impressions for the fabrication of the modified FMA are taken, which allows the implants to be placed in the ideal position. The device is then applied in the post-insertion situation.
After insertion of the mandibular mini-implants, upper and lower alginate impressions and a construction wax bite are taken. The impression of the lower jaw needs to be sufficiently precise to reproduce the position of the mini-implants exactly. The laboratory will then produce a cast design including molar bands, guide planes, and connectors to the mini-implant head (**Fig. 7.43e**). After cementing of the elements, the residual space between the mini-implant head and the connector is filled with a flowable composite.

Case Study 7.16 (Fig. 7.44)

Patient: K.I., female, age 20.
Diagnostic records: models, panoramic radiograph, lateral cephalometric radiograph, intraoral/extraoral photographs.
Main findings: increased overjet, asymmetric occlusion with mandibular midline deviation to the right.
Treatment aims: establish bilateral class I occlusion and coincident midlines using the Functional Mandibular Advancer (FMA).
Appliances: lingual self-ligating brackets, individually fabricated FMA.
Archwire sequence: 0.012 SE and 0.016 SE preformed lingual archwires, 0.016 SS and 0.018 SS custom-bent archwires.
Alternative treatment strategy: different Herbst appliance modifications, orthognathic surgery.
Active treatment time: 14 months.
Retention: vector retention with directional component (for example, retainer with a built-in FMA), bonded retainer.

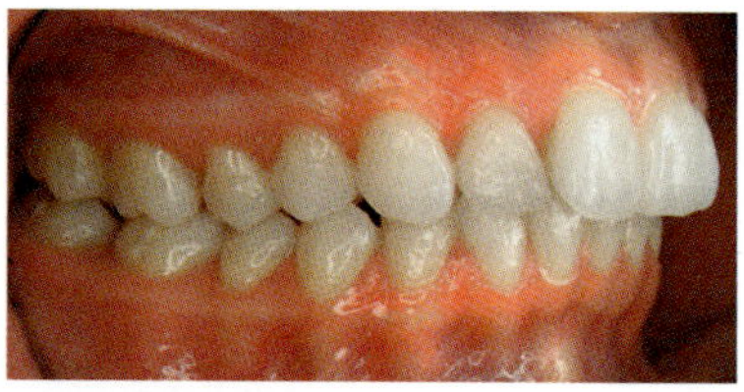
1
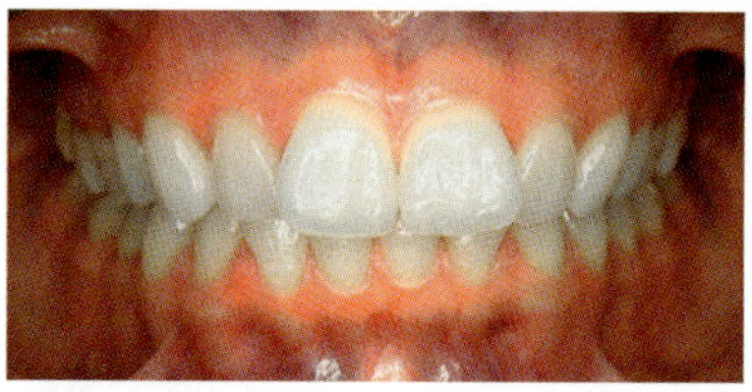
2
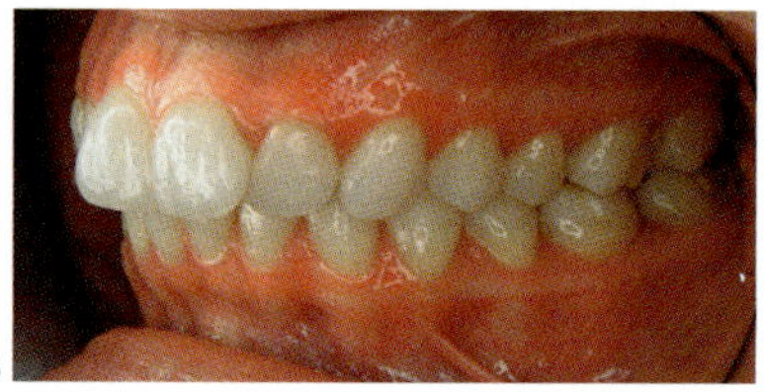
3
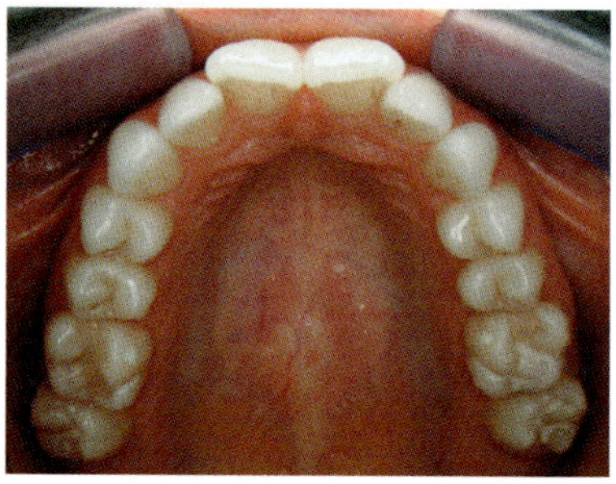
4
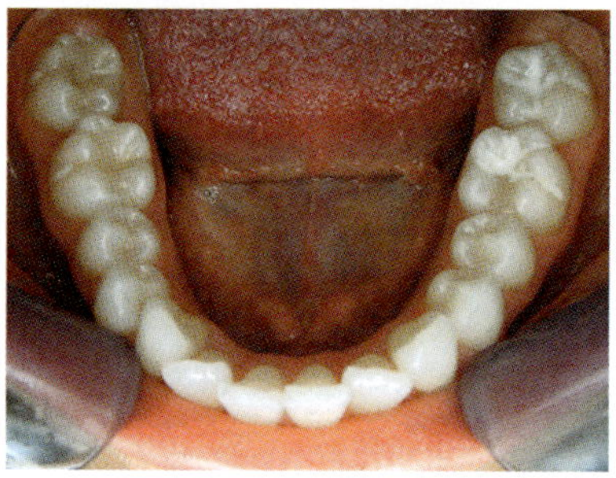
5

Fig. 7.44 1–20
1–5 Before treatment: maxillary and mandibular anterior crowding. Class II on the right, with mandibular shift.

CLINICAL PEARL

Careful diagnosis of the masticatory apparatus, including palpation of the muscles of mastication and the temporomandibular joint, should form part of the initial diagnostic work-up in all patients, particularly when a temporomandibular disorder is suspected. The clinical diagnosis can be supported by diagnostic imaging (magnetic resonance imaging). This patient presented with postero-superiorly directed loading of the joint, leading to anterior disk displacement with reduction, which was revealed by MRI. The treatment aim was stable repositioning of the disk. Anterior repositioning of the mandible should lead to recapturing of the disk.

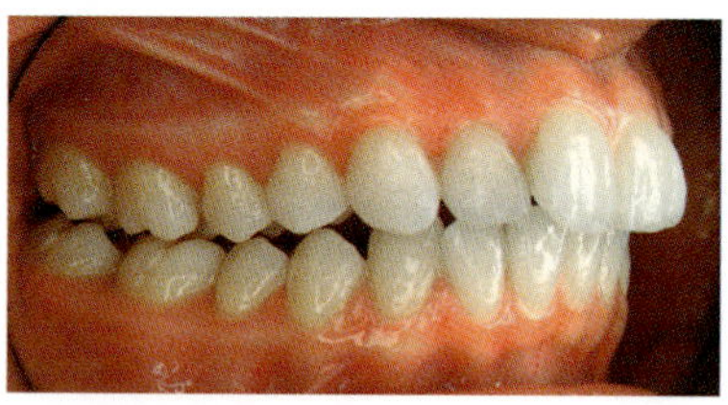
6
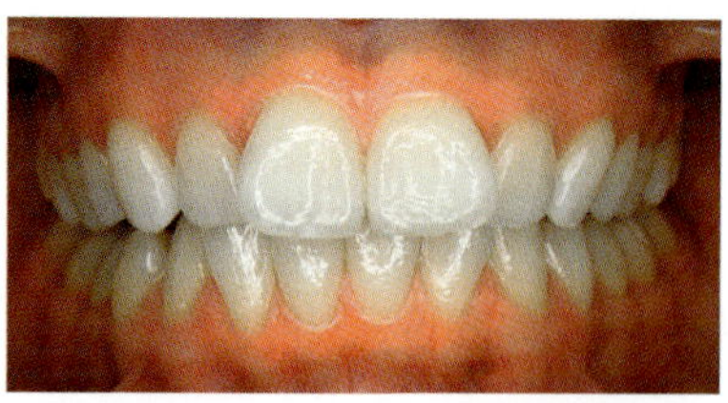
7
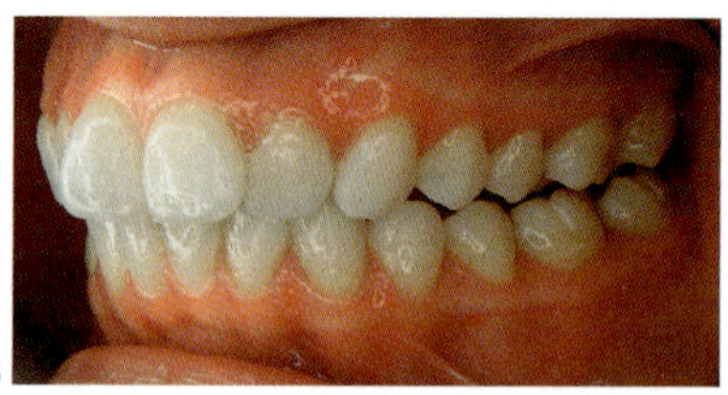
8
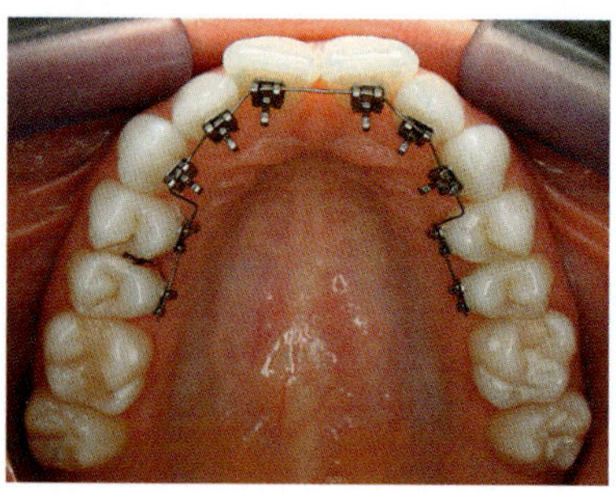
9
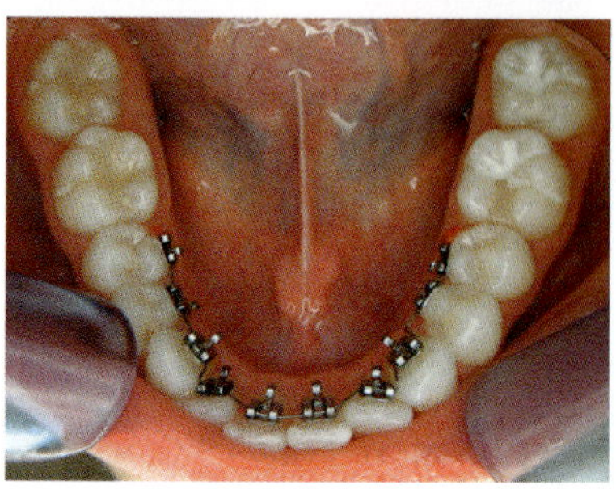
10

6–10 Lingual self-ligating brackets from 5 to 5 with a preformed 0.012 SE lingual archwire.

Clinical pearl:
Initial decompensation through leveling and aligning will reveal the full extent of the underlying skeletal discrepancy. The occlusion is subsequently corrected.

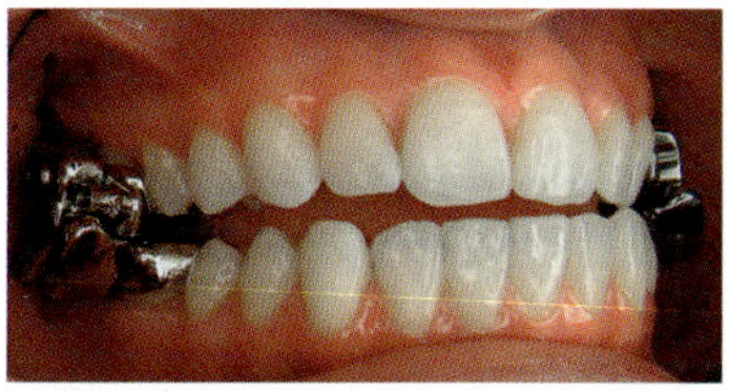
11

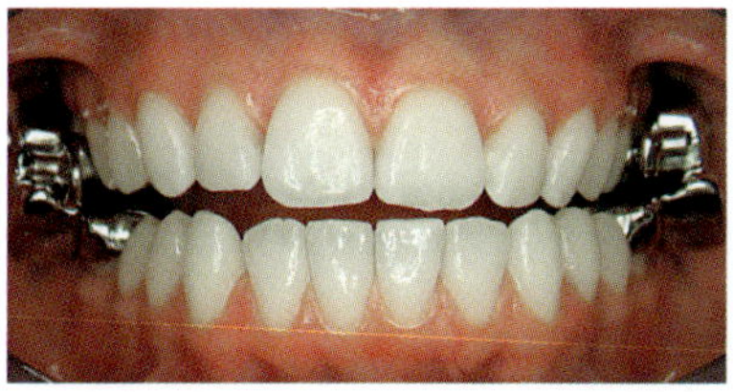
12

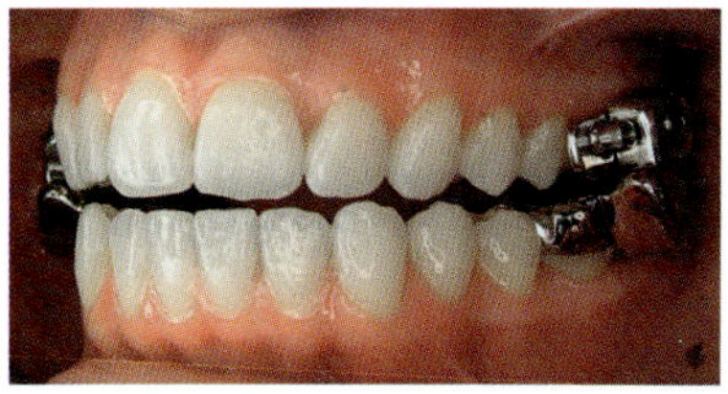
13

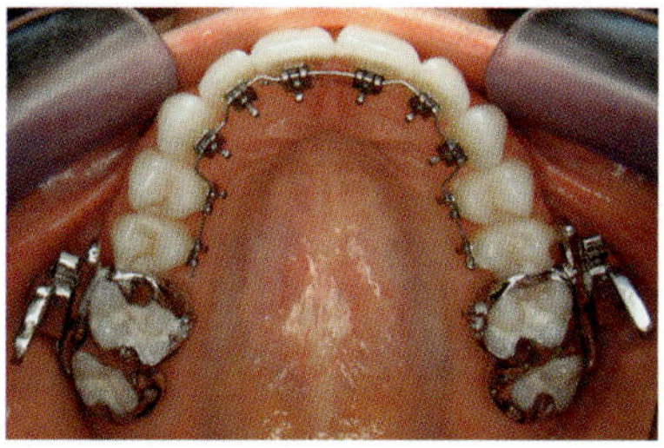
14

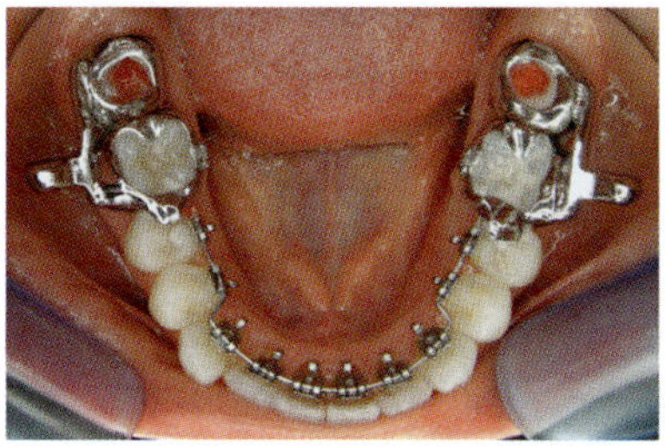
15

11–15 A custom 0.016 stainless-steel archwire.

Clinical pearl:
After insertion of the mandibular advancement appliance, proper function in the protruded position needs to be practiced with the patient.

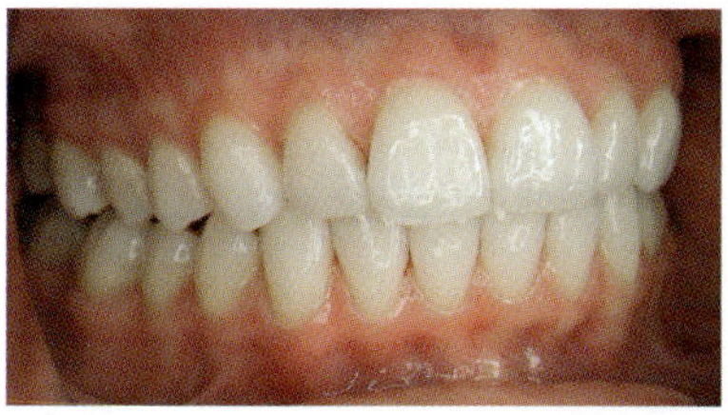
16

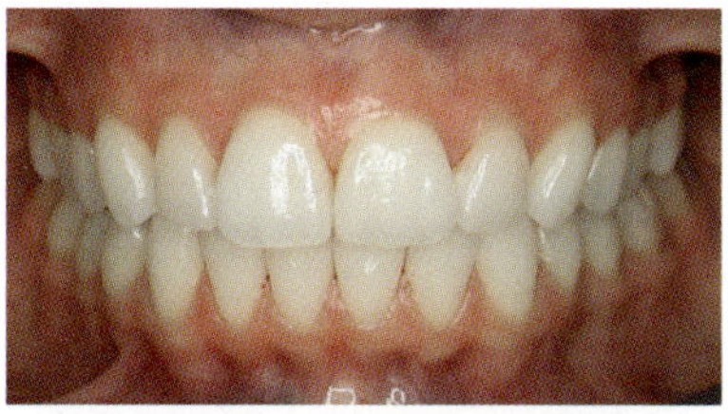
17

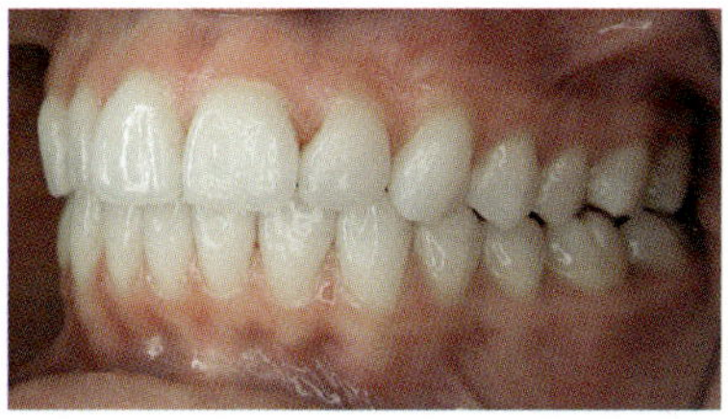
18

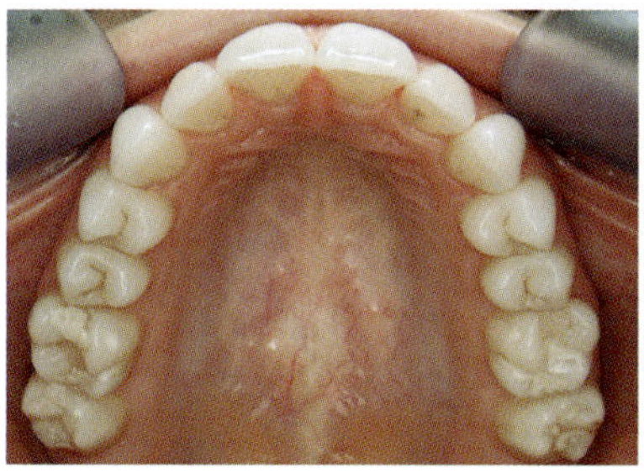
19

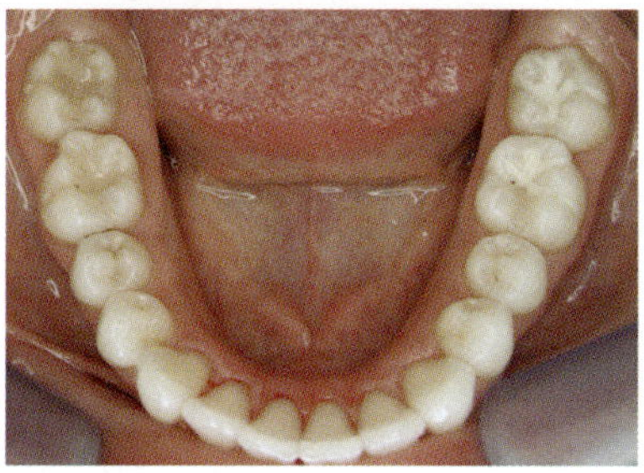
20

16–20 Final result (on the day the appliance was removed).

CLINICAL PEARL

Class II elastics are worn in order to maintain the results. Buccal cleats are bonded to the lower molars, and the elastics are suspended from the lingual brackets on 13 and 23 to the molar cleats which are easy to reach.

Easy-Fit Jumper

Most bite-jumping techniques use prefabricated parts, which are available in a number of sizes to reflect the physiological requirements of individual patients. Recognizing the problem of increased inventory and reactivation, Williams subsequently developed a system with continuous activation in which one size fits all (**Fig. 7.45**). This means that initial measurement of the space requirements is not necessary for fitting the system. The system is marketed as the Easy-Fit Jumper (Forestadent) (see Case Study 7.17). An appliance with similar properties is the SUS 2 (Sabbagh Universal Spring, Dentaurum).

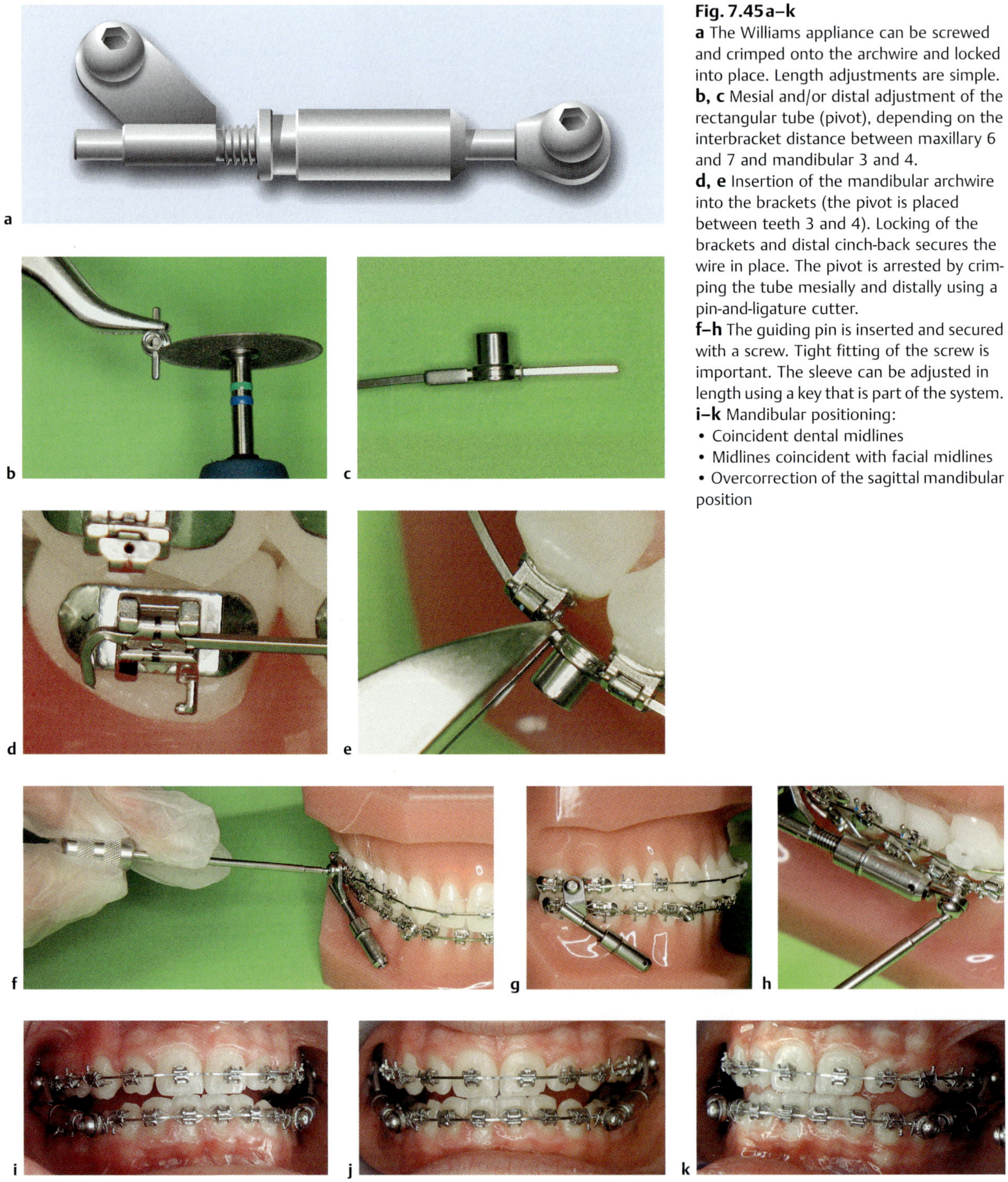

Fig. 7.45 a–k
a The Williams appliance can be screwed and crimped onto the archwire and locked into place. Length adjustments are simple.
b, c Mesial and/or distal adjustment of the rectangular tube (pivot), depending on the interbracket distance between maxillary 6 and 7 and mandibular 3 and 4.
d, e Insertion of the mandibular archwire into the brackets (the pivot is placed between teeth 3 and 4). Locking of the brackets and distal cinch-back secures the wire in place. The pivot is arrested by crimping the tube mesially and distally using a pin-and-ligature cutter.
f–h The guiding pin is inserted and secured with a screw. Tight fitting of the screw is important. The sleeve can be adjusted in length using a key that is part of the system.
i–k Mandibular positioning:

- Coincident dental midlines
- Midlines coincident with facial midlines
- Overcorrection of the sagittal mandibular position

Case Study 7.17 (Fig. 7.46)

Patient: L.P.S, female, age 13.

Diagnostic records: models, panoramic radiograph, lateral cephalometric radiograph, intraoral/extraoral photographs.

Main findings: class $II/_2$, with a 100% deep bite and retrognathic mandible, tooth 42 completely blocked out lingually.

Treatment aims: creating space for tooth 42, deep bite correction, and jumping the bite.

Appliances: self-ligating brackets, molar bands, Easy-Fit Jumper.

Archwire sequence: 0.012 SE, 0.016 SE, 0.016 SS, 0.016 × 0.022 SE, 0.018 × 0.025 SE, 0.019 × 0.025 SS.

Alternative treatment strategy: maxillary first premolar extraction, orthognathic surgery after cessation of growth.

Active treatment time: 15 months.

Retention: functional retention (twin-block modification, later removal of the advancement components possible).

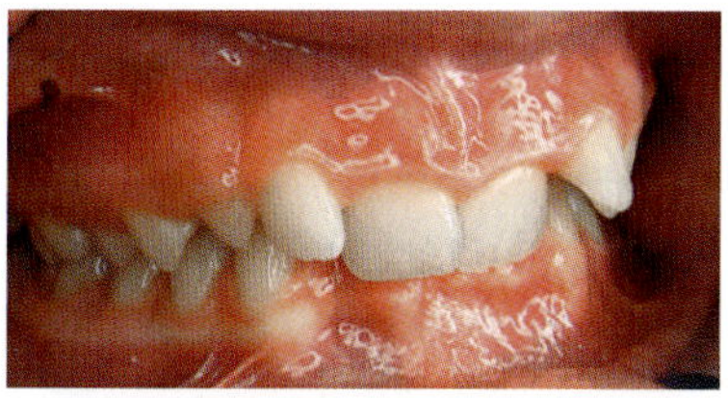
1
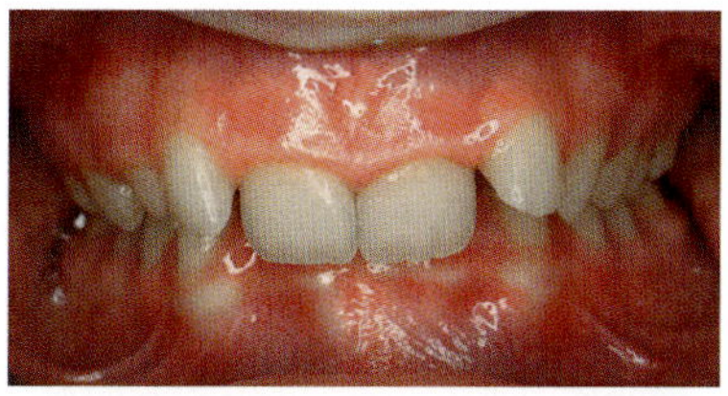
2
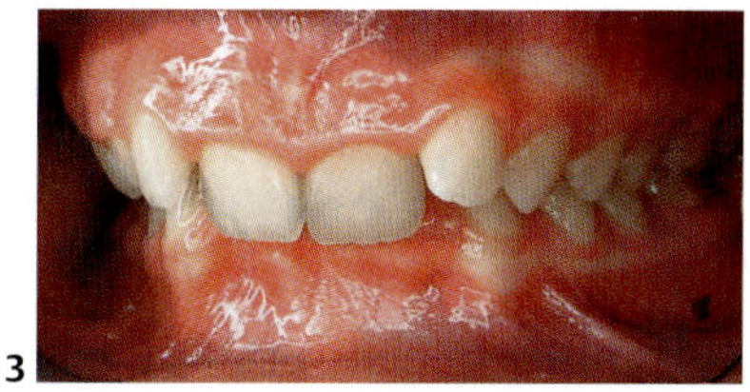
3
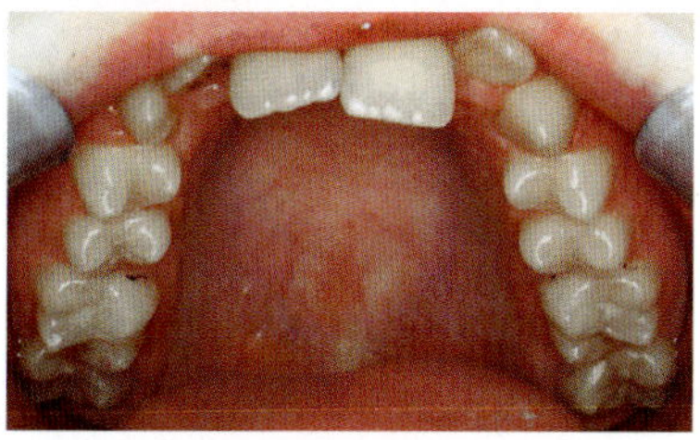
4
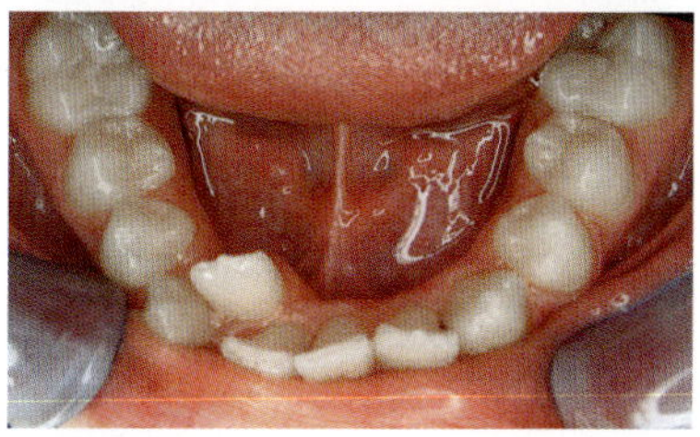
5

Fig. 7.46 1–32
1–5 The situation before treatment: overeruption and retroclination of the maxillary central incisors; mandibular crowding and lingually displaced 42. The dental and skeletal relationships are class II.

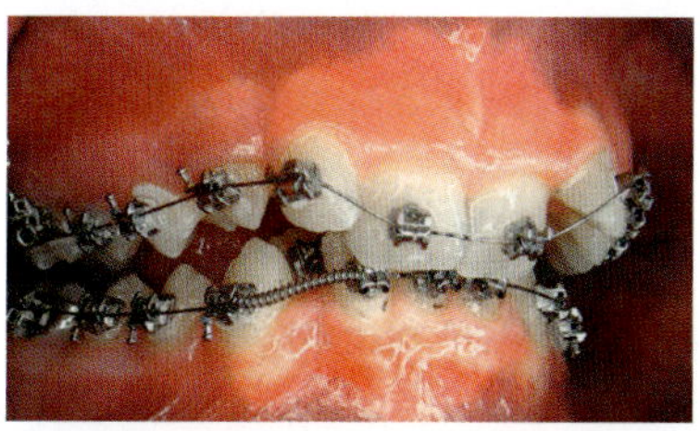
6
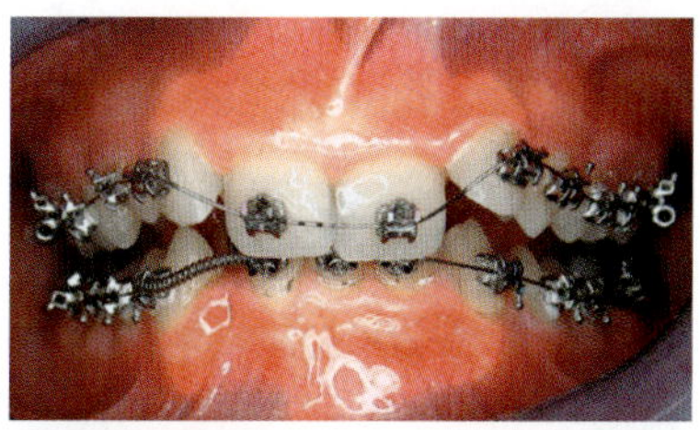
7
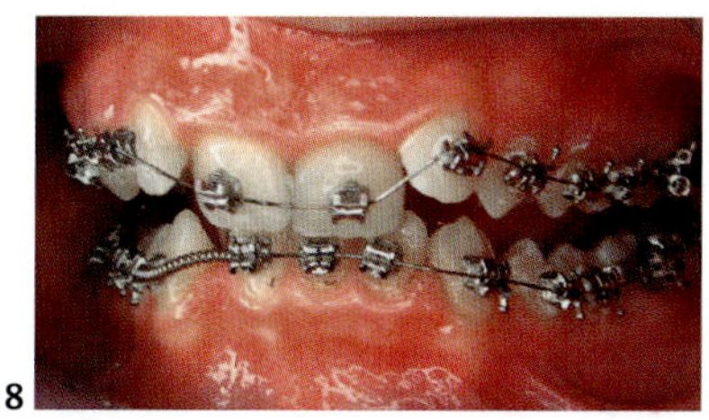
8
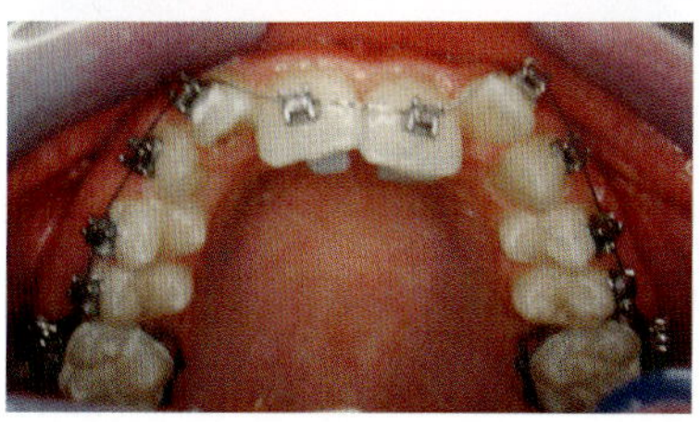
9
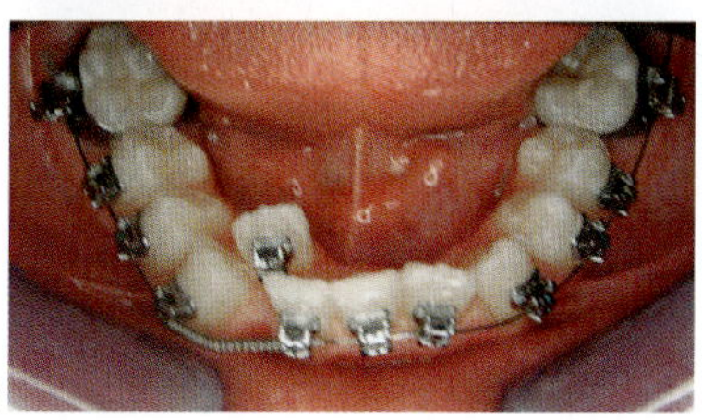
10

6–10 Self-ligating brackets and molar bands; a 0.012 SE archwire is inserted.

11 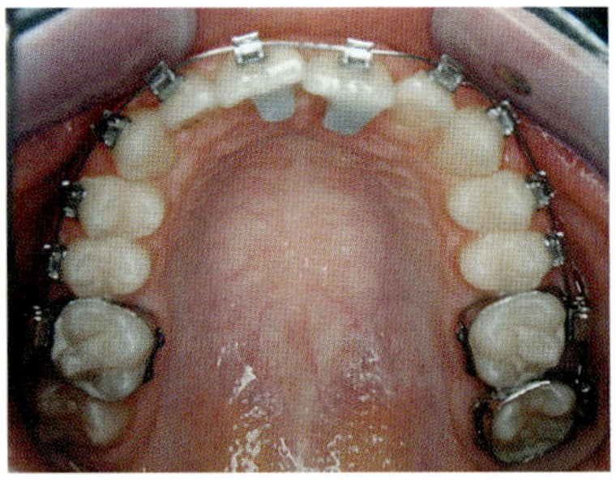
12 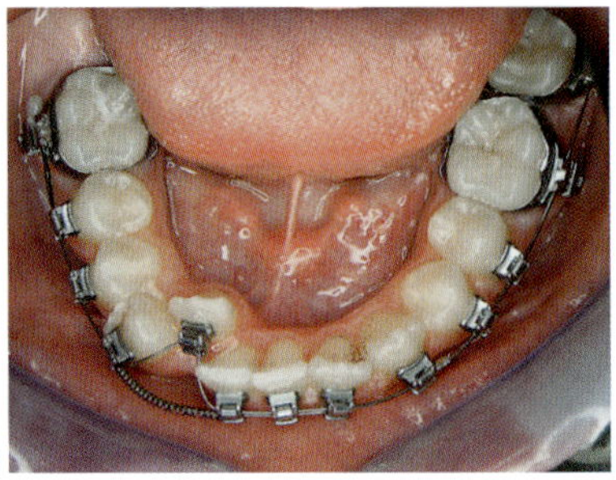
13 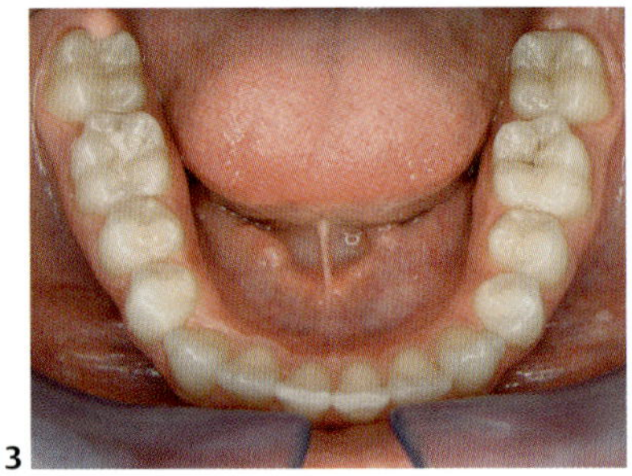

11–13

Clinical pearl:
Apart from "unlocking" the bite, palatal bite-blocks on the maxillary central incisors support protrusion and intrusion of those teeth. A light piggyback archwire brings the mandibular right lateral incisor forward; the space is opened simultaneously with a coil-spring.

14 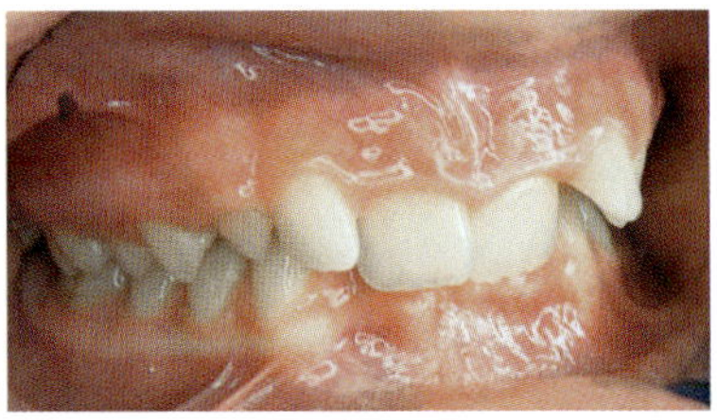
15 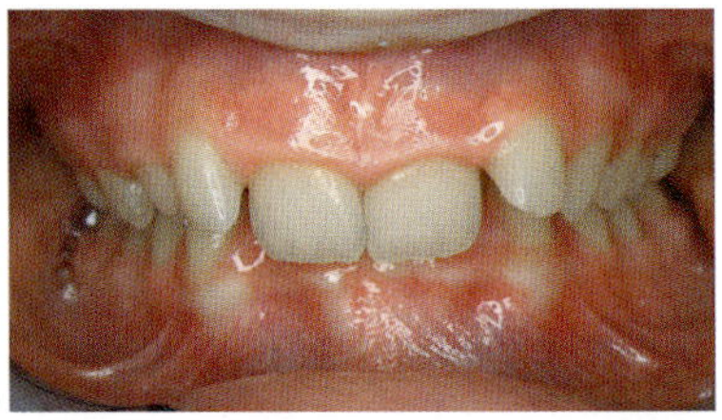
16 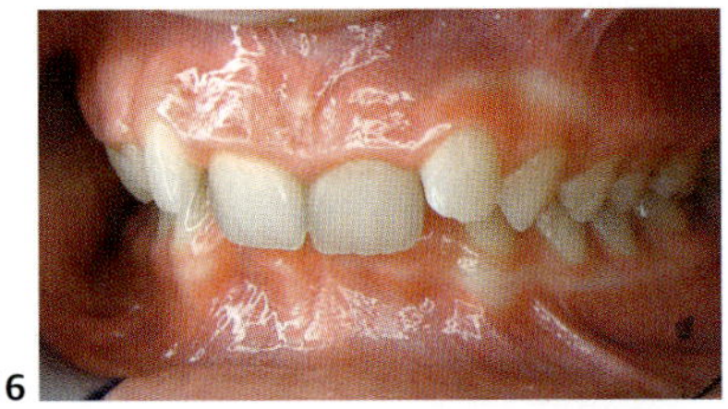
17 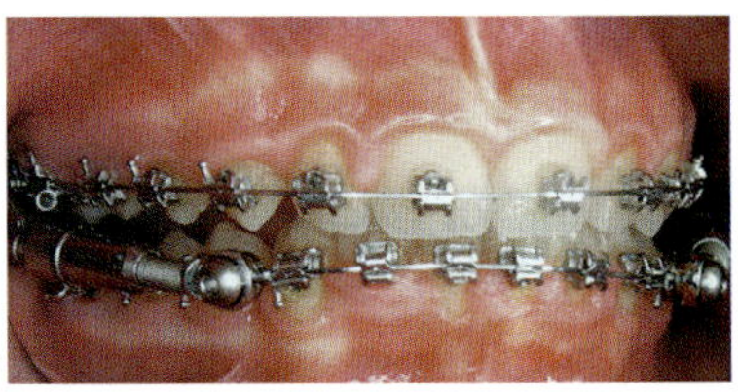
18 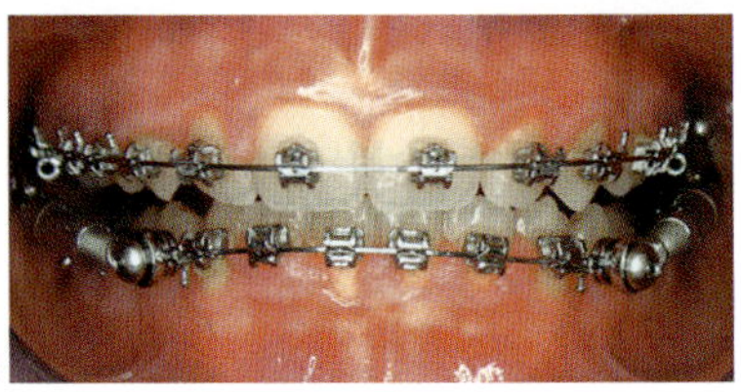
19 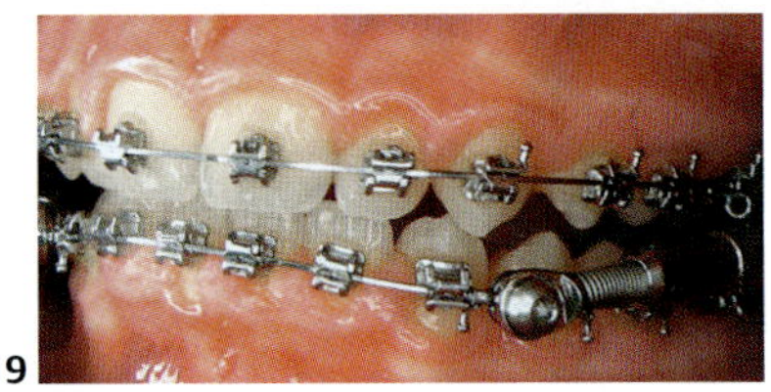

14–19 After initial leveling and alignment, the Easy-Fit Jumper (Williams appliance) was inserted for 6 months.

20 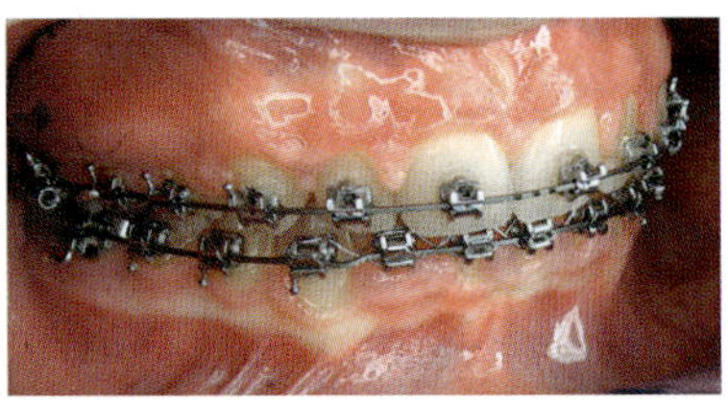
21 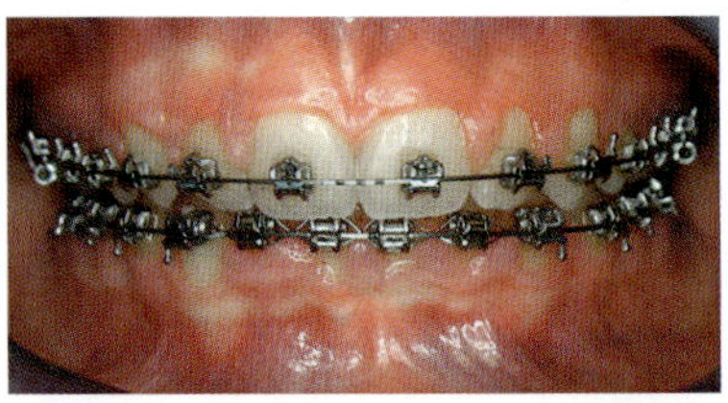
22 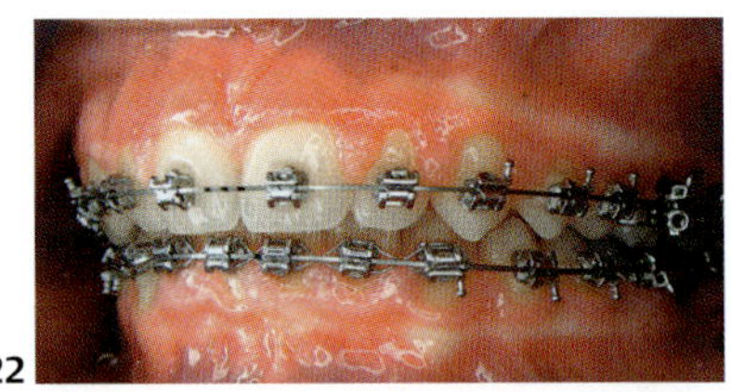
23 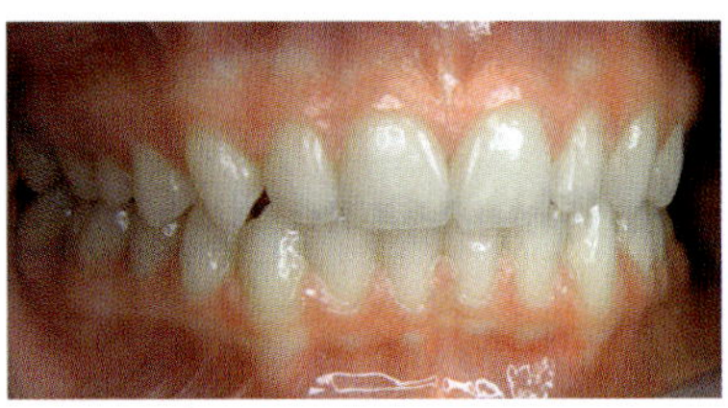
24 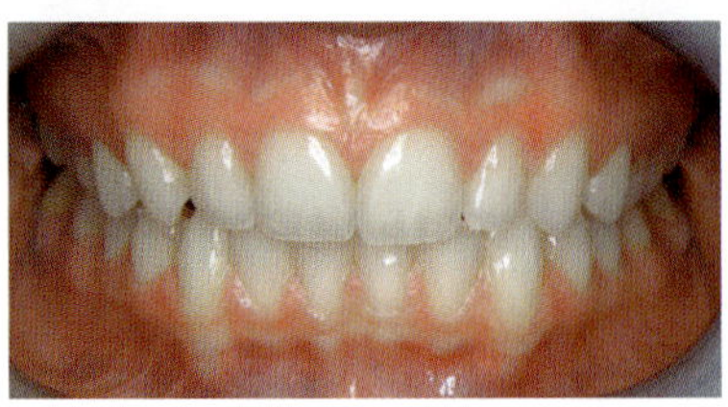
25 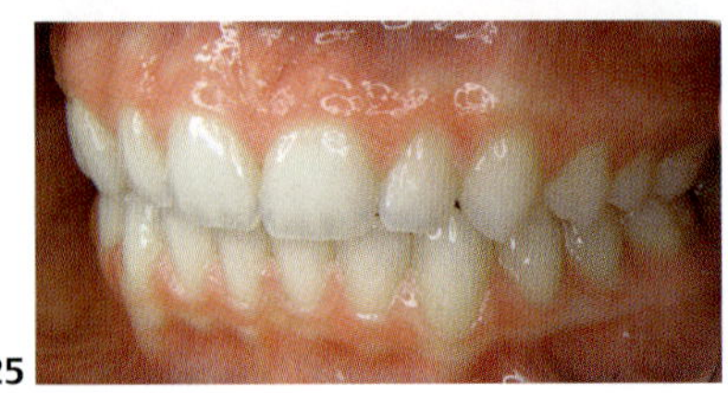

20–25 The final result immediately before debonding, and post-treatment stability due to functional retention with a modified twin-block appliance.

26
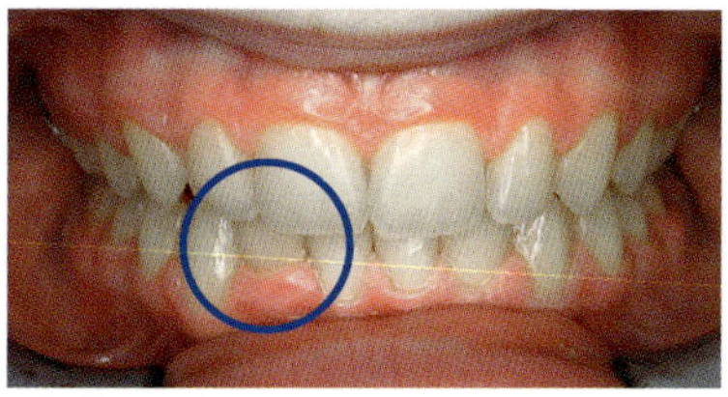
27
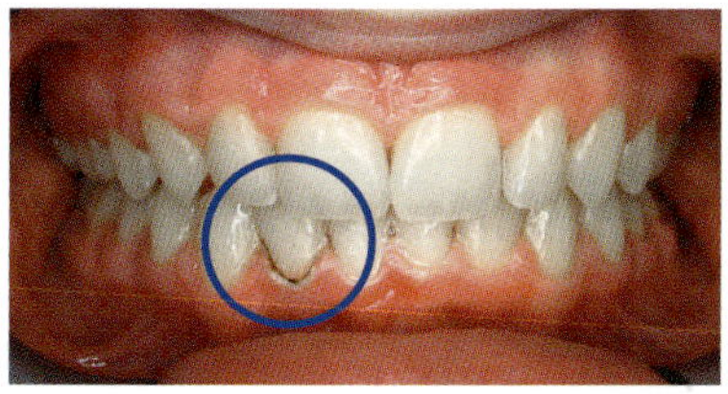
28
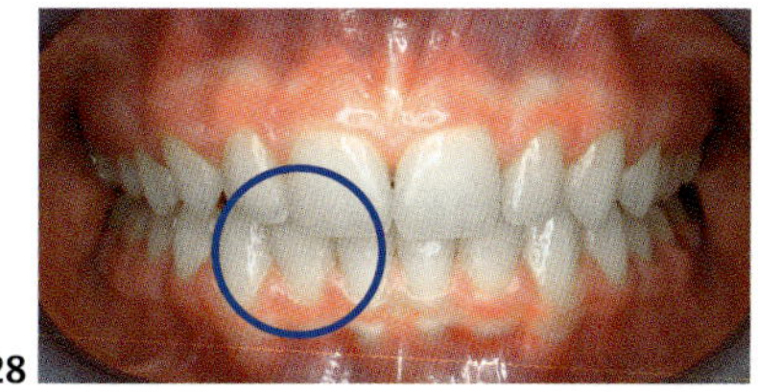

26–28 Esthetic improvement after gingival contouring of the previously lingually excluded 42.

29
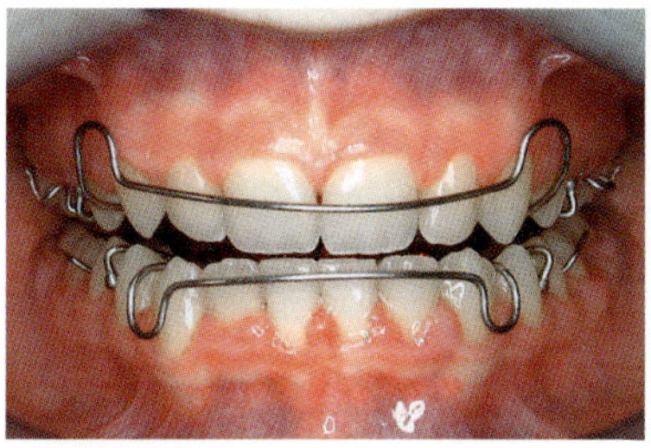
30
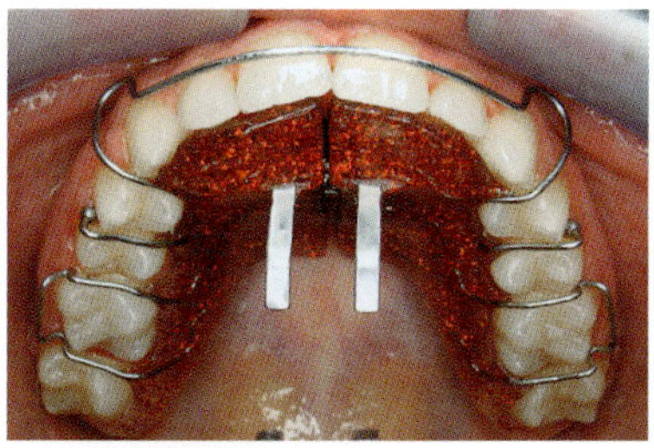

29, 30 Schwarz protusion plate for three-dimensional retention of the final result.

Errors and risks:
A myofunctional appliance was used as a retention device, due to the high risk of relapse of the class II correction.

31
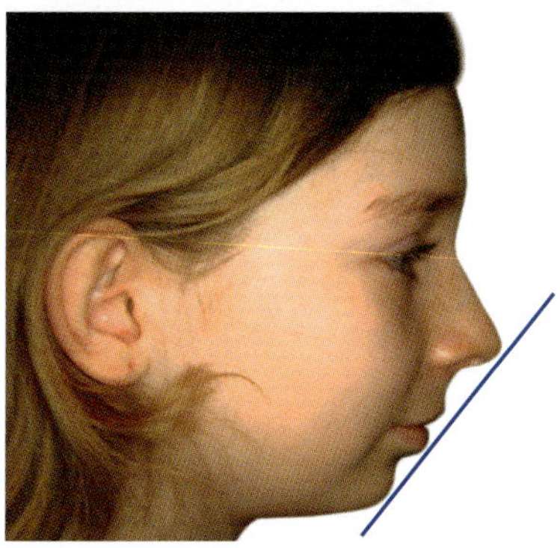
32
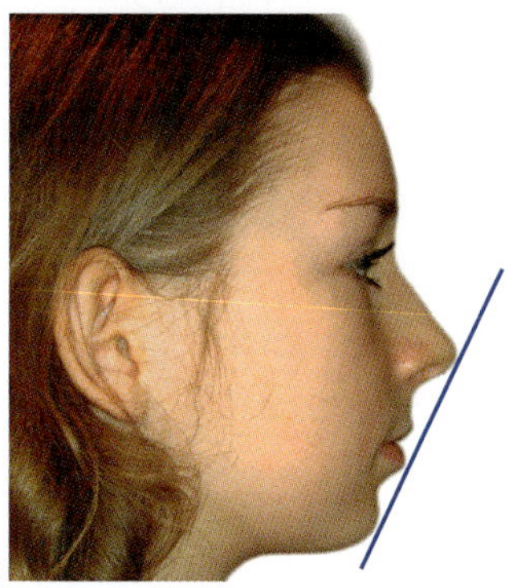

31–32 Marked improvement on both the sagittal and vertical planes.

Correction of Class III Malocclusions

The prognosis of class III treatment needs to be carefully evaluated, as it depends on a number of etiological and hereditary factors. From an etiological point of view, it is important to distinguish whether the class III malocclusion is due to a hypoplastic maxilla, a hyperplastic mandible, or a combination of the two.

Genetically predetermined enlargement of the lower jaw is particularly difficult to treat using orthodontic camouflage. The skeletal relationships often deteriorate during the pubertal growth spurt, and it seems impossible to estimate future mandibular development. In these cases, only serial superimpositions of the cephalogram can determine whether growth is slowing or has stopped. Orthognathic surgery can be considered once growth has largely been completed and the growth spurt has ceased. However, even if a mandibular set-back is planned at a later time point, orthopedic development of the maxilla and midface should be attempted in order to correct problems such as a maxillary transverse deficiency or malar deficiency with reduced cheek prominence.

Transverse discrepancies can be treated using skeletal expansion, as described in the previous section on "Space Creation by Expansion of Arches." This is usually undertaken with a rapid maxillary expansion device such as the hybrid rapid palatal expander. After expansion and distraction of the midpalatal suture, it is thought that all the maxillary sutures will have loosened and that it will be easier to treat a hypoplastic maxilla orthopedically—although this concept has been questioned. The ideal time point for applying a face mask is either during or immediately after expansion of the maxilla. According to a number of studies, mainly based on cephalometrics, a sagittal maxillary traction device can be used in patients up to 12 years of age. However, some operators extend this recommendation to older age groups; patients need to be carefully informed about the potential for relapse, regardless of age group.

Case Study 7.18 (Fig. 7.47)

Patient: Y.M., male, age 14.

Diagnostic records: models, panoramic radiograph, lateral cephalometric radiograph, intraoral/extraoral photographs.

Main findings: skeletal class III with maxillary deficiency.

Treatment aims: rapid palatal expansion and maxillary protraction.

Appliances: self-ligating brackets, molar bands, mini-implants, hybrid rapid palatal enlargement (RPE), Delaire-type protraction facemask.

Archwire sequence: 0.012 SE, 0.016 SE, 0.016 SS, 0.016 × 0.022 SE, 0.018 × 0.025 SE, 0.019 × 0.025 SS.

Alternative treatment strategy: traditional RPE.

Active treatment time: 12 months.

Retention: three-dimensional retention.

1
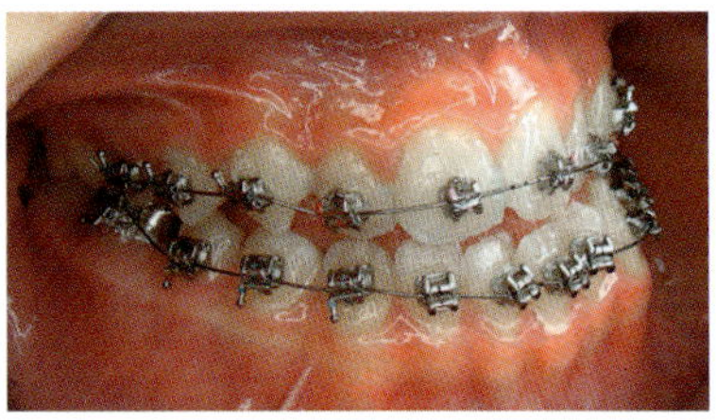
2
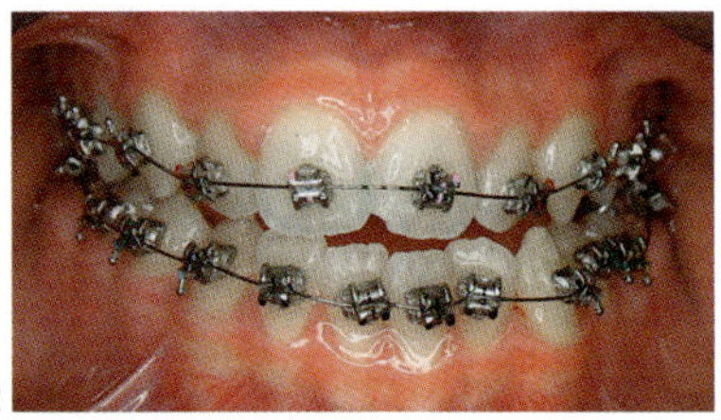
3
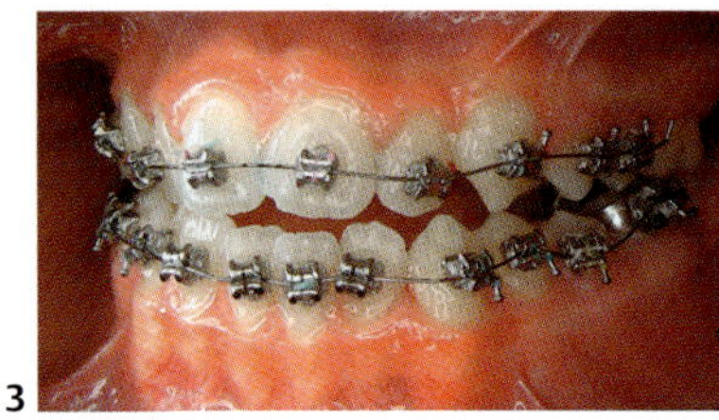
4
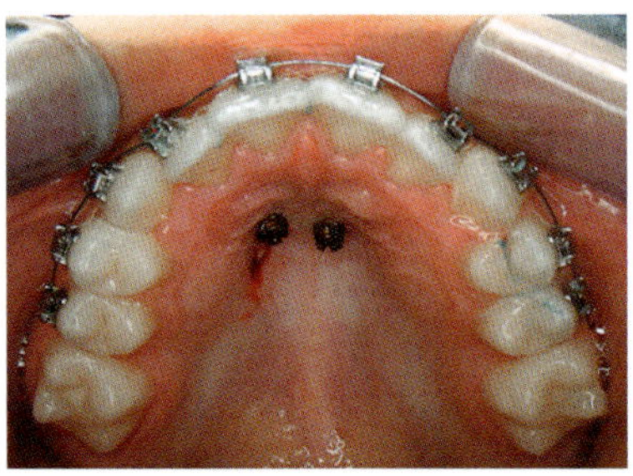
5
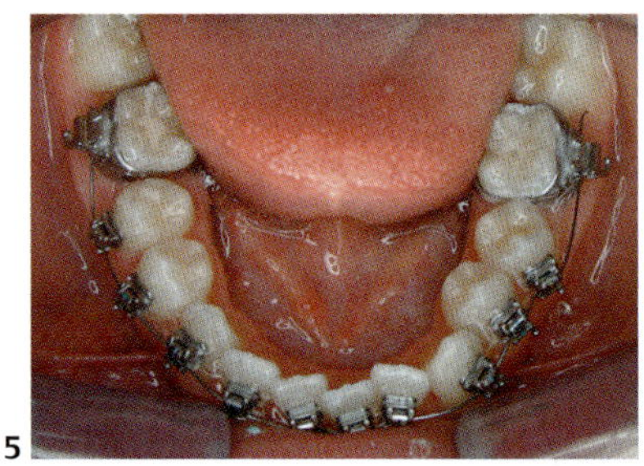

Fig. 7.47 1–23
1–5 Self-ligating brackets, 0.012 SE archwire, mini-implants in place.

6
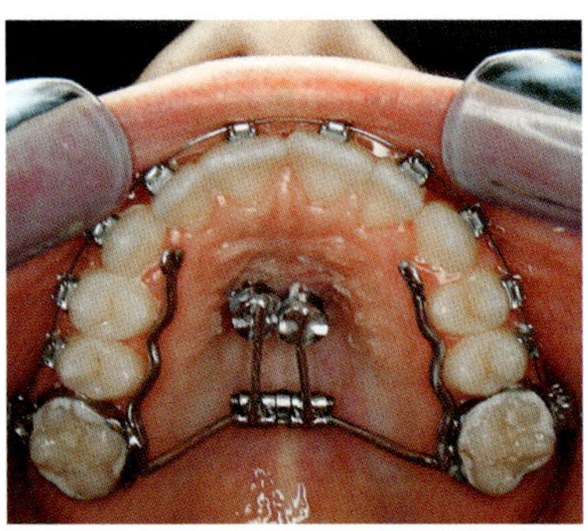
7
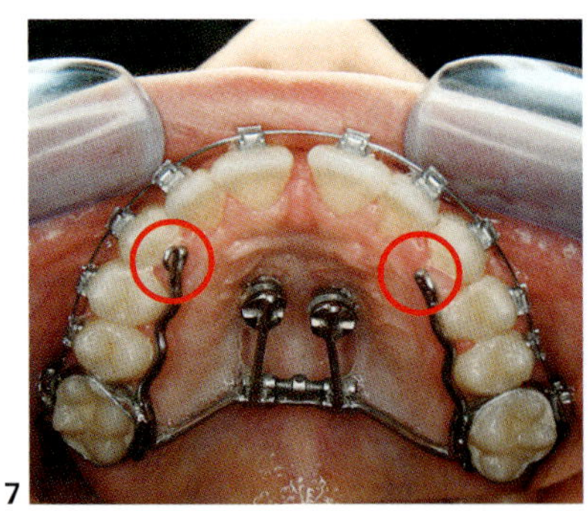
8
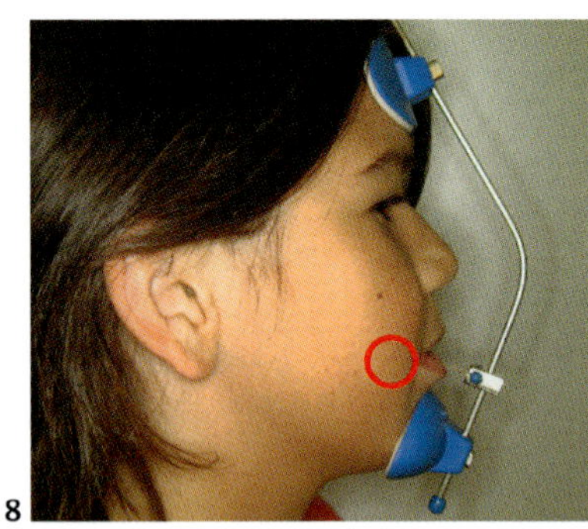

6 Hybrid rapid palatal enlarger (RPE) placed.

7 The hybrid RPE after 12 days of expansion. It has palatal extension arms with anterior hooks welded in place to attach the elastics for maxillary protraction.

8 The protraction facemask is connected to the hybrid RPE (¼, 6 oz) for 24 hours.

ERRORS AND RISKS

Fixed-appliance treatment alone would decompensate the occlusion and would have led to worsening of the class III relationship; the facemask treatment allowed for compensation.

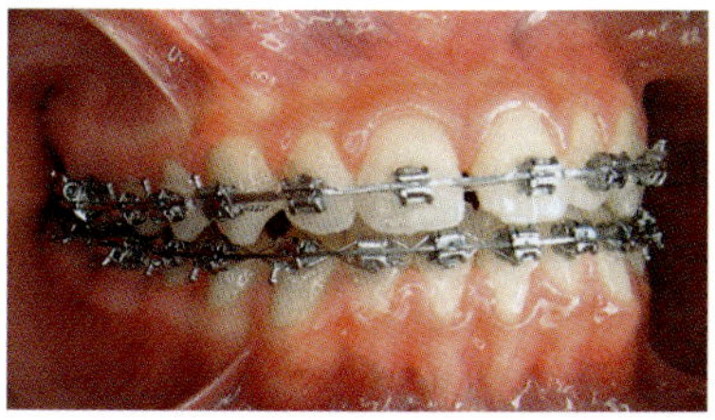
9
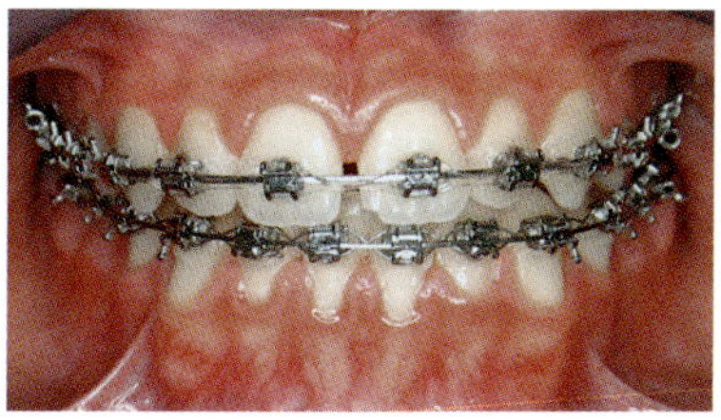
10
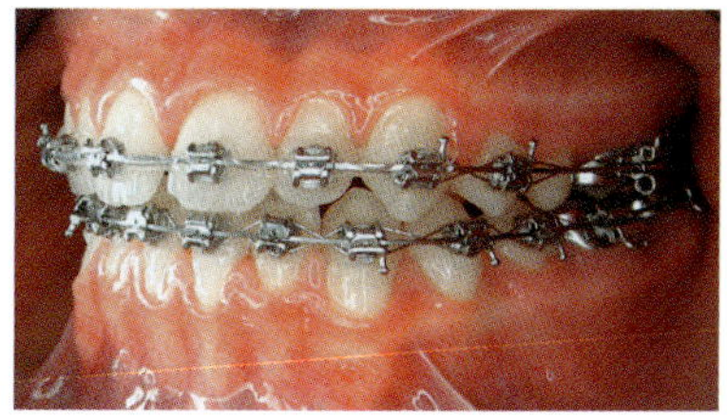
11

9–11 Almost ideal conditions 5 months into treatment.

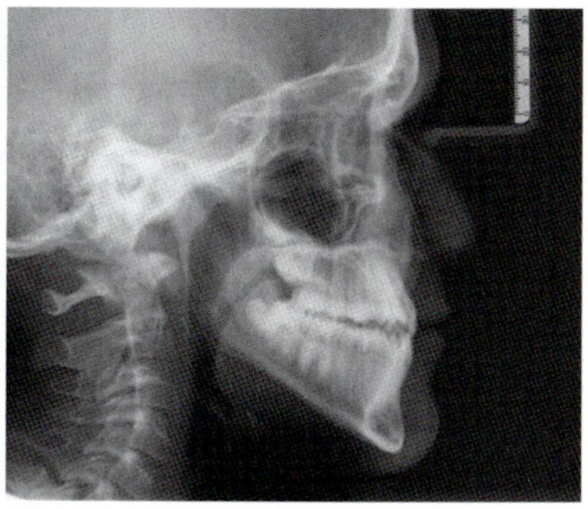
12
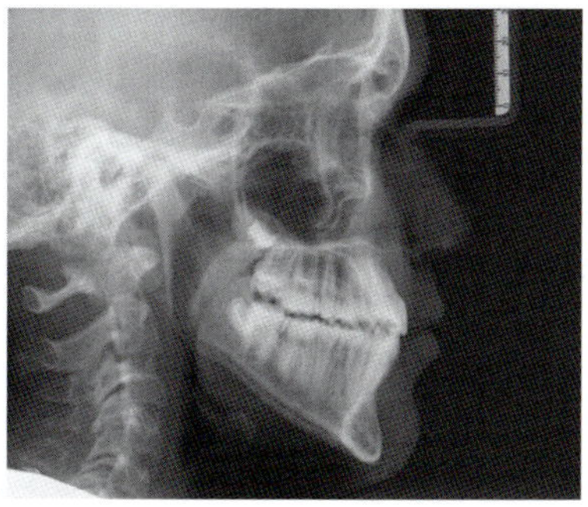
13

12, 13 The maxillary and mandibular incisors were flared as a result of treatment. However, a class I relationship was established with maxillary traction.

ERRORS AND RISKS

The diagnostic records suggest a continuation of the unfavorable growth pattern. Treatment objectives therefore have to be clearly set, and patients need to be informed about the possibility of a compromised result or the need for surgical correction of the skeletal problem.

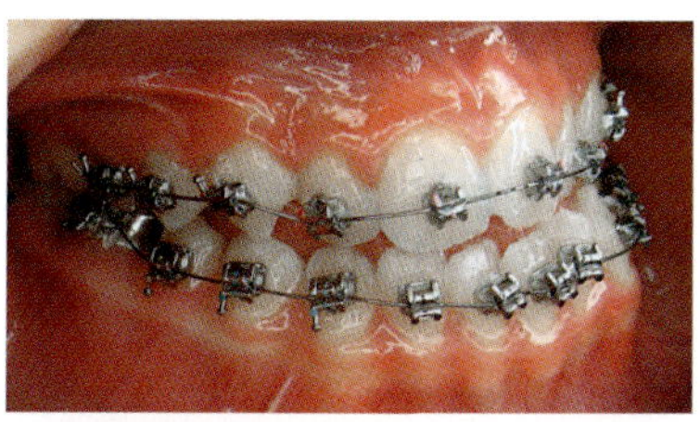
14
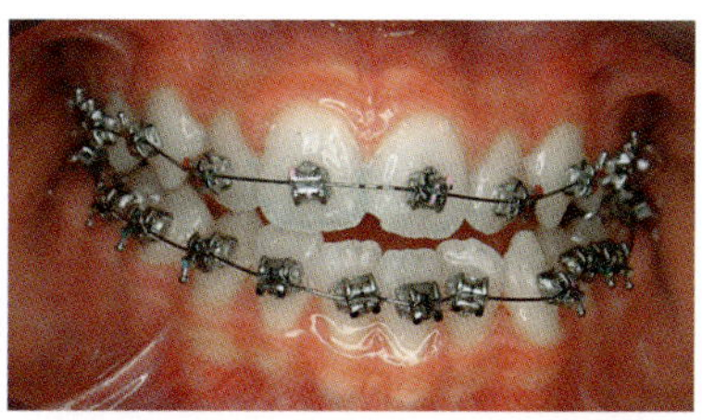
15
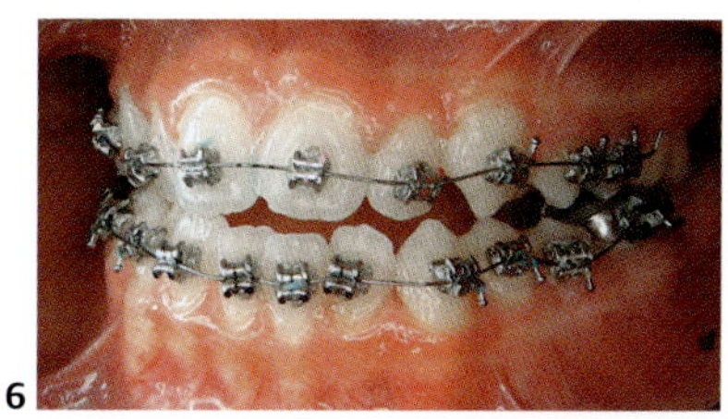
16
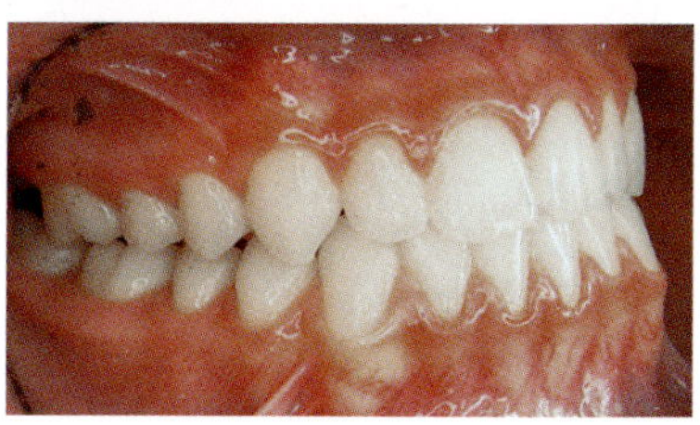
17
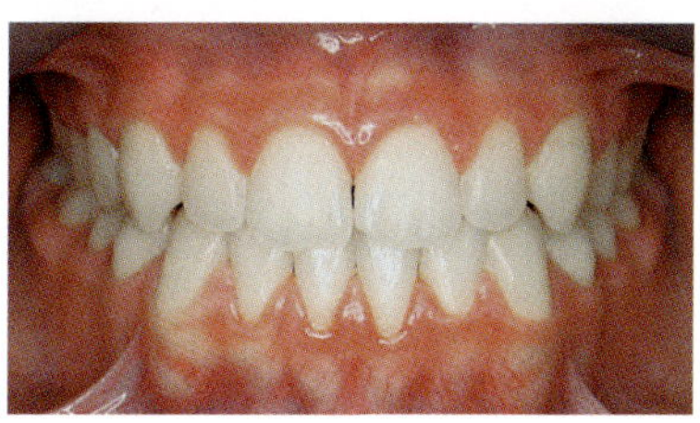
18
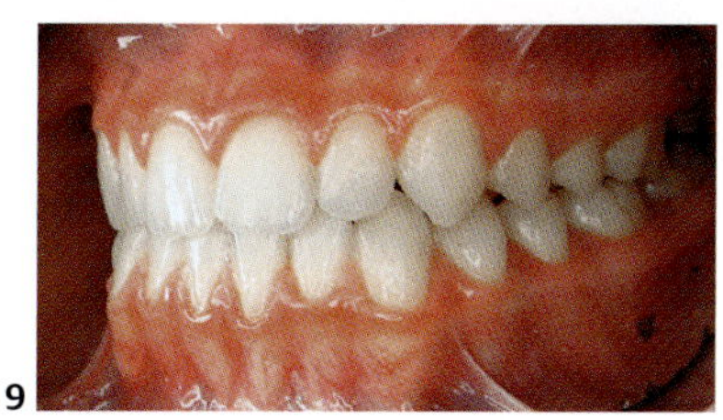
19

14–19 The situation at the start of treatment and after 1 year of retention.

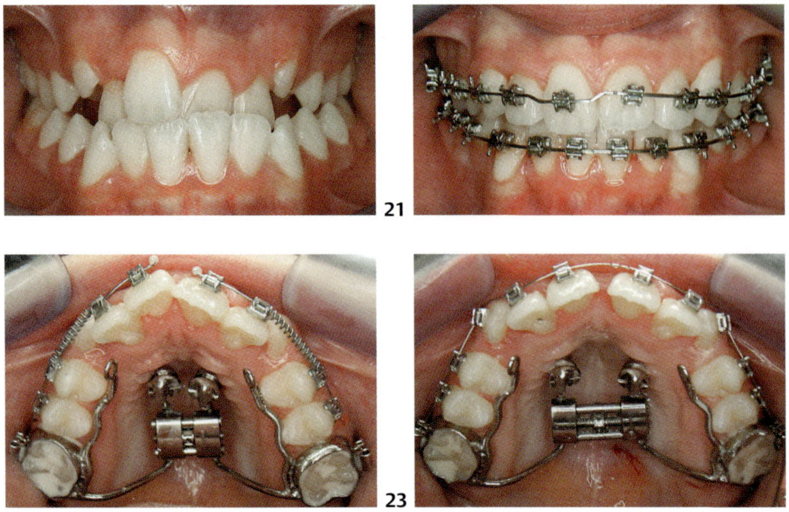

20 21 22 23

20–23 Another example: class III with mandibular prognathism, which was treated with hybrid rapid palatal enlargement and maxillary protraction.
20 Before treatment.
21 At the end of treatment.
22 Before maxillary expansion.
23 12 days after expansion, followed by maxillary protraction.

CLINICAL PEARL

Patients with class III have a propensity to develop mandibular crowding as a consequence of dental compensation. Interproximal enamel reduction, fixed retention, or a combination of the two are often indicated. The extraction of one lower incisor can be a useful alternative.

Esthetic Treatment

Self-Ligating Ceramic Brackets

Although orthodontic treatment in adults is more common now than in the past, adults are often still unwilling to wear particularly noticeable appliances. Esthetic solutions are therefore preferred, and this applies regardless of the ligation mechanism involved. The advantage of using self-ligating esthetic brackets over metal brackets, aside from the biomechanical advantages, lies in their reduced tendency to discolor (which affects the elastomeric element in conventional ligation, particularly when consuming foodstuffs containing colors). The most sensitive area for adults is the "social six"—the anterior labial segment from canine to canine (**Fig. 7.48**). For esthetically demanding patients, most manufacturers produce esthetic self-ligating brackets, which are made of either ceramic or composite material (**Fig. 7.49**). Esthetic archwires may also be considered, but these are not usually available in different tooth colors and can thus be just as visible as metal archwires, so that they do not always offer any marked esthetic improvement.

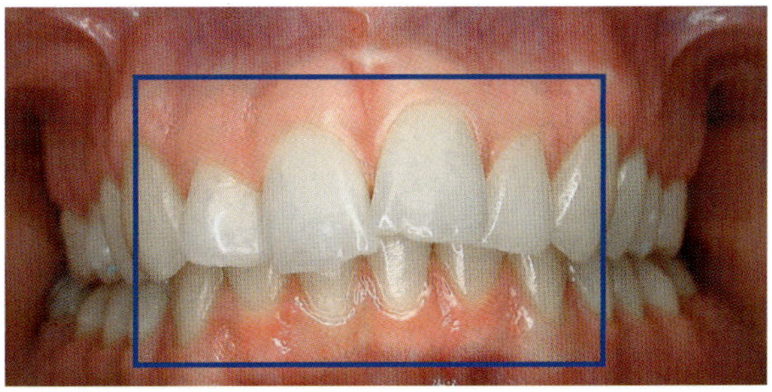

Fig. 7.48 The esthetic zone for orthodontic treatment.

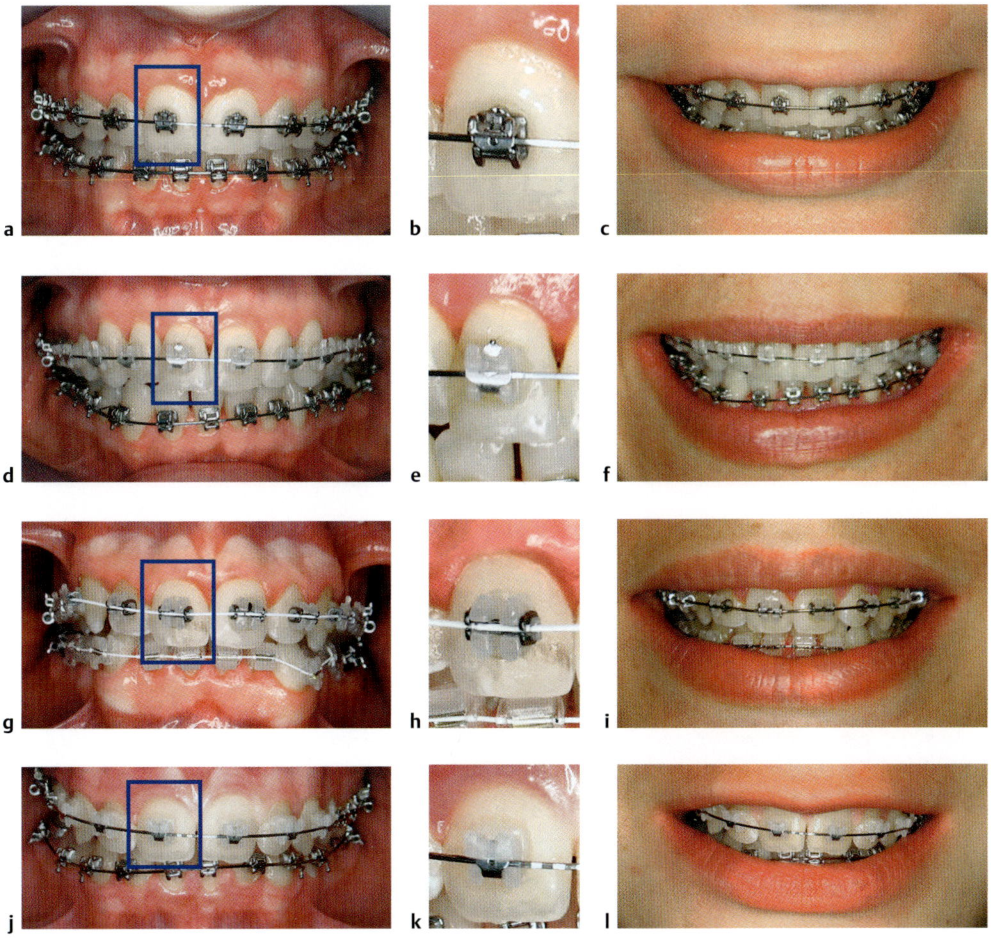

Fig. 7.49 a–l Esthetic self-ligating brackets (SLBs) and their appearance.
a–c A metal bracket for comparison.
d–f Ceramic SLBs (In-Ovation C).
g–i Ceramic SLBs in the maxillary dentition (SmartClip, **g**, **h**) and traditional ceramic brackets in the mandibular dentition (**i**).
j–l Ceramic SLBs in the maxillary dentition (QuicKlear, **j**, **k**) and metal SLBs in the mandibular dentition (**l**).

Case Study 7.19 (Fig. 7.50)

Patient: C.O., female, age 17.
Diagnostic records: models, panoramic radiograph, lateral cephalometric radiograph, intraoral/extraoral photographs.
Main findings: class I occlusion with misalignment of the anterior dentition.
Treatment aims: improving anterior esthetics.
Appliances: Self-ligating brackets, molar bands, interproximal reduction (IPR).
Archwire sequence: 0.012 SE, 0.016 SE, 0.016 × 0.022 SE, 0.018 × 0.025 SE, 0.019 × 0.025 SS.
Alternative treatment strategy: n/a.
Active treatment time: 9 months.
Retention: maxillary and mandibular bonded retainers.

1 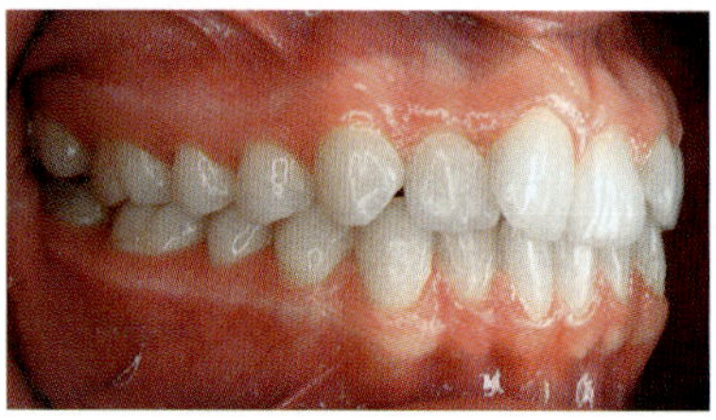
2 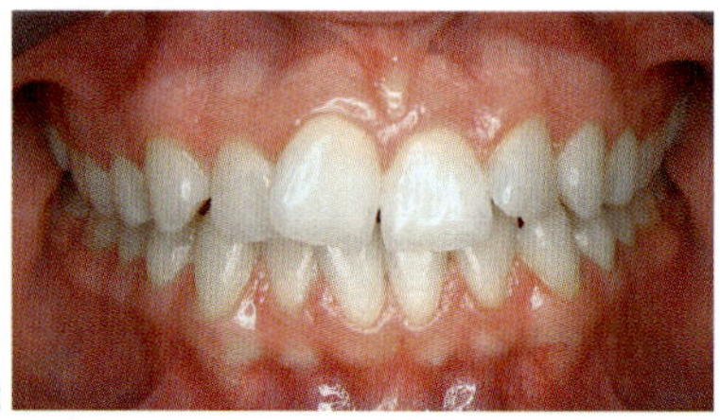
3 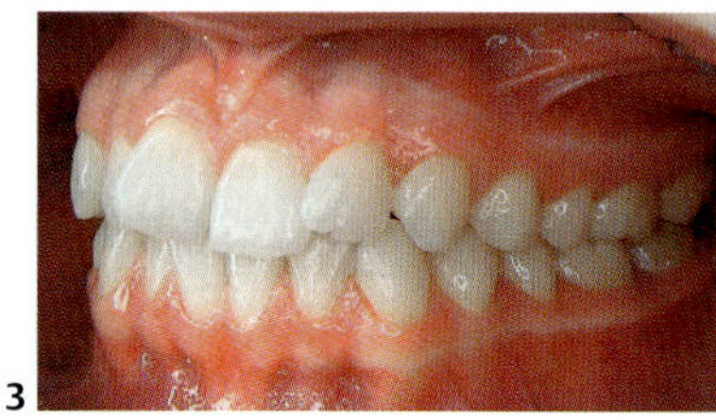
4 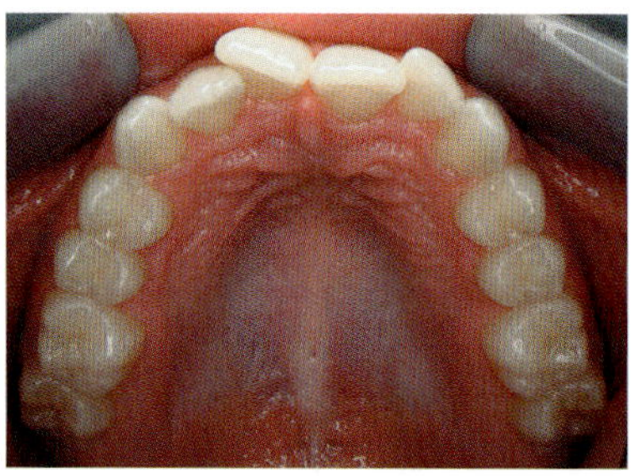
5 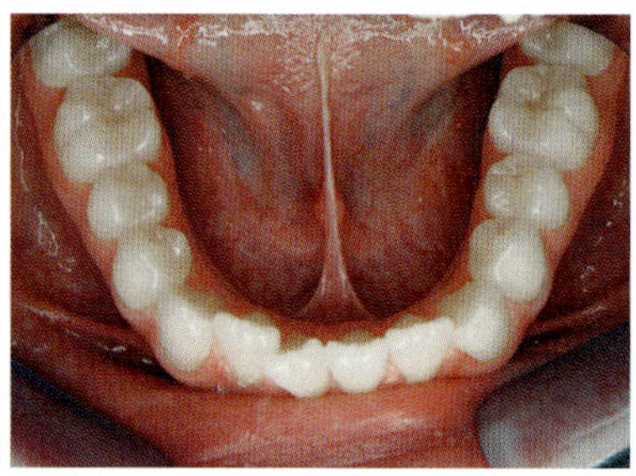

Fig. 7.50 1–25
1–5 Maxillary and mandibular anterior crowding. The patient requested cosmetic improvement.

6 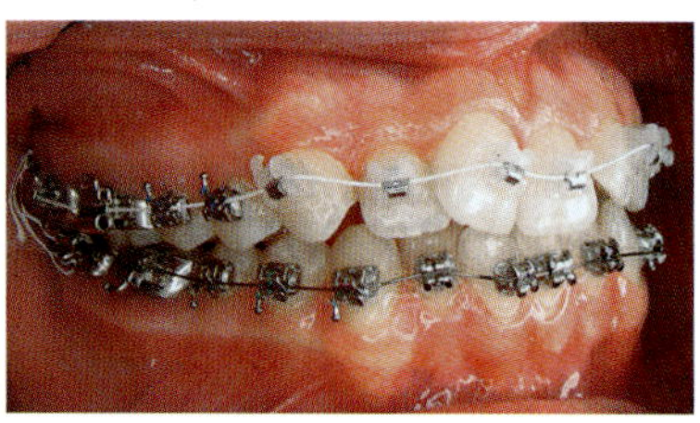
7 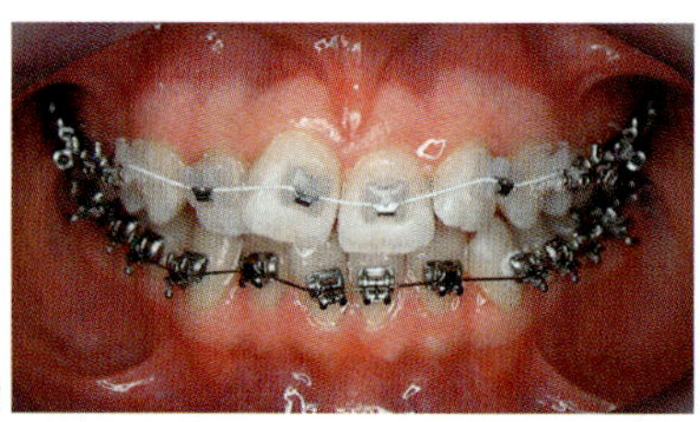
8 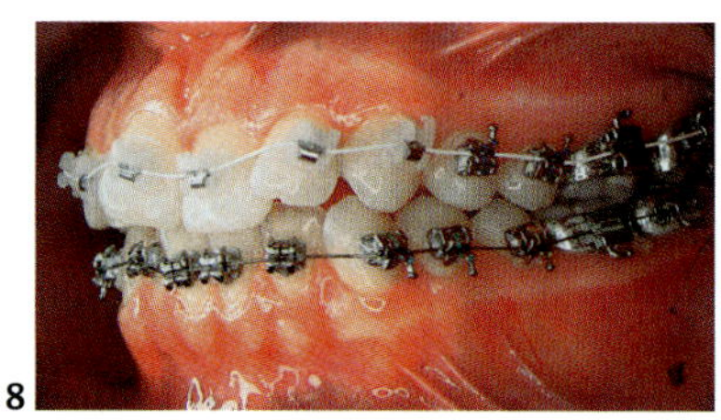
9 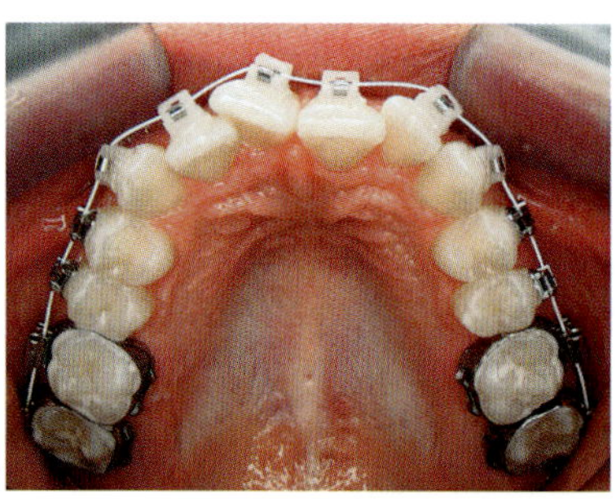
10 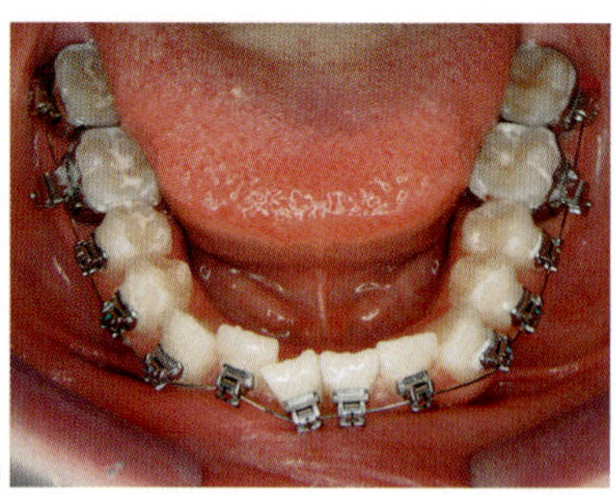

6–10 Self-ligating brackets bonded and a 0.012 esthetic SE archwire in place.

CLINICAL PEARL

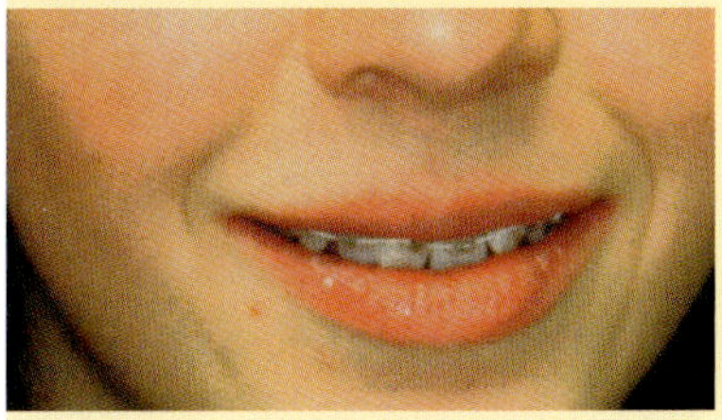

11

11 Ceramic self-ligating brackets from canine to canine and esthetic archwires often improve acceptance by patients, especially in adults.

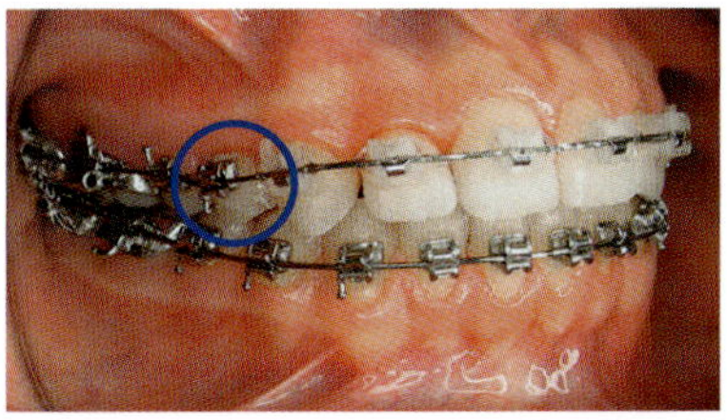

12

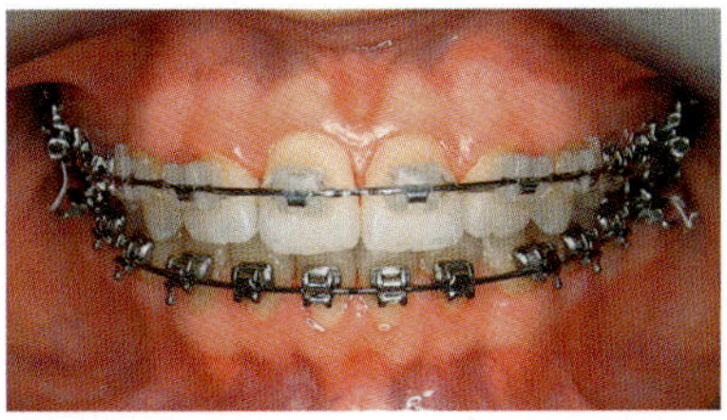

13

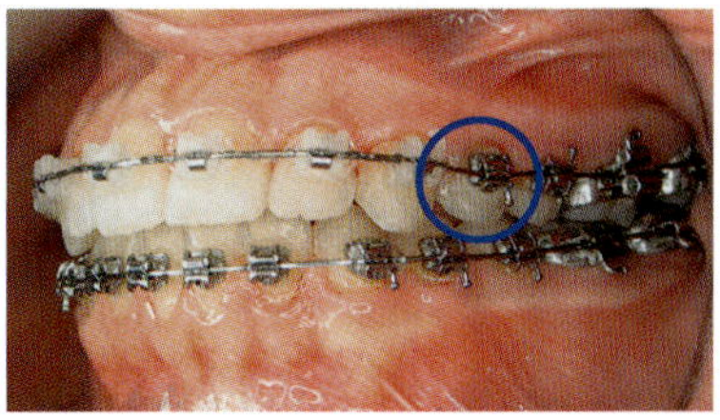

14

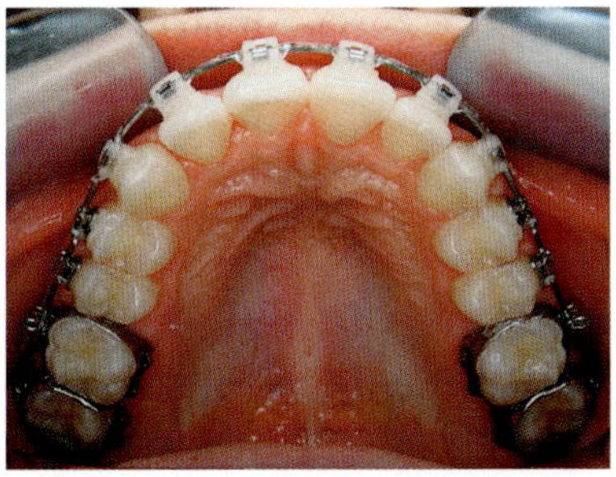

15

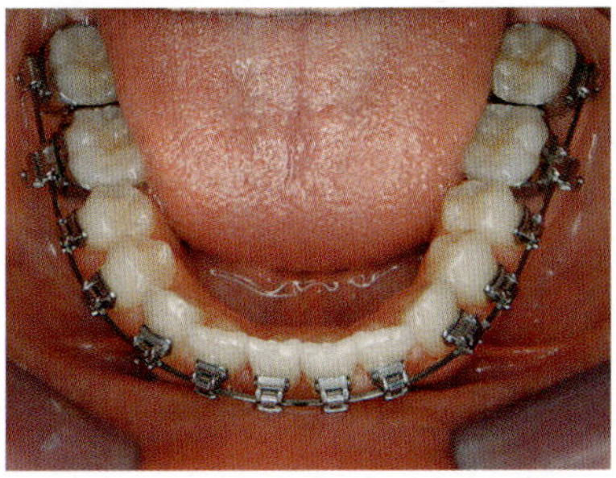

16

12–16

Clinical pearl:
If the treatment aim includes improvement of smile esthetics and reduction of buccal corridors, maxillary first and second bicuspid brackets can be turned upside down, so that the torque value will change from −7° to +7° (Roth prescription).

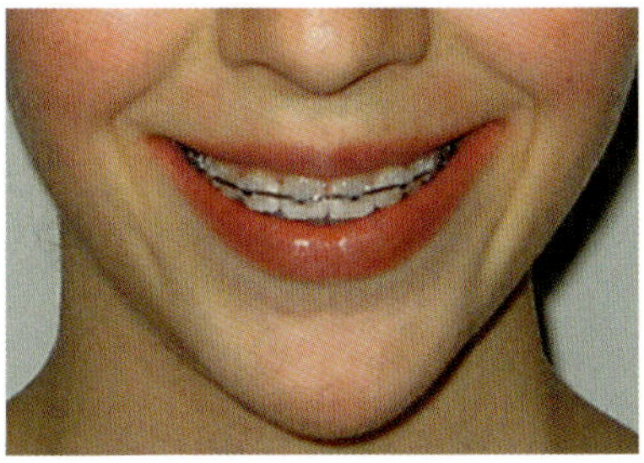

17

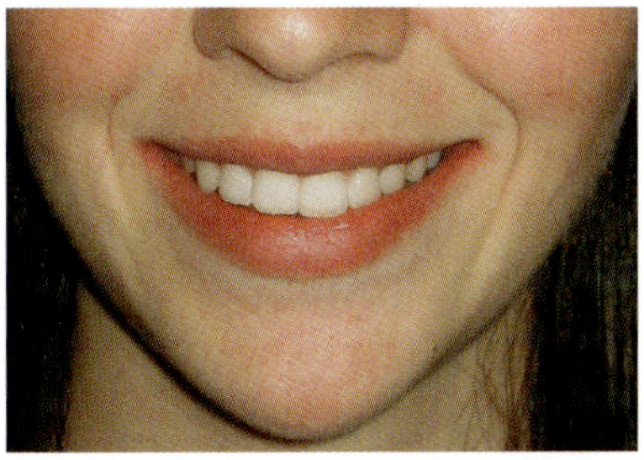

18

17, 18 Comparison of buccal corridors before and after the altered inclination.

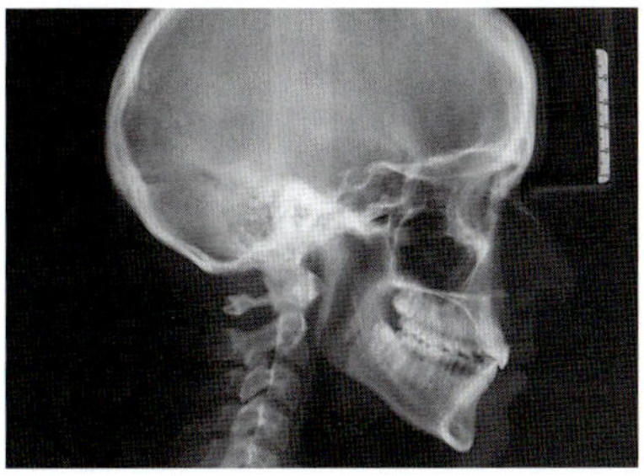

19

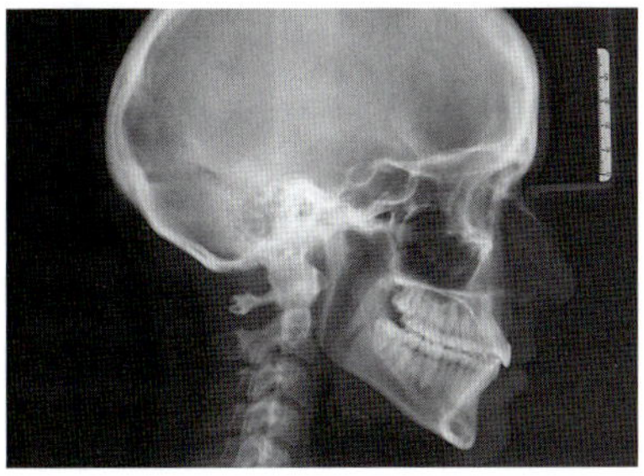

20

19, 20 Comparison of lateral cephalograms before and after treatment. The incisor inclination did not increase markedly, due to interproximal enamel reduction.

21 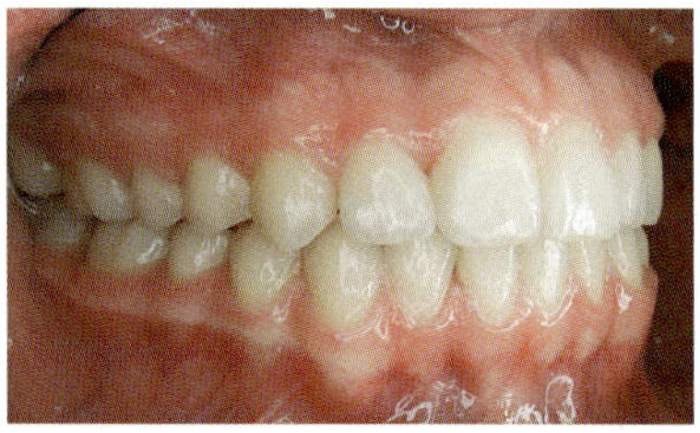
22 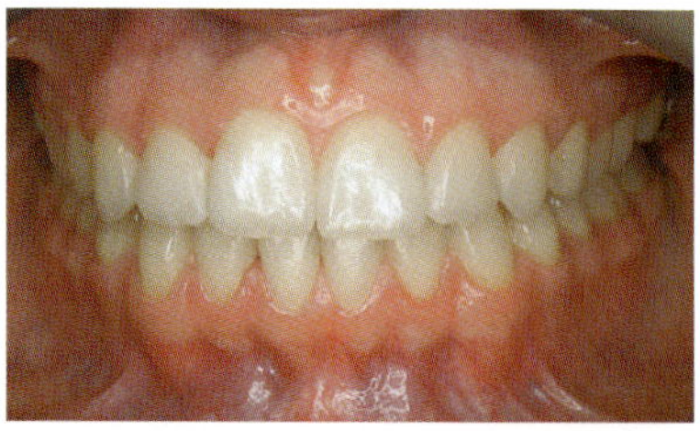
23 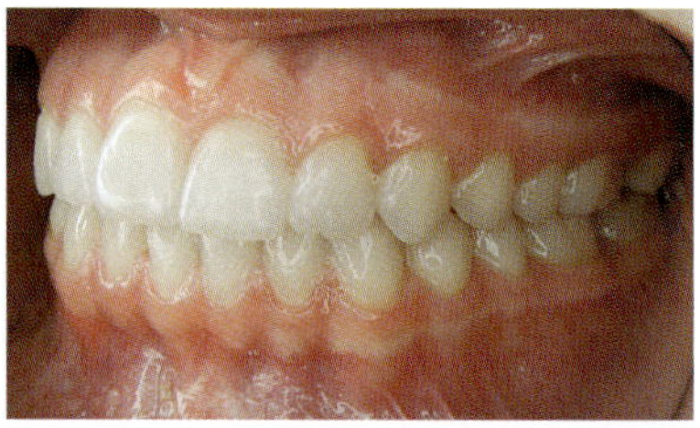
24 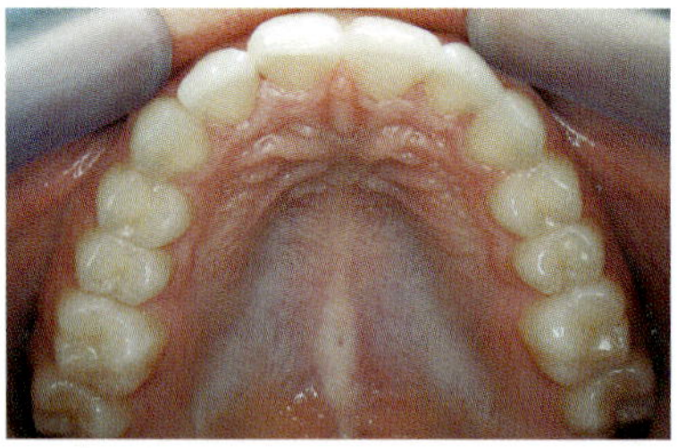
25 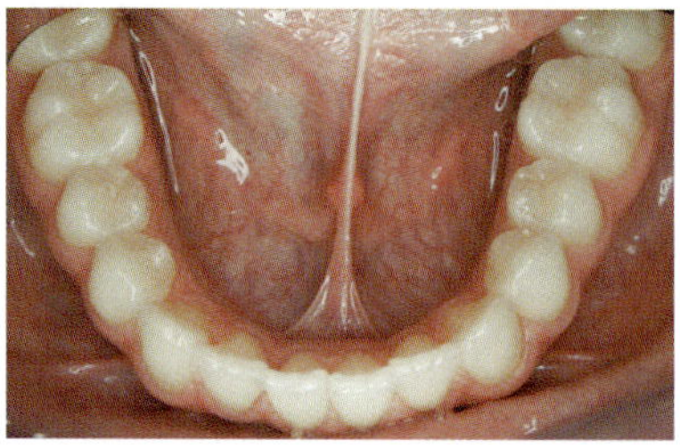

21–25 The final result (before bonding of the fixed retainers).

CLINICAL PEARL

Regardless of whether hybrid rapid palatal expansion, a Frog appliance, or an Easy-Fit Jumper is used, ceramic self-ligating brackets improve the esthetic appearance during treatment and thus increase patient acceptance.

1 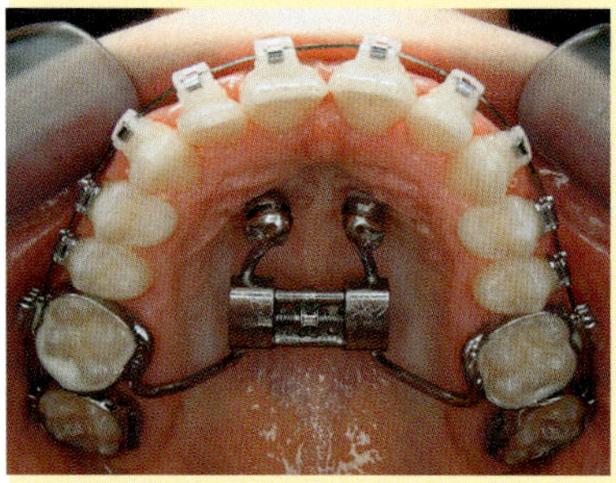
2 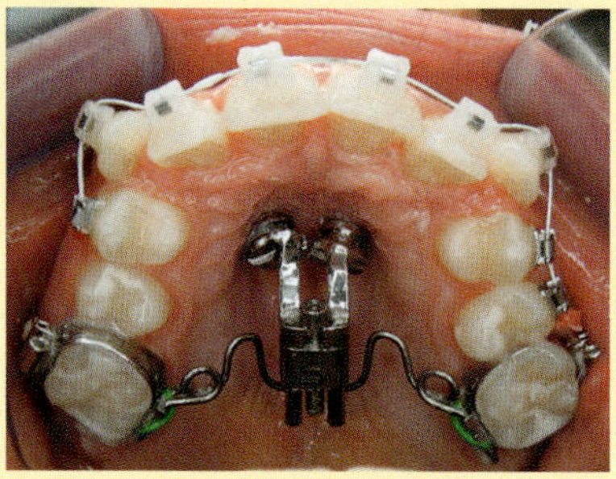
3 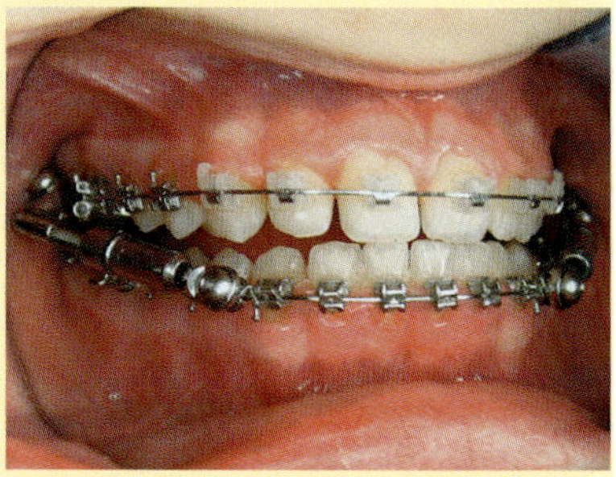

Fig. 7.51 1–3

Lingual Self-Ligating Brackets

Lingual appliances have intermittently been reinvented and further developed during the last 30 years, but they are still not routinely used in orthodontic practices. There are a number of reasons for this, but it is mainly due to the difficulty of bracket placement and archwire changes. The lingual surfaces of the teeth are also much more inconsistent between individuals in comparison with the labial surfaces. In addition, the reduced interbracket distance makes the archwires less efficient. Applying the force lingual to the center of resistance sometimes creates different biomechanical effects from those obtained with traditional labial appliances.[27] For precise three-dimensional programming and patient-specific, individualized treatment, extensive laboratory procedures are necessary, including an individualized set-up for the dentition with manufacturing of individualized brackets and archwires. To allow precise three-dimensional preprogramming of the appliances, laboratory steps are required in which the teeth are measured, set-ups are created, bracket bases are customized, and brackets are transferred to the dentition using transfer aids for indirect bonding.[33]

Simplified lingual techniques have been developed in recent years that avoid the need for complex programming and individualization of lingual appliances. This makes the system a more cost-effective alternative in comparison with fixed labial appliance treatment. These systems are usually designed for alignment of the anterior teeth only and not for treatment of complex problems, which require correction of the occlusion (**Fig. 7.52**). Some lingual brackets have self-ligating mechanisms incorporated. The present authors mainly use the two-dimensional lingual bracket system developed by Philippe. This can often be used as an alternative to the more complex three-dimensional bracket systems and provides good results for limited treatment with minor tooth movement.[22] More recently, this technique has been propagated by Cacciafesta's group.[21] As the name implies, the two-dimensional system only allows two-dimensional control of tooth movement. Leveling and alignment, with correction of rotations and angulation changes in individual teeth, are possible. However, this bracket does not have a rectangular slot, so that controlled torque expression is not possible (**Fig. 7.53**). However, the lack of a rectangular slot and a sophisticated ligation mechanism allows a low-profile design at 1.4 mm. This improves patient comfort, and speech impediments are not as significant as they often are with other lingual bracket types.

These brackets are bonded directly onto the tooth (i.e., without complex laboratory procedures). Vertical positioning of the brackets can be obtained by using a ruler or a gauge (**Fig. 7.54**). Due to the variability of the lingual anatomy of the teeth, it is often necessary to individualize

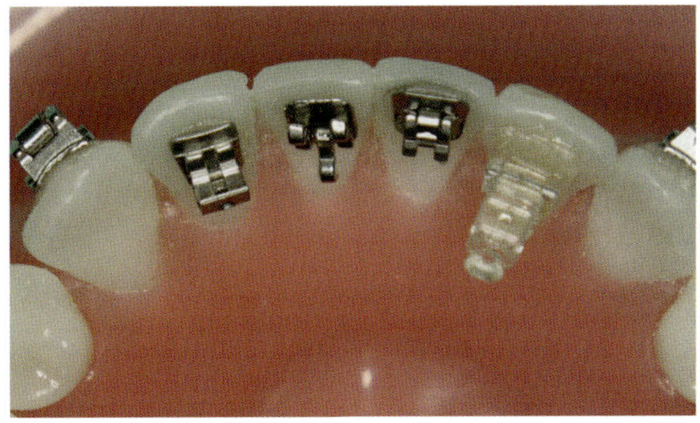

Fig. 7.52 Lingual self-ligating brackets from various manufacturers. Direct bonding without set-up is possible with the In-Ovation L, Phantom, and 2 D Philippe. To ensure appropriate positioning, In-Ovation L has a well-contoured base, while the Phantom bracket comes with a positioning gauge that has to be removed after bonding. The 2 D Philippe can be easily positioned lingually due to its small base. The Evolution LT and 3 D Philippe require a set-up with customization of the bracket base. Displayed from left to right: Evolution LT (Andenta), 2 D Philippe (Forestadent), In-Ovation L (GAC), Phantom (Gestenco).

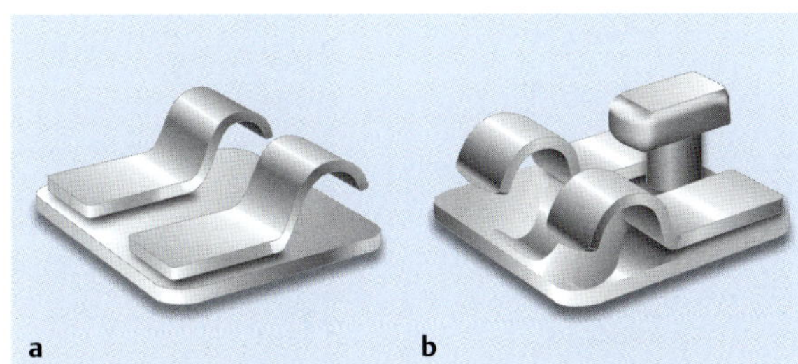

Fig. 7.53a, b The basic configuration of the two-dimensional lingual brackets designed by Philippe. The brackets have self-ligating wings that are closed by bending them toward the bracket base after the wire has been inserted. The inner surface is rounded off, which means that three-dimensional control is not possible.

a 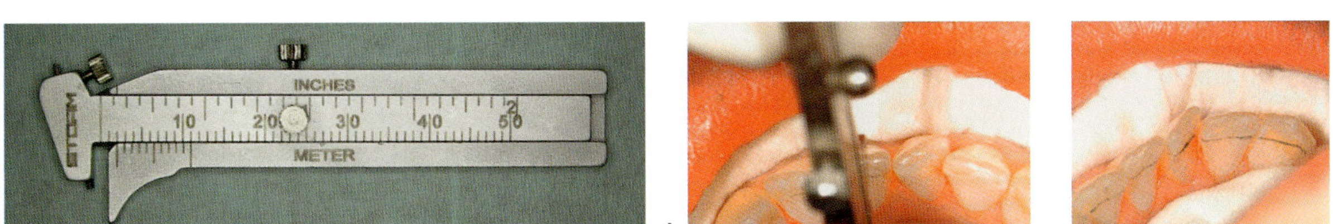

b c

Fig. 7.54a–c Establishing the vertical position for lingual brackets.
a A measurement gauge with 1/10 mm scale and an integrated pencil for marking the height on the conditioned enamel surface.
b, c Intraoral application of the gauge and resulting marks.

the archwire to achieve the best possible alignment. As the bracket only translates two-dimensional information onto the tooth (i.e., rotation, angulation, and height), only one bracket is used for all teeth. Lingual archwires can be individualized using prefabricated mushroom-shaped wires, which are available in a number of sizes (**Fig. 7.55**). The decision on whether to use a two-dimensional approach or a more complex lingual appliance system depends on the diagnosis and the desired treatment outcome. This system is particularly useful for esthetic treatment of anterior crowding, or mild to moderate relapse after previous orthodontic treatment (see also the section on "Management of Relapse" in Chapter 9). If correction of torque values is needed, consideration should be given to using a three-dimensional lingual system, which is more suitable for achieving the desired treatment aims.

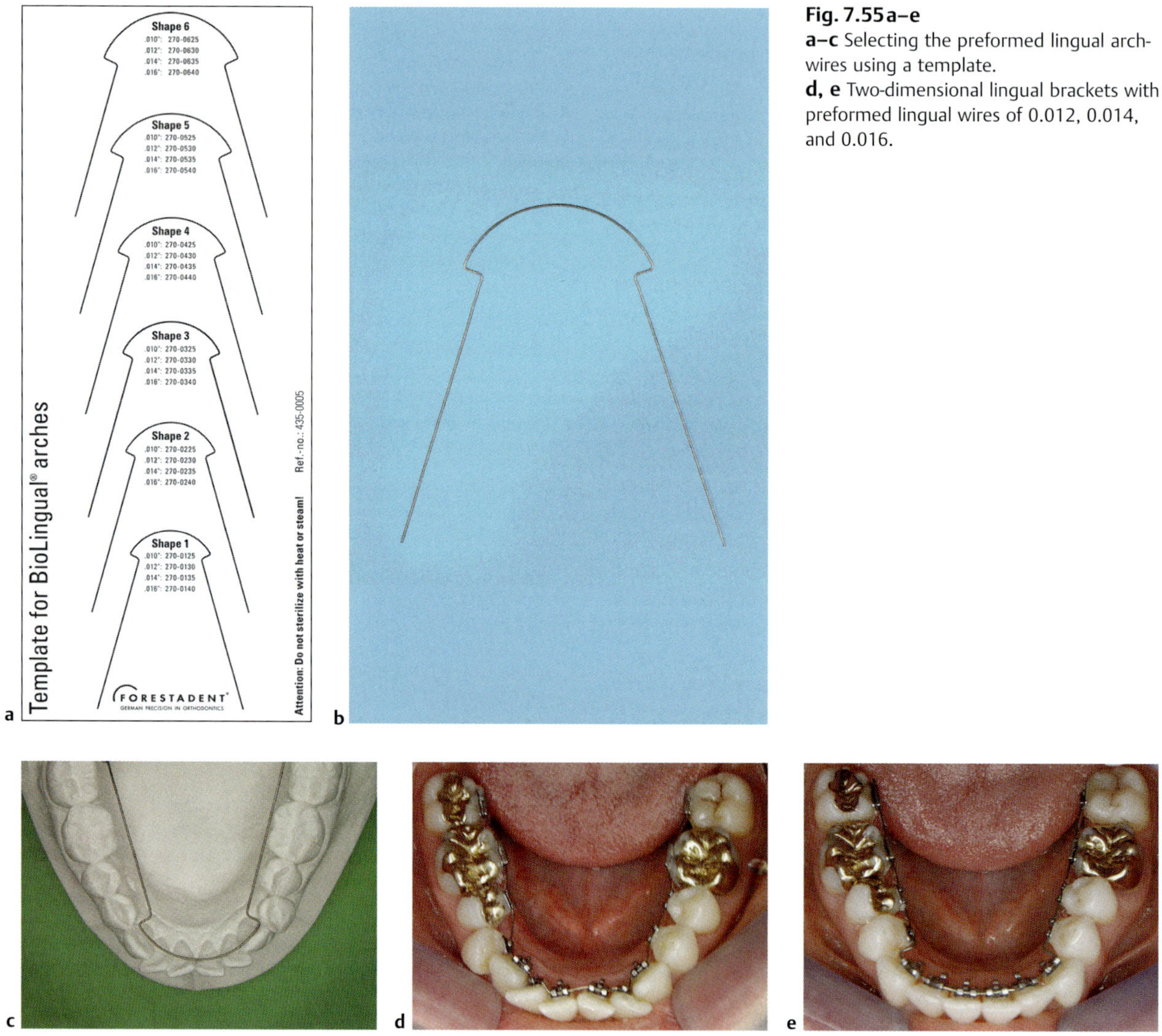

Fig. 7.55 a–e
a–c Selecting the preformed lingual archwires using a template.
d, e Two-dimensional lingual brackets with preformed lingual wires of 0.012, 0.014, and 0.016.

Case Study 7.20 (Fig. 7.56)

Patient: M.S., female, age 17.
Diagnostic records: models, panoramic radiograph, lateral cephalometric radiograph, intraoral/extraoral photographs.
Main findings: retained tooth 63 and impacted tooth 23.
Treatment aims: creating space for tooth 23, exposure, and guided eruption.
Appliances: two-dimensional lingual self-ligating bracket, preformed archwires, later individual archwires.
Archwire sequence: 0.012 SE, 0.014 SE, 0.016 SE, 0.016 SS.
Alternative treatment strategy: n/a.
Active treatment time: 11 months.
Retention: bonded lingual retainer.

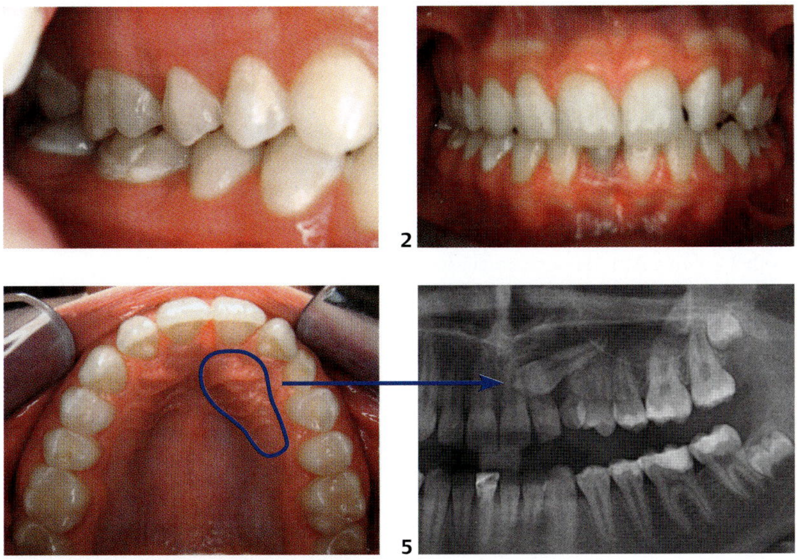

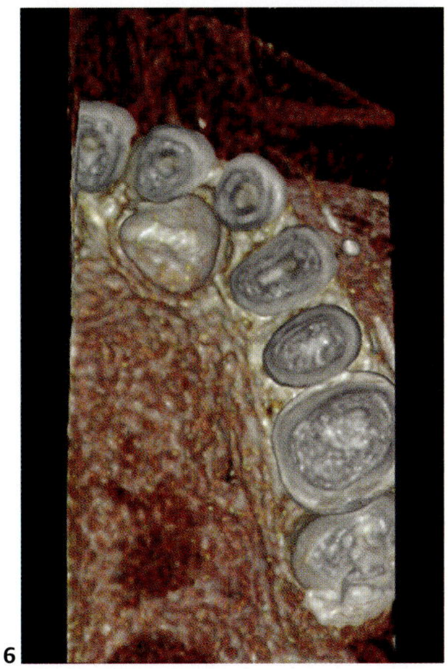

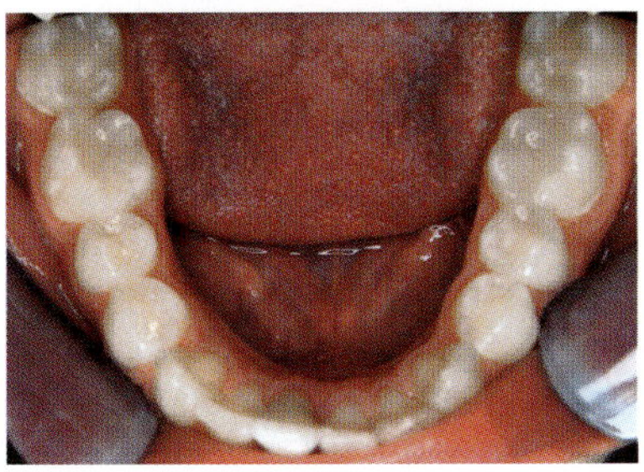

Fig. 7.56 1–18
1–7 The initial situation, with a palatally impacted tooth 23.

NOTE

In **Fig. 7.56**, 5 and 6 show the discrepancy between the perceived canine location on the panoramic radiograph and the actual location as shown in the three-dimensional reconstruction on low-dose computed tomography.

CLINICAL PEARL

Cone-beam computed tomography (CT) or low-dose conventional CT can be useful for accurately establishing the location of impacted teeth, and this additional information is often helpful in treatment planning.

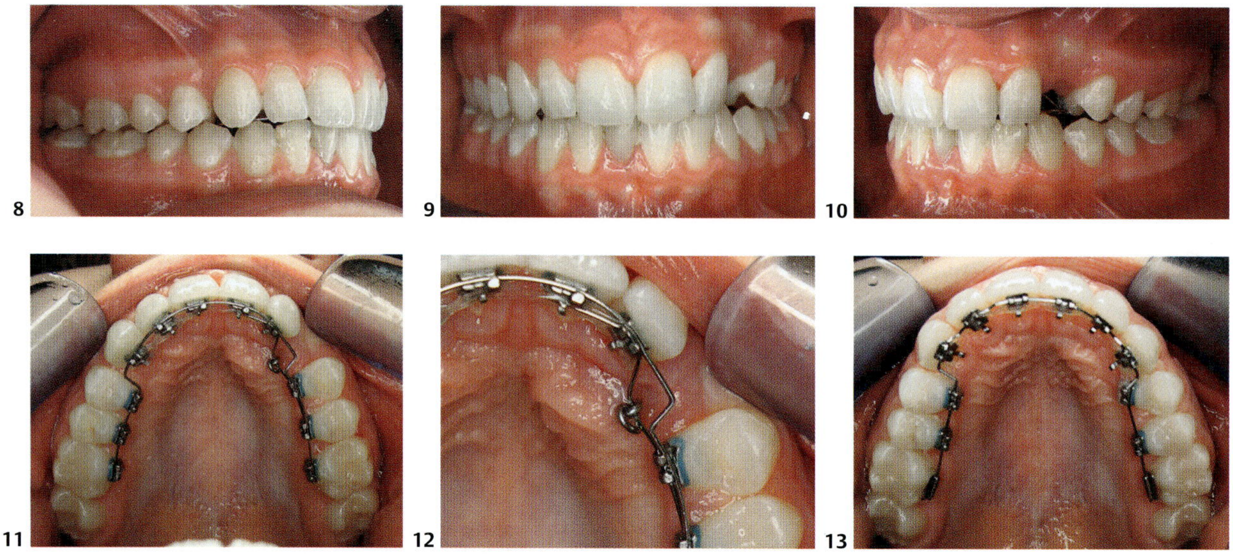

8–13 Piggyback technique for positioning of tooth 23, with a 0.012 SE segmental wire and stainless-steel base arch.

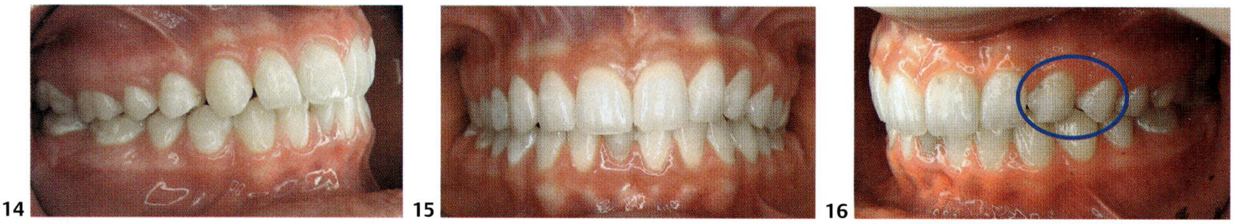

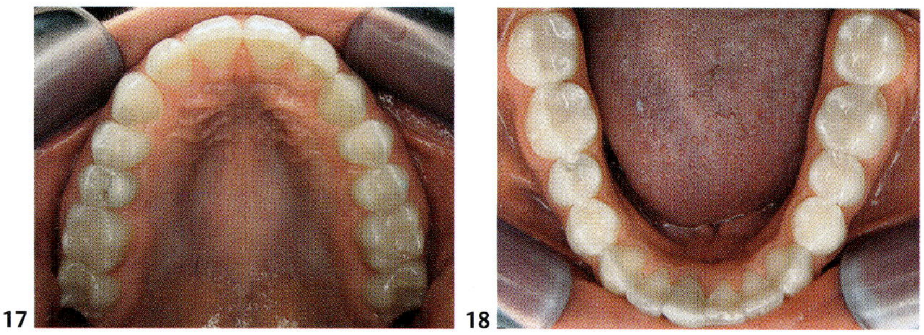

14–18 After 1 year of retention, tooth 23 shows a stable position.

Case Study 7.21 (Fig. 7.57)

Patient: P.D., female, age 44.
Diagnostic records: models, panoramic radiograph, lateral cephalometric radiograph, intraoral/extraoral photographs.
Main findings: mandibular anterior crowding.
Treatment aims: alignment of lower incisors.
Appliances: two-dimensional lingual self-ligating bracket, preformed archwires, later individual archwires, interproximal reduction.
Archwire sequence: 0.012 SE, 0.014 SE, 0.016 SE, 0.016 SS.
Alternative treatment strategy: extraction of a single mandibular incisor.
Active treatment time: months.
Retention: mandibular bonded retainers.

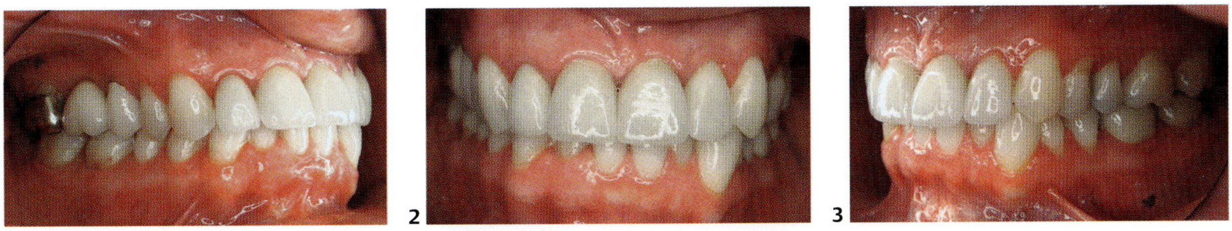

1 2 3

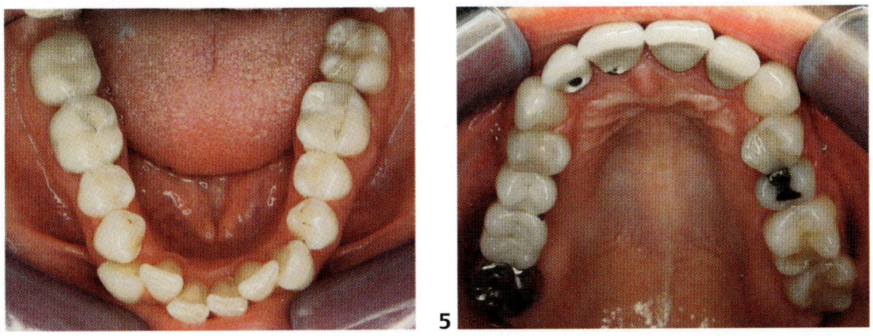

4 5

Fig. 7.57 1–16
1–5 Class I occlusion with mandibular anterior crowding.

ERRORS AND RISKS

In single-arch treatment, it is imperative to avoid changing the arch shape or the incisor inclination, as otherwise the arch coordination can be lost. Interproximal reduction may be needed to create space and resolve crowding.

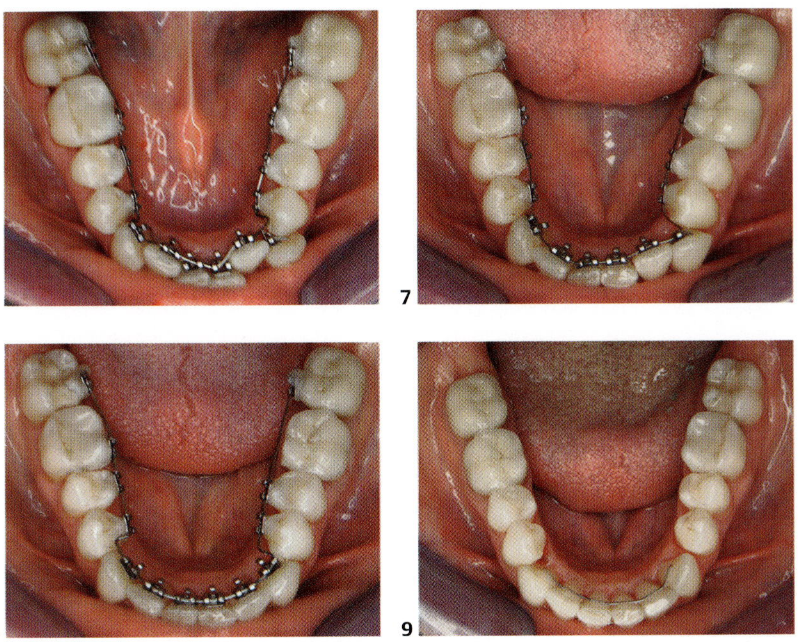

6 7 8 9

6–9 Lingual self-ligating brackets from 7 to 7 and BioLingual archwires in the sequence 0.012 SE, 0.014 SE, and then 0.016 SE stainless steel. At each archwire change, interproximal reduction (IPR) was performed from 5 to 5. Despite the IPR, the final result is potentially unstable and requires permanent retention.

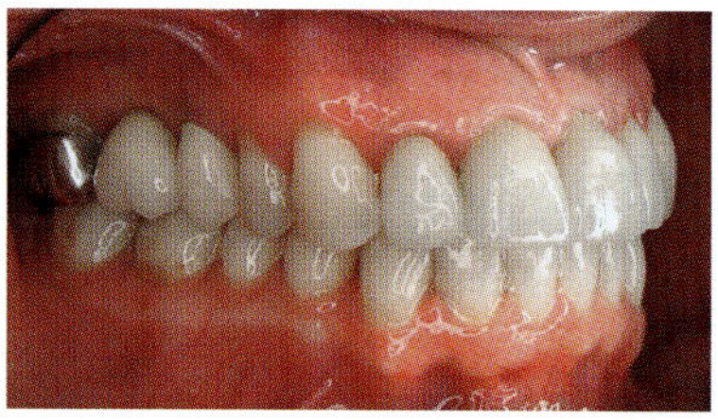
10

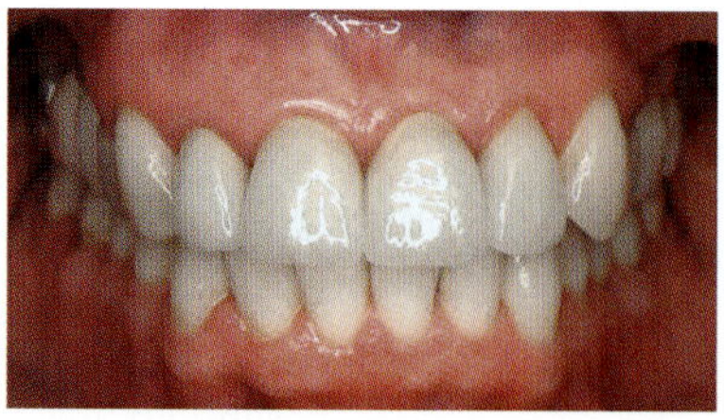
11

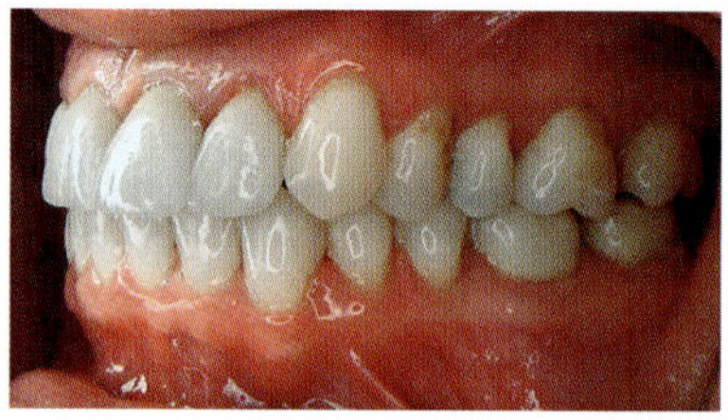
12

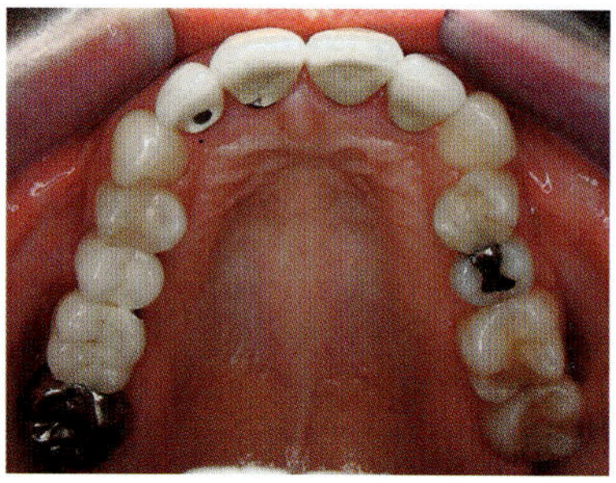
13

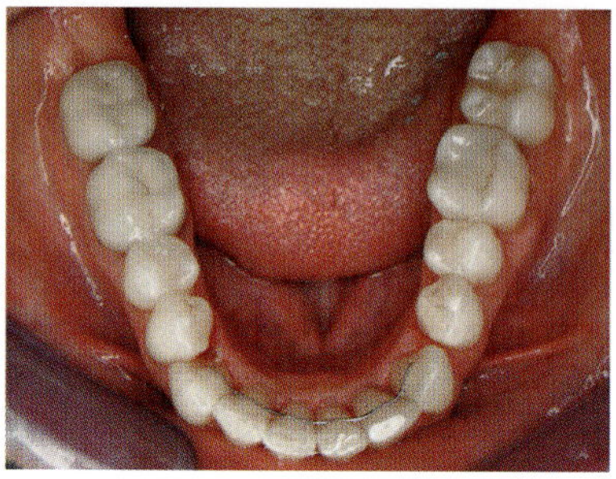
14

10–14 The good occlusion was maintained.

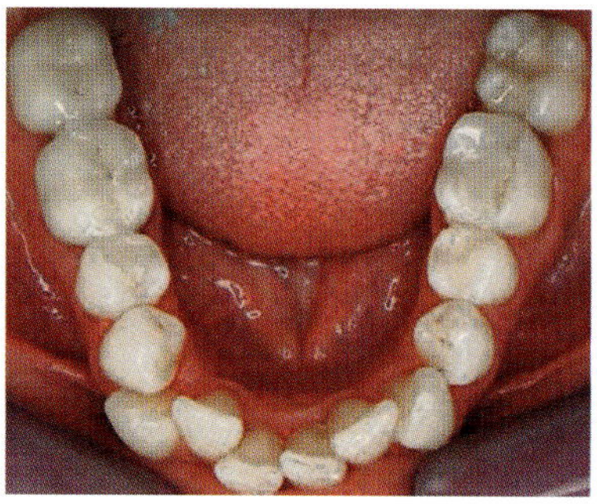
15

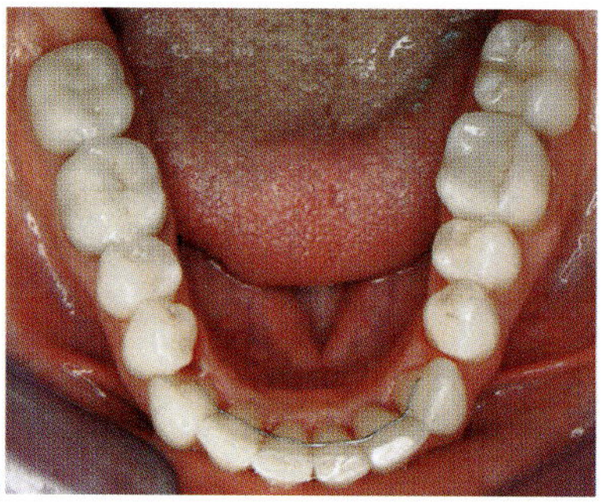
16

15, 16 Before and after treatment.

CLINICAL PEARL

Interproximal enamel reduction (IPR) can be an alternative to extraction treatment. Fluoridation and patient consent need to be observed.

Case Study 7.22 (Fig. 7.58)

Patient: L.S., male, age 23.
Diagnostic records: models, panoramic radiograph, lateral cephalometric radiograph, intraoral/extraoral photographs.
Main findings: esthetically unsatisfactory anterior alignment.
Treatment aims: establishing anterior esthetics.
Appliances: two-dimensional lingual self-ligating bracket, preformed archwires, later individual archwires, interproximal reduction.
Archwire sequence: 0.012 SE, 0.016 SE, 0.016 SS.
Alternative treatment strategy: n/a.
Active treatment time: 19 months.
Retention: vacuum-formed retainer, followed by bonded retainers.

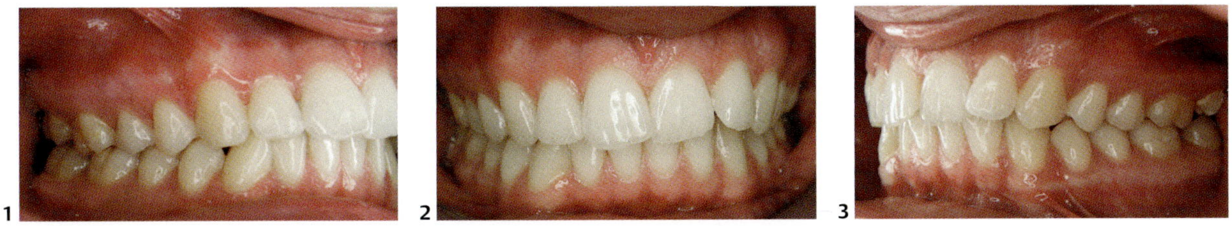
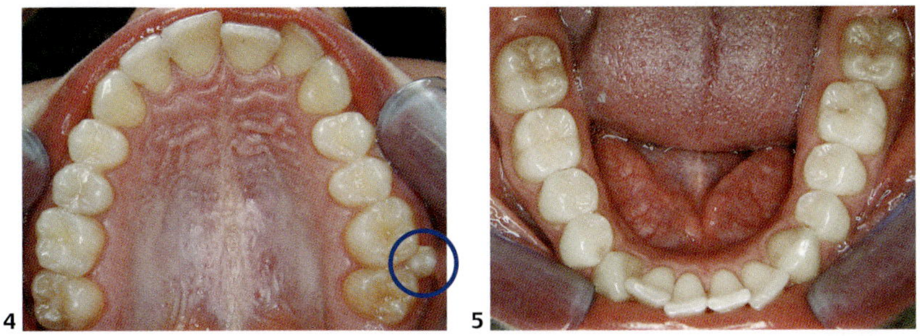

Fig. 7.58 1–20
1–5 Maxillary and mandibular anterior crowding. Class I occlusion on the right side and class II tendency on the left side. There is a supernumerary molar 29.

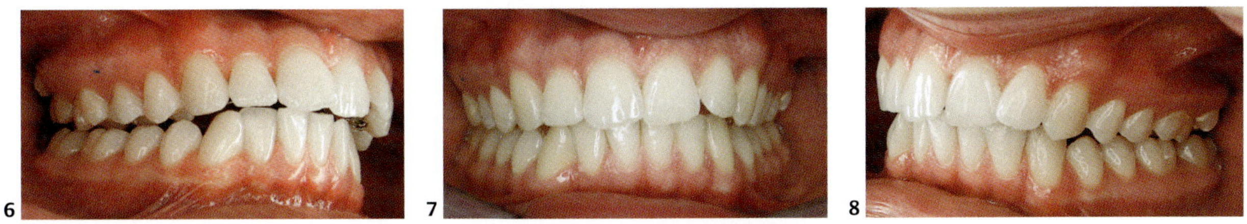
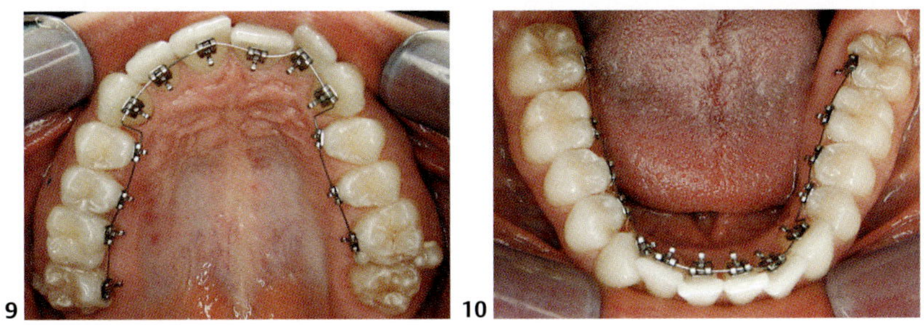

6–10 The initial treatment phase, with 0.012 SE archwires in both arches.

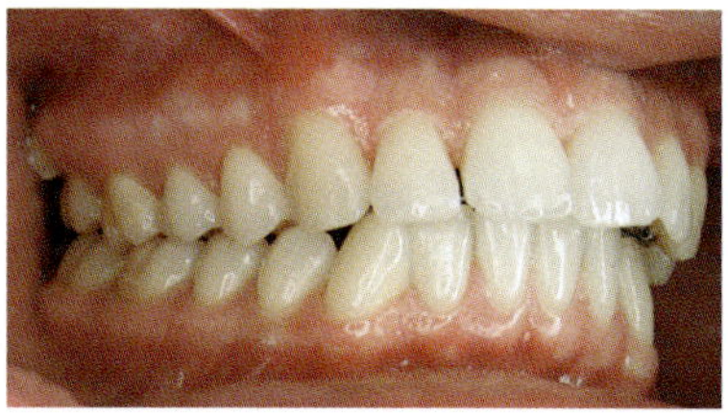
11

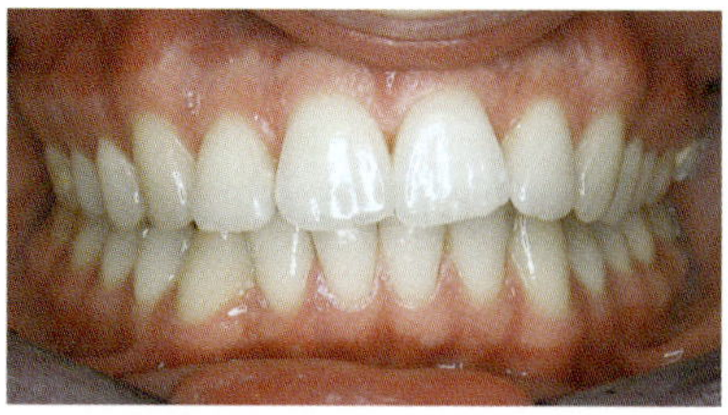
12

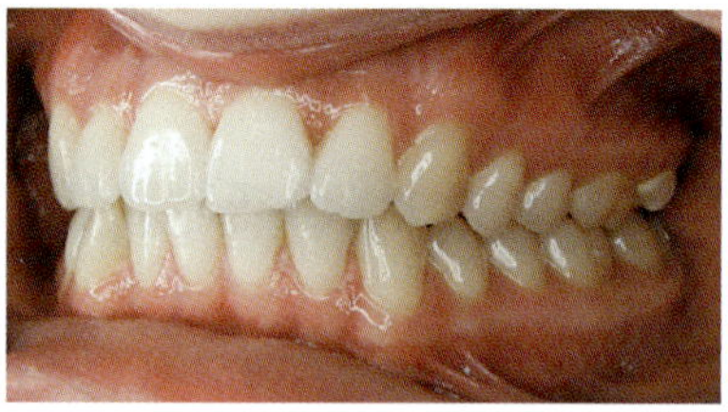
13

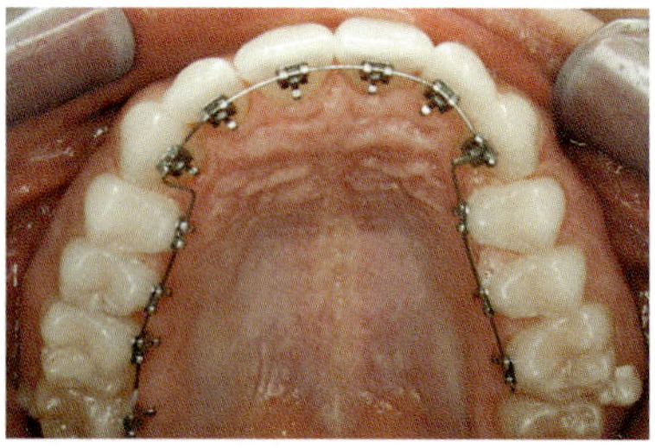
14

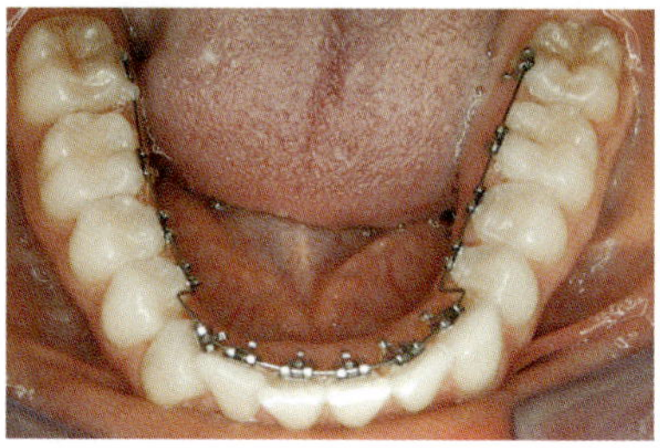
15

11–15 Treatment progress with 0.016 SE archwires in both arches.

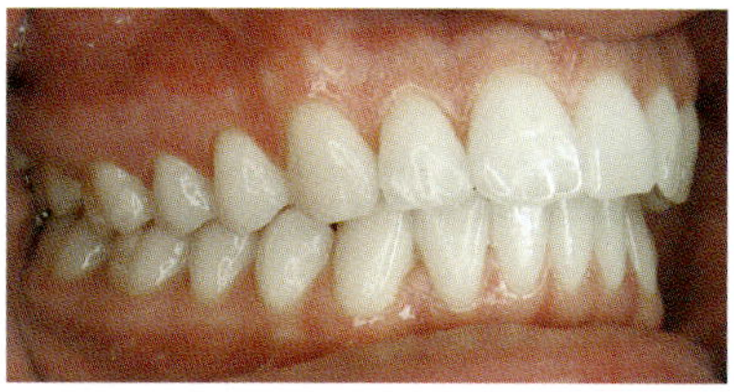
16

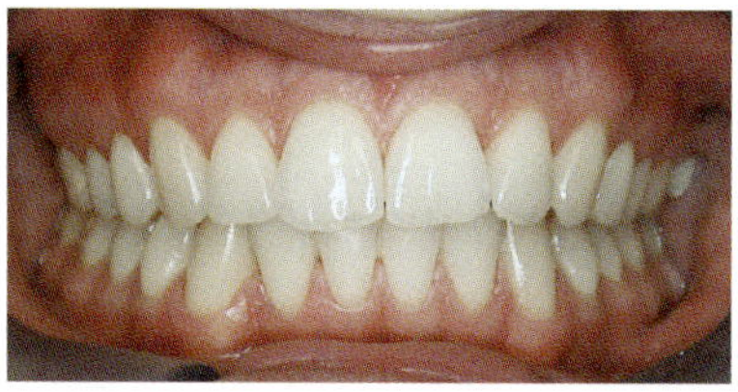
17

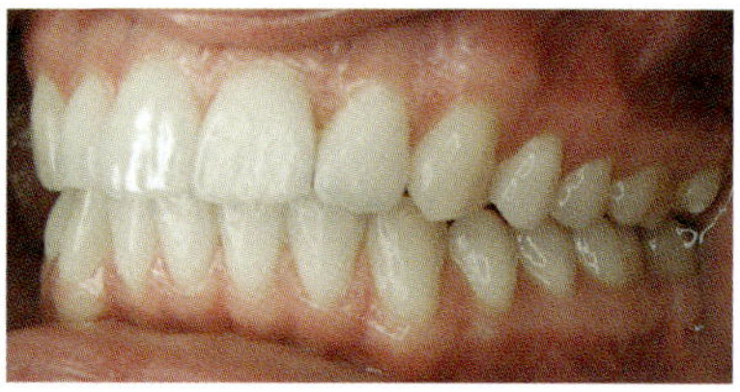
18

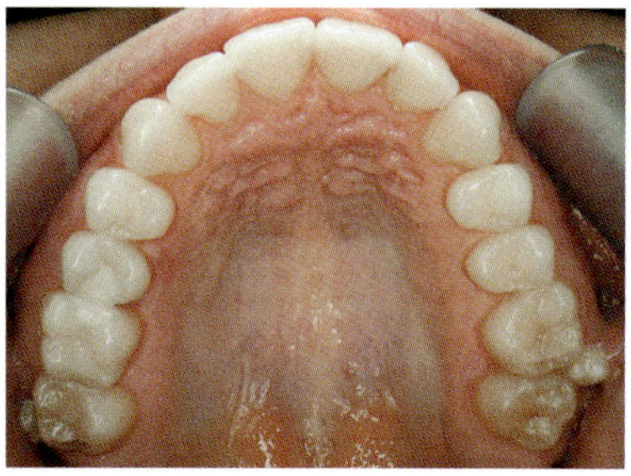
19

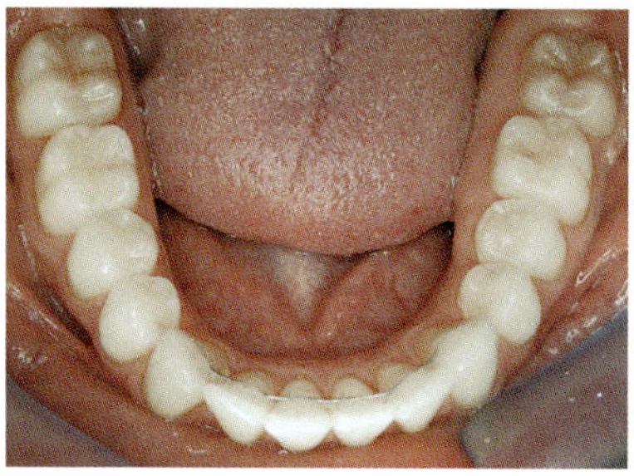
20

16–20 The treatment result after 1 year of retention with a vacuum-formed retainer in the maxilla and a bonded retainer in the mandible. The supernumerary 29 was left in place.

REFERENCES

1. Bednar JR, Gruendeman GW, Sandrik JL. A comparative study of frictional forces between orthodontic brackets and arch wires. Am J Orthod Dentofacial Orthop 1991;100(6):513–522
2. Bock F, Goldbecher H, Stolze A. Klinische Erfahrungen mit verschiedenen selbstligierenden Bracketsystemen. Kieferorthopädie 2007;21:157–167
3. Bourauel C, Höse N, Keilig L, et al. Friktionsverhalten und Nivellierungseffektivität selbstligierender Bracketsysteme. Kieferorthopädie 2007;21:169–179
4. Bussick TJ, McNamara JA Jr. Dentoalveolar and skeletal changes associated with the pendulum appliance. Am J Orthod Dentofacial Orthop 2000;117(3):333–343
5. Cacciafesta V, Sfondrini MF, Ricciardi A, Scribante A, Klersy C, Auricchio F. Evaluation of friction of stainless steel and esthetic self-ligating brackets in various bracket-archwire combinations. Am J Orthod Dentofacial Orthop 2003;124(4):395–402
6. Diedrich P, ed. Kieferorthopädie II. Amsterdam: Elsevier; 2005
7. Drescher D, Bourauel C, Schumacher HA. The loss of force by friction in arch-guided tooth movement. [Article in German] Fortschr Kieferorthop 1990;51(2):99–105
8. Fillion D. Vor- und Nachteile der approximalen Schmelzreduktion. Inf Orthod Kieferorthop 1995;27:64–90
9. Fuziy A, Rodrigues de Almeida R, Janson G, Angelieri F, Pinzan A. Sagittal, vertical, and transverse changes consequent to maxillary molar distalization with the pendulum appliance. Am J Orthod Dentofacial Orthop 2006;130(4):502–510
10. Gelgör IE, Büyükyilmaz T, Karaman AI, Dolanmaz D, Kalayci A. Intraosseous screw-supported upper molar distalization. Angle Orthod 2004;74(6):838–850
11. Gracco A, Lombardo L, Cozzani M, Siciliani G. Quantitative evaluation with CBCT of palatal bone thickness in growing patients. Prog Orthod 2006;7(2):164–174
12. Haubrich J. Praxistipp: Approximale Schmelzreduktion mit dem Ortho-Strips-System. Kieferorthopädie 2007;21:99–102
13. Hilgers JJ. The pendulum appliance for Class II non-compliance therapy. J Clin Orthod 1992;26(11):706–714
14. Hilgers JJ. Die Pendelapparatur — eine Weiterentwicklung. Inf Orthod Kieferorthop 1993;25:20–23
15. Little RM, Wallen TR, Riedel RA. Stability and relapse of mandibular anterior alignment - first premolar extraction cases treated by traditional edgewise orthodontics. Am J Orthod 1981; 80(4):349–365
16. Kinzinger GS, Diedrich PR. Bite jumping with the Functional Mandibular Advancer. J Clin Orthod 2005;39(12):696–700, quiz 715
17. Kinzinger G, Diedrich P. Skeletal effects in class II treatment with the functional mandibular advancer (FMA)? J Orofac Orthop 2005;66(6):469–490
18. Kinzinger GS, Wehrbein H, Diedrich PR. Molar distalization with a modified pendulum appliance - in vitro analysis of the force systems and in vivo study in children and adolescents. Angle Orthod 2005;75(4):558–567
19. Kinzinger G, Gülden N, Roth A, Diedrich P. Disc-condyle relationships during class II treatment with the Functional Mandibular Advancer (FMA). J Orofac Orthop 2006;67(5):356–375
20. Knaup B, Yildizhan F, Wehrbein R. Altersveränderungen der Sutura palatina mediana. J Orofac Orthop 2004;65(6):467–474
21. Macchi A, Norcini A, Cacciafesta V, Dolci F. The use of bidimensional brackets in lingual orthodontics: new horizons in the treatment of adult patients. Orthod 2004;1:1–11
22. Philippe J. L'orthodontie de l'adulte. Paris: Éditions SID; 1989
23. Reitan K. Some factors determining the evaluation of forces in orthodontics. Am J Orthod 1957;43:32–45
24. Reitan K. Biomechanical principles and reactions. In: Graber TM, Swain BF, eds. Orthodontics - current principles and techniques. St. Louis: Mosby; 1985:101–192.
25. Ricketts RM, Bench RW, Gugino CF, Hilgers JJ, Schulhof RJ. Bioprogressive therapy. Denver: Rocky Mountain Orthodontics; 1979
26. Schumacher HA, Bourauel C, Drescher D. The influence of bracket design on frictional losses in the bracket/arch wire system. J Orofac Orthop 1999;60(5):335–347
27. Scuzzo G, Takemoto K. Invisible orthodontics. Berlin: Quintessenz; 2003
28. Sheridan JJ. Air-rotor stripping. J Clin Orthod 1985;19(1):43–59
29. Sheridan JJ. Air-rotor stripping update. J Clin Orthod 1987;21(11): 781–788
30. Stroud JL, English J, Buschang PH. Enamel thickness of the posterior dentition: its implications for nonextraction treatment. Angle Orthod 1998;68(2):141–146
31. Timms DJ. Forcierte Gaumennahterweiterung. Berlin: Quintessenz; 1986
32. Walde KC. The simplified molar distalizer. J Clin Orthod 2003;37(11):616–619, quiz 626
33. Wiechmann D, Rummel V, Thalheim A, Simon JS, Wiechmann L. Customized brackets and archwires for lingual orthodontic treatment. Am J Orthod Dentofacial Orthop 2003;124(5):593–599
34. Wilmes B. Anwendungsgebiete von Mini-Implantaten. In: Mini-Implantate in der Kieferorthopädie - Innovative Verankerungskonzepte. Berlin: Quintessenz; 2007:89–120
35. Yildizhan F. Strukturparameter des medianen Gaumens und orthodontische Verankerungsimplantate. Dissertation. Aachen, 2004
36. Zachrisson BU, Nyøygaard L, Mobarak K. Gesundheitszustand unterer Frontzähne über 10 Jahre nach approximaler Schmelzreduktion. Inf Orthod Kieferorthop 2007;39:103–110
37. Zhong M, Jost-Brinkmann PG, Zellmann M, et al. Clinical evaluation of a new technique for interdental enamel reduction. J Orofac Orthop 2000;61(6):432–439
38. Zöller J, Ullrich H. Combined surgical-orthodontic palatine suture expansion in adulthood. [Article in German] Fortschr Kieferorthop 1991;52(2):61–65

Auxiliary Equipment and Techniques

Bjoern Ludwig, Bettina Glasl, and Thomas Lietz

8

The following advertising slogan appears in a brochure highlighting the advantages of self-ligating systems: "Everything's simpler and you save on everything!" Other advertising materials are more specific, and the following list details the main advantages claimed by manufacturers of self-ligating systems:

- Increased patient comfort
- Ease of operator handling
- Mechanism that is easy to open and close
- Allows faster ligation than conventional brackets
- Better oral hygiene
- Reduced friction characteristics leading to shorter treatment times
- Shorter appointment times (less chairside time)
- More efficient treatment (fewer appointments and increased intervals between appointments)

Clearly, self-ligating brackets cannot produce any of these advantages unless they are used by an experienced clinician who understands the basic principles and the strengths and weaknesses of the bracket systems. Some cases involve a degree of difficulty at which self-ligating brackets (SLBs) and wires alone are insufficient for solving the problem. Even in the hands of the most experienced operator, SLBs may need to be supplemented with auxiliaries. As SLBs are only one of the many tools available to contemporary orthodontists, it is the operator's responsibility to establish the most suitable way to treat a malocclusion and to select the most appropriate strategies and tools. This chapter presents supplementary information on adjuncts and auxiliary techniques, which may be helpful when treating different malocclusions using self-ligating brackets.
The use of self-ligating brackets does not redefine the principles of orthodontics. Most of the treatment approaches that are already known still apply—to move a tooth into a desired spot, you require time, anchorage, and space. Treatment should only be contemplated once these three parameters have been considered carefully and the treatment objectives have been designed around them.

Practical Application of Self-Ligating Brackets

"Open the door, insert the archwire, close the door!" That is how simple the use of an SLB should be. However, this may be more wishful thinking than reality. There are two main weaknesses that affect the use of self-ligation in orthodontics—the ligating mechanism itself and the operator who uses it.
Self-ligating brackets are difficult to manufacture. The materials used, particularly for the locking mechanism, have to be able to withstand masticatory forces as well as the stress that normally occurs during orthodontic treatment, while at the same time they have to have the ideal properties to allow precise fabrication. Assembling the ligation mechanism and coupling it to the rest of the bracket is a challenging manufacturing process. The mechanism needs to be manufactured to extremely high standards, and this is particularly difficult because different materials are used for the bracket base and the locking mechanism, and by default their respective tolerances differ. The resulting bracket is a delicate device that requires careful and diligent handling.
There is no single self-ligating bracket available today that is capable of tolerating inept and "forced" handling by the operator. The opening of the locking mechanism, insertion of the archwire, and closure of the locking mechanism have to be undertaken carefully and require an understanding of the locking mechanism itself as well as careful tactile handling. Most operators experience a steep learning curve associated with the use of self-ligation. Regardless of which

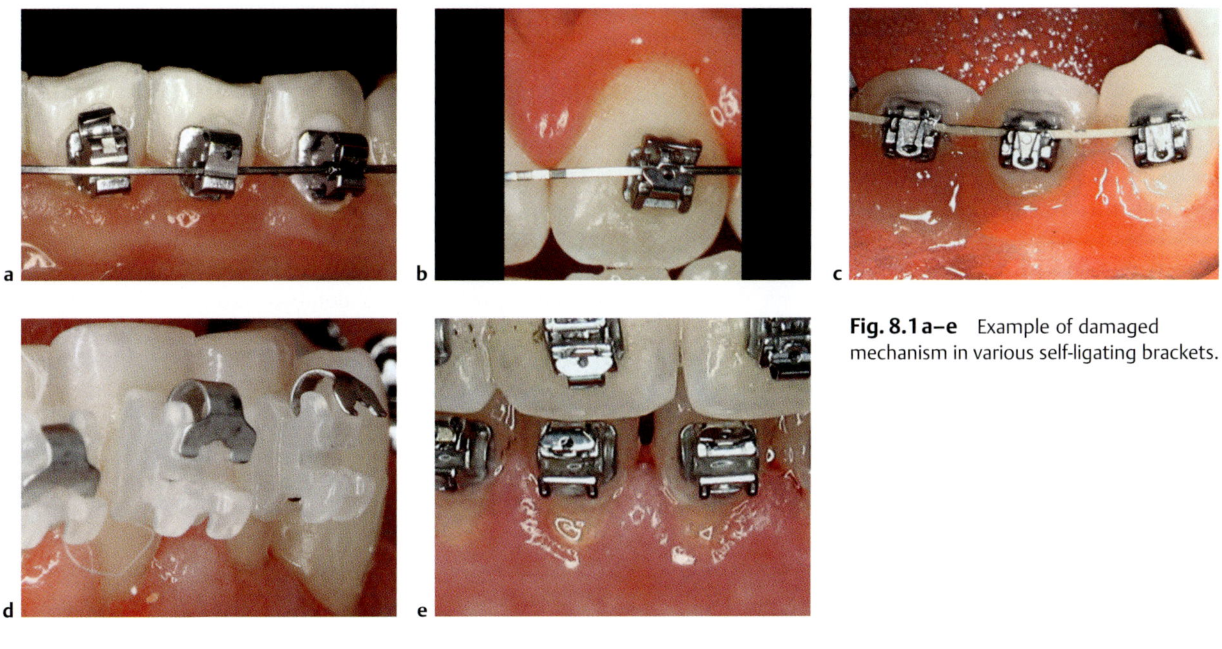

Fig. 8.1 a–e Example of damaged mechanism in various self-ligating brackets.

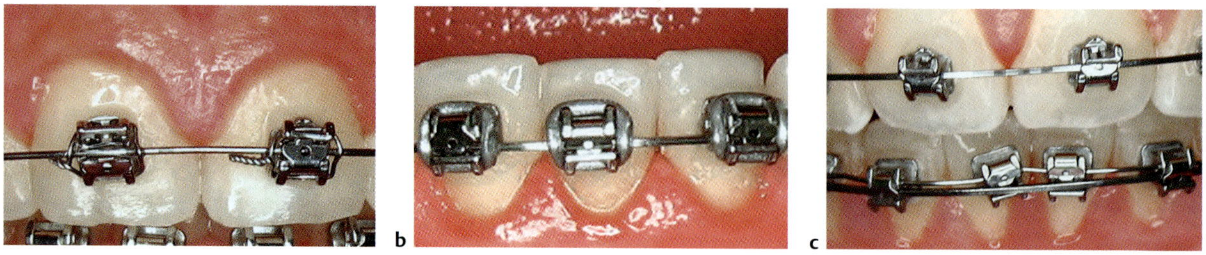

a b c

Fig. 8.2a–c A damaged self-ligating mechanism does not necessarily require replacement of the bracket. Treatment can often be continued using a wire ligature (**a**) or elastic ligature (**b**). A third option is to use the auxiliary slot (if present) instead (**c**).

Table 8.1 The learning curve for an untrained layperson using traditional brackets (red) and self-ligating brackets (blue). Even after some practice, elastic ligation took three times longer than self-ligation

Method	Attempt 1	Attempt 2	Attempt 3	Attempt 4	Attempt 5	Attempt 6
Time in minutes						
Clip 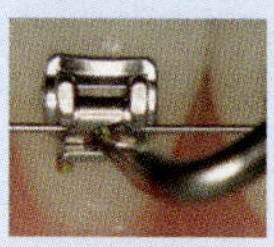	2.14	1.45	1.25	1.21	1.23	1.37
Elastic 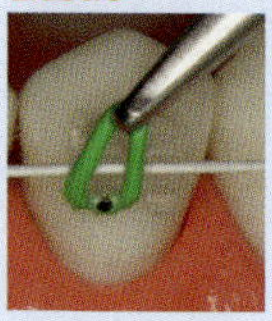	7.26	5.15	4.50	3.08	4.07	4.57

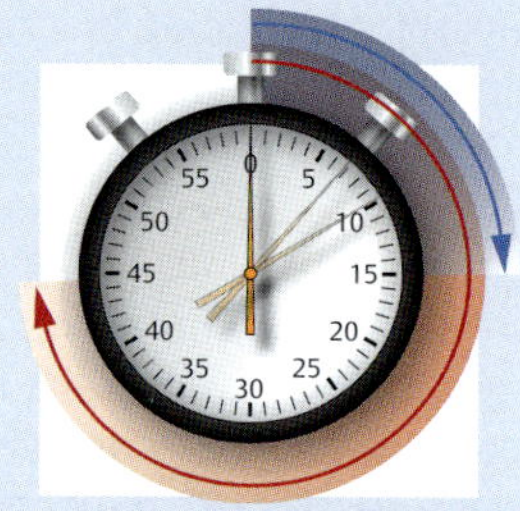

system is used, operators need to understand the exact details of the locking mechanism so that they can use it effectively. This is the first step in the successful use of SLBs. Most manufacturers produce large models of the self-ligating bracket, usually made of acrylic. These models are designed to train operators (dentists and staff) how to open and close the locking mechanism. Poor manipulation techniques by the operator may irreversibly damage the locking mechanism and render the bracket useless for the remainder of the treatment (**Fig. 8.1**).

Some manufacturers used to offer replacements for the locking mechanism itself (e.g., for the Speed System); the mechanism can be repaired intraorally once it has been inadvertently damaged. It requires some expertise to change this delicate mechanism without damaging the bracket itself or debonding it. Also, the costs of brackets are much lower now, so it is questionable whether the time spent repairing a bracket justifies the procedure. It is often easier to continue to use the damaged bracket with conventional ligation (elastomeric ring or steel ligature) or to replace the bracket (**Fig. 8.2**). Lightly tied stainless-steel ligatures have similar frictional characteristics to self-ligating brackets (7). However, this assumes that there are tie-wings present on the bracket that can be used for conventional ligation. Not all brackets, however, are designed in this way (see Chapters 2 and 3).

It is not always possible to assess the user-friendliness of a particular self-ligating bracket system after training on a demonstration model. Whatever the system, it takes considerable time for the operator to become accustomed to self-ligation and to no longer using wire or elastomeric ligatures. However, there is also a learning curve when conventional ligation is used. Comparisons of the learning curves for previously untrained personnel show that self-ligation is actually learned more quickly than ligation with elastomeric elements or tie-wings, and that it takes less time to ligate the wire using SLBs, even for inexperienced operators. In the authors' experience, however, it appears to be difficult for operators to learn the effective use of self-ligation once they have previously been trained in the use of conventional ligation techniques (**Table 8.1**).

As mentioned above, a detailed understanding of self-ligating mechanisms is often the key to using the system successfully. It is mandatory to have the recommended instrumentation for opening and closing the brackets. It may be useful to remember that closure of most mechanisms can be undertaken without instrumentation using gloved fingers, which often proves to be more efficient than religating conventional brackets with elastomeric ligatures. Manufacturers produce instruments specifically designed for their own bracket systems, most of which are not compatible with other systems.

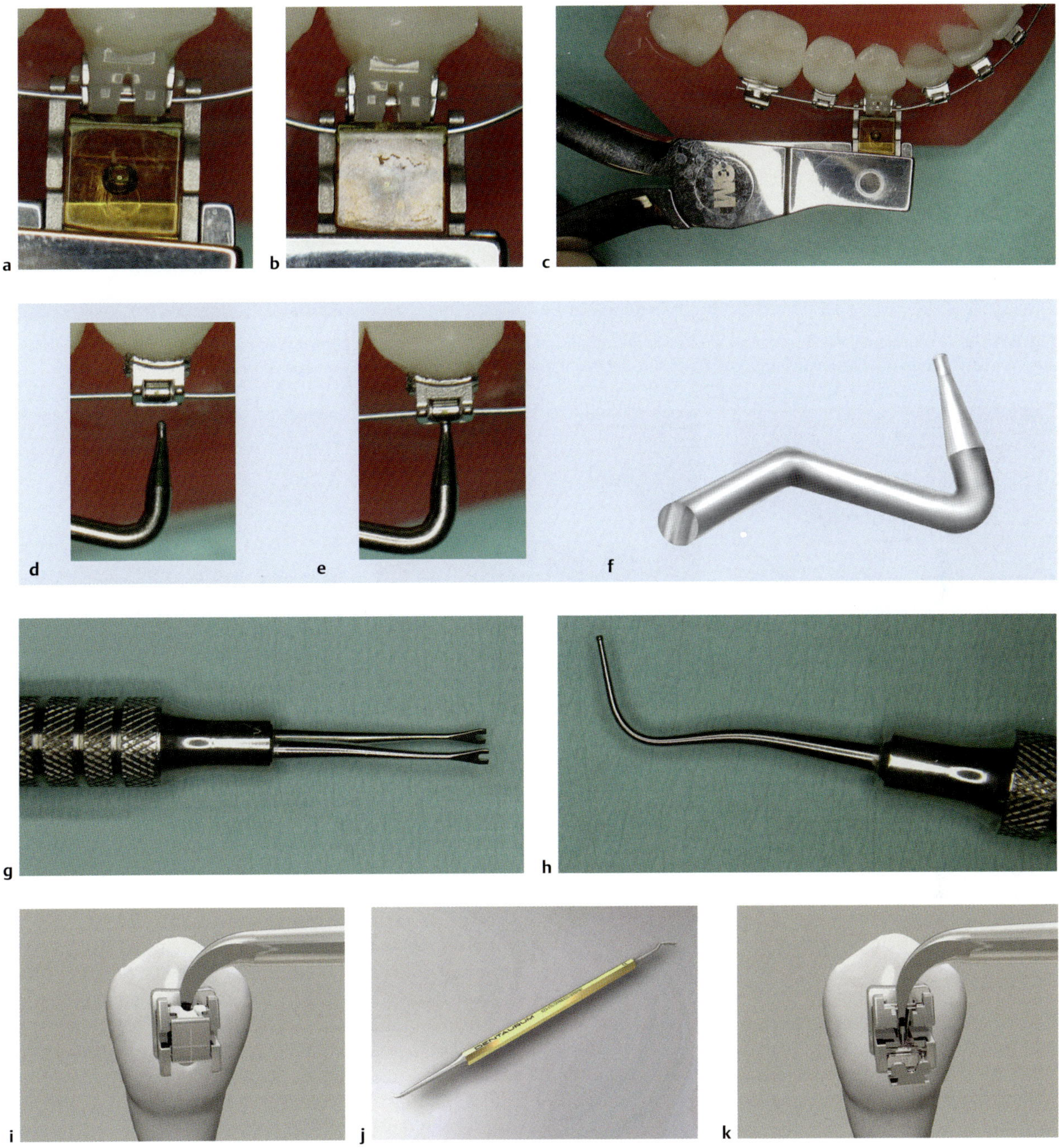

Fig. 8.3a–k Different types of instruments for opening the mechanism in self-ligating brackets.
a–c The SmartClip bracket (3 M Unitek) with special pliers.
d–f The Quick bracket instrument (Forestadent), similar to a dental probe.
g–h The In-Ovation instrument (GAC).
i–k The Discovery SL instrument (Dentaurum), resembling a scaler (images with kind permission from Dentaurum).

CLINICAL PEARL

Although the dedicated adjuncts appear expensive, it is advisable to use the instruments recommended by the manufacturer (**Fig. 8.3**).

Specifically, the probe-like instruments for self-ligating brackets can be easily confused between different manufacturers or indeed between various systems produced by the same manufacturer. It may be advisable to mark the various instruments for particular systems if several self-ligating systems are used in the same practice.

The locking mechanism itself is a fine-tuned mechanical device that is likely to fail if it is handled inappropriately and with too much force (**Fig. 8.4**).

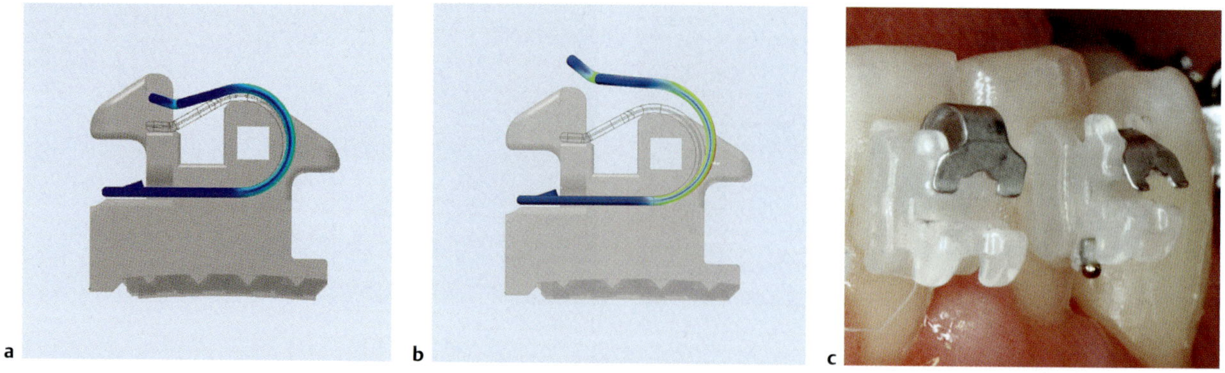

Fig. 8.4a–c Finite-element (FEM) analysis of stresses and strains on the self-ligating bracket clip: correct handling (**a**), incorrect handling (**b**), pivoting motion (**c**). The color transition shows the stresses that cause to irreversible deformation at the curvature of the clip.

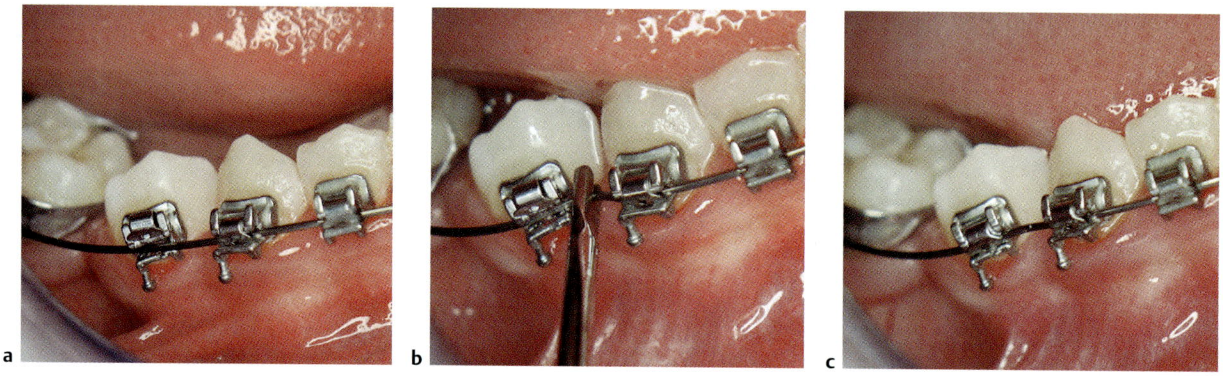

Fig. 8.5a–c A bifid wire director aids in pushing the archwire into the bracket slot and achieving full engagement.

ERRORS AND RISKS

Once a lid or locking mechanism has been bent or distorted, it cannot be repaired. It is often best to use conventional ligation on the damaged bracket (if possible) or to replace the bracket.

The locking mechanism will also fail if composite finds its way into the mechanism, particularly during the bonding procedure. This can often be avoided if the correct amount of bonding agent is carefully applied in the middle of the bracket base.

CLINICAL PEARL

Excess bonding material should ideally be removed immediately after seating the bracket, to prevent the bonding material from interfering with the self-ligating mechanism.

The self-ligating mechanism can also be damaged during chewing, particularly when there are strong masticatory forces; this is often the case in patients with a deep bite. This type of damage can often be prevented by using bite-opening devices (see the following section on "Bite Planes," p. 183).

Another reason for irreversible damage to the locking mechanism occurring is forced engagement of the archwire in the bracket slot. This can be a problem particularly if large or excessively stiff wires are used. The fit of the archwire needs to be carefully checked before the operator attempts to close the locking mechanism. The lid can be irreversibly damaged during closure of a poorly fitting archwire. The propensity to cause damage depends on the wire size and material, the position of the tooth, and the position of the bracket on the tooth itself. Any of the above parameters are important, as they can lead to the archwire not being fully engaged in the bracket slot. The lid may subsequently not shut properly if the wire cannot be seated properly in the bracket slot and this may lead to ineffective treatment. Additional instruments (such as a wire director) are often useful for engaging the archwire properly into the bracket slot before closing the locking mechanism (**Fig. 8.5**). Several manufacturers now also offer self-ligating molar brackets. These can be useful, as they allow extraoral preparation of the archwire for detailing or cinch-back bends, with subsequent easy insertion into molar SLBs. This reduces the risk of debonding the bracket or otherwise damaging it in comparison with creating the bends intraorally (**Fig. 8.6**). **Table 8.2** highlights the potential reasons for damage to the locking mechanisms and offers suggestions for ways to prevent these problems.

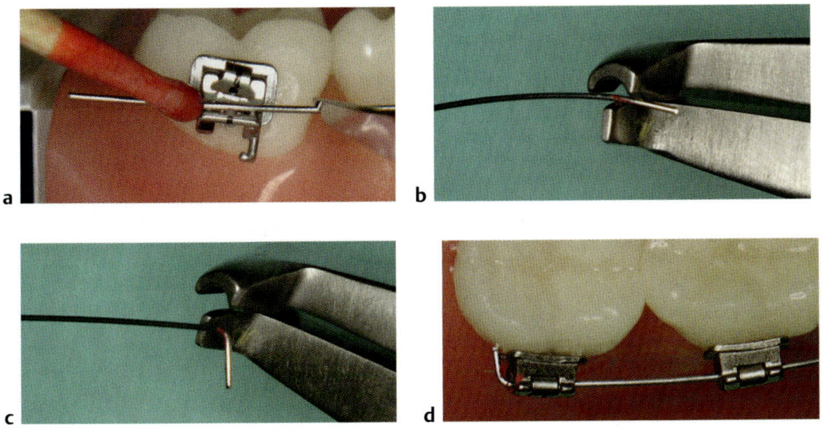

Fig. 8.6a–d Self-ligating molar brackets can be used instead of traditional tubes. The correct archwire length is marked intraorally (**a**), the cinch-back bend is then placed extraorally (**b, c**), and the wire is inserted afterwards (**d**).

Table 8.2 Typical errors that can increase the risk of a clip defect and ways to prevent them

Reason for mechanism defect	Preventative measure	Solution
Direct occlusal forces	Bite planes: • Anterior • Posterior	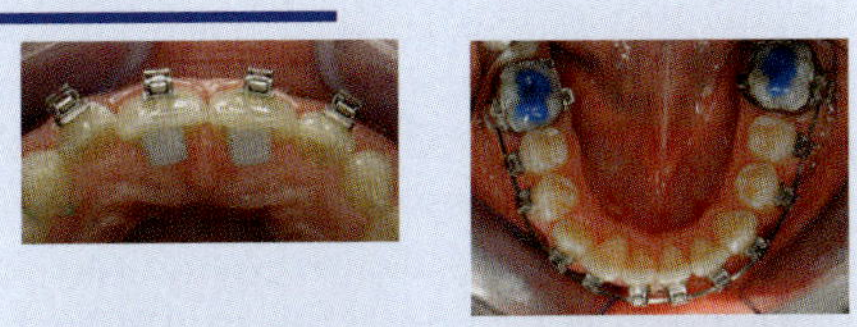
Archwire prevents complete locking of the clip	• Use smaller SE archwire, be patient • Full engagement of the SE wire with a wire director	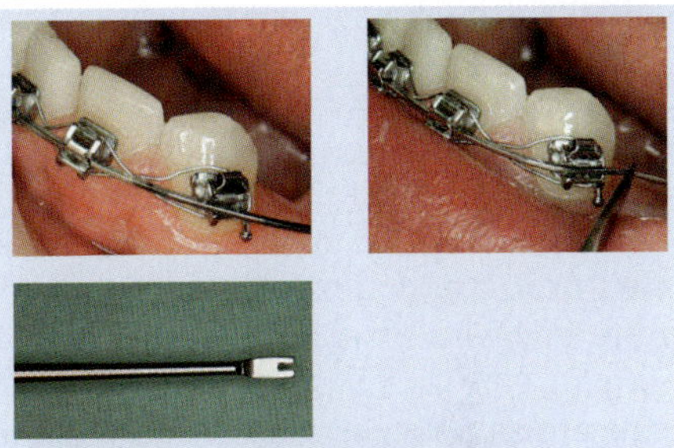
Use of a noncompatible instrument (e.g., dental probe)	Use of the appropriate instrument	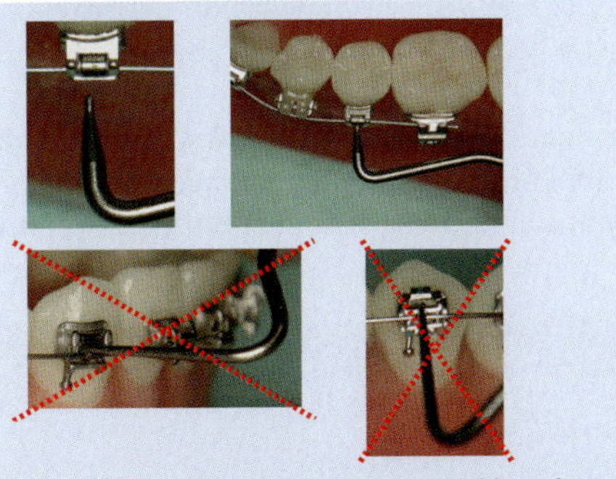 Caution: the dental probe can act like a lever arm, distorting the self-ligating mechanism
Operator error	• Training on the typodont • Follow manufacturer's instructions	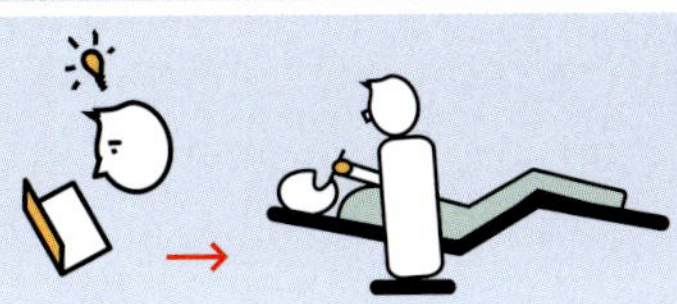

SE, superelastic.

Archwire Shift

Slippery Archwires

Low-friction systems allow shifting (swivelling) of the archwire, particularly if initially very thin wires are used during the leveling and alignment phase. This is a very common occurrence in an orthodontic practice and is often the reason for emergency appointments, as it can lead to pronounced soft-tissue irritation (**Fig. 8.7**). Shifting of larger archwires can lead to distortion of the dental arch and arch asymmetry. It is therefore very useful to stop the archwires from shifting and sliding freely in the brackets. **Table 8.3** summarizes the methods and materials necessary to prevent shifting of archwires.

Annealing. Annealing the distal ends permanently changes the elastic properties of the archwires, as they become formable. This is particularly useful for modern superelastic alignment wires. A conventional cigarette lighter or a blowtorch can be used for this. Following annealing at the desired spot, the wires are cinched back. It appears advisable to turn the ends lingually rather than to the gingival side, as this may prevent trauma to the gums and patient discomfort.

Changing the archwire shape. The shape of a superelastic archwire can be changed without permanently altering its physical properties by using devices such as the Memory Maker, which warms up the archwire in a controlled way using an electric current. This can be applied either to the entire archwire or only to a section of it. During the warming, the archwire can be permanently deformed using appropriate pliers; the original mechanical properties of the wire itself will not change, however. This is particularly useful for initial alignment wires.

Permanent deformation using special instruments. A number of instrument manufacturers offer special instruments for bending wires back, such as hammerhead pliers (originally developed by Hu-Friedy, Inc.). Tuckers can also be used to permanently deform archwires, as can birdbeak pliers, and with some limitations, Weingart pliers as well. However, these tools work best if the wires have previously been annealed—particularly with superelastic wires. Turning archwires back without annealing them is usually only possible with stiff nonresilient wire types such as stainless steel and titanium–molybdenum alloy (TMA).

Application of stops. To secure an archwire's position, the cinch-back bend should be placed bilaterally, distal of the most distal bracket or tube. Annealing and cinching archwires can be time-consuming, uncomfortable for the patient, and may also lead to inadvertent debonding of brackets, especially when molar tubes are used and the bends are made intraorally. Often, archwires need to be inserted intraorally, cut to size, removed, and then annealed before they can be reinserted and cinched. Cinched archwires can be difficult to remove, as the bent ends usually have to be cut off first. An alternative method is to use stops, which should be placed mesial and distal to a bracket. This prevents shifting of the archwire in a predictable way and at the same time allows the archwire to be removed easily. A number of prefabricated crimpable stops are available on the market. They can be picked up with either ligature cutters or specific crimping pliers. The stops are placed over the archwire using these instruments and then crimped down. A number of manufacturers produce these stops so that the inside is serrated or roughened, which gives them a more secure grip. However, crimpable stops work best on rectangular archwires. They often still slip on small round wires. An alternative to using crimpable stops is to apply light-cured composite on the archwire. It is also sometimes advisable to add composite to a crimpable stop, as these can sometimes feel rough to the patient. Composite is used to give the stop a smooth surface and secure it at the same time. Both of the above composite techniques are suitable for all types and sizes of archwire.

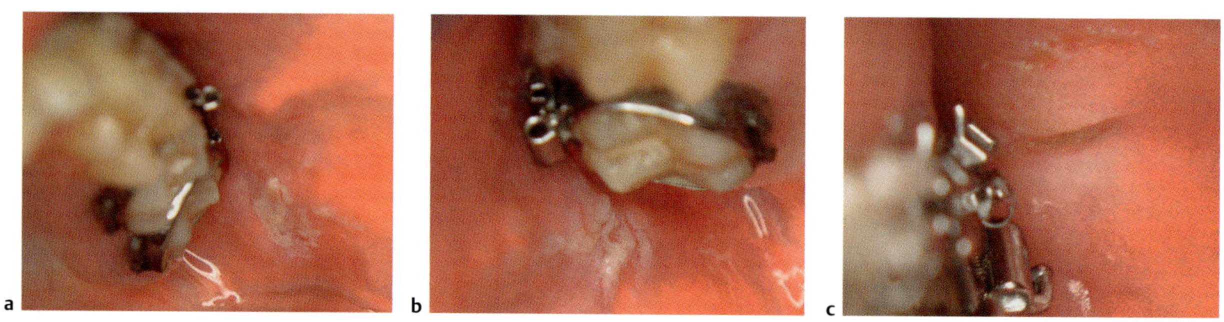

Fig. 8.7a–c Mechanical irritation of the mucosa caused by a continuous wire that has slipped distally. The protruding wire part can cause considerable soft-tissue irritation.

Table 8.3 Methods of securing the archwire to avoid sliding

Method	Illustration	Material	Advantages	Disadvantages
Annealing the distal ends	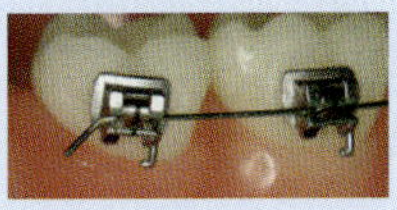	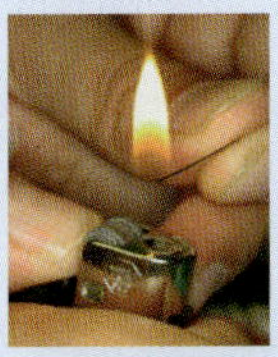 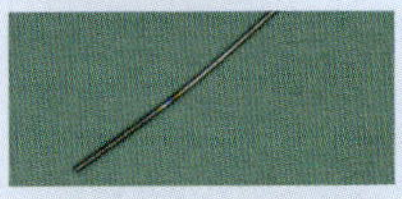	• Inexpensive • Quick • Simple	• Uncontrolled effect • Only applicable extraorally
Shape change using the Memory Maker	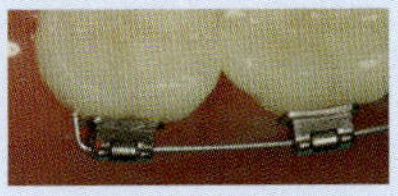	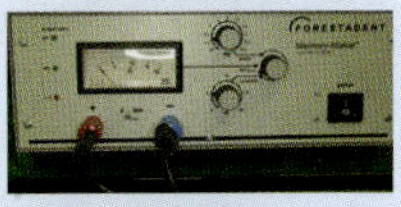 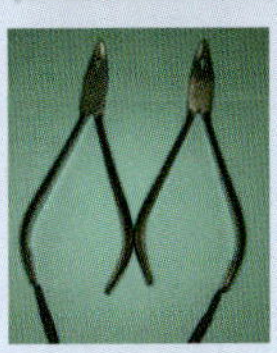	• Precise • Does not affect the properties of other archwire areas	• Expensive • Only applicable extraorally
Hammerhead pliers	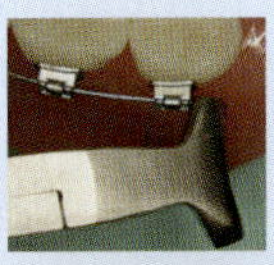 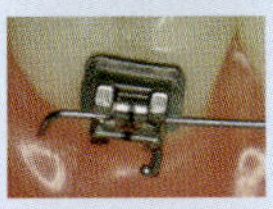	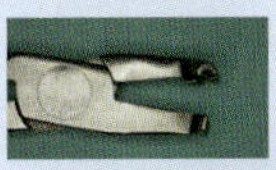 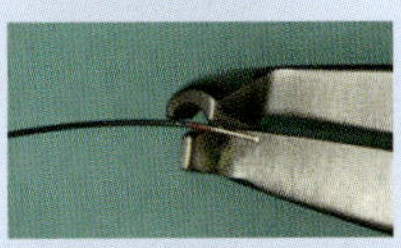	• Specially designed for NiTi wires • Intraorally applicable • No annealing required	• Cinch not flush • Does not work on SE wires unless these are annealed
Cinching tool	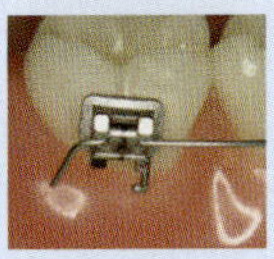	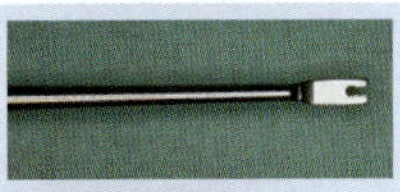 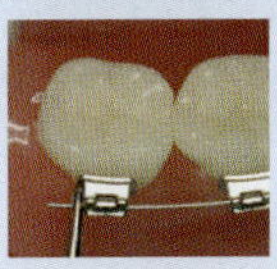	• Leads to a flush cinch • Intraorally applicable • Ideal for annealed NiTi wires	• Not suitable for NiTi wires that are not annealed
Composite stops	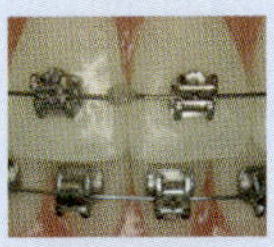	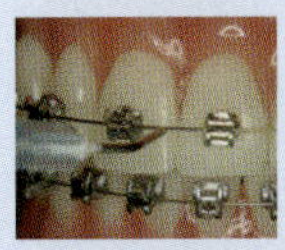	• Quick • Intraorally applicable • Inexpensive • Comfortable	• Can come loose
Crimpable stops	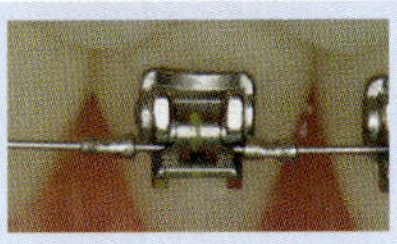	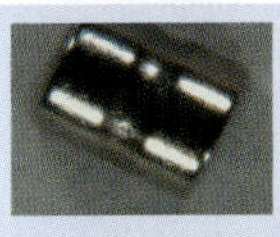 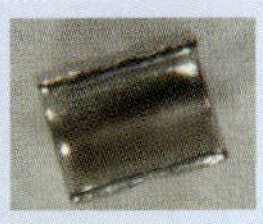 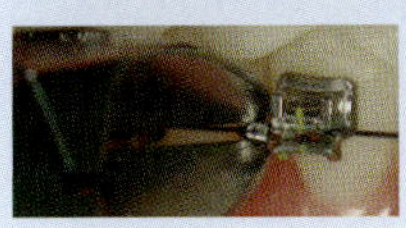	• Quick • Intraorally applicable	• Expensive • Special pliers advisable • A ligature cutter can inadvertantly cut through the archwire and become blunt

Detailing Bends

Individualized Arches

All of the desired tooth movements are already preprogrammed into the preadjusted straight-wire bracket. At least in theory, it should therefore be possible to achieve a good orthodontic result by simply inserting a sequence of straight wires into the precisely positioned brackets. In clinical practice, however, this does not always appear to be the case. Shortcomings in ideal bracket positioning, as well as technical and anatomical issues, may require modification and individualization of archwires to address the desired treatment outcome (**Fig. 8.8**). This applies to any type of ligation—conventional or self-ligating. Usually, intrusion and extrusion bends, in and out bends, and torque adjustments are used, while rotations are better corrected by repositioning the brackets.

NOTE

Superelastic archwires can only be permanently deformed using the Memory Maker. The ideal wires for detailing bends are stainless steel and TMA wires.

Detailing bends have to be very precise when used with SLBs. Inappropriate or incorrect placement of detailing bends stands out much more with SLBs than with conventional ligation, as the doors will no longer shut or will start to distort after forced closure. The operator should therefore avoid closing the mechanism with significant force and should modify the bends if necessary. What might initially appear to be a disadvantage is therefore actually advantageous, as it ensures that controlled light forces are used. This should be beneficial in relation to inadvertent damage to the teeth, leading to root resorption.

NOTE

Operators should avoid placing detailing bends intraorally with the archwire still engaged. This can lead to damage to the self-ligating mechanism. We recommend removing the archwire from the mouth, placement of the detailing bends, followed by coordination of the archwires and then reinsertion.

To mark the location of the detailing bends on the wire, we recommend hygienic, single-use wax markers (**Fig. 8.9**).

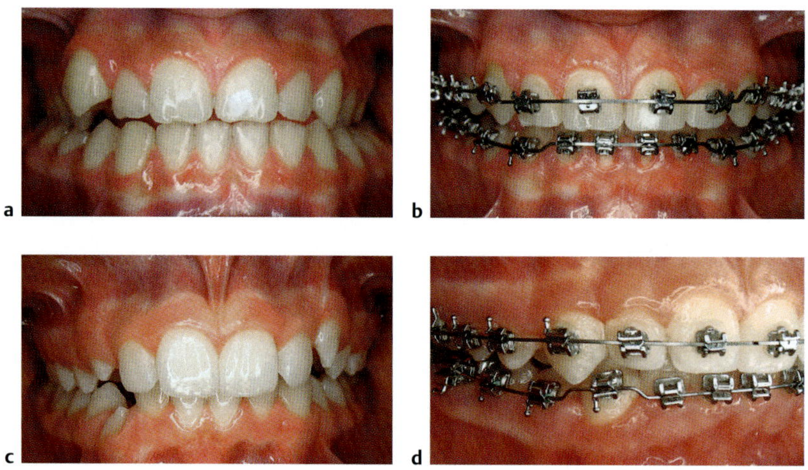

Fig. 8.8a–d A customized archwire using step-up bends for an entire arch segment or a single tooth. To increase the overbite (**a, b**) a step-up artistic bend was placed along the mandibular incisors. The second patient (**c, d**) presented with delayed eruption of tooth 43. As soon as a bracket could be bonded, the tooth was included in the orthodontic appliance. However, the bracket was not in the appropriate position. This had to be compensated for by a single-tooth step-up bend.

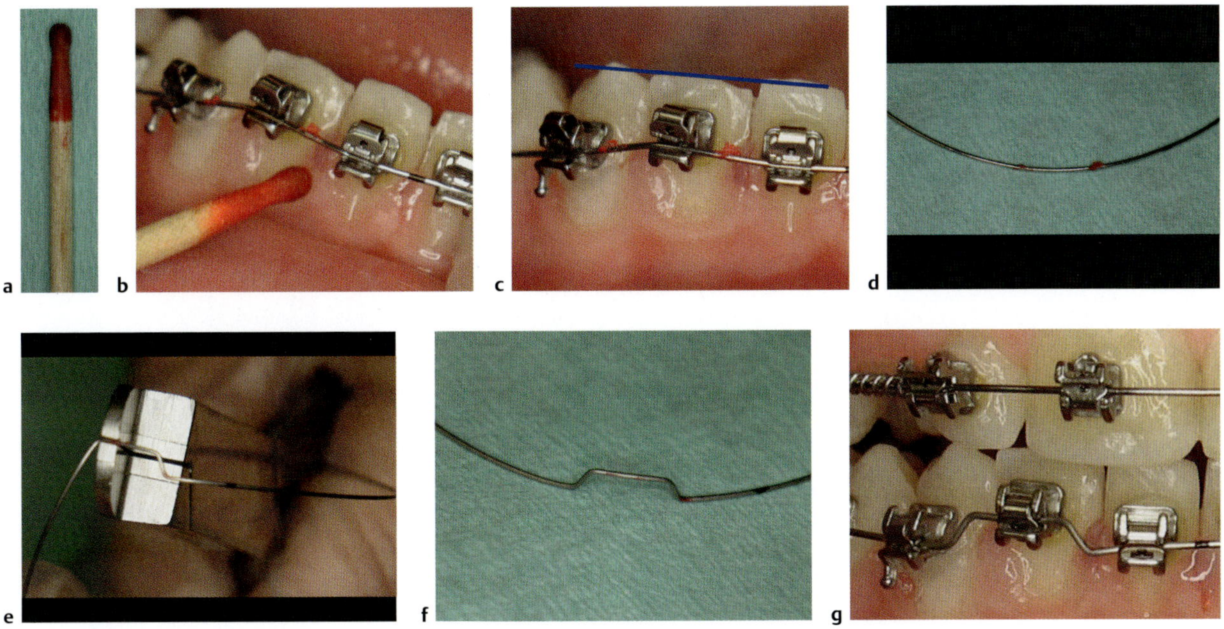

Fig. 8.9a–g The following steps are recommended to customize an archwire: the positions of the bends are marked intraorally with a disposable wax marker (**a–d**), the bends are placed (**e**) and verified on a flat surface (**f**). The customized wire can then be inserted (**g**).

Correction of the Occlusion

Most patients will require the use of elastomeric elements, at least on a temporary basis, and these can be applied in an intramaxillary or intermaxillary fashion. Intramaxillary elastics can be applied easily if the bracket resembles the traditional twin design. Brackets with a single-block design may make it more difficult to use elastomeric chains. These usually need to be placed underneath the archwire, which will mean reduced friction but makes replacing the modules difficult, as the wire has to be removed each time the archwire needs to be changed. Replacing the elastomeric chains with elastic thread is another alternative, but thread is less efficient than chain.

Intermaxillary elastic elements (class II, class III, or vertical elastics) are often necessary to achieve the desired treatment outcome. The authors prefer to use brackets with incorporated hooks for the buccal segments, which makes the use of elastics easy. The alternative—using Kobayashi ties to add hooks—is cumbersome and often requires repair. **Table 8.4** shows the most important ways of engaging intermaxillary elastics. The literature describes many—often ingenious—applications for elastics. In our experience, however, we find that using such innovations can be misunderstood by the patient, and this can occasionally lead to negative effects on the treatment outcome. We therefore prefer the simple application of elastomeric elements, which allows patients to follow the instructions easily.

Table 8.4 Example arrangements for various intermaxillary elastics

Vector	Elastic size/force	Graphic	Typodont
Mainly sagittal Class II Class III	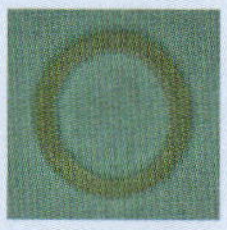 ¼" 4 oz	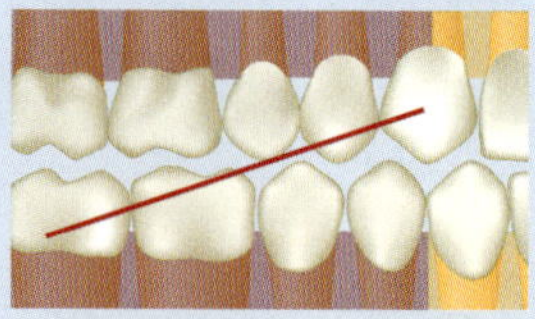	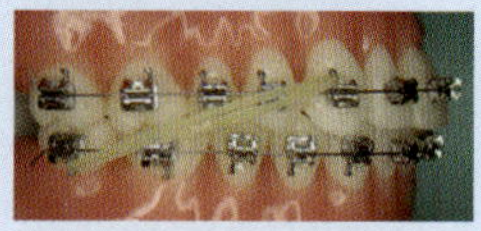
	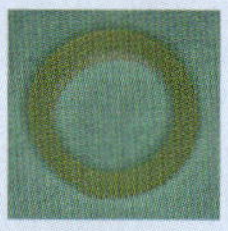 ¼" 6 oz	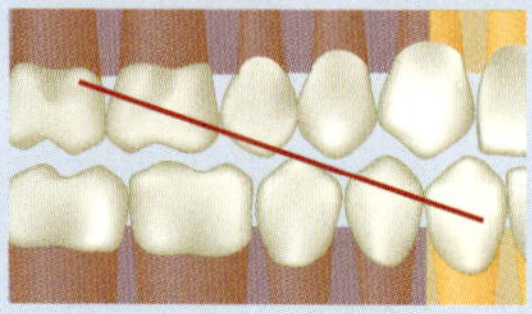	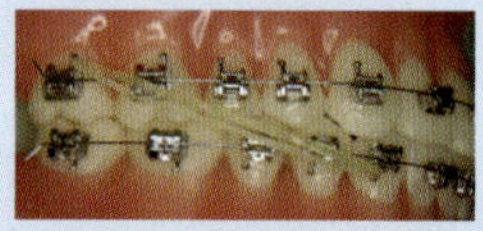
Mainly vertical	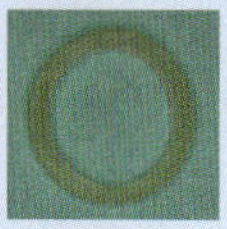 ⅛" 3.5 oz	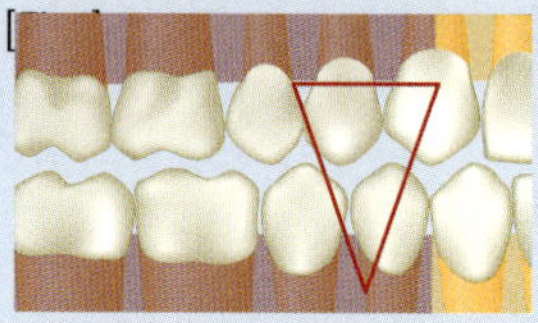	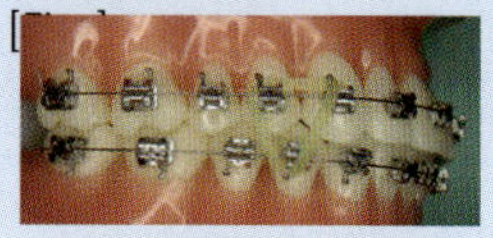
	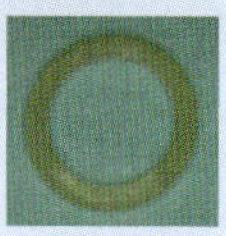 ³⁄₁₆" 6 oz	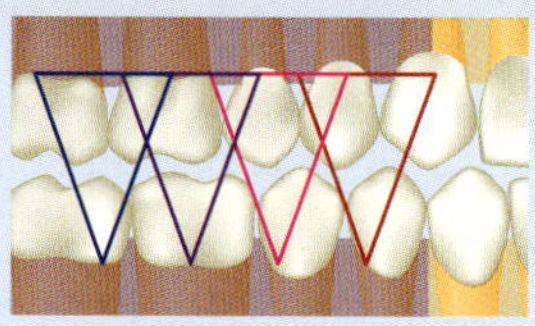	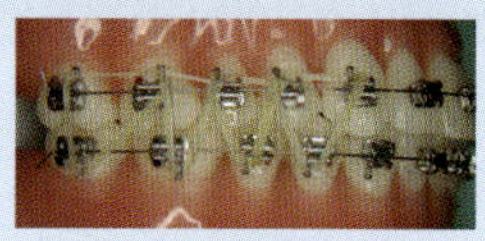
Combined forms of sagittal and vertical vectors. All of the elastic formations can be used with a class II or class III component.		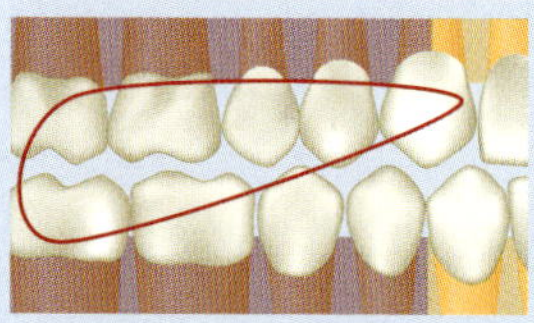	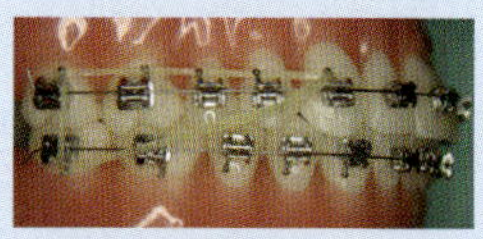
		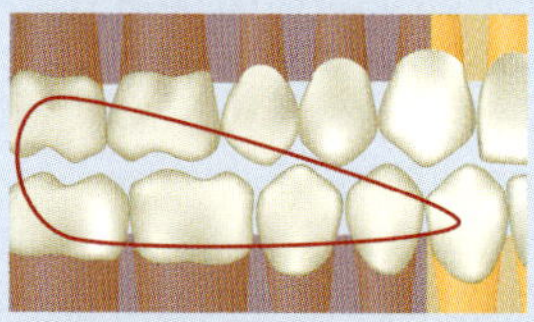	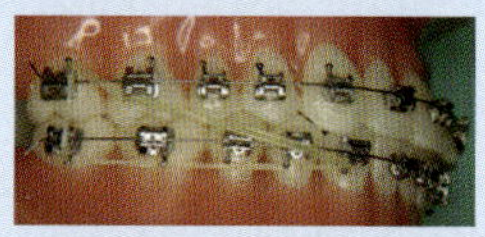
		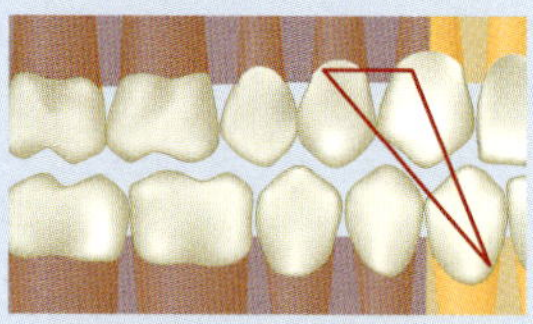	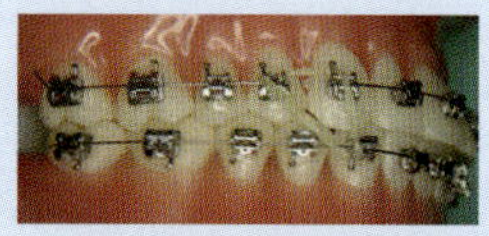
		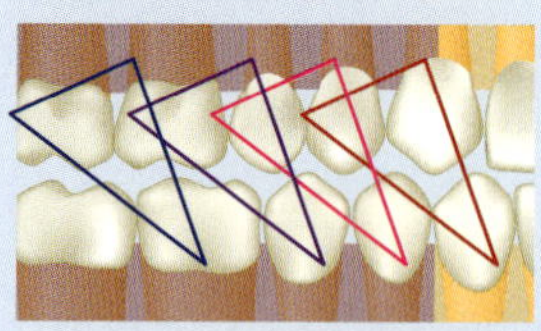	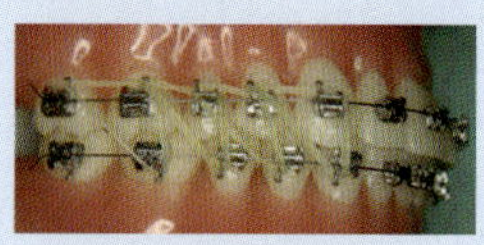
		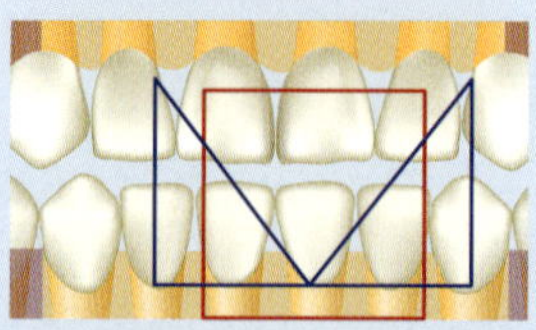	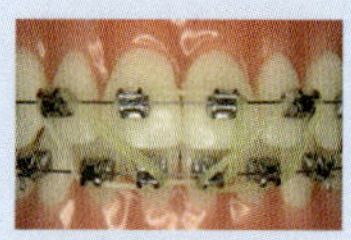
		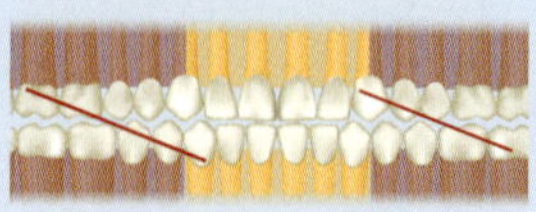	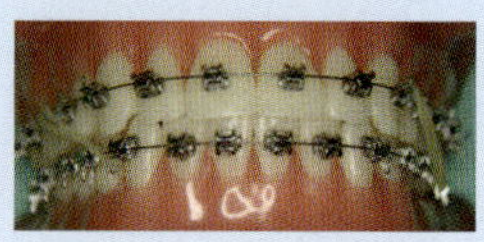

Other Useful Auxiliaries

Spikes

Leveling and alignment can be associated with anterior and lateral bite opening. If the tongue starts to interpose in the space, resolve of the opposite can be difficult and tongue habits may develop and may become permanent. An initially simple habit can potentially create a difficult treatment situation. For patients presenting with a habitual tongue thrust, we find that one of the more efficient ways of dealing with this to use prefabricated pads with spikes attached (**Fig. 8.10**). We recommend using a continuous ligature, which is fitted around each individual attachment; this prevents inadvertent swallowing or aspiration of the lingual attachments.

The spikes may initially be uncomfortable for the patient, and it is advisable to inform and instruct the patient accordingly. Each time the tongue assumes its potentially harmful position the patient is made aware of the spike due to the discomfort. Over time, this leads to the tongue being trained to adopt a different, corrected position. In our experience, the tongue interposition tends to disappear after a short time, but we find it best to leave the spikes in place for at least several months in order to prevent relapse of the tongue interposition.

Bite Planes

The locking mechanism in SLBs can be damaged if excessive force is used. This also applies, with occlusal forces when patients bite on brackets in centric occlusion or during mastication. The operator should therefore carefully check for any occlusal interference, particularly if teeth directly occlude on the SLB's locking mechanism. If this is the case, we recommend either using an anterior bite plane or a posterior bite elevator. Careful evaluation of the temporomandibular joint is advisable before these auxiliaries are applied. When planning bite opening with auxiliaries, it is also advisable to consider the growth pattern. A patient with a brachycephalic deep bite will benefit more from anterior bite elevators, as these allow molar extrusion, while posterior bite elevators invade the leeway space and can cause relative intrusion of the molars.

Bite elevators attached to the palatal surfaces of the upper front teeth are very useful adjuncts. By disoccluding the posterior teeth (**Fig. 8.11**), they allow uninhibited vertical development of the alveolar processes. Anterior bite planes are particularly useful for patients with class II/$_2$ malocclusions, as they allow simultaneous alignment of both upper and lower arches and bite opening. A reduced lower anterior facial height can be corrected with this approach, especially in combination with a mandibular reverse curve of Spee alignment wire or vertical elastics. The anterior bite planes need to be checked at each appointment, as they may have become ineffective. The proclination of the upper front teeth that is often associated with treatment for a class II/$_2$ incisor relationship may move the attachments anteriorly and thus make them ineffective. Subsequently, the protective function for the lower front teeth may have been lost. The lower labial segment may actually fall behind the bite planes in such a way that alignment of the lower front teeth is prevented, as the posterior aspect of the bite planes constantly pushes the lower labial segment lingually.

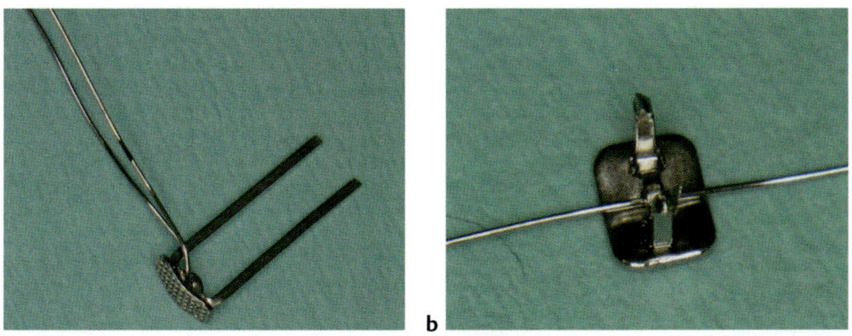

Fig. 8.10 a, b A spike pad with a steel ligature to avoid ingestion/aspiration (PhD C. Sander) (**a**). The spike length can be customized with a heavy-duty wire cutter, which creates tapering ends (**b**).

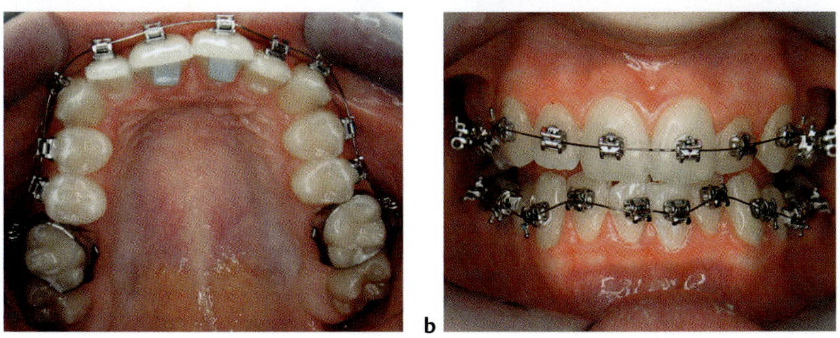

Fig. 8.11 a, b Lingual bite planes to unlock the occlusion, allowing undisturbed tooth movement.

PROCEDURE

Bite planes should not have a negative impact on the patient's occlusion. If not used correctly, bite planes may force the lower jaw distally, preventing alignment of the lower labial segment, on the one hand, and worsening the sagittal discrepancy on the other. Bite planes may also increase stress on the temporomandibular joint. At the same time, the bite planes should be adjusted to prevent patients from shifting laterally on contact. We find that anterior bite planes can be an extremely useful adjunct to self-ligation treatment, particularly if the above recommendations are followed.

In our experience, the following two techniques have proved useful for manufacturing bite planes.

Anterior Bite Planes

Anterior bite planes can be purchased prefabricated from a number of manufacturers (e.g., Bite Turbo, Ormco), or they can be made to suit the patient's individual needs. In our practice, we use a preformed mold system known as the Mini-Mold (Ortho Technology), which makes it very easy to fabricate and apply anterior bite planes.

Figure 8.12 is a step-by-step guide on how to fabricate and use the Mini-Mold system. Initially, the enamel surface has to be conditioned. The mold is then filled with the composite and positioned at the desired location on the

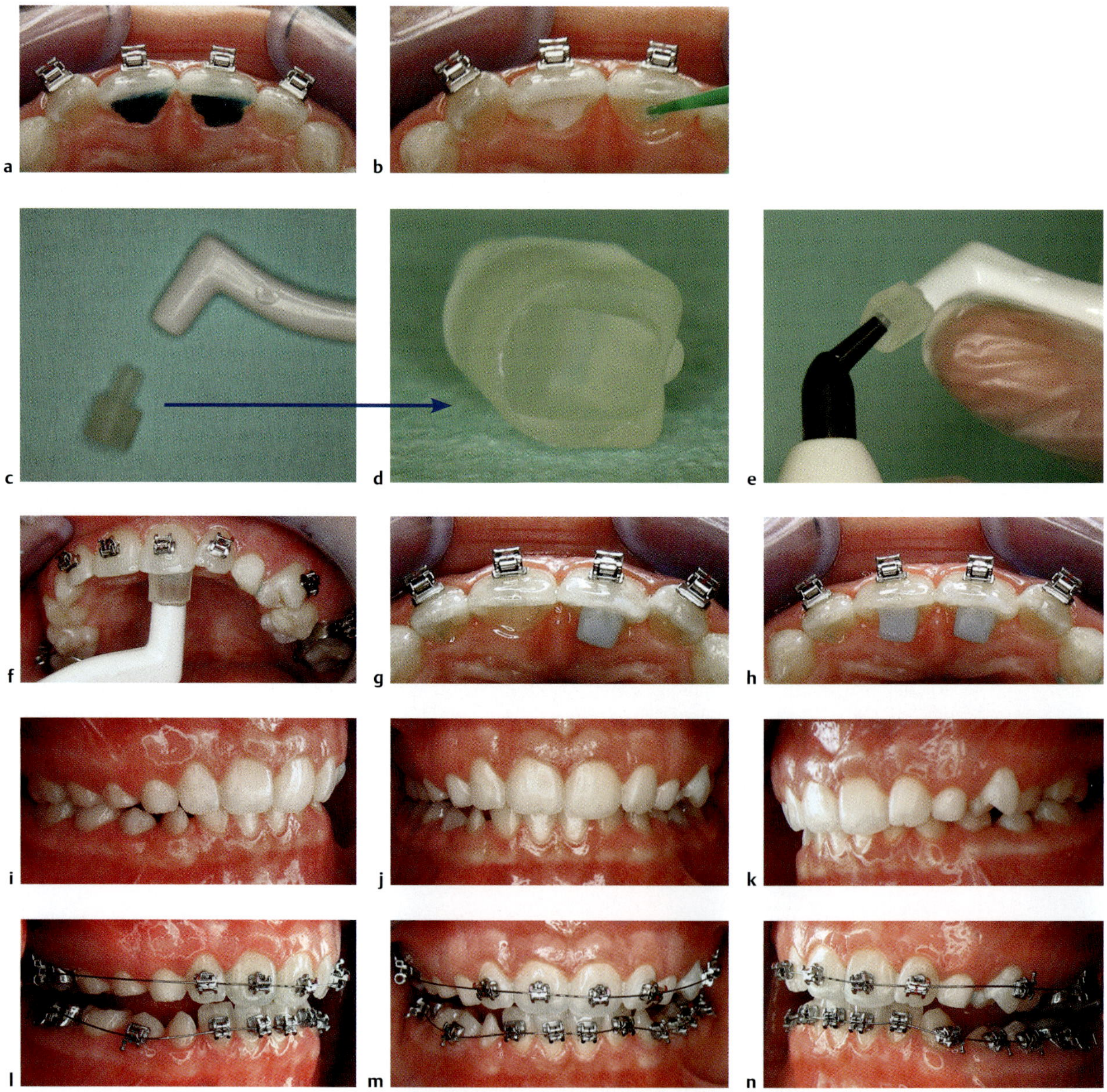

Fig. 8.12 a–n Clinical steps with the Mini-Mold system. The patient presents with a deep bite and buccal crossbite on tooth 24, which is locked into its position by the occlusion. The lingual bite planes allow immediate bonding of both arches and correction of the scissors bite without occlusal interference.

palatal site of the upper anterior teeth. The composite is then light-cured. Bite planes that have been manufactured in this way are usually stable and do not break or debond. They can be easily adjusted and are also relatively easy to remove. Due to the color of the material, it is easy to recognize residual composite on the palatal surface of the teeth so it can be completely removed following bite opening. Added advantages of this technique in comparison with premanufactured bite-opening appliances (such as bite turbos) are its lower cost and the reduced risk of swallowing or aspiration.

Lateral Bite Planes

Lateral bite planes can be added to the occlusal surface after appropriate conditioning. Either glass ionomer materials or composite materials are suitable for this purpose. In our experience, we have found that a blue glass ionomer cement, Band Lok Blue (Reliance Orthodontics), or Triad VLC Gel (Dentsply) works quite well. The latter is available in a number of different colors. The coloring makes it easier to remove the composite at the end of treatment. Independent of the material and bonding choice, removal of posterior bite planes can often be time-consuming and cumbersome, especially if they have been applied directly to the mandibular occlusal surface.

Omitting the enamel conditioning makes composite removal easier, but the molars have to be banded when this technique is used. The bands are used for fixation of posterior bite planes in the following way: a long wire ligature is threaded around lingual cleats, and the wire runs over the occlusal surface and is then fixed around the buccal tube. Triad VLC Gel, a flowable composite, is then applied (**Fig. 8.13**). To remove composite, the wire ligature is cut buccally and the posterior bite plane is lifted off the molar together with the ligature.

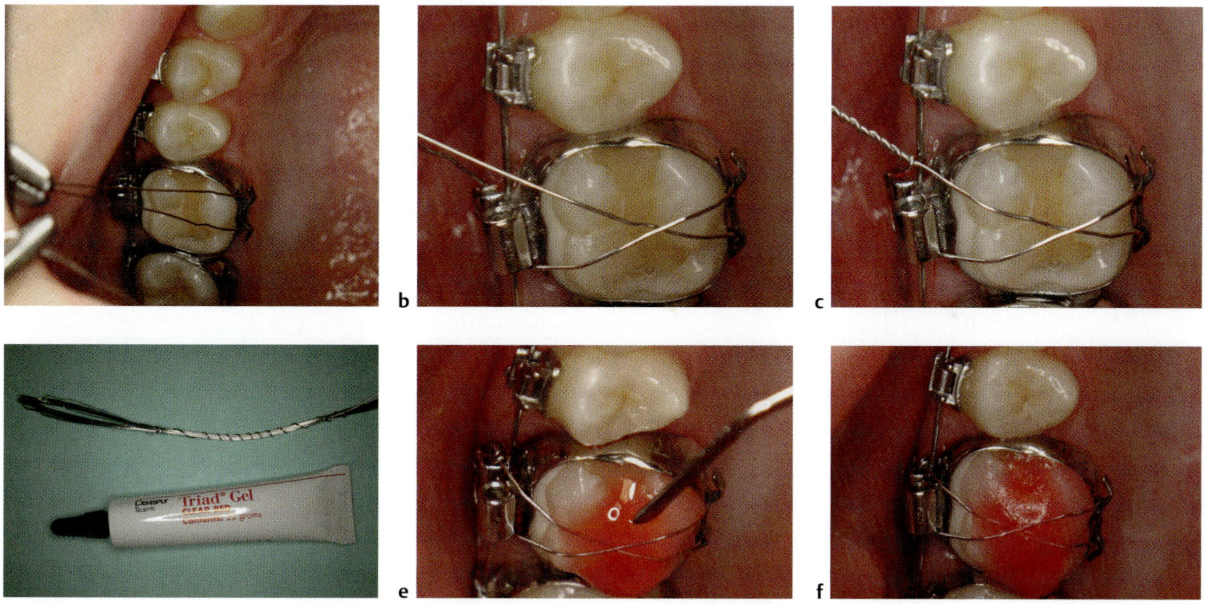

a b c d e f

Fig. 8.13 a–f Clinical steps for fabricating posterior bite elevators without prior enamel conditioning. A crossed-over steel ligature (**a–c**) provides retention for the flowable composite (**d–f**).

Case Study 8.1 (Fig. 8.14)

Patient: J.Z., male, age 13.
Diagnostic records: models, panoramic radiograph, lateral cephalometric radiograph, intraoral/extraoral photographs.
Main findings: palatally erupted tooth 13 in crossbite.
Treatment aims: alignment of the canine and correction of the crossbite, alignment of the mandibular incisors.
Appliances: self-ligating brackets, molar bands, posterior bite elevators.
Archwire sequence: 0.012 SE, 0.016 SE, 0.016 × 0.022 SE, 0.018 × 0.025 SE, 0.019 × 0.025 SS.
Alternative treatment strategy: n/a.
Active treatment time: 10 months.
Retention: three-dimensional retention followed by fixed retention.

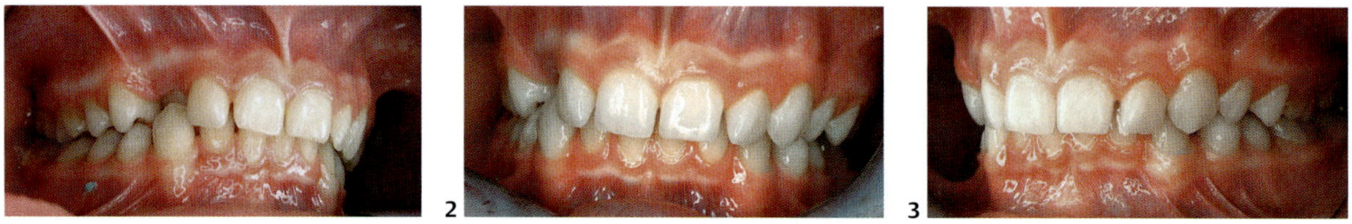
1 2 3

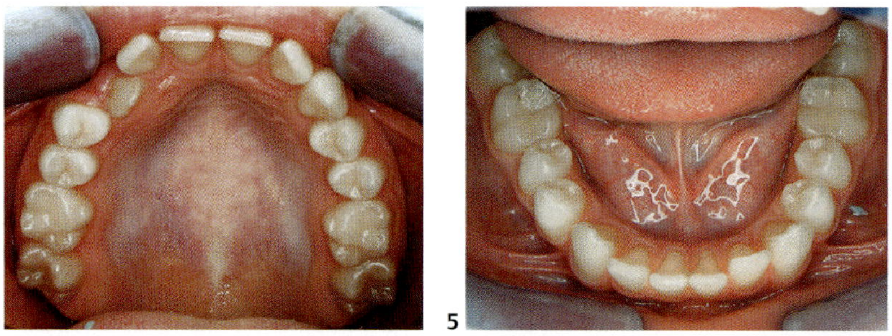
4 5

Fig. 8.14 1–20
1–5 Crossbite on teeth 13/43.

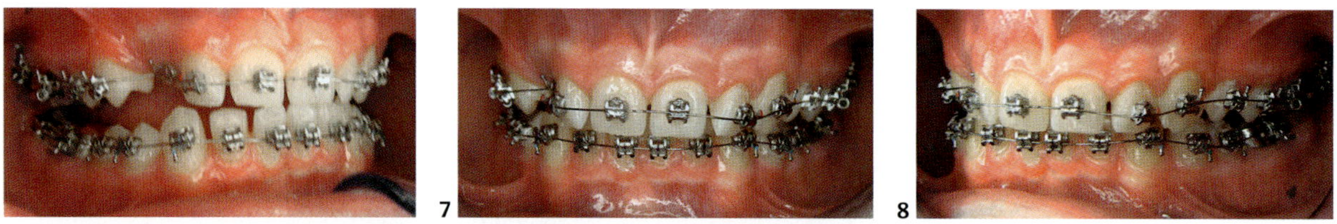
6 7 8

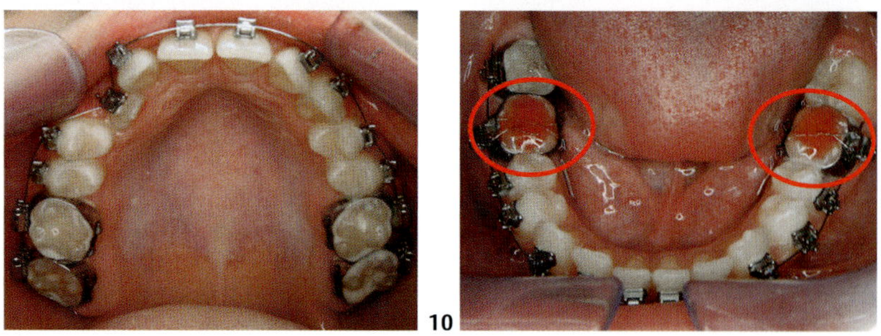
9 10

6–10 Full bonding with self-ligating brackets and 0.012 SE archwires. Posterior bite elevators on teeth 36 and 46.

CLINICAL PEARL

Bite-opening using a posterior bite plane can be easily achieved by applying a ligature from the lingual to the buccal side. The composite is then added for bite opening. Using a flowable composite is ideal for this purpose. Removing the composite is relatively easy, as the bite plane is removed together with the ligature used to fix it to the occlusal surface.

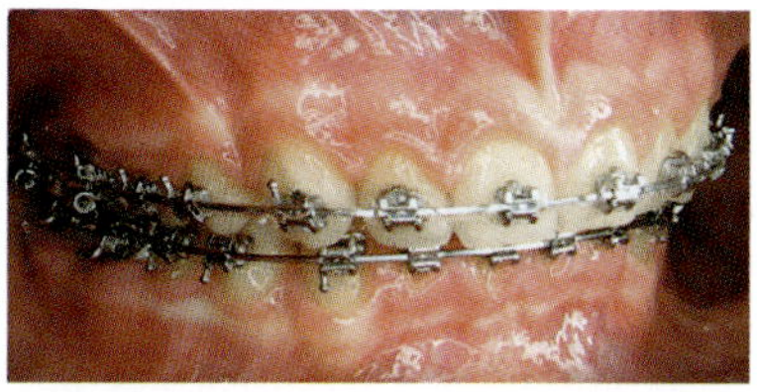
11

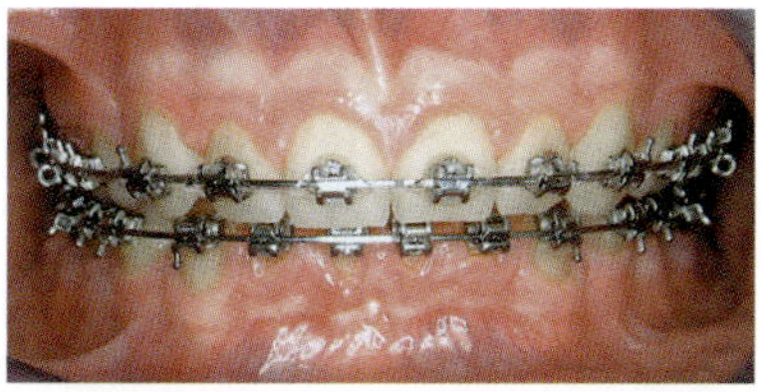
12

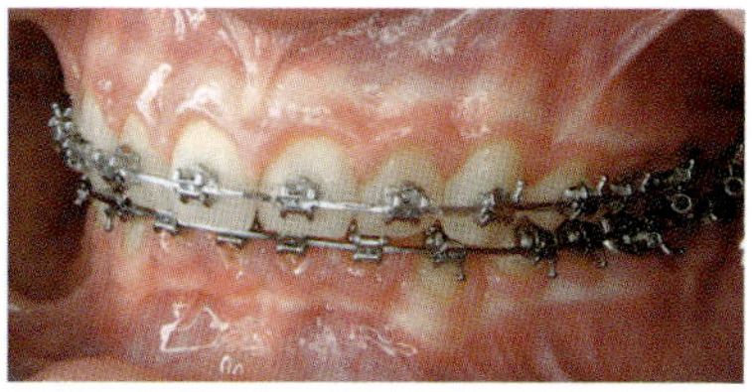
13

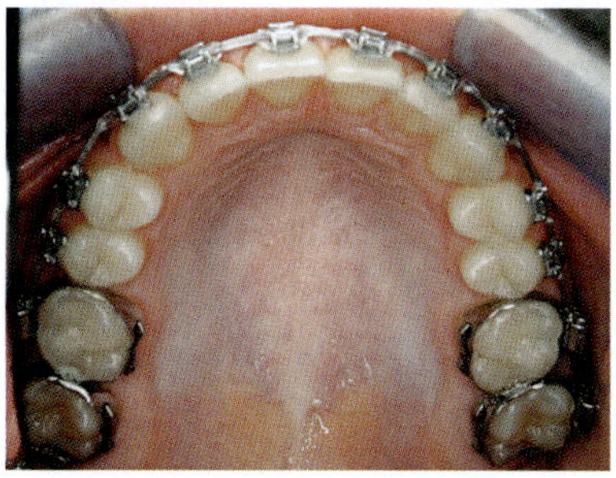
14

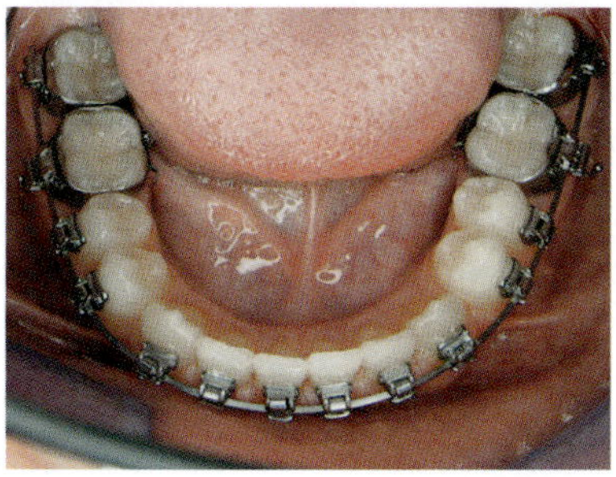
15

11–15 0.018 × 0.025 SE archwires; crossbite corrected.

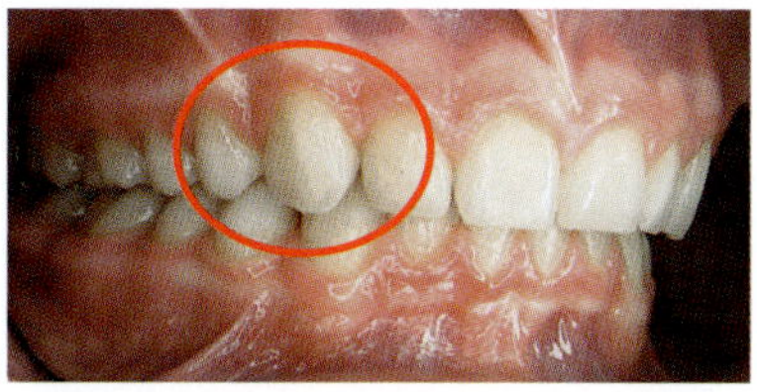
16

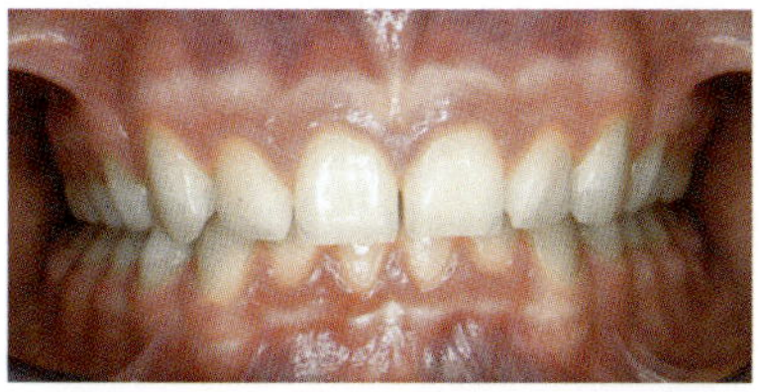
17

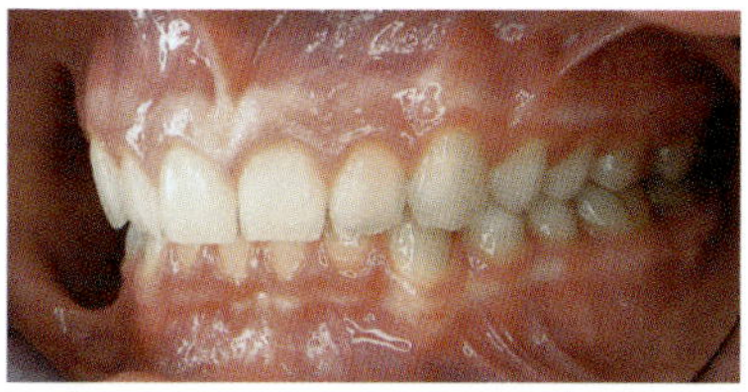
18

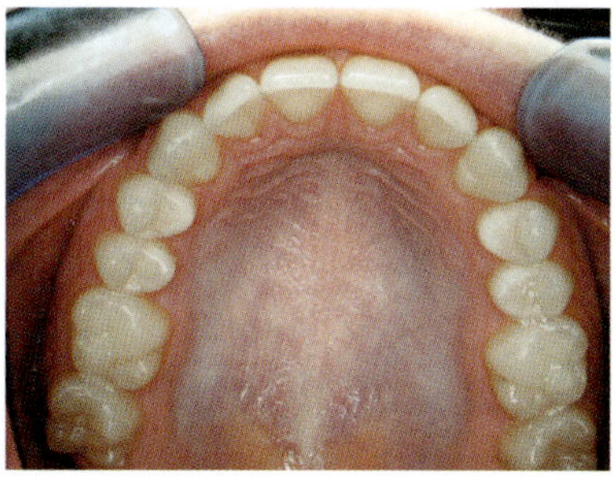
19

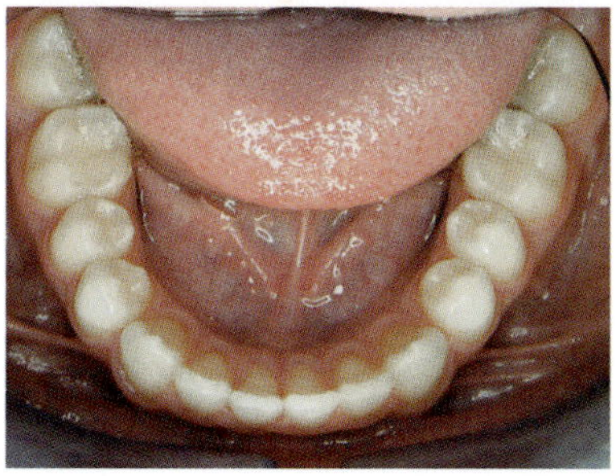
20

16–20 After 1 year of retention.

Combination of Buccal and Lingual Brackets (Hybrid Appliance)

Significantly displaced, severely crowded, and rotated teeth often do not have enough space to be aligned in the dental arch. The situation can often be so difficult that it is not even possible to place brackets on the buccal tooth surface. Traditionally, this situation is treated by using a compressed open coil spring to create the space needed. This can add treatment time and may shift teeth or midlines in undesired directions. An alternative method of aligning severely displaced teeth is to apply a lingual bracket to the severely misaligned tooth. Using this technique, very irregular arches can often still be treated with continuous archwires (see Case Studies 8.2 and 8.3). Lingual brackets are easily placed on the palatal side of very ectopic teeth, particularly canines. The normal archwire can be ligated fully, as shown in Case Study 8.2, **Fig. 8.15**. The archwire runs via the palatal tooth surface of the ectopic tooth to the buccal side and pulls it into place. This approach also prevents occlusal interference with the bracket, avoiding the bond failures that would be likely to occur had a buccal bracket been used.

Lingual brackets can also be used on the buccal side and can be very useful there. Extremely rotated and crowded teeth are often not easily accessible with conventional-sized brackets. If a tooth cannot be bonded with a regular attachment but if the operator decides to include it in the fixed appliance, he or she could contemplate using a temporarily placed two-dimensional bracket, for example. These brackets are extremely flat and narrow, so they can be fitted even on the most severely crowded teeth (see Case Study 8.3 and **Fig. 8.16**).

Case Study 8.2 (Fig. 8.15)

Patient: C.D., male, age 18.
Diagnostic records: models, panoramic radiograph, lateral cephalometric radiograph, intraoral/extraoral photographs.
Main findings: palatal position of tooth 23, crossbite, deep bite.
Treatment aims: alignment of tooth 23, correction of crossbite and deep bite.
Appliances: self-ligating brackets, molar bands, posterior bite elevators.
Archwire sequence: 0.012 SE, 0.016 SE, 0.018 SE, 0.016 × 0.022 SE, 0.019 × 0.025 SS.
Alternative treatment strategy: n/a.
Active treatment time: 12 months.
Retention: fixed retainer.

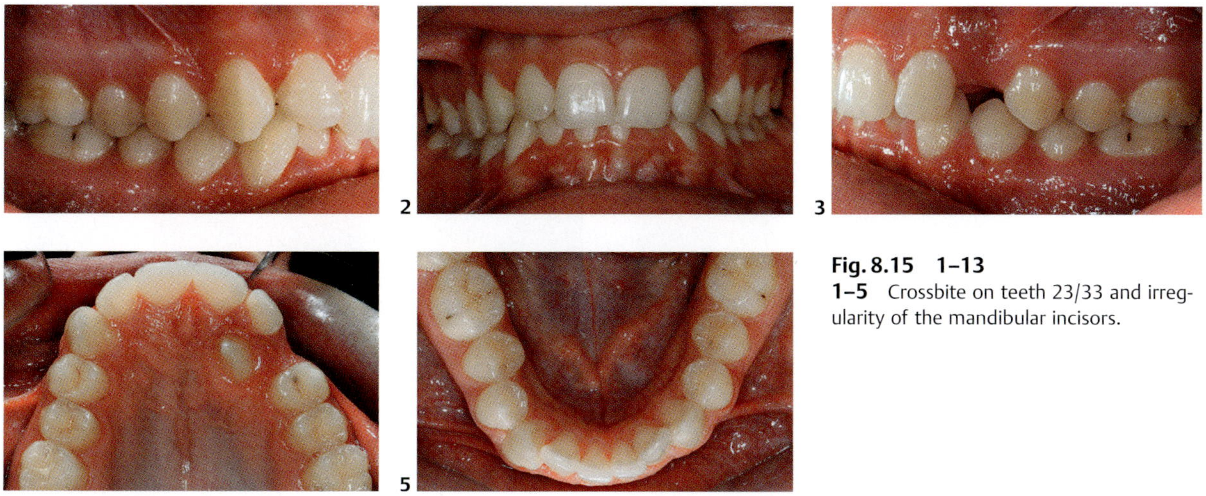

Fig. 8.15 1–13
1–5 Crossbite on teeth 23/33 and irregularity of the mandibular incisors.

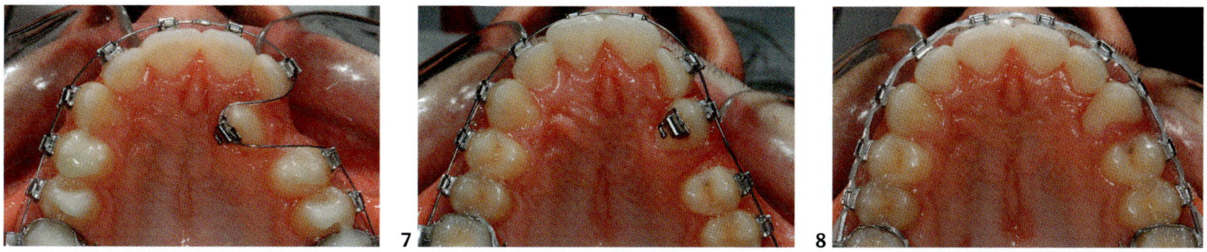

6 A self-ligating bracket bonded to the palatal surface of tooth 23, with a fully engaged 0.012 SE archwire.

7 Self-ligating bracket with a 0.016 SE archwire.

8 0.018 × 0.025 SE archwire for three-dimensional tooth positioning.

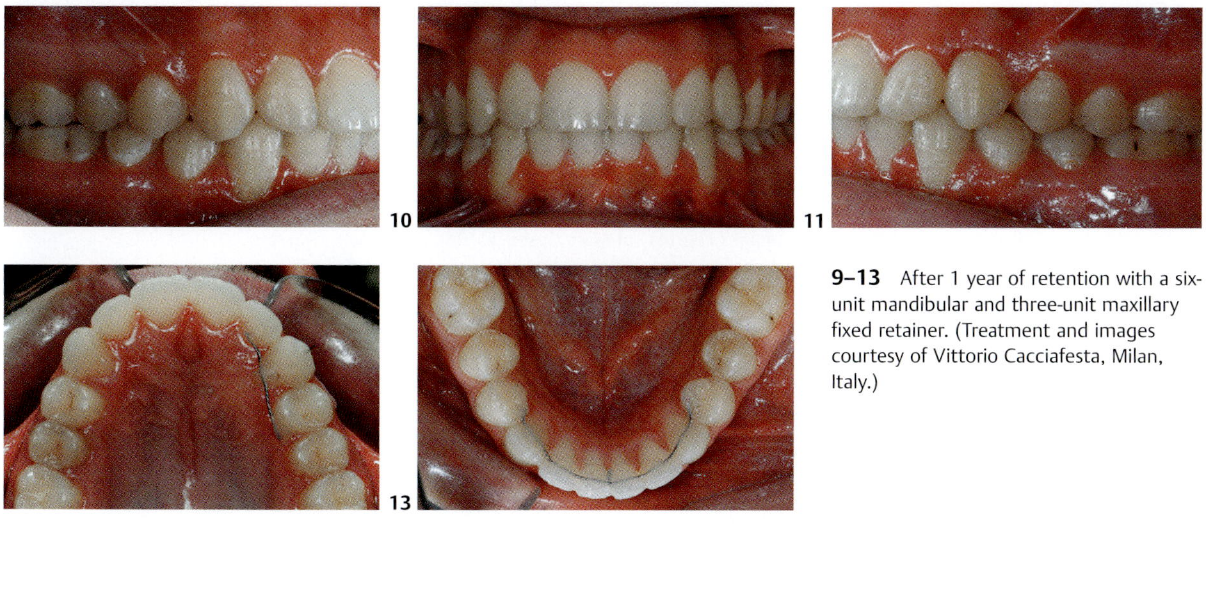

9–13 After 1 year of retention with a six-unit mandibular and three-unit maxillary fixed retainer. (Treatment and images courtesy of Vittorio Cacciafesta, Milan, Italy.)

Case Study 8.3 (Fig. 8.16)

Patient: M.M., female, age 12.
Diagnostic records: models, panoramic radiograph, lateral cephalometric radiograph, intraoral/extraoral photographs.
Main findings: lingually blocked-out tooth 42.
Treatment aims: opening of space and alignment of tooth 42.
Appliances: self-ligating brackets for mandibular arch only, molar bands, posterior bite elevators, two-dimensional lingual bracket for tooth 42.
Archwire sequence: 0.012 SE, 0.016 SE, 0.018 SE, 0.016 × 0.022 SE, 0.018 × 0.025 SE, 0.019 × 0.025 SS.
Alternative treatment strategy: n/a.
Retention: fixed retainer.

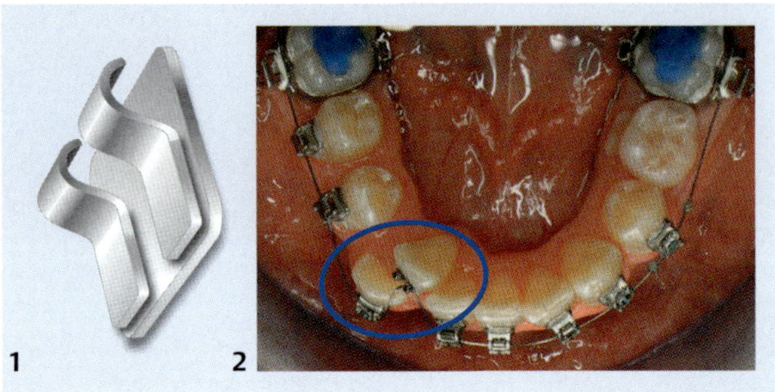

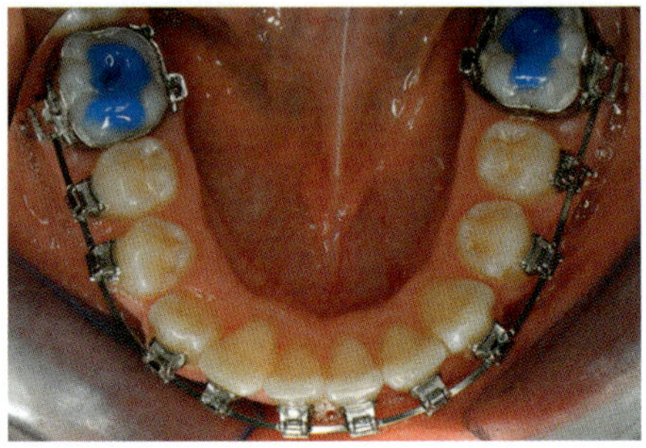

Fig. 8.16 1–6
1–2 A lack of space in the area of teeth 42 and 43 and a lingually blocked-out tooth 42.

3 Teeth 42 and 43 are aligned. Three-dimensional torque control with a 0.018 × 0.025 SE archwire.

CLINICAL PEARL

The small, low-profile two-dimensional bracket (Forestadent) can be bonded to buccal tooth surfaces even in severely crowded conditions, the crowded tooth can be included in the fixed appliance from the start. The resilience of the superelastic archwire will work like a push-coil and create space while aligning the tooth.

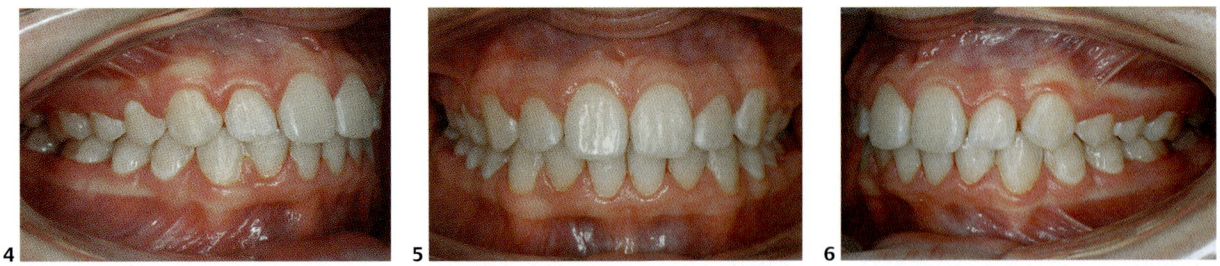

4–6 After 1 year of retention. (Treatment and images courtesy of Marc Geserick, Ulm, Germany.)

Auxiliary Slots

A number of manufacturers offer self-ligating brackets that have an auxiliary slot. For this slot to be useful, it should have a size of at least 0.4 × 0.4 mm (0.016 × 0.016 inches).

The auxiliary slot can be used to align late erupting teeth in the overlay technique (**Fig. 8.17**). We find that it can also be used for uprighting springs, intrusion or extrusion springs, derotational springs (**Fig. 8.18**), and for applying the Sander leveling spring (**Fig. 8.19**).[22]

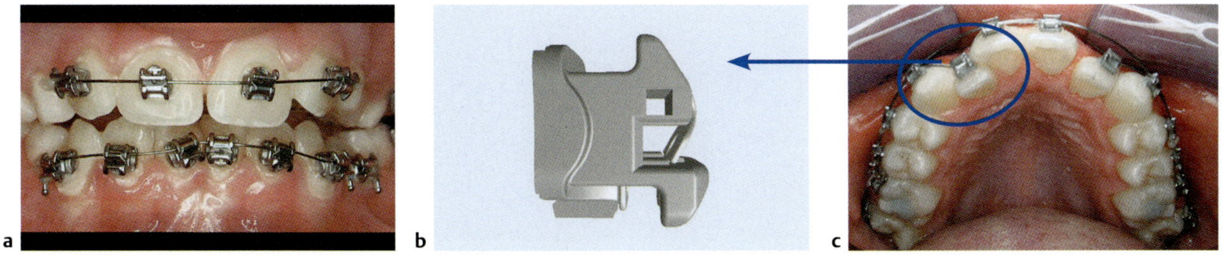

Fig. 8.17 a–c Leveling using the auxiliary slot. Severely rotated teeth can be derotated very effectively using a 0.010 SE segmental wire in the auxiliary slot (**a**). The normal archwire progression takes place in the main slot. Teeth with delayed eruption or severely displaced teeth can be aligned using the auxiliary slot and a light leveling wire (for example, 0.012 SE), while the base archwire remains unchanged (**b, c**).

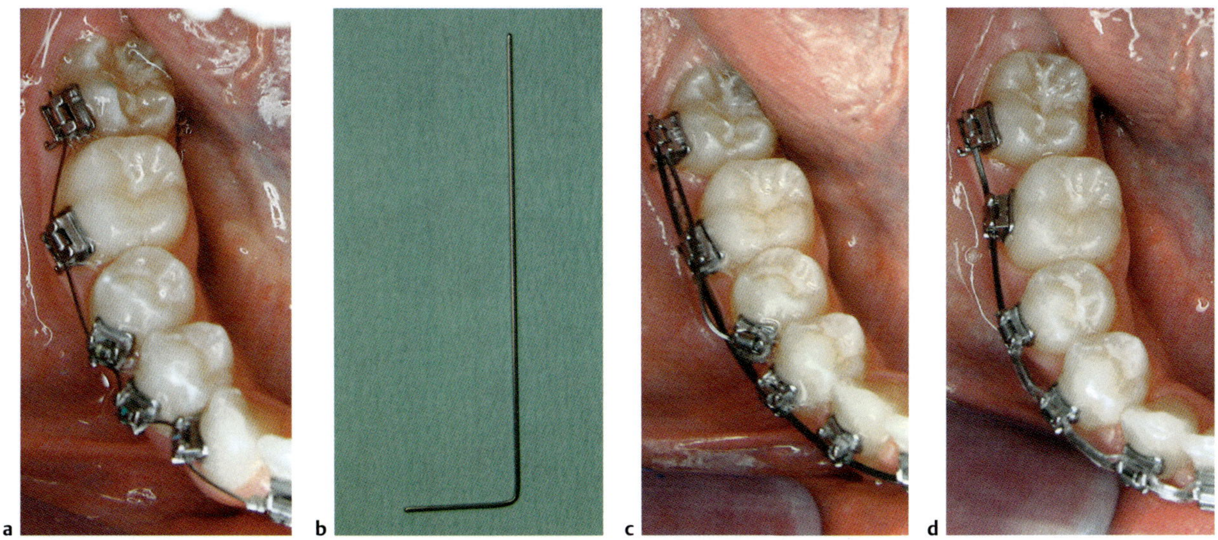

Fig. 8.18 a–d Use of a derotation spring. Tooth 45 presents with severe mesial rotation, which the leveling archwire was unable to correct (**a**). While in a rigid base arch, the rotation was corrected using the derotation spring (whip spring), which was inserted into the auxiliary slots on teeth 45 and 47 (**b–d**).

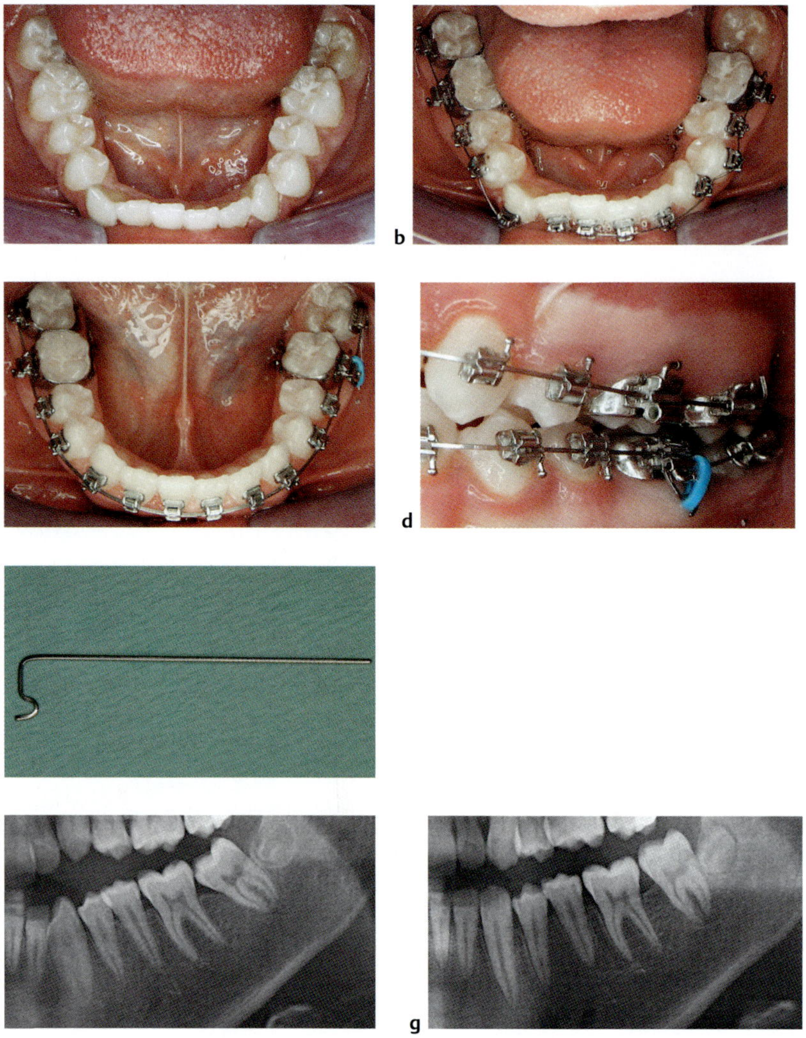

Fig. 8.19 a–g The Sander uprighting technique.[22] Teeth with up to 20° inclination to the occlusal plane can be effectively uprighted using the NiTi uprighting spring (0.016 × 0.016, Forestadent). The spring is inserted from the mesial into the auxiliary slot of the band or bracket, an elastic ligature is placed on the spring, and it is then engaged into the bracket of the tipped tooth. The spring is secured by attaching the ligature mesially to the hook on the uprighting spring.

Case Study 8.4 (Fig. 8.20)

Patient: L.K., female, age 14 years.
Diagnostic records: models, panoramic radiograph, lateral cephalometric radiograph, intraoral/extraoral photographs.
Main findings: retained tooth 53 and impacted tooth 13.
Treatment aims: open space, exposure, and guided eruption of tooth 13.
Appliances: self-ligating brackets, molar bands.
Archwire sequence: 0.012 SE, 0.016 SE, 0.016 × 0.022 SE, 0.018 × 0.025 SE, 0.019 × 0.025 SS, 0.012 SE and 0.016 SE as segmental piggy-back wires for eruption and alignment of tooth 13.
Alternative treatment strategy: n/a.
Active treatment time: 16 months.
Retention: fixed retainer.

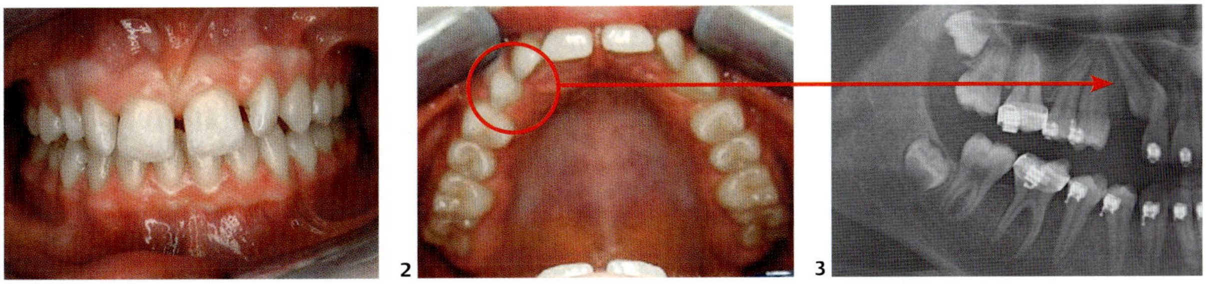

1 2 3

Fig. 8.20 1–21
1–3 An impacted tooth 13 with a persisting deciduous predecessor.

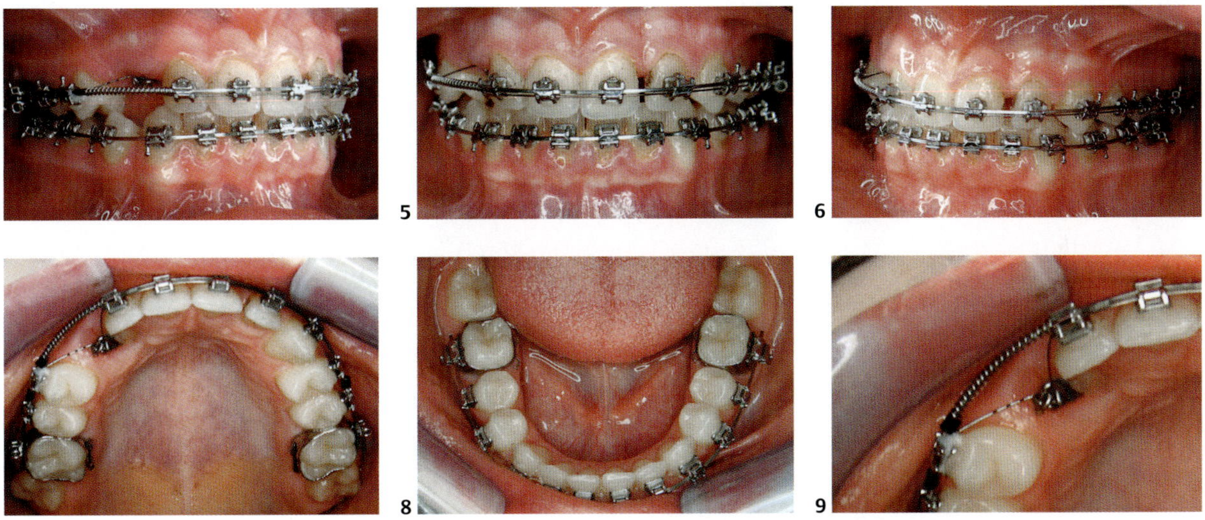

4 5 6 7 8 9

4–9 Self-ligating brackets with a stainless-steel base arch and 0.012 SE piggyback wire for eruption of tooth 13.

CLINICAL PEARL

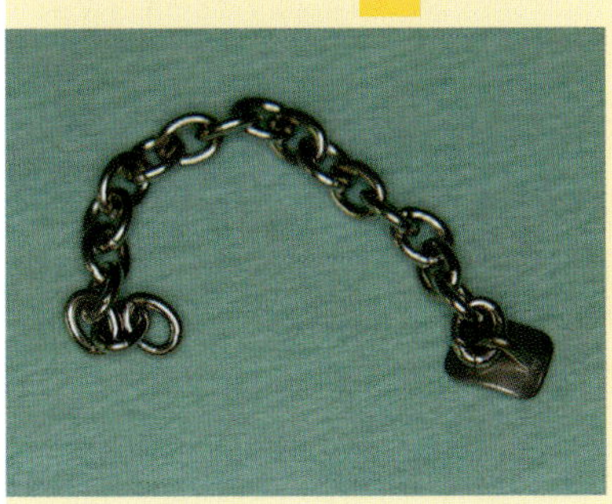

10

The impacted canine has been bonded with a gold chain. A titanium chain can also be used. The chain can be shortened as the tooth emerges and the successive removal of the links is useful for confirming tooth movement.

11
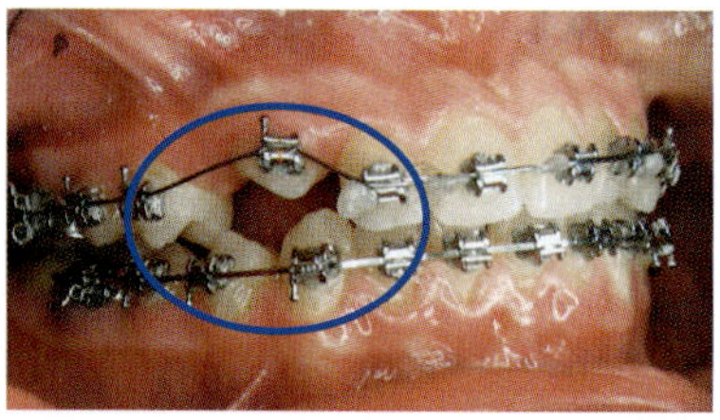
12
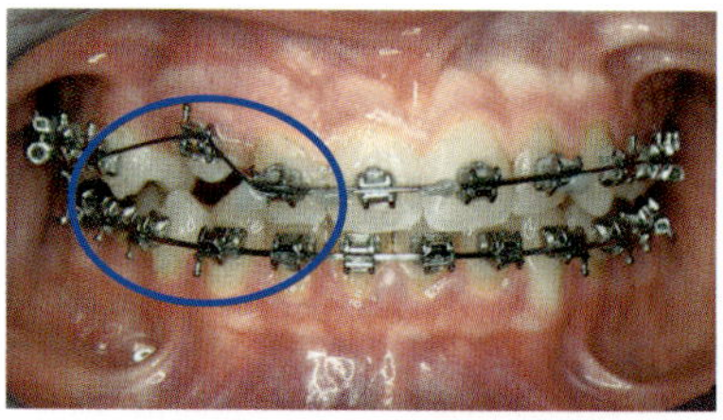
13
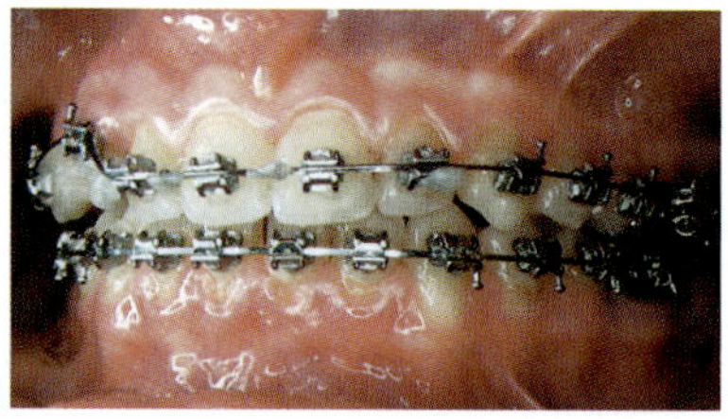
14
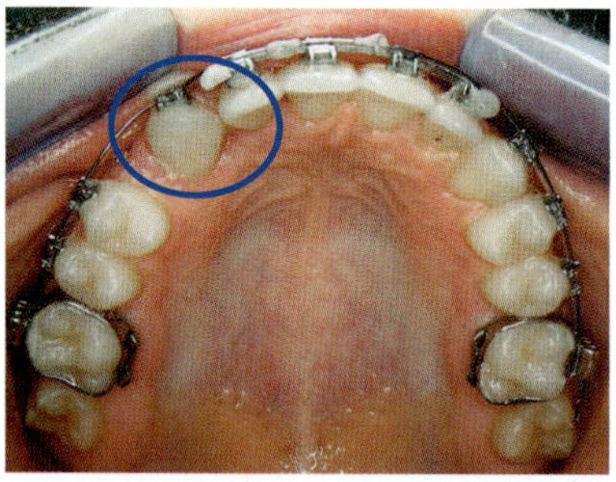
15
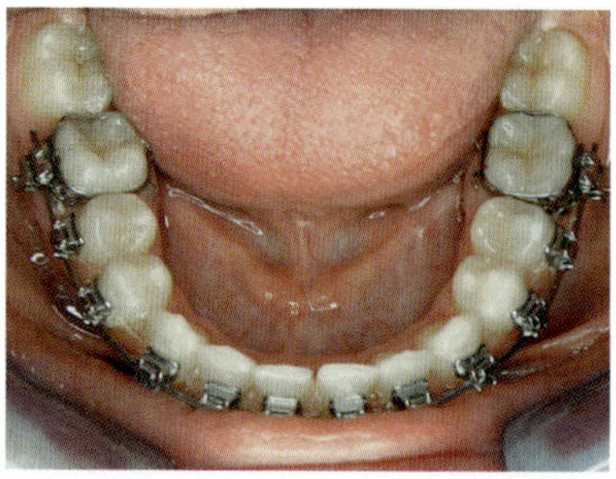

11–15 Tooth 13 (now bonded with the appropriate bracket).

Clinical pearl:
The arch shape is preserved with a rigid rectangular wire, while the ectopic canine is moved using a 0.012 superelastic segmental arch (piggyback archwire).

16
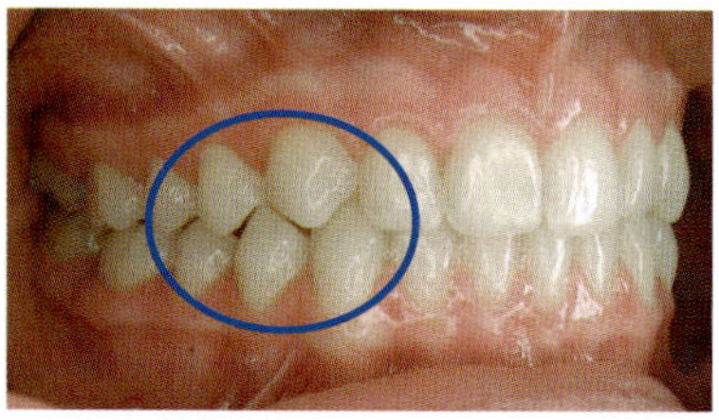
17
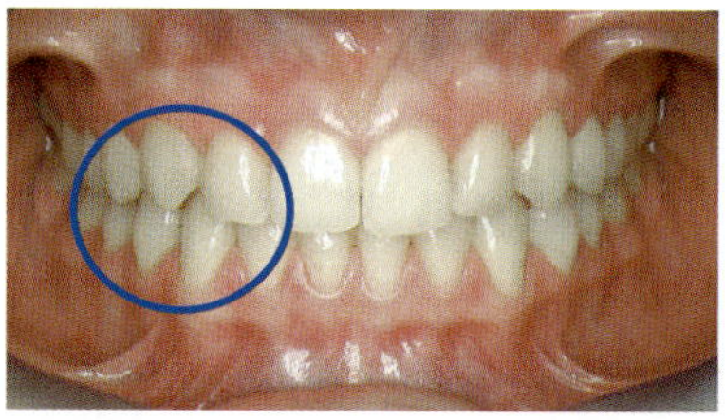
18
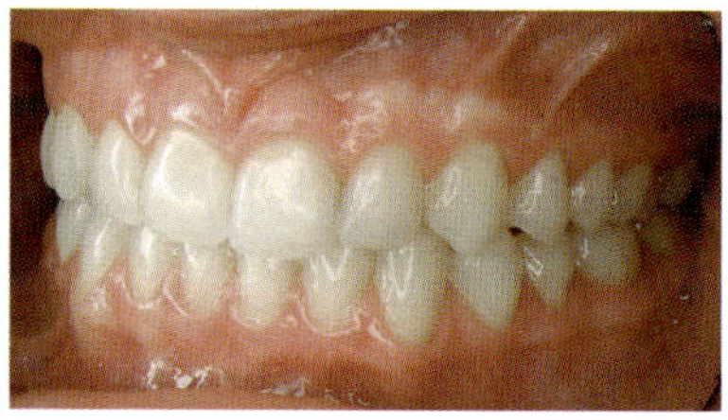
19
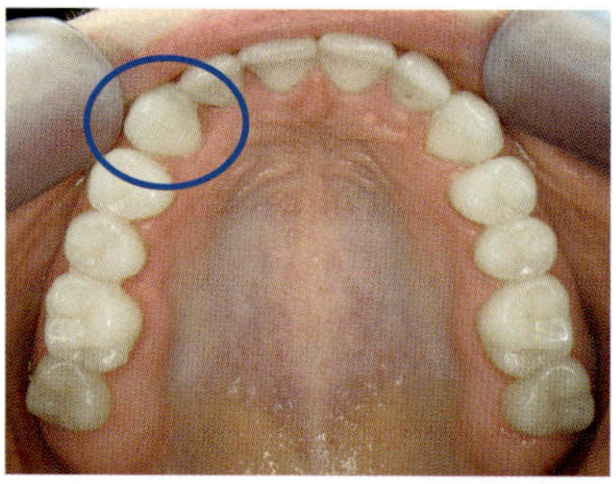
20
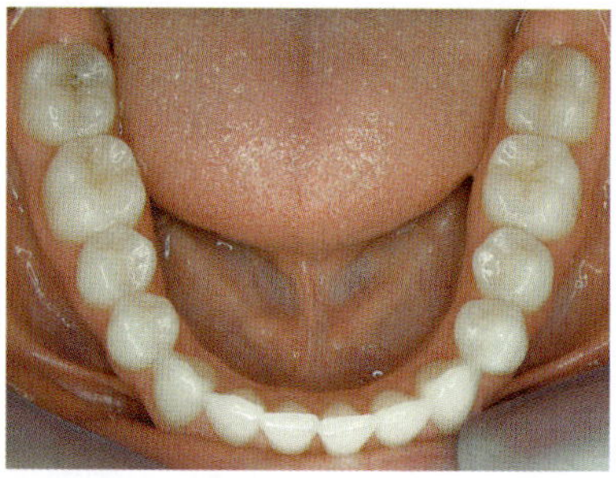
21
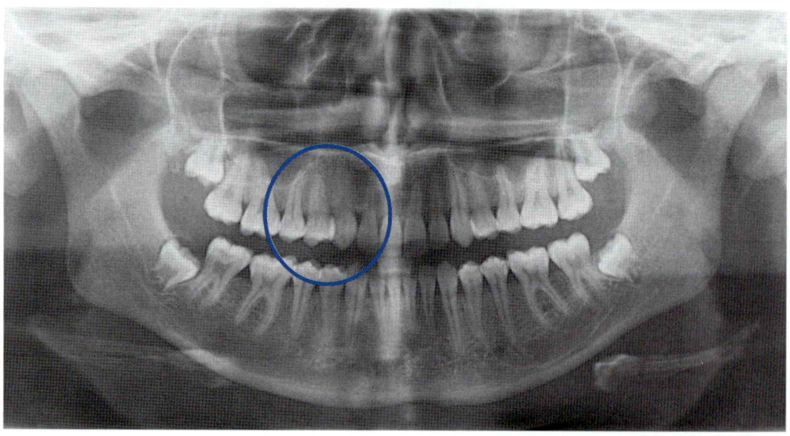

16–21 After 1 year of retention.

CLINICAL PEARL

- A gold or titanium chain should be used for forced eruption of impacted or ectopic teeth.
- The chain links can be shortened successively as the tooth approaches the desired position.
- Simple attachment, simple activation.
- SLBs with an adequate auxiliary slot size can be used to accommodate larger piggyback wires.

Interproximal Enamel Reduction (Stripping)

Space creation is an important part of orthodontic treatment. Interproximal enamel reduction is a long-established alternative treatment to extraction. A number of terms are used in the orthodontic literature to describe this technique, and this can sometimes be confusing: interproximal reduction (IPR) of enamel, stripping, tooth size reduction, recontouring, reshaping, slenderizing, slicing, and trimming of teeth are all used to describe this technique.

Contemporary orthodontics has moved away from the very clearly defined extraction and nonextraction approaches that were predominant for many years. Symmetrical extraction of two premolars, which creates between 14 and 16 mm of space, often leaves the balance heavily lopsided towards space creation. This can in turn lead to prolonged residual space closure, retroclination of incisors, and sometimes the creation of a tooth-sized discrepancy, leading to small extraction spaces remaining at the end of fixed-appliance treatment. However, interproximal enamel reduction can deal with a number of space requirements in a predictable way.

Advantages and Disadvantages

Interproximal enamel reduction has several advantages:

- There is only minimal loss of tooth substance (in comparison with extraction treatment in particular)
- Less overall tooth movement is often necessary (in comparison with space closure in an extraction approach).
- Treatment times are usually shorter.
- There is potentially better stability of the arches (due to establishment of contact surfaces rather than contact points).
- Residual extraction spaces after orthodontic treatment are avoided.

Although some of the potential side effects are not confirmed in the scientific literature, it is important to carefully inform patients and obtain their consent, in view of the following potential issues associated with tooth size reduction:

- Interproximal cleaning can be more difficult following the procedure and special adjuncts may become necessary in order to maintain good oral hygiene.
- There may be cosmetic issues such as a squarer appearance of the teeth.
- There is a potential for all the enamel to be removed down to the dentine, with subsequently increased sensitivity of the teeth.
- There is potentially an increased risk of decay (caries).

CLINICAL PEARL

It is advisable to document the patient consultation, with special emphasis on the discussion of IPR.

Indications and Amount of Space Creation

IPR is particularly useful in patients with primary or secondary crowding. It is also used in patients with significant tooth size discrepancies between the arches and those with abnormally shaped teeth and to reduce or eliminate triangular-shaped spaces in the gingival tissues in patients with an increased distance from the dental contact point to the alveolar crest. The overall space that is made available has been extensively described in the literature, but with significant variations between authors. Most references suggest removing no more than 50% of the existing enamel thickness. This will lead to space creation between 6.5 and 9 mm per arch.[5,6,10,23,24] Up to 11 mm of space may be created if all of the teeth including the second molars are slenderized.[26] **Table 8.5** gives an indication of the values for amounts of enamel that can be reduced for each individual tooth. The lower incisors should only be slenderized by approximately 0.2 mm on each side, so that no more than 50% of the enamel is reduced.[8,11,25]

Table 8.5 Recommended guidelines for enamel reduction for each tooth surface. The enamel on the lower incisors should not be reduced by more than 0.2 mm per tooth surface

Tooth (reduction in mm)	I1		I2		C		P1		P2		
	Mesial	Distal	Mesial	Distal	Mesial	Distal	Mesial	Distal	Mesial	Distal	
Maxilla	0.3	0.3	0.3	0.3	0.3	0.6	0.6	0.6	0.6	0.6	
	0.6		0.6		0.9		1.2		1.2		Σ 9.0 mm
Mandible	0.2	0.2	0.2	0.2	0.2	0.3	0.6	0.6	0.6	0.6	
	0.4		0.4		0.5		1.2		1.2		Σ 7.4 mm

Instrumentation

Most of our patients accept enamel size reduction as a treatment, particularly when the only other alternative for space creation involves the extraction of teeth. As mentioned above, however, it is very important to inform the patient appropriately and to obtain consent. A number of methods of reducing enamel size are described in the literature: hand files, rotational instruments, disks (rotating or oscillating), and conventional rotational handpieces using tungsten-carbide or diamond-coated burs. The oscillating blades and the disks can be coated on one side or both sides, depending on the clinical need to reduce the enamel thickness on one side of a particular tooth in one stage or two teeth simultaneously. Whichever instrument is used, the goal should be to achieve a smooth tooth surface at the end of the procedure, to avoid discolorations or carious decay.

Motor-driven devices are often more efficient for enamel size reduction and less uncomfortable for the patient. Other rotational instruments, such as disks, can be purchased with a guard to reduce the likelihood of inadvertent soft-tissue damage. However, these are rather bulky and are not easy to use in the buccal segments in particular.

Newly developed oscillating systems, such as the Ortho-Strips or O-Drive system (**Fig. 8.21**), have blunt edges and are therefore less likely to cause inadvertent trauma to the soft tissues than any of the other instruments mentioned above. Other advantages of these systems are that they are easy to insert into the interdental spaces and offer secure and easy handling of enamel reduction between the teeth (**Fig. 8.22**).

A number of publications confirm that enamel reduction with oscillating systems can be carried out safely, with little roughness remaining.[4,13] However, it is still important to polish the newly created interproximal spaces to prevent discoloration (e.g., with Sof-Lex-XT disks, 3 M Unitek). This can produce an enamel surface comparable with that of natural enamel.[4] It is also advisable to apply topical fluoride immediately after the procedure. The additional loss of enamel due to the polishing is less than 0.1 mm.[13]

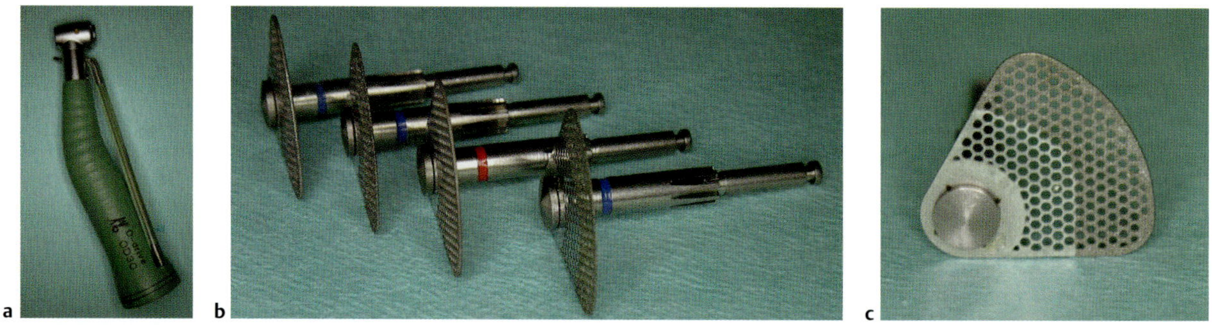

Fig. 8.21 a–c An oscillating contra-angle handpiece with built-in irrigation (KaVo O-Drive, **a**) and diamond-coated perforated disks with different coarseness levels (Komet, **b, c**). The disks oscillate at an angle of 30° and are available in thicknesses of 0.15–0.45 mm with medium and fine coarseness.

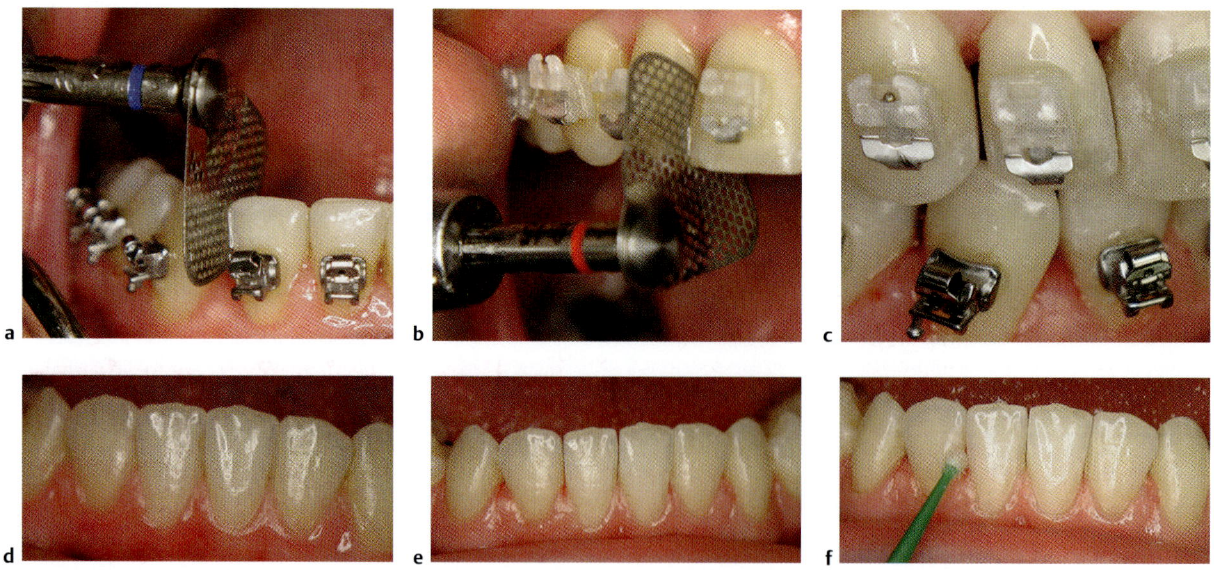

Fig. 8.22 a–f Clinical steps with the O-Drive system. The disk oscillates at an angle of 30° and at approximately 5500 vibrations/minute. It is inserted into the interproximal site from the occlusal direction under constant irrigation (**a–c**). The oscillating movement reduces the likelihood of slipping and damaging adjacent structures. After the subsequent polishing, the surface should be sealed with a highly concentrated fluoride varnish (for example, Elmex Fluid, Gaba, or Fluorprotector, Vivadent) (**d–f**).

Recontouring of Incisal Edges

Recontouring of teeth includes additive as well as subtractive measures. Reshaping of teeth mostly benefits the visible aspect of the anterior teeth and is therefore regarded as a cosmetic procedure. Enamel reshaping of ragged or chipped incisal edges of the anterior front teeth, particularly on the incisors and canines (**Fig. 8.23**), is the most commonly used procedure.

Additive procedures such as composite veneers or incisal edge build-ups can be used to treat enamel defects (see Case Study 8.5) or conical tooth shapes; it is also useful in adults, in whom widening of teeth can reduce or eliminate triangular-shaped spaces at the gingival level or restore microdontic teeth to better proportions (**Fig. 8.24**). Additive measures can also be useful for restoring tooth shape in substitution cases (e.g., canine for lateral incisor).

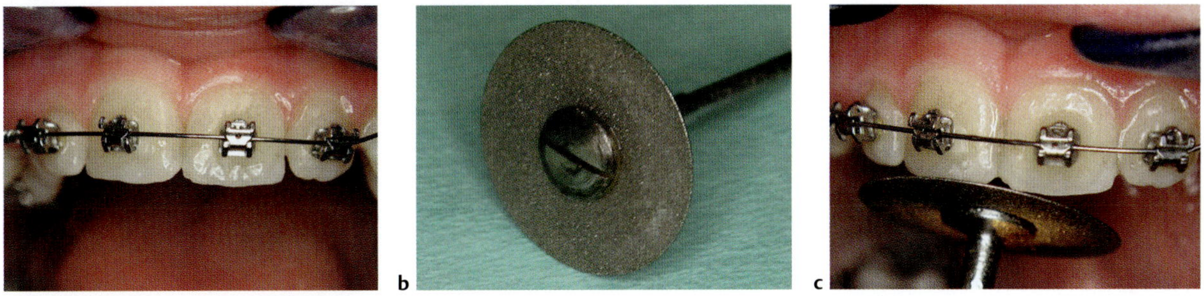

a b c

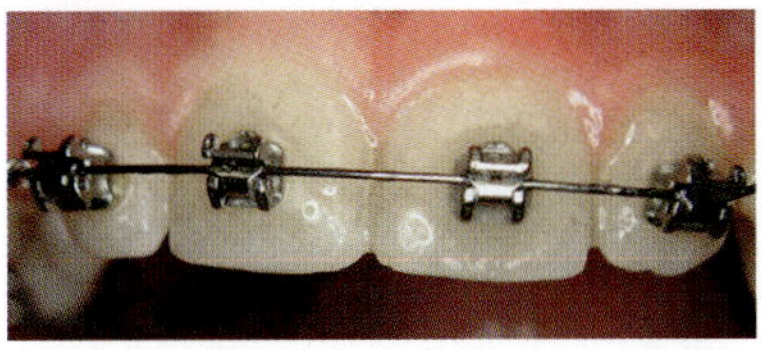

d

Fig. 8.23 a–d Correction of incisal wear at the maxillary incisors. Persistent malocclusion can lead to unphysiological, asymmetric wear patterns on teeth that become particularly evident after the teeth have been properly positioned (**a**). Correction of minor defects can usually be achieved subtractively, by polishing with a diamond disk (**b–d**). The larger surface area of the flat disk prevents the instrument from becoming caught in the notch and accentuating the irregularity, as may happen when a conventional bur is used.

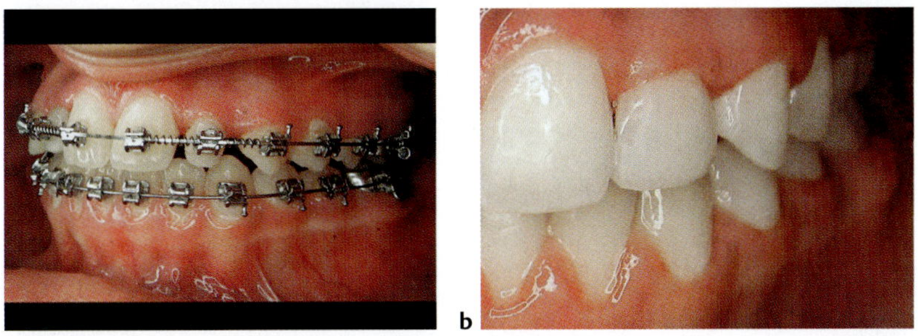

a b

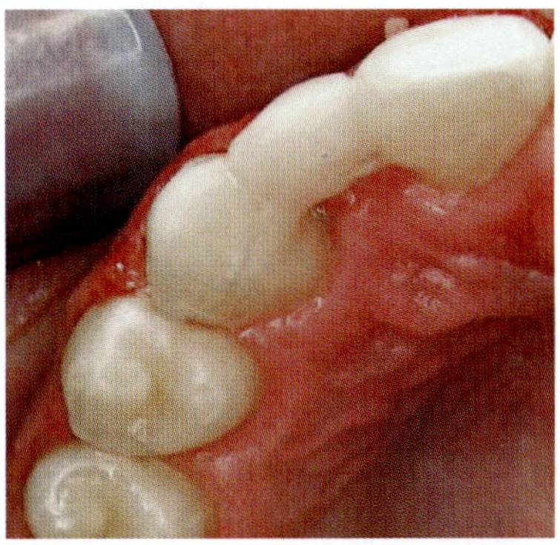

c

Fig. 8.24 a–c The final result of orthodontic treatment. The microdontic tooth 22 was built up directly with composite (**a, b**). The edentulous site 12 was restored with a fiber-reinforced adhesive bridge (Everstick, Stick Tech) (**c**).

Case Study 8.5 (Fig. 8.25)

Patient: S.K., female, age 13.
Diagnostic records: models, panoramic radiograph, lateral cephalometric radiograph, intraoral/extraoral photographs.
Main findings: amelogenesis imperfecta, early loss of severely decayed first molars, lack of arch coordination.
Treatment aims: interdisciplinary goal: to establish a stable occlusion and archwire coordination; restoration of malformed enamel surfaces.
Appliances: self-ligating brackets, molar bands.
Archwire sequence: 0.012 SE, 0.016 SE, 0.016 × 0.022 SE, 0.019 × 0.025 SE.
Alternative treatment strategy: n/a.
Active treatment time: 5 months.
Retention: three-dimensional retention.

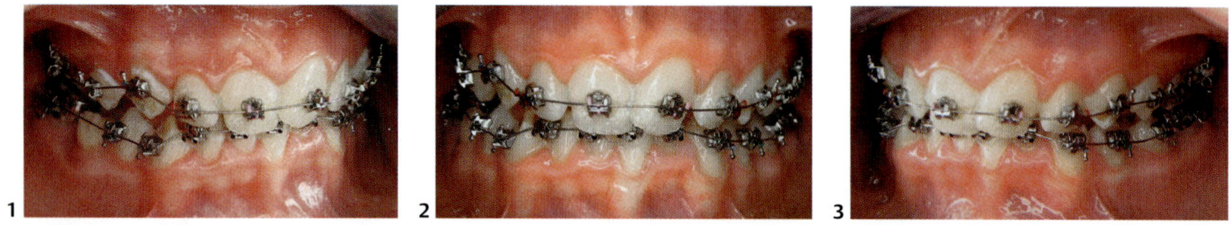

Fig. 8.25 1–12
1–3 Self-ligating brackets in place and an initial SE wire for leveling, alignment, and arch development.

CLINICAL PEARL

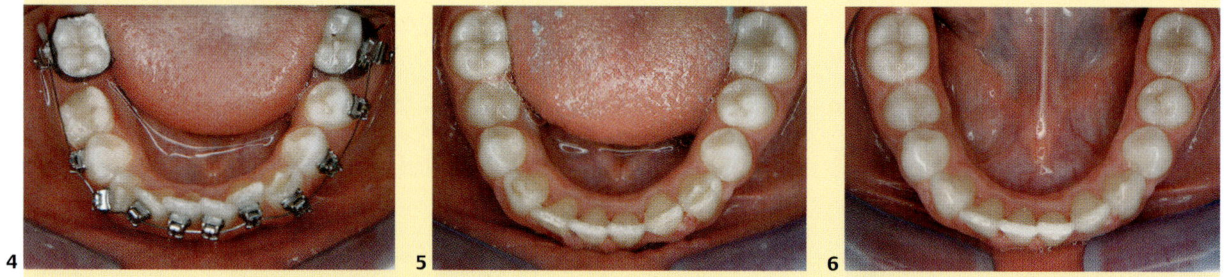

4–6 Self-ligating brackets allow rapid and gentle alignment of teeth. This can be particularly useful for patients with preexisting medical conditions, when short treatment times are indicated.

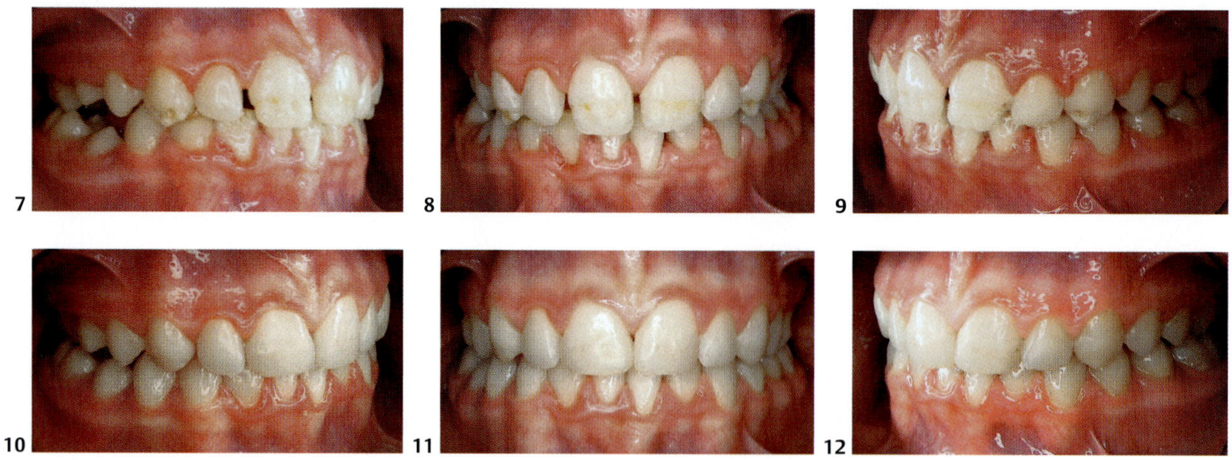

7–12 The final treatment result and subsequent restoration of enamel defects.

Mini-Implants

Anchorage is defined as resistance to undesired tooth movement. Every tooth movement requires anchorage. In particular, physical movements of teeth over long distances involve significant anchorage requirements. The forces generated should ideally be pitched against a stationary anchorage point. According to Newton's Third Law of Motion, every application of a force creates an equal and opposite force. If this force acts on other teeth (the dental anchorage units), it tends to create undesired tooth movement—i.e., anchorage loss. This is true for any appliance, whether removable or fixed. The extent to which these dental anchorage units move (and how much anchorage is lost) depends on:

- The combined root surface in the direction of tooth movement of the teeth included in the anchorage segment
- The quality and quantity of the surrounding bone

Fixed appliances can move teeth without the often need for patient compliance. However, compliance is needed to ensure that the teeth move in the right direction. The above principles are the same whether the operator uses self-ligating brackets or conventional ligation.

NOTE

Self-ligating brackets by themselves cannot resolve all anchorage issues, although this has been claimed by a number of manufacturers.

Depending on the treatment goals, three anchorage categories can be defined:

1. Minimum anchorage (space closure : anchorage = 1:2)
2. Moderate anchorage (space closure : anchorage = 1:1)
3. Maximum anchorage (space closure : anchorage = 2:1)

These three different types of anchorage are illustrated in **Fig. 8.26**. The treatment aim encompasses space closure following extraction of the lower first premolars. This resembles a minimum anchorage scenario, in which the space would close at a ratio of 1 : 2 (1 mm canine retraction for every 2 mm of premolar protraction), if the treatment aim mainly includes mesial movement of the lower second premolar rather than distal movement of the lower canine (**Fig. 8.26a**). "Moderate anchorage" would be defined as reciprocity of the forces, with equivalent movement of both units resulting in a space-closing ratio of 1 : 1 (1 mm canine retraction for every 1 mm of premolar protraction). In this scenario, it would be advisable to add at least one molar to the second premolar to bolster anchorage (**Fig. 8.26b**). Traditionally, maximum anchorage is defined as space closure with a ratio of 2 : 1 (2 mm of canine retraction for every 1 mm of premolar protraction). In this case maximum anchorage requires a maximum amount of anterior retraction. Due to biomechanical shortcomings, however, it was traditionally not possible to ensure that anchorage units remained completely stationary. For a "true maximum anchorage" or absolute anchorage scenario, a mini-implant can be used to reinforce the anchorage (**Fig. 8.26c**). This means that the anchorage units will remain stationary, as the forces are distributed to skeletal structures and will allow complete retraction of the canine without mesialization of the posterior teeth.

In addition to quantitative amounts, anchorage can also be defined in terms of quality. The following classification can be a useful guide for treatment planning:

1. *Tissue-borne anchorage:* intraoral appliances can be used to provide anchorage involving the soft tissues, such as a lip bumper.
2. *Tooth-borne anchorage:* this can be divided into intramaxillary and intermaxillary anchorage.
   - *Intramaxillary anchorage* can be provided by transpalatal arches or lingual arches and by modifying fixed appliances—e.g., by adding buccal root torque in the archwire and augmenting the anchorage unit (by joining teeth together, for example).

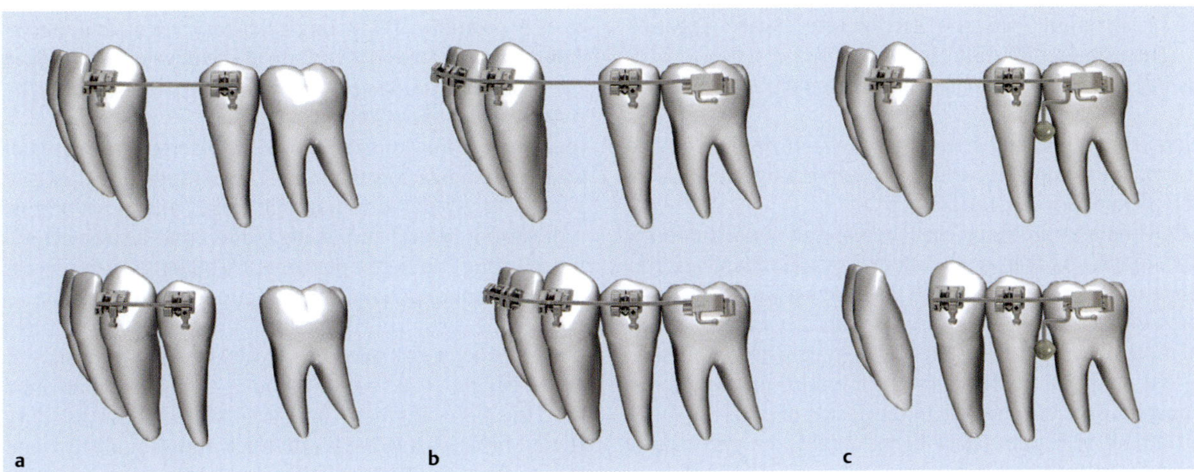

Fig. 8.26a–c After extraction of the first premolar, the canine needs to be retracted. Minimal (**a**), medium (**b**), and maximum (**c**) anchorage create different outcomes. (Images courtesy of Dentaurum.)

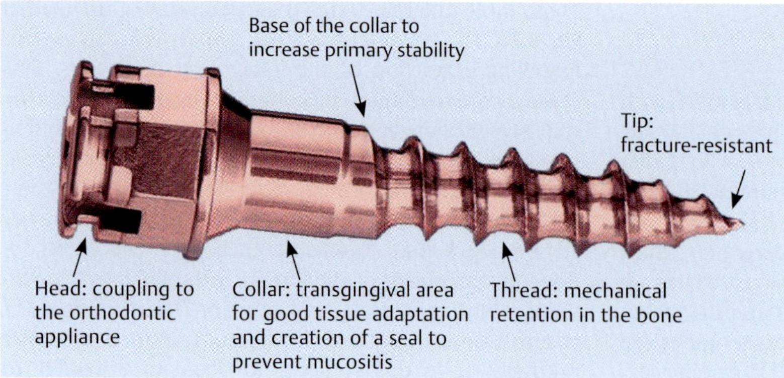

Fig. 8.27 Components of an orthodontic miniscrew implant using Ortho Easy as an example. (Image courtesy of Forestadent.)

- *Intermaxillary anchorage* is usually provided by using teeth on the opposing jaw (such as intermaxillary class II or class III elastics or fixed-functional appliances such as the Herbst appliance and its derivatives).

3. *Extraoral anchorage*, such as headgear and a facemask.
4. *Endosseous anchorage*, such as mini-implants, miniplates, or dental implants. This type of anchorage is also referred to as "absolute anchorage."

The following discussion provides examples highlighting the importance of mini-implants in contemporary orthodontics. However, this is not intended as a comprehensive summary of the extensive literature on mini-implants.[3,15]

Uses and Choices of a Mini-Implant System

There are a large number of indications for the use of mini-implant anchorage, particularly in combination with self-ligating brackets:

1. For space closure
2. For intrusion
3. For uprighting of molars
4. To provide temporary support for a crown (to replace a missing tooth until a full-sized implant can be placed (see the section on "Tooth Morphology" in Chapter 9)
5. Distalization (see the section on "Space Creation Through Distalization" in Chapter 7)
6. Rapid maxillary expansion (see Chapter 7)

Numerous books and articles are available on the detailed use of mini-implants, which can serve as guidelines for the inexperienced clinician.[3,12,27,28]
Mini-implants are being used increasingly for orthodontic anchorage, and at least 45 different mini-implant systems were on the market in 2008. This makes it very difficult to provide a systematic overview, particularly as the features of most systems are constantly changing; parameters such as the shape of the head size of the mini-implant are in constant flux. With regard to the design of mini-implants, a number of features have been found to be particularly useful (**Fig. 8.27**):

- Thread: self-tapping, drill-free design
- Length of the screw: either 6.8 mm or 10 mm
- Outer diameter of the thread: approximately 1.6 mm
- Shape of the implant body: slightly conical or cylindrical
- A "multifunctional head": ideally with a cross-slot and undercut for inserting auxiliaries
- Material: titanium 6 aluminum 4 vanadium ($TiAl_6V_4$)
- Low inventory

These parameters are useful for choosing a mini-implant system that can be applied in most clinical scenarios, while at the same time keeping inventory and ordering easy.[14]

Planning the Biomechanics and Area of Insertion

Only the usual orthodontic diagnostic records are required for planning biomechanics and insertion of an orthodontic mini-implant—such as study models, photographs, and panoramic and lateral cephalometric radiographs.
Generally, mini-implants can be inserted at any site that offers sufficient bone. The only area that appears to have an extremely high failure rate is the lingual side of the lower jaw.[2] However, this site should also be avoided due to the position of the lingual artery, vein, and nerve. Another area to avoid is the site of the developing wisdom teeth in the maxilla and mandible. The area around the palatal artery should also be avoided.
Ideally, the mini-implant should be inserted in an area of attached gingiva (**Fig. 8.28**).[1,21] The planned insertion site should be evaluated radiographically (with a panoramic radiograph) beforehand. Study models may also be helpful for selecting the site of placement. The long-term success of an implant depends on the amount of bone available, as well as the distance from adjacent anatomical structures that may be at risk such as vessels, nerves, and adjacent teeth. Poggio et al.[21] and Maino et al.[20] have confirmed that the bone required for successful implant stability should be at least 0.5–1.0 mm thick and should surround the implant on all sides. When planning the position of

the mini-implant, the operator should be careful to avoid blocking the movement of adjacent teeth by choosing an insertion site that is not too close to the tooth to be moved. The ideal insertion sites can be identified by marking the mucogingival border and dental long axis on study casts. The areas suitable for insertion are also referred to as "safe zones" by Poggio et al.[21] (**Fig. 8.29**). Panoramic radiographs are usually sufficient for preoperative planning of the insertion site, as they make it possible to estimate the interradicular distance and assess the proximity to other important structures in relation to the desired insertion site.

In dental implantology, stents are often used for precise positioning of the implants in the preoperatively determined position. For planning the position of mini-implants, small metal wires can be used for preoperative assessment of the insertion point. Alternatively, marking pins inserted in the area of the selected insertion site can also be used. These pins are only 1 mm long and are retained in the gingiva.[9,15,16,18] Usually, a piece of dental floss is attached to the head to prevent swallowing or aspiration (**Fig. 8.30**). The conical shape allows insertion with Weingart or Howe pliers, under topical anesthesia, and the pin is large enough to be easily identified on any radiograph (**Fig. 8.31**).

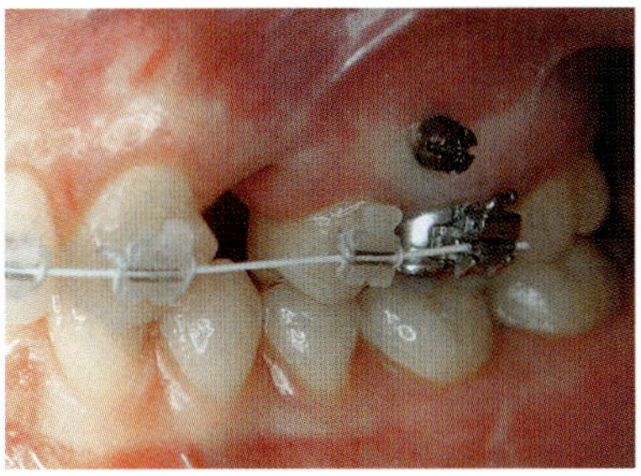

Fig. 8.28 The head of the miniscrew implant should be positioned in the attached gingiva.

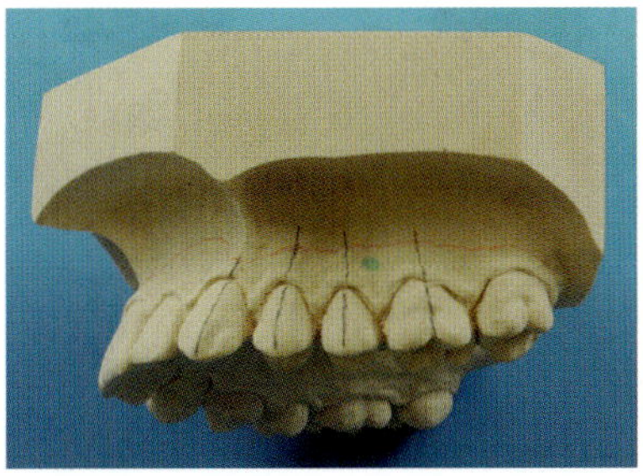

Fig. 8.29 Marking the dental long axis and the mucogingival junction on the model allows precise location of the insertion site.

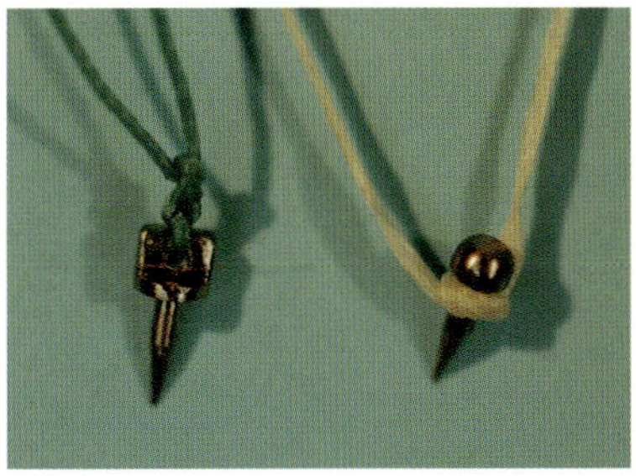

Fig. 8.30 Two radiographic pins are currently available: the Tomas X-marker (Dentaurum, left) with a preattached security thread, and the Radiographic Pin (Forestadent, right), with floss attached to prevent ingestion/inhalation.

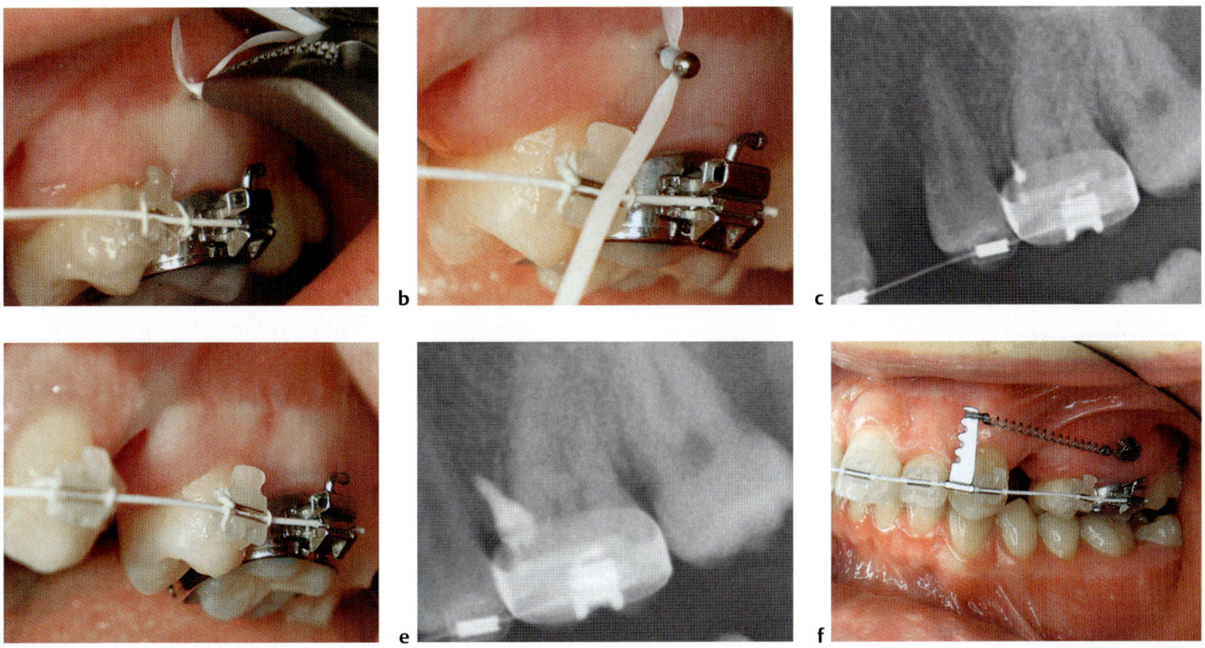

Fig. 8.31 a–f Application of the Radiographic Pin. Placement at the preplanned insertion site (**a**), ready for imaging (**b**), radiograph (**c**), insertion site marked in the gingiva (**d**), miniscrew implant inserted (radiographic follow-up, **e**) and loaded (**f**).

Table 8.6 Overview of pre-fabricated auxiliaries which need minor modifications before use

Auxiliary	Indication	Characteristics	Product name	Used with …
Power arm	En-masse retraction/ indirect anchorage	Crimpable split tube with laser-welded wire for custom hooks. Can also be used to couple the mini-implant to the archwire	Tomas power arm, square	Tomas pin
			Tomas power arm, round	Tomas pin
			Hook	A-1
Wire elements	Indirect anchorage	Prefabricated wire elements to couple the orthodontic appliance with the mini-implant	Tomas t-wire	Tomas pin
			L-anchor	Ortho Easy
			U-anchor	Ortho Easy
			Pin hook	M.A.S.
Uprighting springs	Molar uprighting along with extrusion or intrusion if desired	NiTi spring connected to stainless-steel wire using sliding connection	Tomas uprighting spring	Tomas pin
			Titanol uprighting spring	Ortho Easy

It is important to remember that the information provided by radiographic aids has a high level of uncertainty. Depending on the position of the tube, the film, and the pin, the radiograph may show significant distortion. Interpretation of the resulting radiograph may lead to false-positive or false-negative conclusions. However, joint assessment of the clinical findings along with the study model and the existing pretreatment radiographs usually provides enough useful information for accurate mini-implant placement.

In summary, the site of insertion for a mini-implant is selected by taking numerous factors into account—biomechanical considerations as well as anatomical and physiological aspects. The precise operative procedure is not described here, as it is beyond the scope of this chapter. Reference can be made to the relevant literature.[3,12,17] The implants are usually immediately loaded following insertion.

Attachments

Even with a successful mini-implant, the anchorage of the teeth and the predictability of tooth movement are only as good as the connection between the mini-implant and the teeth. The auxiliaries and connectors that establish the link between mini-implants and teeth thus play a very important role in the use of mini-implants. The attachments or connectors are often standard components for fixed-appliance treatment (such as round and rectangular wires, springs, elastic chains, expansion screws) or custom-made appliances. The versatility of the mini-implant allows clinicians to follow their desired strategy, taking advantage of cortical anchorage. However, a number of specially designed attachments are available that make the connection between the mini-implant and the fixed appliance easier and more efficient.

Most manufacturers of mini-implants provide these adjuncts to mini-implant treatment as part of their armamentarium. It is often very useful to keep all these auxiliaries on one tray, as this facilitates the treatment flow. Auxiliary sets specifically designed for use with a particular implant system are also commercially available (for example, the Tomas Auxiliary Kit from Dentaurum). These are often sold separately from the implant system itself. Some of these elements can be used for direct anchorage, while others can be used for indirect anchorage. The adjuncts can be classified into three groups:

- *Standard parts* (not prefabricated): these are usually wires (round or rectangular) in various sizes and materials. These wires are used to manufacture the auxiliaries individually.
- *Partly prefabricated parts* (**Table 8.6**): these are auxiliaries that are supplied by the manufacturer nearly ready to use. However, they have to be adapted (usually in a chairside procedure) to the patient's individual situation. The cost of these adjuncts is usually low and the time needed to modify them is minimal.
- *Prefabricated parts* (**Table 8.7**): this group includes a large number of very diverse attachments, which all have one aspect in common: they are ready to use and do not require any individualization. However, the added ease and efficiency are usually counterbalanced by high costs.

Most of these attachments (for details, see **Table 8.7**)[19] are not new and have been successfully used in orthodontics for many years. Several of the auxiliaries have been modified for use with mini-implants. The operator should be

Table 8.7 Overview of prefabricated auxiliaries for immediate use without any modification

Auxiliary	Indication	Characteristics	Product name	Used with ...
Crimpable hook	En-masse retraction	Crimpable split tube with welded hook for the attachment of elastic elements (elastic chains, coil springs)	Tomas crimp hook	Tomas pin
			Power arm crimpable	Ortho Easy
			DISCOpender	Orthodontic Mini-implant
			Crimpable hook	Dual-top anchor screw
			Crimpable hook	AbsoAnchor
Open coil springs	Distalization Mesialization	Superelastic NiTi compression springs	Tomas compression spring	Tomas pin
			TruFlex nickel titanium spring	Spider pin
Closed coil springs	Mesialization Distalization En-masse retraction	Superelastic NiTi springs with eyelets that fit the mini-implant head	Tomas coil spring	Tomas pin
			Tomas–Nikodem spring	Tomas pin
			Spring	Ortho Easy
			VectorTAS delta spring	VectorTAS
			Ortho locking closed coil spring	Ortho Implant
			NiTi closed spring	Dual-top anchor screw
			NiTi closed coil spring	AbsoAnchor
			Gentle NiTi closed coil spring	AbsoAnchor
			Coil spring	A-1
Hooks for elastics or other elastic modules	Mesialization Distalization En-masse retraction Guided eruption	Small hooks that fit onto the mini-implant head and allow secure attachment of elastic modules	Tomas hook	Tomas pin
			Tomas monkey hook	Tomas pin
			Monkey hook	M.A.S.
			Screw hook	A-1
Sliding hook	Mesialization Distalization En-masse retraction	Rectangular tube with extension for attachment of elastic modules	Power arm sliding	Ortho Easy
			VectorTAS Power arm	VectorTAS
			Sliding hook	A-1
Stops	Miscellaneous applications, e.g.: activation of open coil springs	Metal tubes with screws or crimpable split tubes	Tomas stop screw	Tomas pin
			Tomas slotted stops	Tomas pin
			Crimpable stop	Ortho Easy
			Crimpable stop	AbsoAnchor
Cross-tubes	Indirect anchorage	Cross-tubes to connect two wires together	Tomas cross-tube	Tomas pin
			Cross-tube	Ortho Easy

Continued ▷

Table 8.7 Overview of prefabricated auxiliaries for immediate use without any modification (continued)

Auxiliary	Indication	Characteristics	Product name	Used with...
Abutments	Distalization Rapid palatal expansion (RPE)	Attachments that fit the mini-implant head and serve as connectors to lab-made appliances, for example for distalization or rapid palatal expansion	Labor abutment	Ortho Easy
			BENEFIT standard abutment	BENEFIT
			BENEFIT abutment with slot	BENEFIT
			BENEFIT abutment with bracket	BENEFIT
			BENEFIT abutment with wire	BENEFIT
			BENEFIT connector plate with fixation screw	BENEFIT

aware of compatibility issues between the auxiliaries and the corresponding mini-implant. A number of the auxiliaries cannot be used with mini-implants from different manufacturers. Nevertheless, it is generally possible to adapt individual parts to many different types of mini-implants. Numerous combinations are possible, and in general, the larger the number of auxiliaries that can be used with a particular implant system, the more versatile the implant system.

NOTE

Mini-implants are a reliable method of providing anchorage that is suitable for a large number of orthodontic treatment aims. Combining them with SLBs also opens up completely new orthodontic treatment possibilities, which can be particularly useful for preprosthetic orthodontic treatment.

Example Applications for Mini-Implants

Case Study 8.6 (Fig. 8.32)

Patient: M.G., male, age 19 years.
Diagnostic records: models, panoramic radiograph, lateral cephalometric radiograph, intraoral/extraoral photographs.
Main findings: recently extracted tooth 26.
Treatment aims: protraction of teeth 27, 28.
Appliances: self-ligating brackets, molar bands, two-dimensional lingual bracket, NiTi closed coil springs, miniscrew implant.
Archwire sequence: 0.018 SS, 0.017 × 0.025 SS.
Alternative treatment strategy: n/a.
Active treatment time: 11 months.
Retention: bonded retainer for teeth 25, 27, 28.

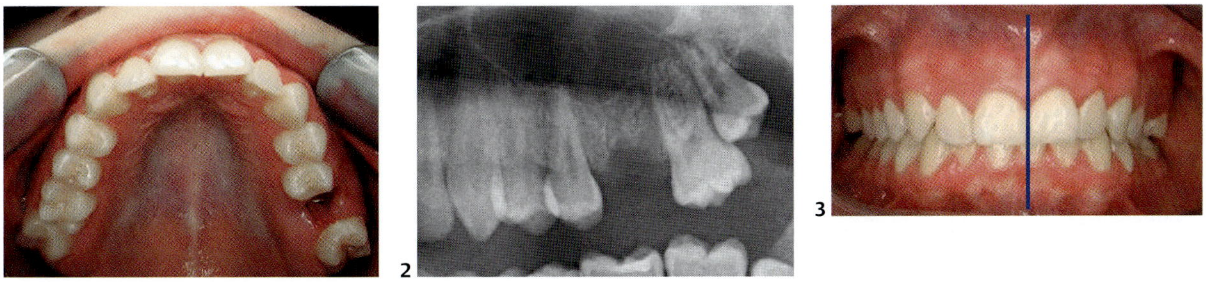

Fig. 8.32 1–10
1–3 Space closure in the area of 26 is the only treatment objective in an otherwise well-aligned dentition.

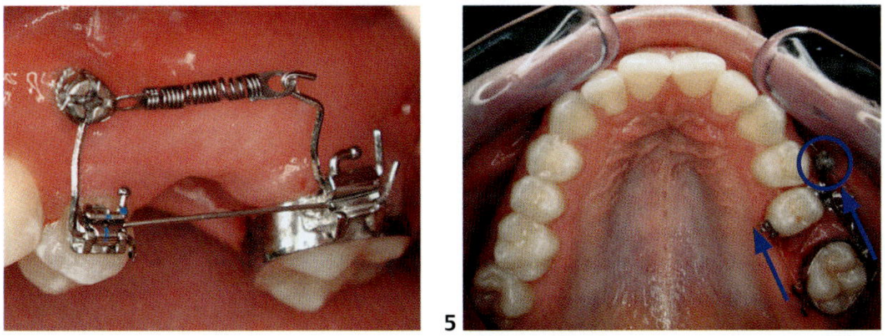

4, 5 Segmental space closure using a sectional orthodontic appliance consisting of an orthodontic miniscrew implant for indirect anchorage of tooth 25 and direct protraction of tooth 27.

CLINICAL PEARL

A power arm was inserted into the auxiliary tube of the molar band. This raises the point of force application to the level of the molar's center of resistance.

Result: improvement of tooth movement, with reduction of vertical side effects due to ideal force vectors.

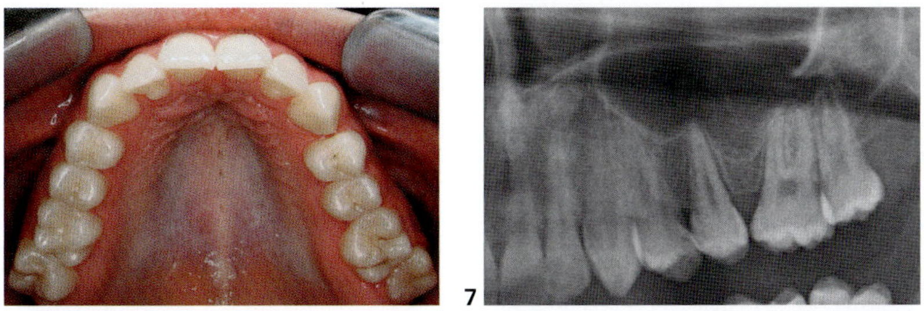

6–10 The sinus prevented complete protraction of 27. The roots were not parallel at the end of orthodontic treatment. However, a clinically satisfactory occlusion was achieved, despite the radiographically visible angulation of tooth 27.

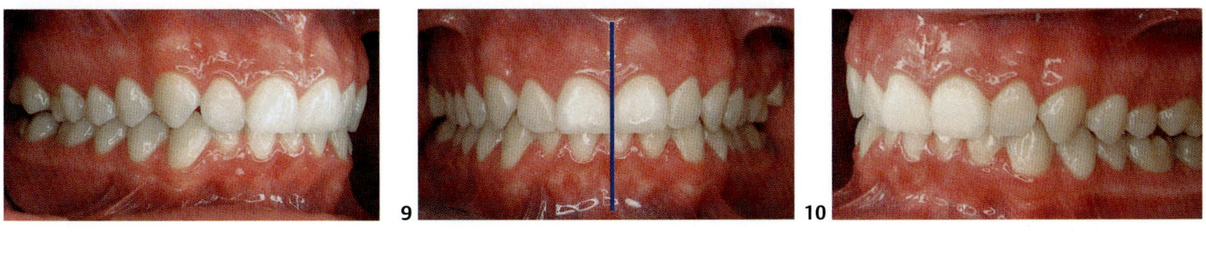

Case Study 8.7 (Fig. 8.33)

Patient: M.Z., male, age 17.
Diagnostic records: models, panoramic radiograph, lateral cephalometric radiograph, intraoral/extraoral photographs.
Main findings: congenitally missing teeth 35 and 41, deep bite, skeletal class II tendency.
Treatment aims: It was decided to remove the lower left second deciduous (75) and to mesialise the first and second molar on that side to create space and allow for eruption of the impacted lower left third molar.
Appliances: self-ligating brackets, molar bands, Space-Jet, miniscrew implant.
Archwire sequence: 0.012 SE, 0.016 SE, 0.016 SS, 0.016 × 0.022 SE, 0.019 × 0.025 SS.
Alternative treatment strategy: n/a.
Active treatment time: 15 months.
Retention: three-dimensional retention with a Hawley retainer.

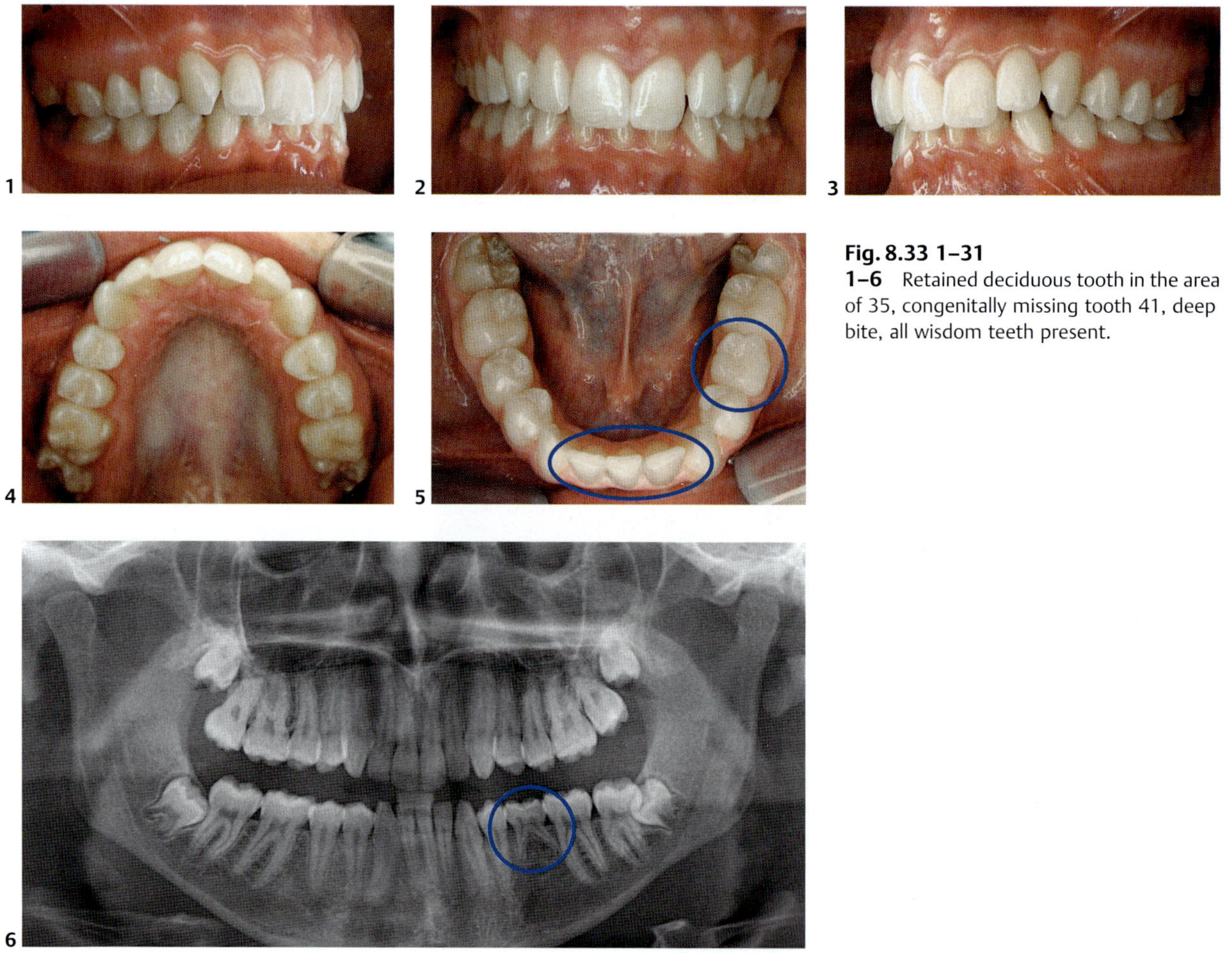

Fig. 8.33 1–31
1–6 Retained deciduous tooth in the area of 35, congenitally missing tooth 41, deep bite, all wisdom teeth present.

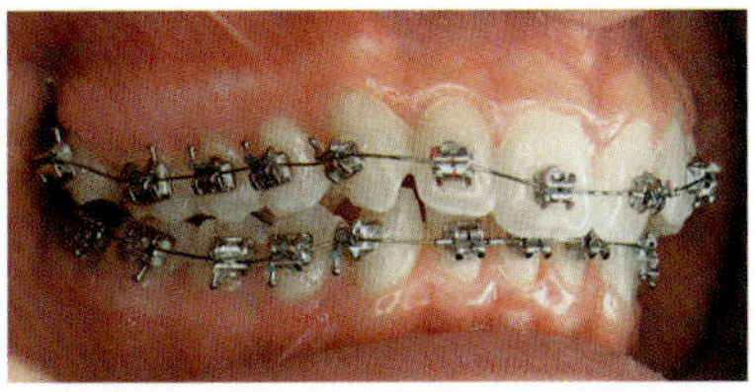
7

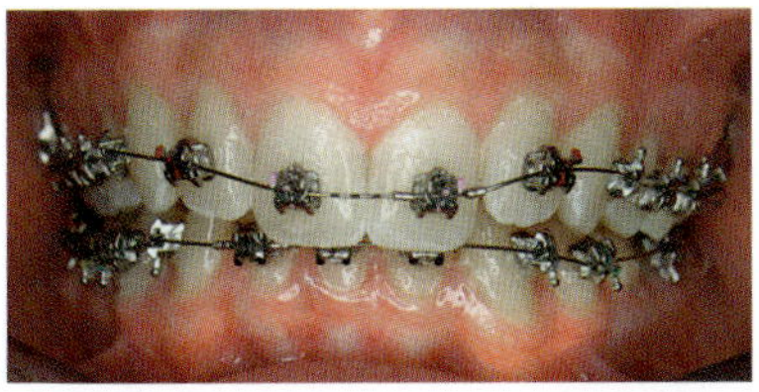
8

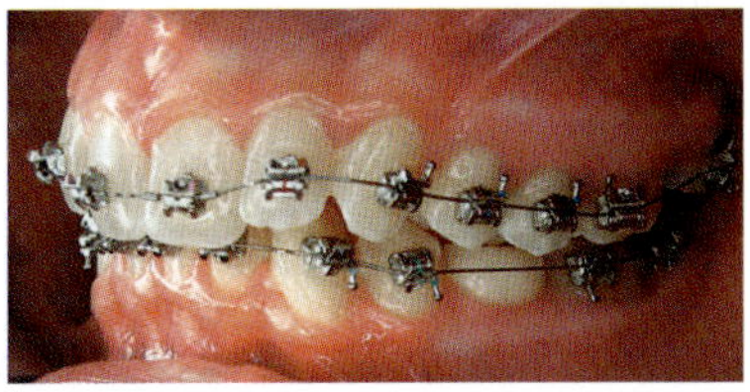
9

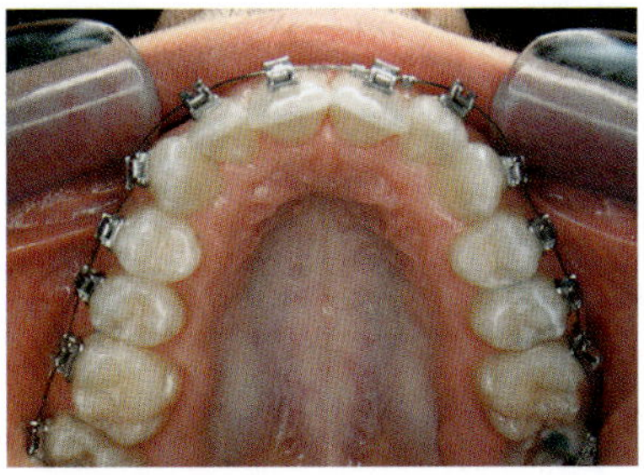
10

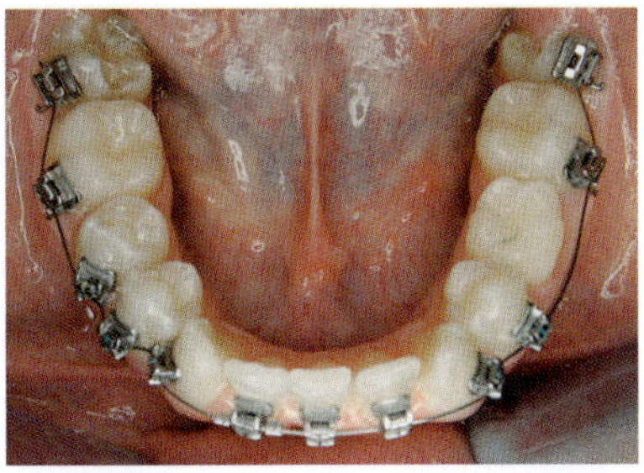
11

7–11 Self-ligating brackets and 0.012 SE archwire in place.

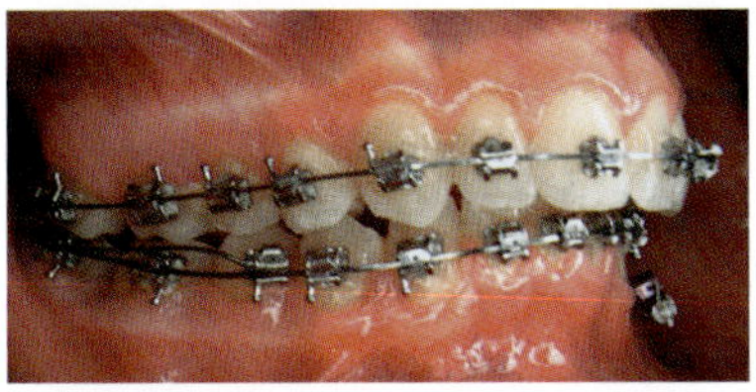
12

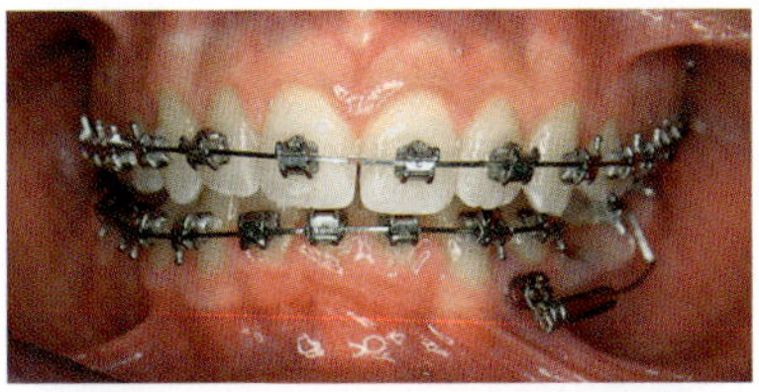
13

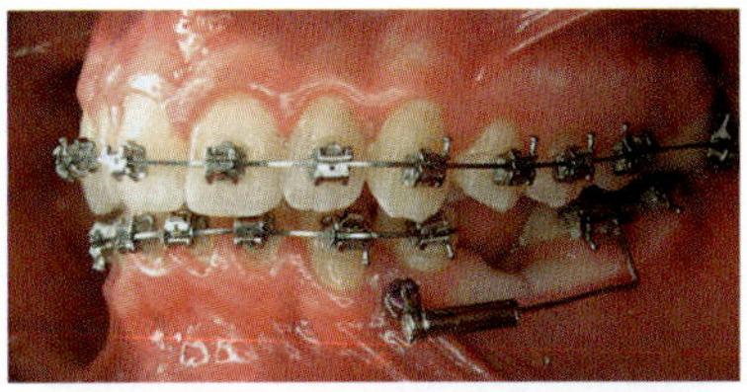
14

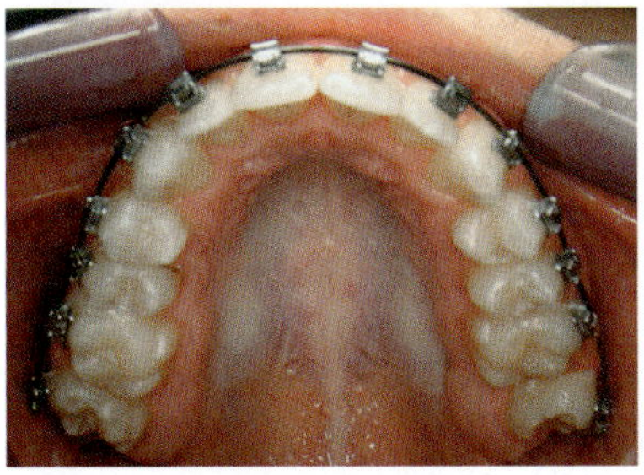
15

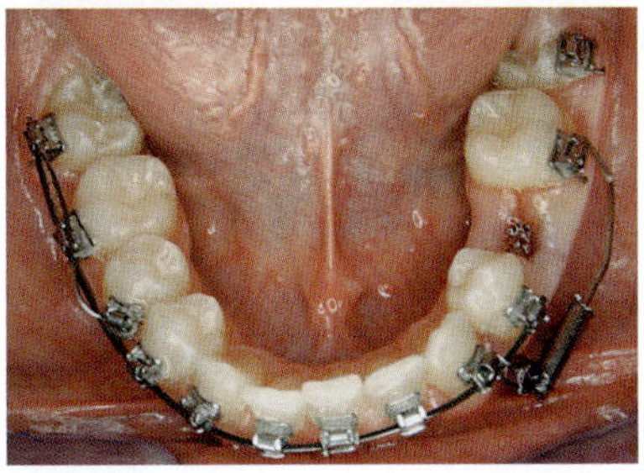
16

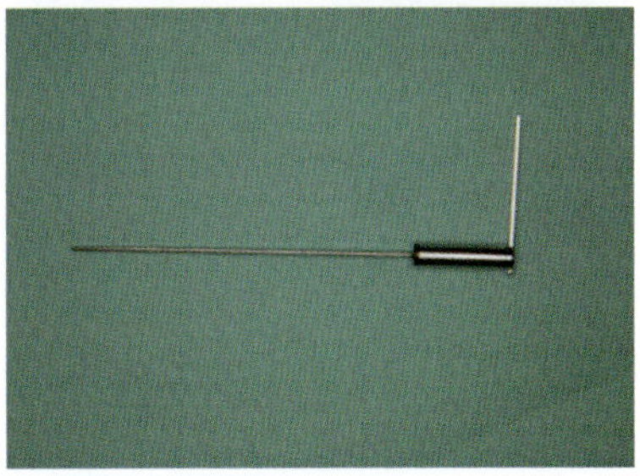
17

12–17 Rectangular stainless-steel base arches, NiTi derotation spring for tooth 45, miniscrew implant for direct space closure of the edentulous site 35. The Space-Jet (Forestadent) is a prefabricated protraction spring for use with orthodontic miniscrew implants. The wire ends are connected to a protraction spring at an angle of 90° and serve as connectors to both the miniscrew implant and the tooth requiring protraction.

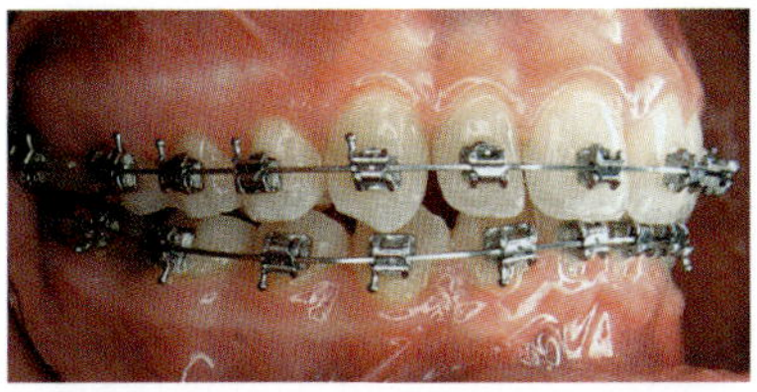
18

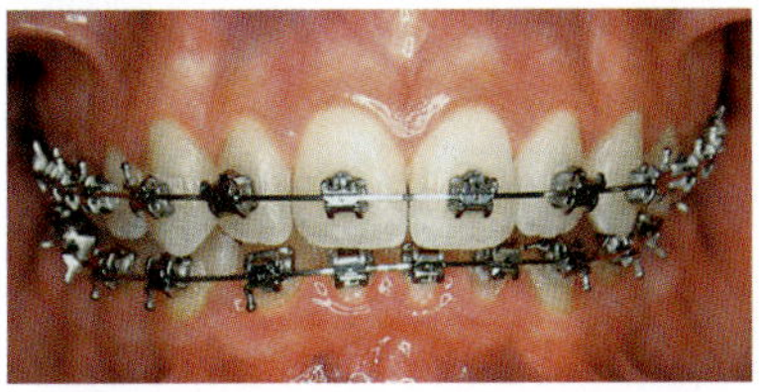
19

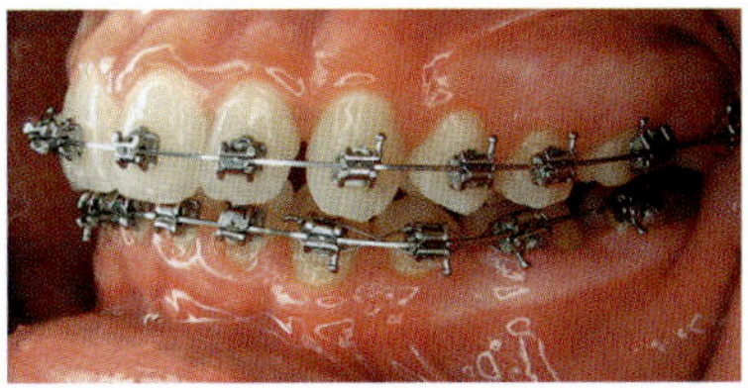
20

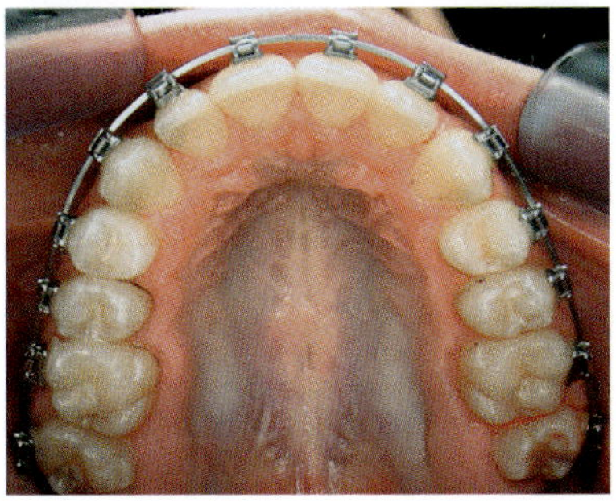
21

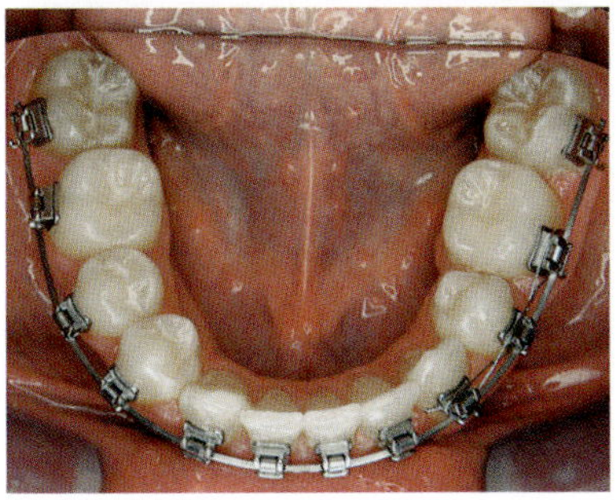
22

18–22 Completed protraction of teeth 36 and 37.

23
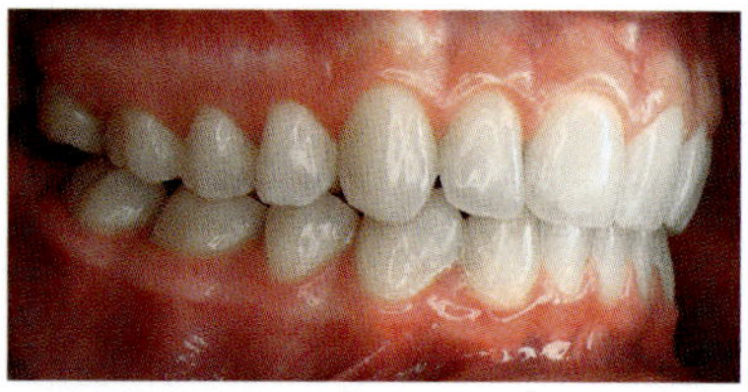
24
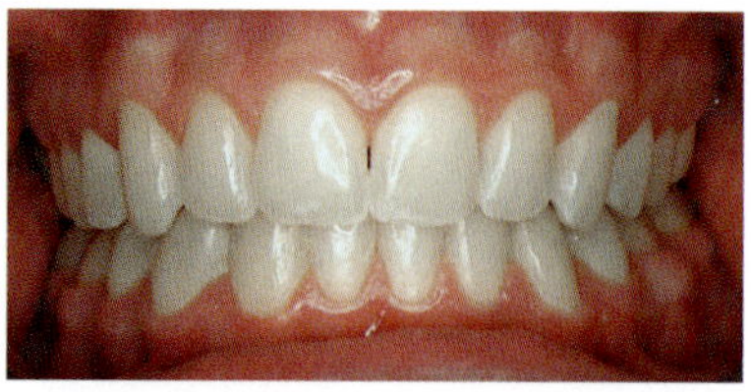
25
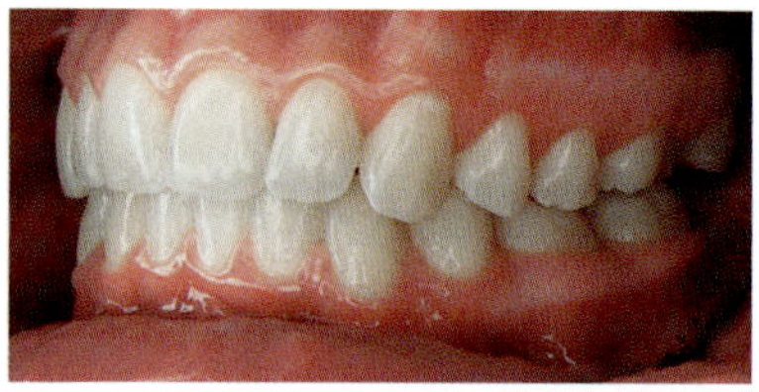
26
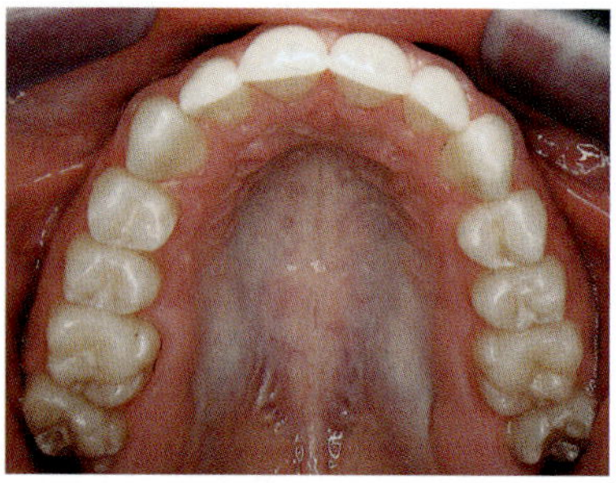
27
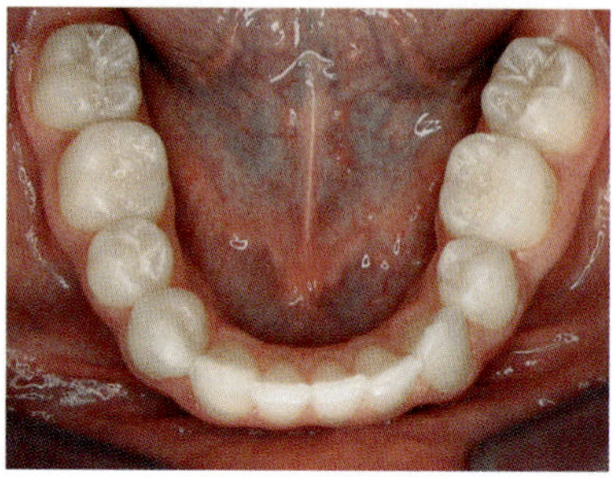

23–27 The result after 1 year of retention; coincident midlines, class III occlusion on the right side due to missing tooth 41, and space closure.

Clinical pearl:
Slight recontouring of the incisal tip of tooth 43 may be required.

28
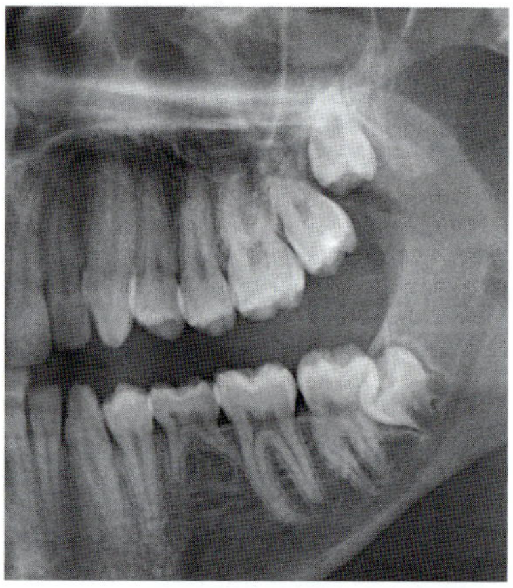
29
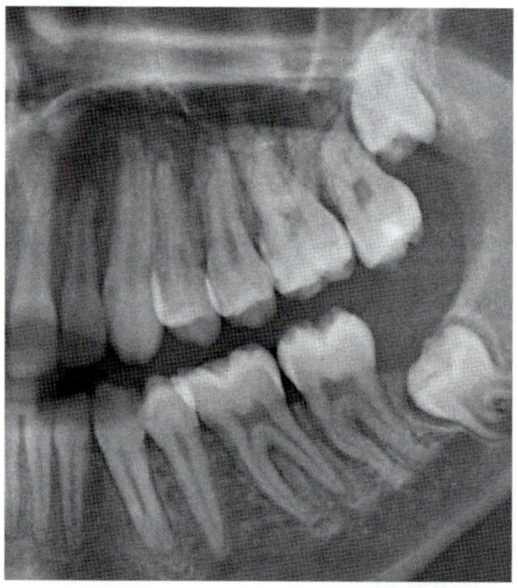

28, 29 After space closure in the third quadrant, the wisdom tooth now has sufficient space for spontaneous eruption, to act as an antagonist for the opposing maxillary dentition.

30
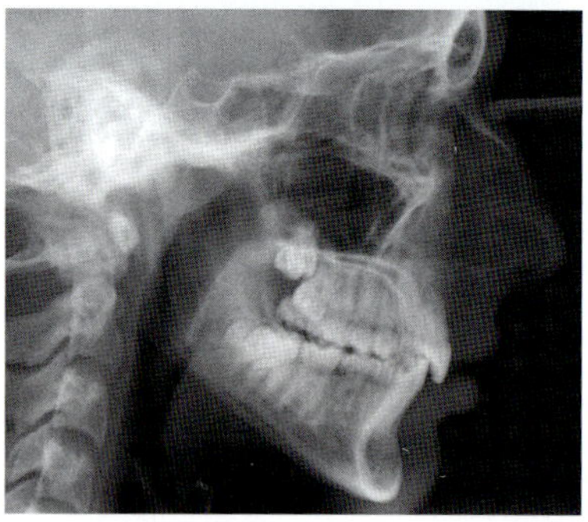
31
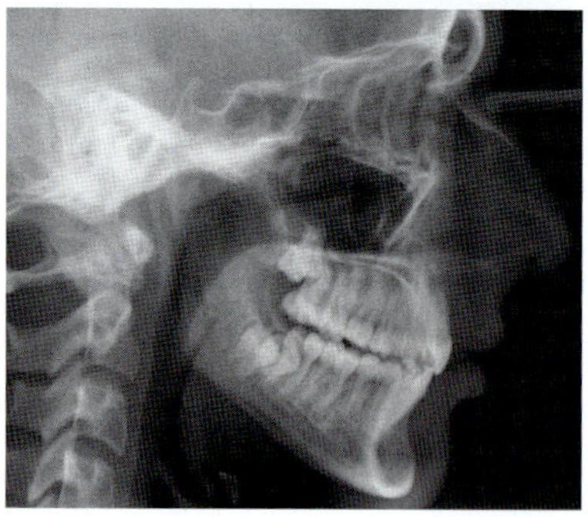

30, 31 Cephalometric radiographs: the slightly retrognathic mandibular position at the beginning of treatment (**30**) should be compared with the improved post-treatment position (**31**).

NOTE

The upper left second molar must not be left to overerupt while the opposing lower third molar emerges. This can be achieved using a bonded retainer.

Case Study 8.8 (Fig. 8.34)

Patient: C.M., female, age 16.
Diagnostic records: models, panoramic radiograph, lateral cephalometric radiograph, intraoral/extraoral photographs.
Main findings: skeletal open bite, tongue thrust.
Treatment aims: dental compensation of the skeletal problem.
Appliances: self-ligating brackets, molar bands, intrusion spring, miniscrew implant, transpalatal arch.
Archwire sequence: 0.012 SE, 0.016 SE, 0.016 SS, 0.016 × 0.022 SE reverse curve of Spee, 0.017 × 0.025 SE reverse curve of Spee.
Alternative treatment strategy: orthognathic surgery.
Active treatment time: 14 months.
Retention: three-dimensional retention, spikes as needed (see Chapter 9).

Fig. 8.34 1–11 Stepwise closure of the open bite.

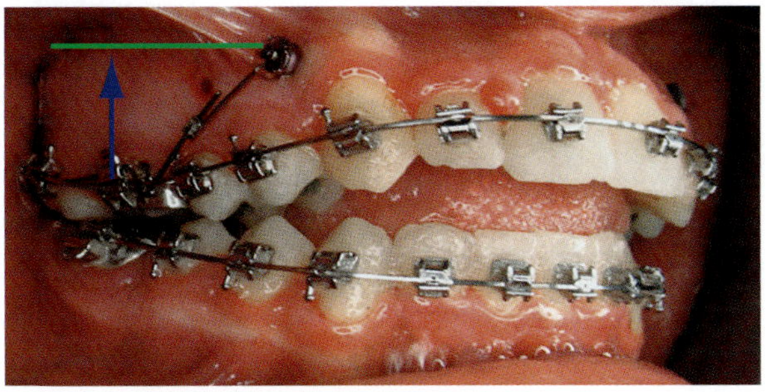
1

1 Step 1. Skeletally anchored intrusion springs to reduce posterior contact. Activation of the TMA (**T**itanium **M**olybdenum **A**lloy) arm at 1.5 N.

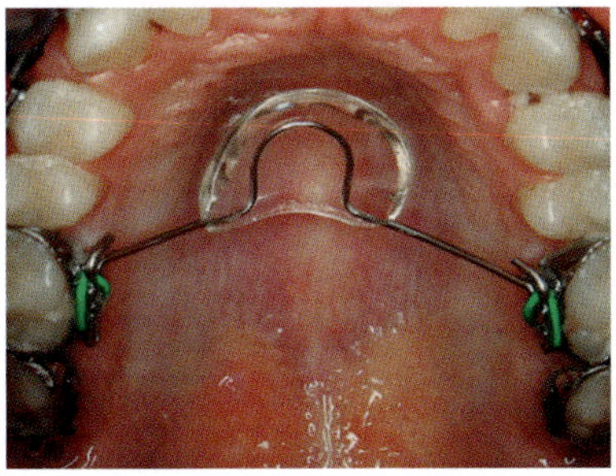
2

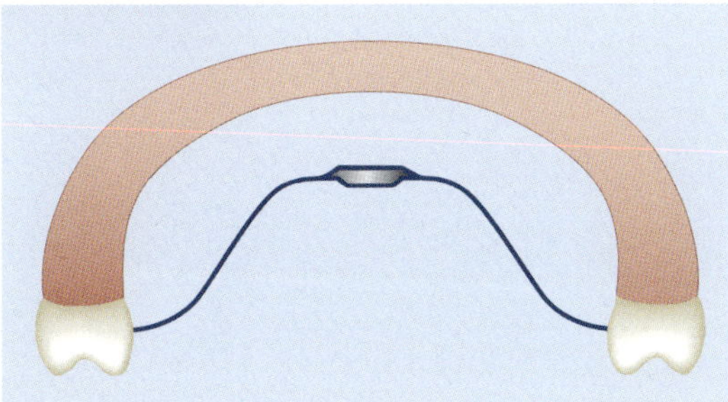
3

2, 3 Step 2. The transpalatal arch has sufficient clearance to the palate to avoid buccal flaring of the molars. The acrylic button allows the tongue pressure to support molar intrusion.

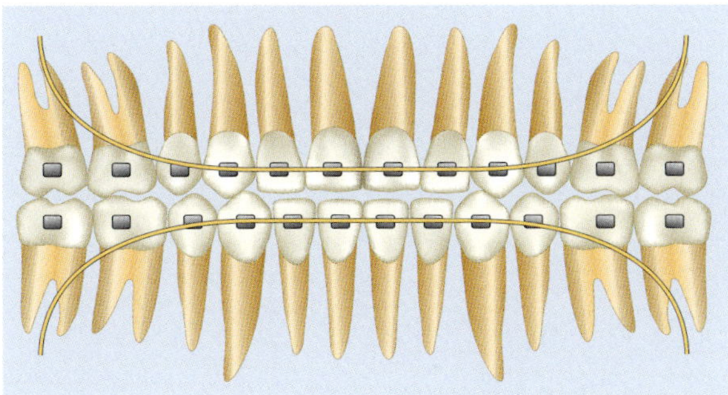
4

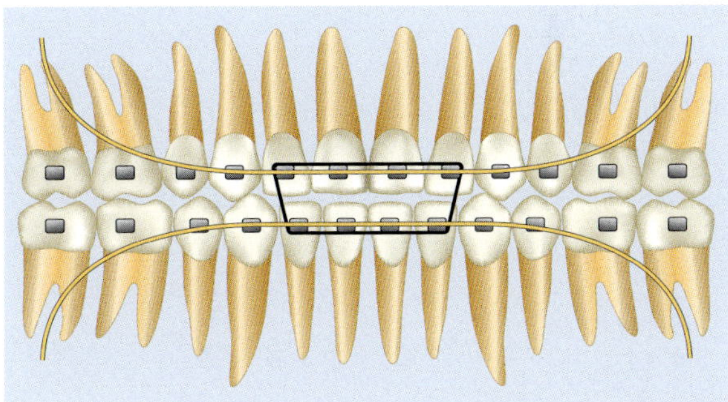
5

4, 5 Step 3. The Kim/Sato technique: reverse curve of Spee wires are inserted in both jaws and programmed for anterior extrusion and posterior intrusion using anterior box elastics.

NOTE

Anterior box elastics have to be worn 24 hours a day (Kim/Sato Mechanics). This avoids further anterior bite opening and promotes posterior intrusion (with the curve of Spee in the upper arch and the reverse curve of Spee in the lower arch). The patient must be informed about the consequences if the box elastics are not worn: worsening of the anterior open bite. This technique is only recommended for highly motivated and compliant patients.

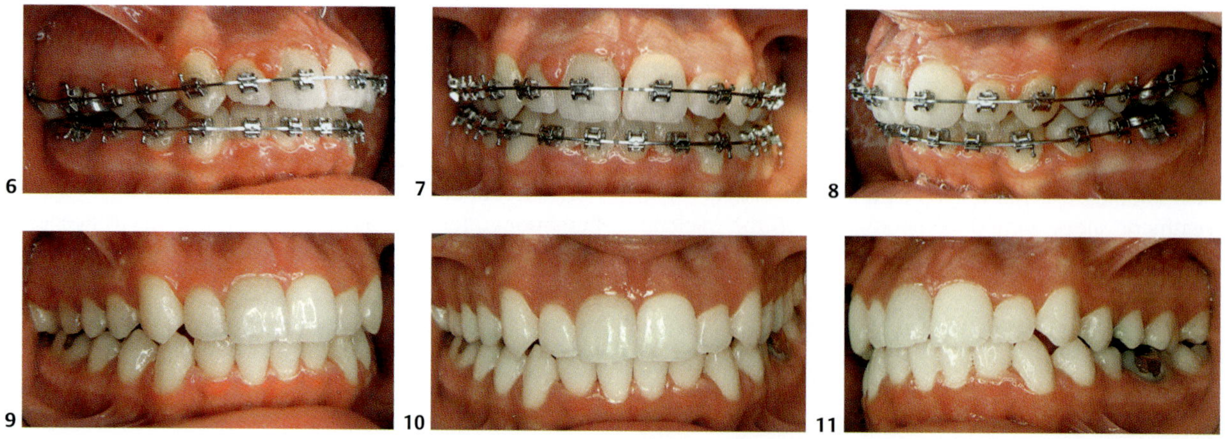

6–11 The treatment result immediately before debonding and after 2 years of retention. This borderline orthognathic case was treated successfully without surgery. Despite a persistent slight midline deviation, the overbite was corrected with a more stable result. The healthy gingiva, which was irritated and inflamed before treatment, serves as an indication that the patient's mouth-breathing habit has also improved.

Case Study 8.9 (Fig. 8.35)

Patient: D.F.H., male, age 16.
Diagnostic records: models, panoramic radiograph, lateral cephalometric radiograph, intraoral/extraoral photographs.
Main findings: mandibular second molars mesially impacted.
Treatment aims: uprighting of teeth 37 and 47.
Appliances: self-ligating molar tubes, uprighting springs, miniscrew implant.
Alternative treatment strategy: extraction of teeth 37 and 47 with alignment of teeth 38 and 48.
Active treatment time: 8 months.
Retention: three-dimensional retention with a Hawley retainer.

1 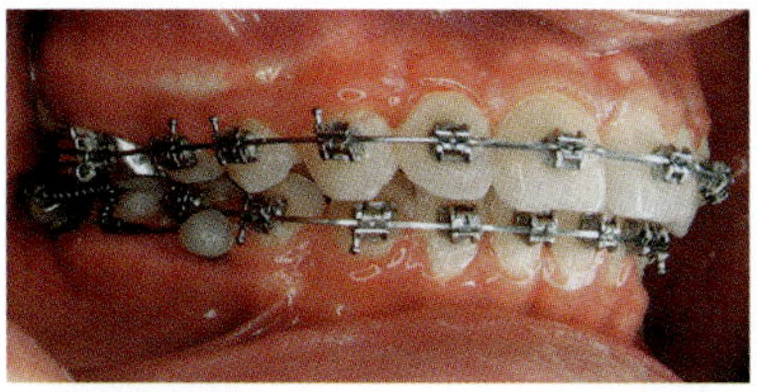

2 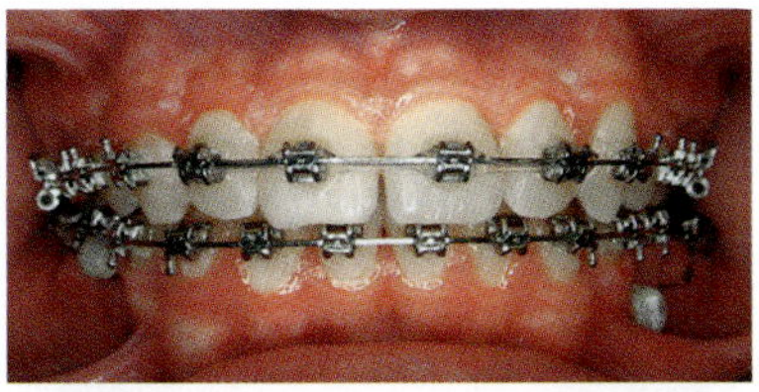

3 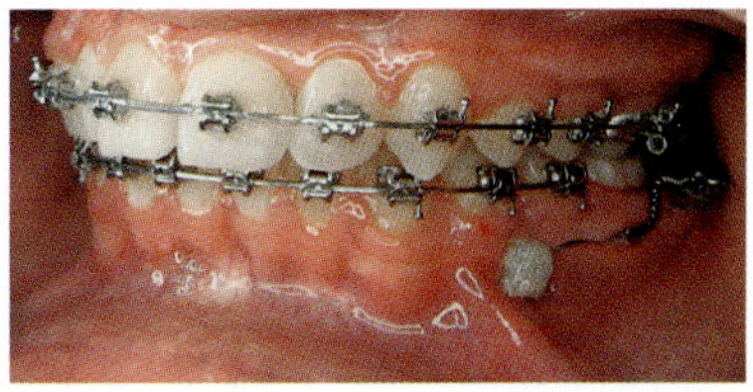

4 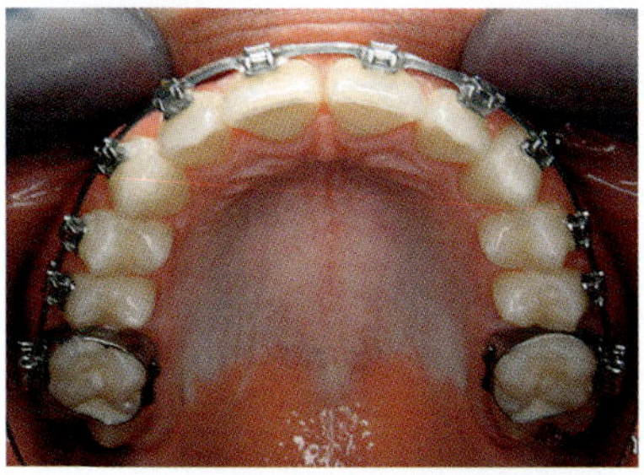

5 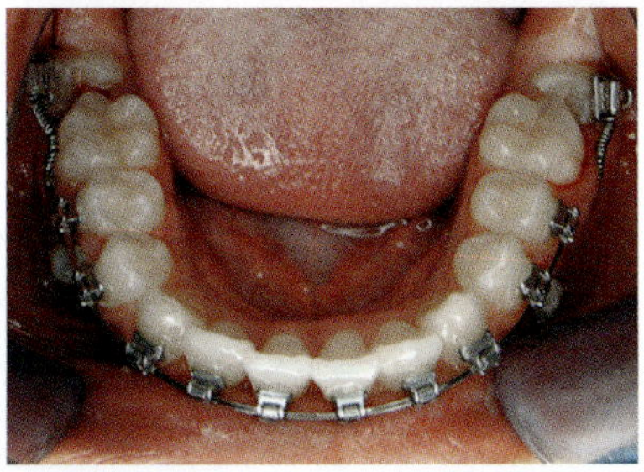

6 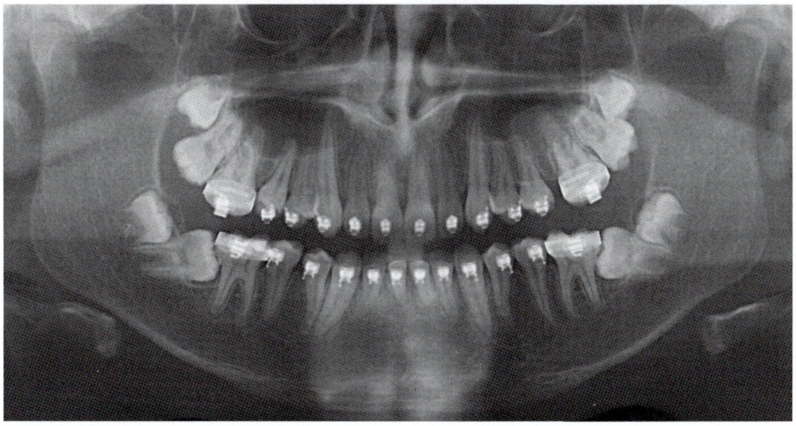

Fig. 8.35 1–15
1–6 Well-progressing treatment with self-ligating brackets. The progress panoramic radiograph shows mesially impacted mandibular second molars. After extraction of teeth 38 and 48 and surgical exposure of teeth 37 and 47, brackets were bonded and miniscrew implants were placed to allow molar uprighting with an uprighting spring and to avoid reciprocal side effects. The springs were activated to allow distalization and uprighting at the same time.

7 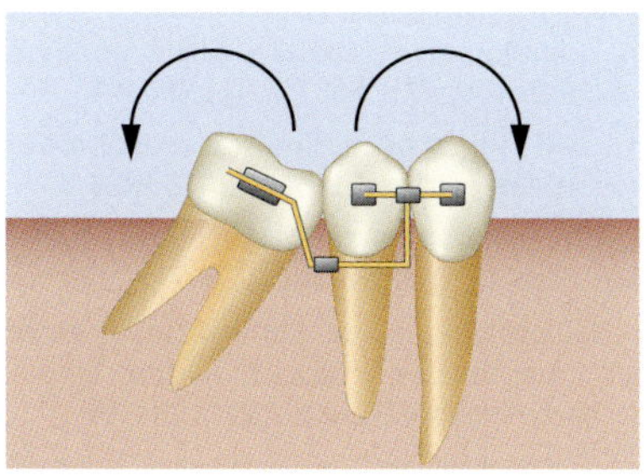

8 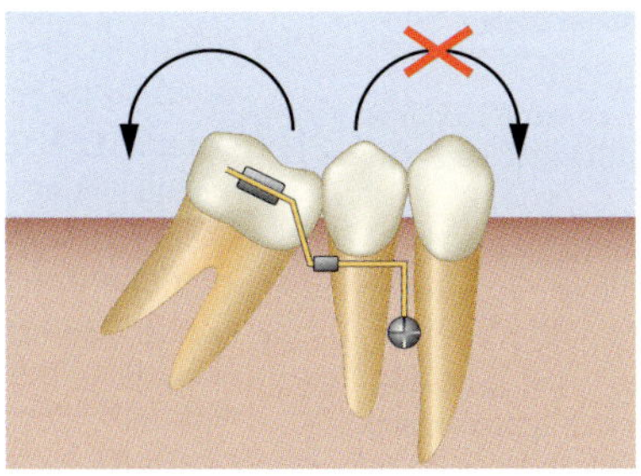

7, 8 Uprighting a molar creates momentum that may have an undesired effect on the anterior dentition. Use of a miniscrew implant can absorb the undesired reciprocal momentum.

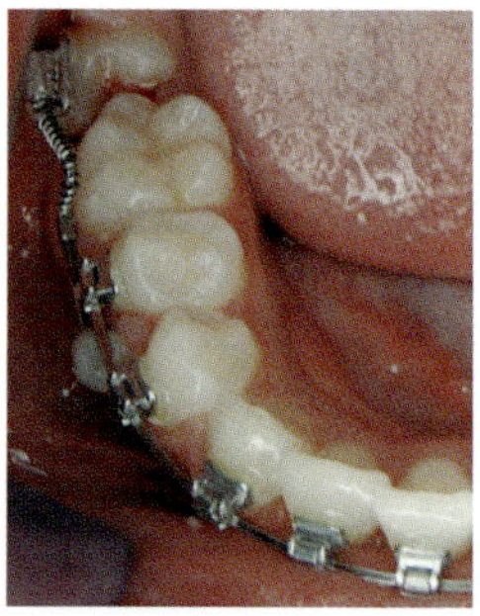
9
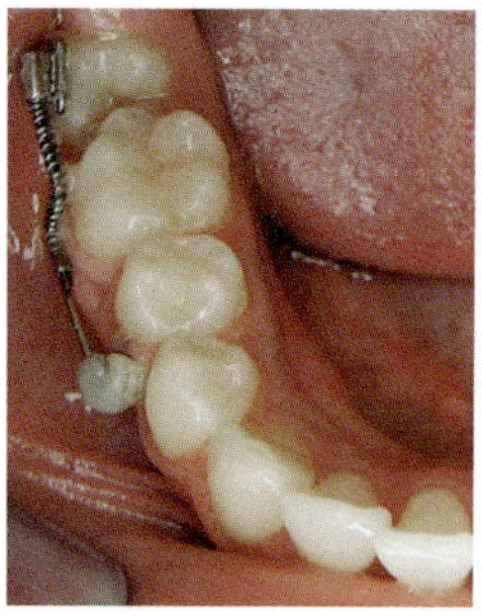
10
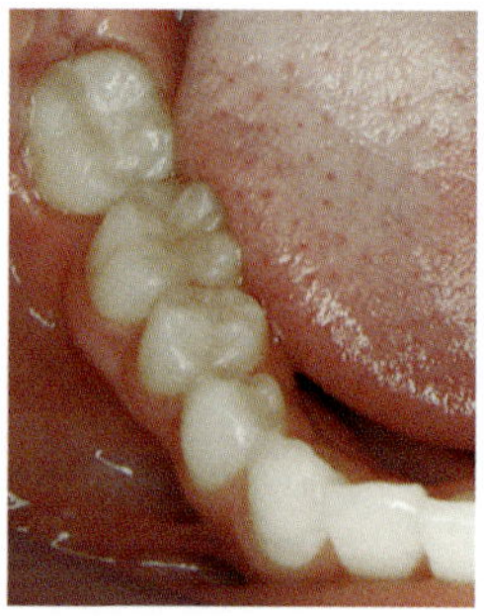
11

9–11 The initial uprighting phase (9). The front teeth of the patient were debonded after alignment of the dentition was completed (10). Posterior sectional mechanics were used for continuation of the molar uprighting. A mini-implant which was inserted between 44 and 45 was used for anchorage.

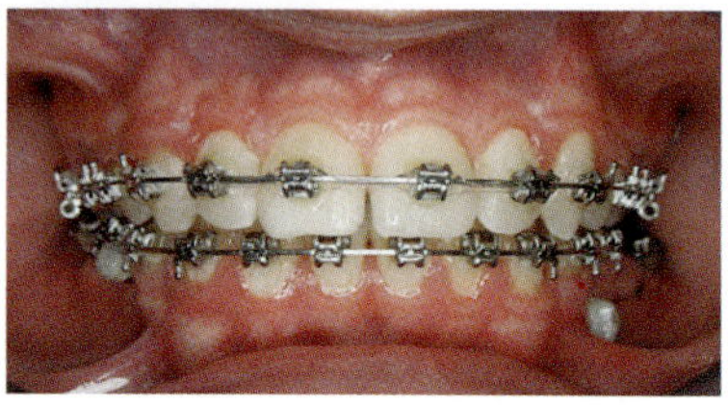
12
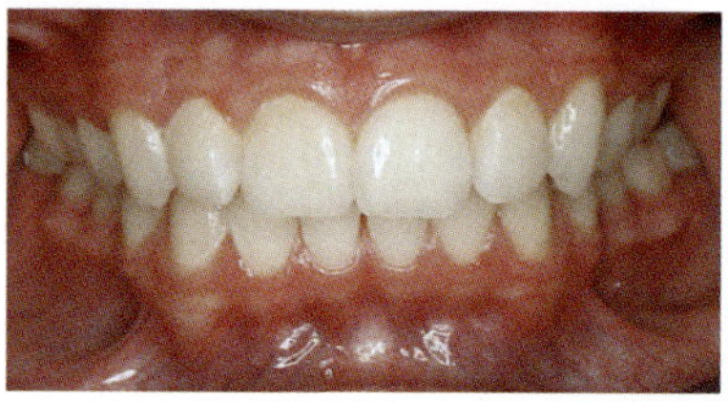
13

12, 13 The miniscrew implant absorbs reactive forces and prevents negative biomechanical effects on the anterior dentition during molar uprighting.

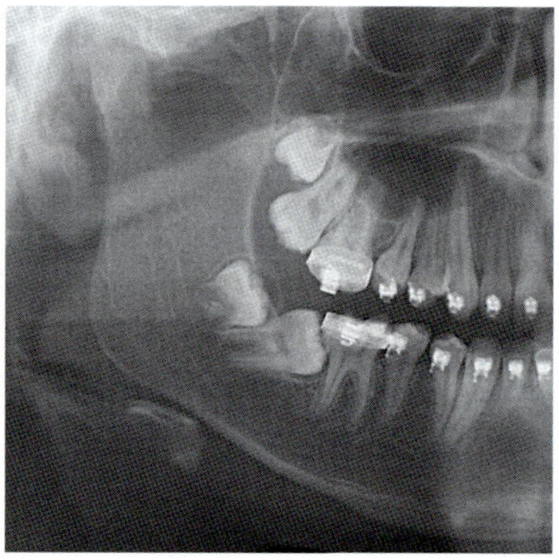
14
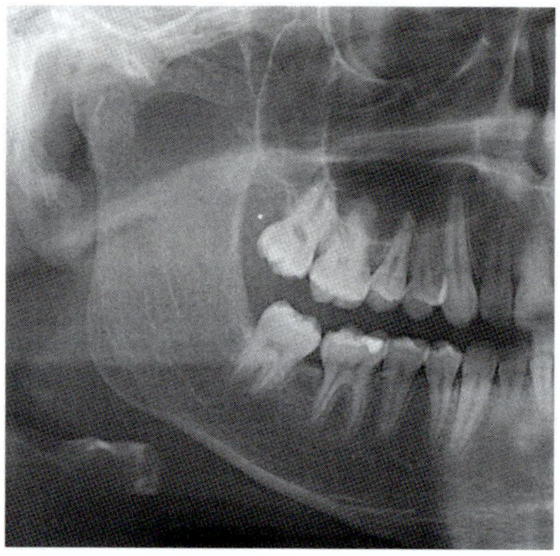
15

14, 15 Panoramic radiographs before and after successful molar uprighting.

REFERENCES

1. Berens A, Wiechmann D, Rüdiger J. Skeletal anchorage in orthodontics with mini- and microscrews. Int Orthod 2005;3:235–243
2. Berens A, Wiechmann D. Mini- und Mikroschrauben als skelettale Verankerung in der Kieferorthopädie. Optimierung des klinischen Vorgehens. Kieferorthopädie 2006;20(3):167–174
3. Cope JB. OrthoTADs. The Clinical Guide and Atlas. Dallas: Under Dog Media; 2007
4. Danesh G, Hellak A, Lippold C, Ziebura T, Schafer E. Enamel surfaces following interproximal reduction with different methods. Angle Orthod 2007;77(6):1004–1010
5. Fillion D. Zur approximalen Schmelzreduktion in der Erwachsenenkieferorthopädie. Teil 2: Vor- und Nachteile der approximalen Schmelzreduktion. Inf Orthod Kieferorthop 1995;27:64–90
6. Fillion D. Zur approximalen Schmelzreduktion in der Erwachsenenkieferorthopädie. Teil 3: Grundprinzipien der approximalen Schmelzreduktion und Vorgehensweise anhand dreier Fälle. Inf Orthod Kieferorthop 1995;27:91–105
7. Fuck LM, Wilmes B, Gürler G, et al. Friktionsverhalten selbstligierender und konventioneller Bracketsysteme. Inf Orthod Kieferorthop 2007;39(1):6–17
8. Gillings B, Buonocore M. An investigation of enamel thickness in human lower incisor teeth. J Dent Res 1961;40:105–118
9. Grüner W. Der Einsatz von Minischrauben in der täglichen Praxisroutine. Kieferorthop Nachr KN 2007;5(9):9–10
10. Haubrich J. Praxistipp: Approximale Schmelzreduktion mit dem Ortho-Strips-System. Kieferorthopädie 2007;21(2):99–102
11. Hudson A. A study of the effects of mesiodistal reduction of mandibular anterior teeth. Am J Orthod 1956;42:615–624
12. Lee JS, Kim JK, Park YC, Vanarsdall RLJ. Application of Orthodontic Mini-Implants. Hanover Park, IL: Quintessence; 2007
13. Ley M, Koussah RA, Radlanski RJ, et al. Untersuchung einer neuartigen Technik zur approximalen Schmelzreduktion. Ergebnisse einer Pilotstudie. Kieferorthopädie 2007;21(2):91–96
14. Lietz T. Minischrauben – Aspekte zur Bewertung und Auswahl der verschiedenen Systeme. In: Ludwig B, ed. Mini-Implantate in der Kieferorthopädie. Innovative Verankerungskonzepte. Berlin: Quintessenz; 2007:11–71

15. Ludwig B. Mini-Implantate in der Kieferorthopädie. Innovative Verankerungskonzepte. Berlin: Quintessenz; 2007

16. Ludwig B, Glasl B, Kopp S. Neue Röntgenhilfe zur präoperativen Diagnostik für Miniimplantate. Kieferorthopädie Nachrichten 2007;9:5–6

17. Ludwig B, Glasl B, Landes C, Lietz T. Insertion von Minischrauben. In: Ludwig B, ed. Mini-Implantate in der Kieferorthopädie. Innovative Verankerungskonzepte. Berlin: Quintessenz; 2007:73–88

18. Ludwig B, Glasl B, Lietz T, et al. Radiological location monitoring in skeletal anchorage: introduction of a positioning guide. J Orofac Orthop 2008;69(1):59–65

19. Ludwig B, Glasl B, Lietz T, et al. Minischrauben – Fixpunkt in der Praxis. Teil 5: Hilfsmittel für die Therapie. Kieferorthopädie Nachrichten 2008;6(5):1,8–13

20. Maino BG, Bednar J, Pagin P, Mura P. The spider screw for skeletal anchorage. J Clin Orthod 2003;37(2):90–97

21. Poggio PM, Incorvati C, Velo S, Carano A. "Safe zones": a guide for miniscrew positioning in the maxillary and mandibular arch. Angle Orthod 2006;76(2):191–197

22. Sander C, Sander FM, Sander FG. Leveling of the second molar with a superelastic spring. J Orofac Orthop 2006;67(3):186–195

23. Sheridan JJ. Air-rotor stripping. J Clin Orthod 1985;19(1):43–59

24. Sheridan JJ. Air-rotor stripping update. J Clin Orthod 1987;21(11):781–788

25. Shillingburg HT Jr, Grace CS. Thickness of enamel and dentin. J South Calif Dent Assoc 1973;41(1):33–36, passim

26. Stroud JL, English J, Buschang PH. Enamel thickness of the posterior dentition: its implications for nonextraction treatment. Angle Orthod 1998;68(2):141–146

27. Sung JH, Kyung HM, Bae SM et al. Microimplants in orthodontics. Daegu: Dentos; 2006

28. Wilmes B. Insertion von Minischrauben. In: Ludwig B, ed. Mini-Implantate in der Kieferorthopädie. Innovative Verankerungskonzepte. Berlin: Quintessenz; 2007:89–120

Retention and Stability

Bettina Glasl and Bjoern Ludwig

9

Every orthodontic treatment can be divided into two phases: the active treatment phase, during which the malocclusion is corrected, and the retention phase, in which the orthodontic result has to be maintained. Lasting esthetic quality and long-term stability of the achieved treatment outcome are the general aim, and also the reason why most patients wish to undergo orthodontic treatment. Maintaining the esthetic result is therefore one of the core requirements in orthodontics and this has been the main focus of attention for more than 100 years. Edward H. Angle (1855–1930)—the founder of fixed orthodontic treatment as we use it today and the inventor of the Edgewise appliance—realized at a very early point in his 43-year career as an orthodontist that post-treatment stability is often an issue. He recommended a number of retentive measures following orthodontic treatment. One of his pupils, A.J. Oppenheim, summarized this view in a statement that is still valid today: "Retention is the most important problem in orthodontics; in fact, it is *the* problem."

There is still no scientific or practical consensus on how relapse can be prevented, except for wearing retainers and some movement of teeth may occur even when these are used. The etiology of tooth movement after orthodontic treatment (relapse or otherwise) is not clear, and a number of factors have been discussed in the literature. The present authors consider that tooth movement after orthodontics is a multifactorial event and that there are no known parameters that could reliably predict the tendency to relapse and the amount of tooth movement for individual patients.[9–11] A large body of published evidence appears to suggest that the occlusion undergoes lifelong changes whether orthodontic treatment has been undertaken or not.[10] Most of the recommendations regarding retention techniques and protocols are based on empirical parameters rather than on sound scientific evaluation.[4,15,18]

CLINICAL PEARL

As there are no reliable predictors for the individual risk of tooth movement after orthodontics and a long-term, individualized retention plan should be considered. The patient needs to be aware of the requirements and limitations of retention.

Biological Basis

There is evidence that specific types of malocclusion are associated with particular relapse patterns. Independently of the original malocclusion and completed therapy, however, the following four general factors that determine the stability of the orthodontic outcome can be identified.

Active Tooth Movement

Orthodontic movement of teeth has an impact on the surrounding gingival, periodontal, and bony structures of the teeth. Applying force to teeth leads to periodontal changes that result from a number of complex processes and adaptive responses at molecular level.[14] Subsequent to active orthodontic treatment, consolidation of the result in terms of tissue changes at the cellular level occurs after 3–4 months. Adaptation of the elastic fibers and collagen network of the gingiva takes longer, however. It takes between 6 months and 1 year for these to reorganize, depending on the patient's age.[18,20]

NOTE

The supracrestal fibers are able to induce postorthodontic tooth movement for up to 2 years.[18,20]

Functional Parameters of the Orovestibular System

Orthodontic treatment has an immediate impact on the stomatognathic system, particularly when the treatment is undertaken during growth; a fine-tuned and highly individual interplay between the functionality of the chewing apparatus, the tongue, and the facial musculature develops during this period in particular. All kinds of orofacial functions and dysfunctions, such as parafunctions or habits, can have an impact on the stability of a patient's postorthodontic occlusion. In particular, functional changes in habitual tongue positioning can be a challenge for the stability of the final orthodontic result; the tongue is a relatively powerful, subconsciously controlled muscle (**Fig. 9.1**). The section on "Retention Following Treatment for Anterior Open Bites" below provides suggestions for retention strategies that are largely compliance-free.

Patient's Age

Some authors claim that a patient's residual growth may influence the orthodontic treatment results. Particularly in treatment for patients with underlying skeletal problems, there is often a need for greater retention until the end of the active growth period.[3] As growth patterns are genetically predetermined, there is a risk of long-term relapse. In fact, growthlike changes in the maxillofacial skeleton appear to persist well into adulthood.

Although growth changes do not appear to be a predominant factor for relapse in adult patients, it is important to remember that this group has a reduced ability to respond to orthodontic stimuli. Cellular activity is reduced in comparison with adolescent patients, and the individual cellular response to orthodontic treatment tends to decrease with increasing age. This appears to be the case for both hard and soft tissues. Orthodontists need to be aware that when treatment for adult patients is being planned, the stability of the desired result will be affected by the patient's reduced ability to adapt to the changes achieved. In addition, all orthodontic treatment changes are also affected by a reduced capability of tissue repair (with all the associated consequences) as the patient gets older.

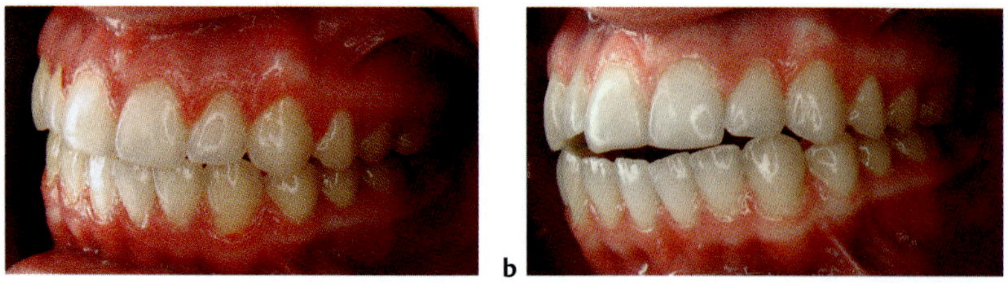

a b

Fig. 9.1 a, b Parafunctional habits contributing to relapse.
a The patient had a class II occlusion and an open bite due to tongue interposition at the beginning of treatment. During the course of treatment, the situation improved and the tongue thrust disappeared, possibly due to simultaneous speech therapy. At the conclusion of treatment, the patient was given information about the risk of relapse. The result remained stable 1 year into retention.
b The return of the parafunctional tongue habit led to a relapse of the open bite, with marked proclination of the incisors.

Tooth Morphology

Morphological aspects of the tooth, such as length and cusp inclination, can constitute a determining factor for amount, and duration of retention. Well-defined occlusal anatomy allows good interdigitation and geometric locking of the occlusion and can therefore contribute to the overall stability of the final occlusion (**Fig. 9.2**). Hypoplastic lateral incisors with absent or insufficient interproximal contact points may compromise the stability at the end of active treatment and should therefore ideally be treated immediately after the removal of the fixed appliances, at least with temporary restorations. Poor contact-point morphology is well known to decrease the likelihood of stability of orthodontic alignment. This is even more so in cases in which spaces have been maintained for prosthetic replacement of teeth. Patients who are affected by hypodontia are often treated during adolescence, but dental implants should not be placed until growth has ceased. This means that the orthodontic result has to be maintained until the implants can be placed. It used to be customary to use removable appliances that incorporated the missing teeth and acted as a denture. An alternative to this concept is to place resin-bonded bridges. However, contemporary orthodontic treatment provides the alternative of placing mini-implants (which are normally used as temporary anchorage devices) in the edentulous site and using them as an abutment to fit a temporary crown, which in turn acts as the prosthetic replacement for the missing tooth or teeth (see the section on "The Spaced Dentition" below, p. 226). This allows very secure tooth replacement for the intermediate phase until the patient reaches an age at which conventional implants can be placed. An additional advantage of this method of prosthetic replacement is that it is also independent of patient compliance. While the method provides functional continuity of the dental arches and esthetic rehabilitation, it is still slightly controversial, and it remains unclear how the bone at these sites develops with continued growth.

Bolton tooth-size discrepancies, usually caused by decreased mesiodistal widths in the maxillary anterior teeth, will also affect space requirements on the opposing jaw as well. These can be corrected in two ways. Small teeth can be made wider by means of composite build-ups

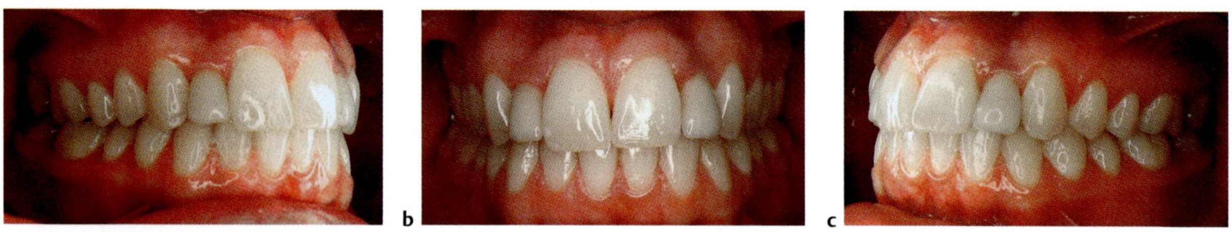

a b c

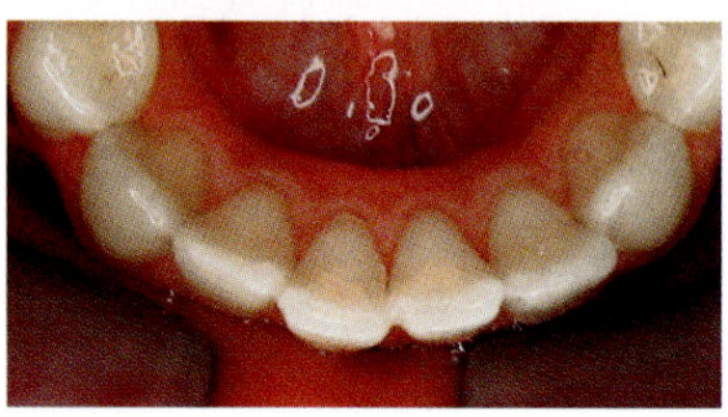

d

Fig. 9.2 a–d Occlusion status 7 years into retention.
a–c The lateral incisors were congenitally missing and were replaced by dental implants after growth had stopped. Up to that point, full-time retention was required with a removable retainer containing pontics. The edentulous sites and hence the implant-supported crowns are slightly narrow in comparison with the mandibular incisors. As a result, the mandibular incisors are slightly retroclinal.
d After a 7-year retention period, slight mandibular incisor contact point slippage becomes apparent. At this point, fixed retention is indicated. The patient was treated with a SOX retainer to correct the minor relapse, followed by fixed retention (see also the section on "Management of Relapse," p. 230).

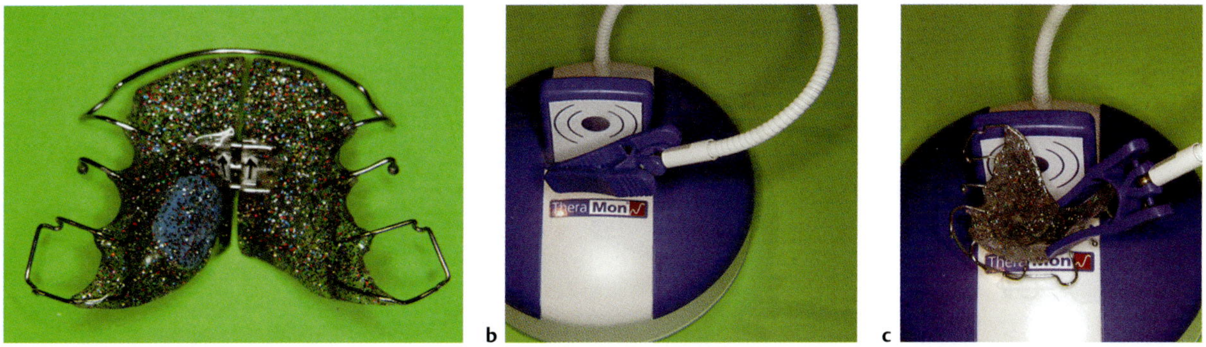

a b c

Fig. 9.3a–c A modified Hawley retainer with a built-in microchip (**a, c**) and reading unit (**b, c**) for downloading data. The microchip is temperature-sensitive and responds to the temperature in the oral cavity. As the device tracks the range of physiological temperature variation in the oral cavity, storing it near a constant heat source as an alternative to wearing it does not work.

or veneers. On the other hand, teeth that are relatively large in comparison with the teeth in the opposing dentition can be reduced in size by interproximal reduction. The decision on which jaw to correct should be based on the size of the discrepancy, esthetics, and tooth shape. For patients in whom the tooth-size discrepancy has not been addressed appropriately, prolonged retention needs to be carefully planned, as there is an increased risk of relapse after active orthodontic treatment, particularly in the arch that has the larger teeth (see the section on "Retention after Correction of Significant Rotations and Severe Crowding," p. 224) (**Fig. 9.2 d**).

Concepts of Retention

A basic distinction is made between retention of limited duration and long-term retention. The definitions relate to the duration of the retention, rather than to the mode of the retention (such as removable or fixed).

Retention Protocol

A general rule of thumb suggests that the duration of retention should be equal to or longer than the duration of active treatment. However, most contemporary orthodontists recommend that for shorter treatment durations in particular, long-term retention is advisable. Long-term retention with removable appliances can be difficult to achieve, however, as it relies heavily on patient compliance. Aids for monitoring the patient's retainer wear have long been sought, and many attempts have been made to enhance or monitor patient compliance. A modern, cost effective option is available in the form of a microchip that is polymerized into the retainer acrylic (TheraMon, **Fig. 9.3**). TheraMon is an abbreviation of "therapeutic monitoring." A thermosensitive microchip records the amount of time spent in the oral cavity. The information can then be read wirelessly and downloaded to a computer.

Relapse Prevention Based on the Original Malocclusion

Although there are no scientific data on the potential for relapse to the original malocclusion, it appears empirically sound to incorporate the pretreatment situation into the design of the retention protocol.

Standard Retainers

Following correction of dental alveolar discrepancies, retention with standard removable appliances, such as a Schwartz plate or Hawley or Van der Linden retainers, is generally sufficient. These retainers allow good settling of the occlusion, as they involve only little interocclusal interference, if any. Settling can be satisfactorily achieved with these appliances while at the same time maintaining the alignment of the labial segments (**Figs. 9.4** and **9.5**).

Case Study 9.1 (Fig. 9.4)

Patient: G.B., female, age 14.
Diagnostic records: models, panoramic radiograph, lateral cephalometric radiograph, intraoral/extraoral photographs.
Main findings: buccally positioned tooth 13 and right-sided unilateral open bite.
Treatment aims: alignment of tooth 13 and establishment of solid occlusion.
Appliances: Self-ligating brackets.
Archwire sequence: 0.012 SE, 0.016 SE, 0.016 × 0.022 SE, 0.018 × 0.025 SE, 0.019 × 0.025 SS.
Alternative treatment strategy: n/a.
Active treatment time: 11 months.
Retention: three-dimensional retention, allowing settling.

1 2 3
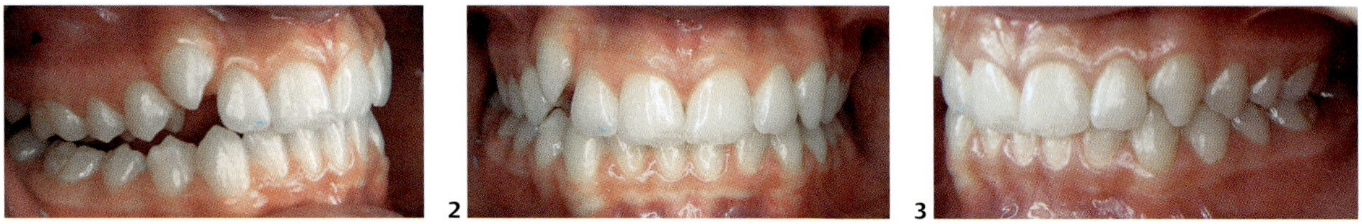

4 5
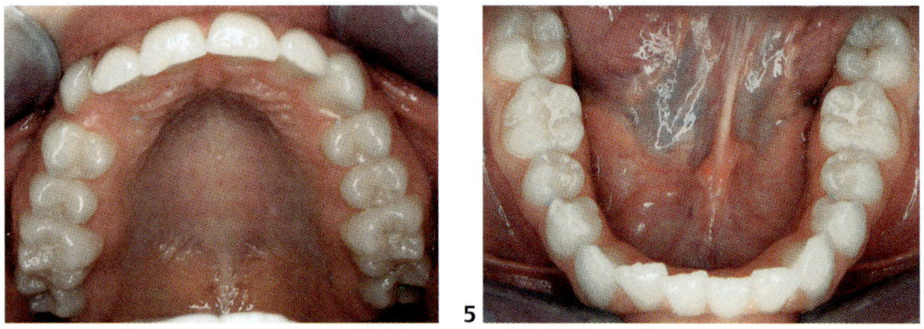

Fig. 9.4 1–24
1–5 The pretreatment situation, with tooth 13 positioned buccally and a right-sided open bite.

6 7 8
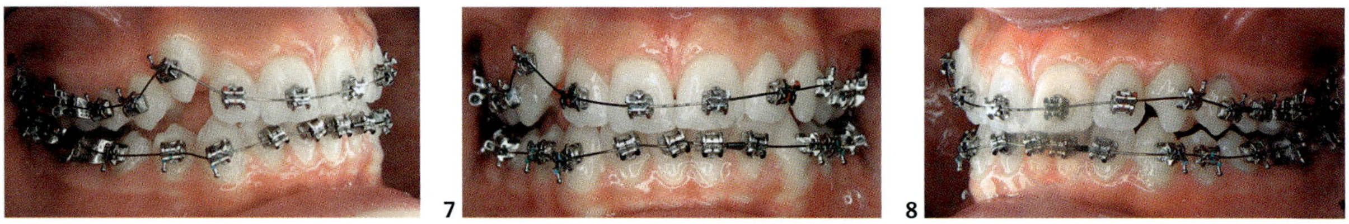

9 10
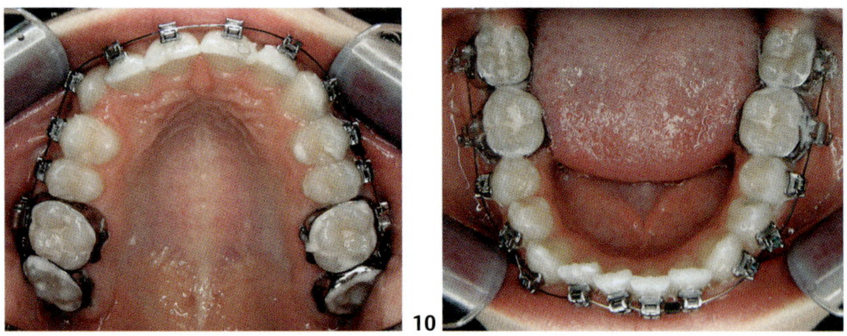

6–10 Self-ligating brackets with full initial 0.012 SE archwire, immediately fully engaged in all brackets.

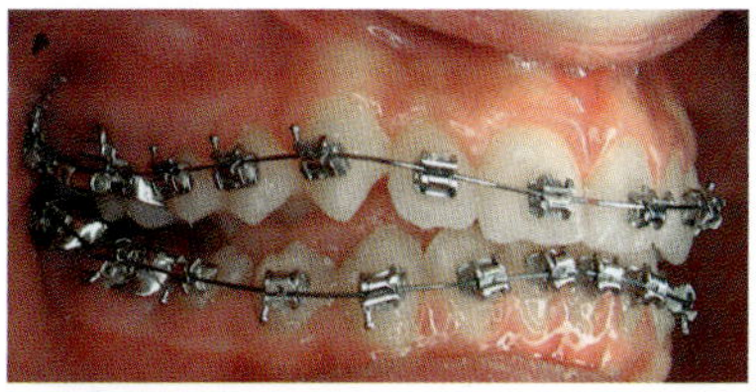
11
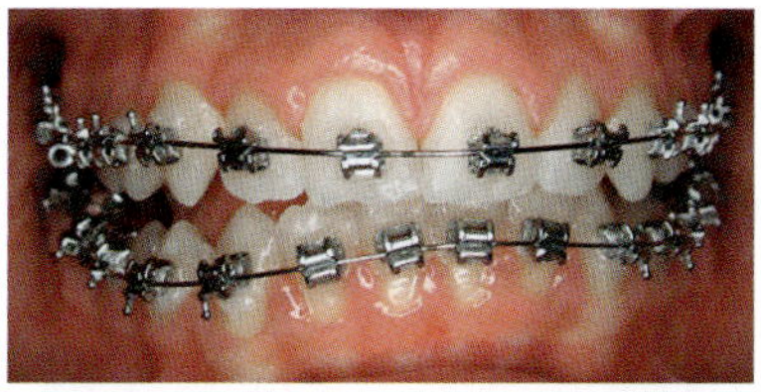
12
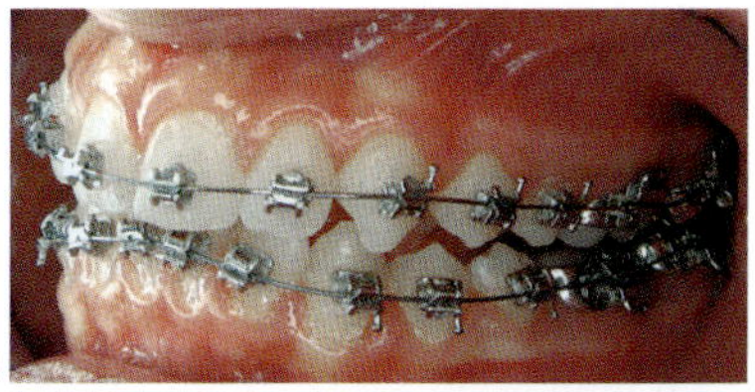
13
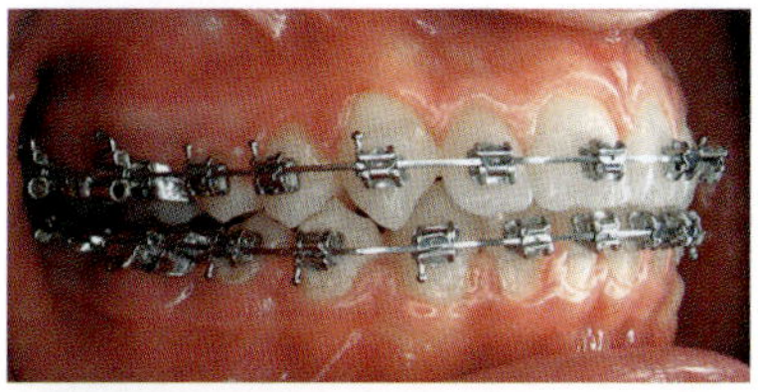
14
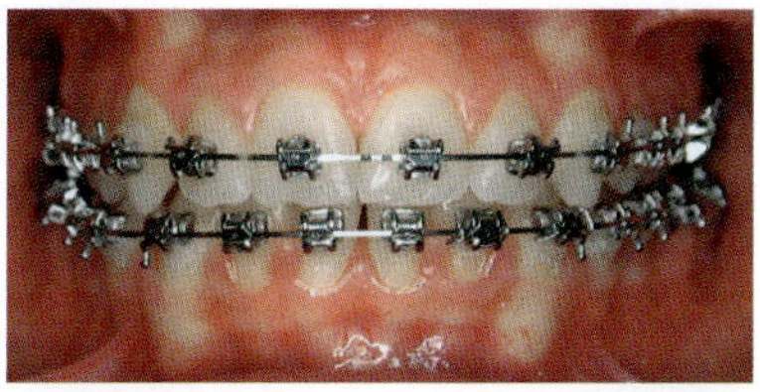
15
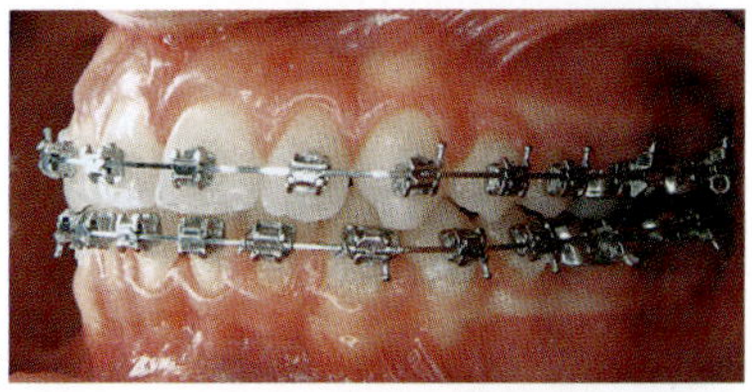
16
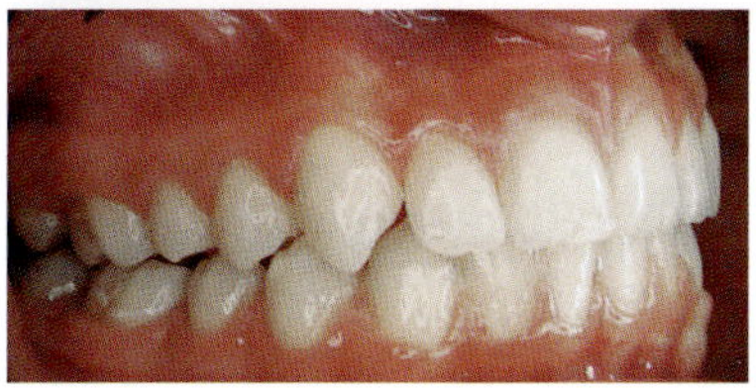
17
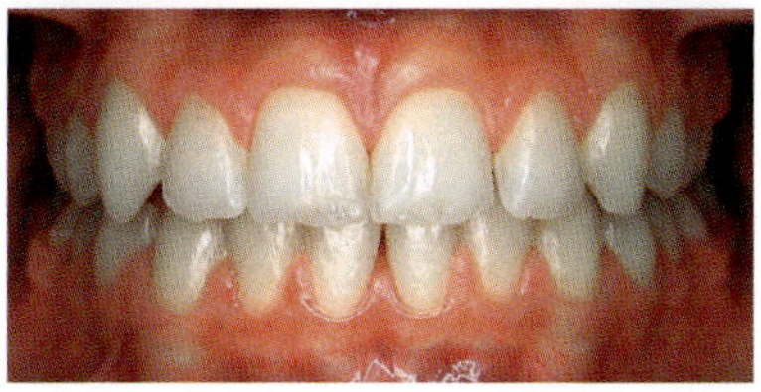
18
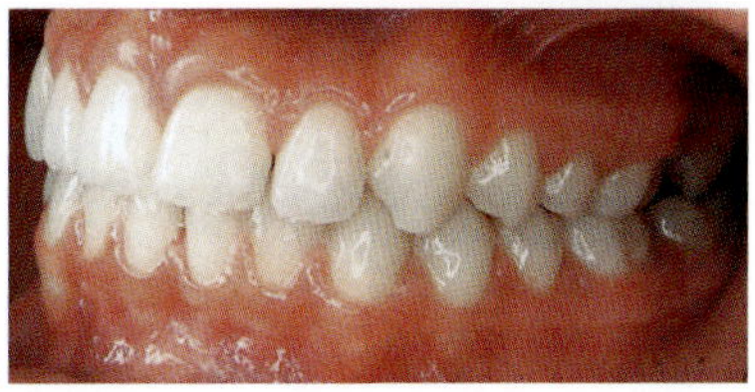
19

11–19 Treatment progress with alignment of tooth 13 (top), subsequent settling of the occlusion (center), and the final result (bottom).

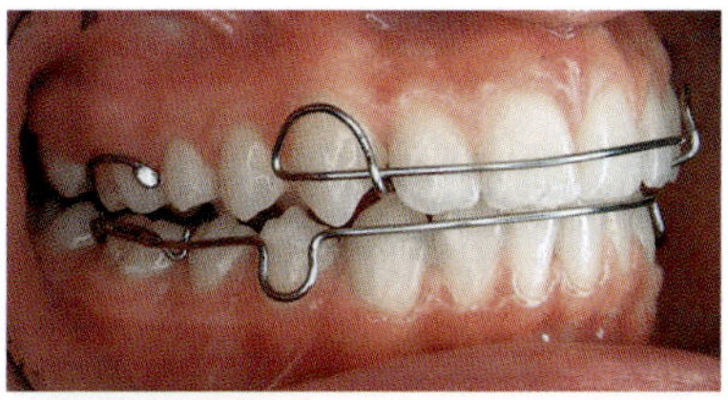
20
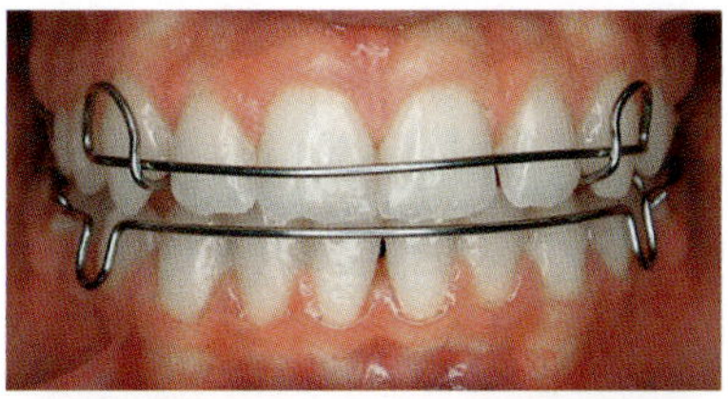
21
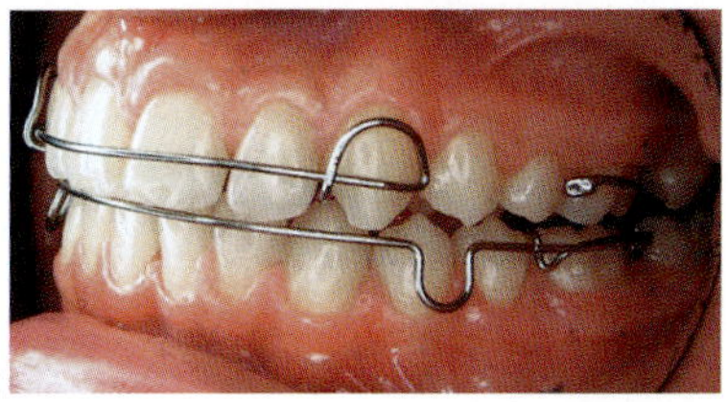
22
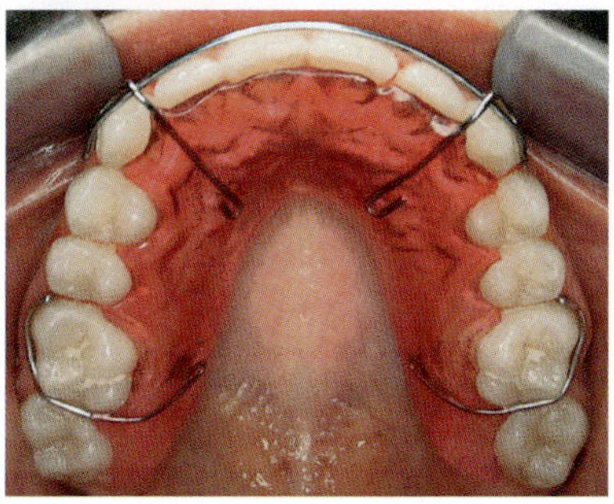
23
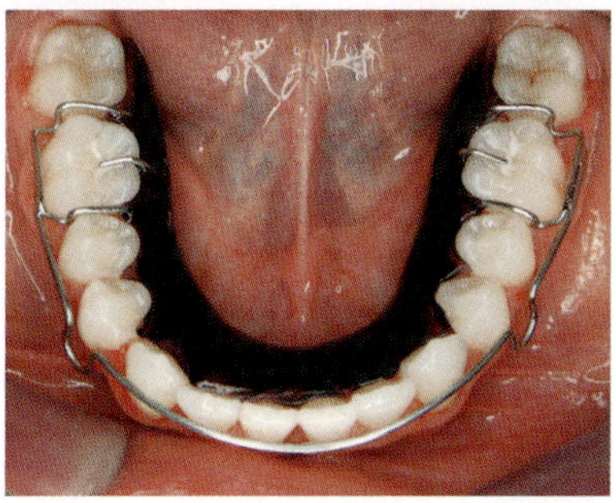
24

20–24 Retention was achieved with a Van der Linden retainer in the maxilla and a modified Hawley retainer in the mandible. The Van der Linden retainer makes it possible to correct the position of the canine during retention if necessary. The residual space in the area of 22 can be closed by activating the labial bow. The appliance is retained by two c-clasps at the first molars. This design allows vertical settling of the occlusion.

The modified Hawley retainer has two Adams clasps on first molars to which the labial bow is soldered. This design shortens the labial bow and makes it more resistant to deformation in comparison to a Begg retainer but yet allowing settling of the posterior occlusion.

Case Study 9.2 (Fig. 9.5)

Patient: J.H., female, age 13.
Diagnostic records: models, panoramic radiograph, lateral cephalometric radiograph, intraoral/extraoral photographs.
Main findings: deep bite and class II tendency with maxillary and mandibular anterior crowding.
Treatment aims: bite opening and alignment.
Appliances: Self-ligating brackets, anterior bite elevators.
Archwire sequence: 0.012 SE, 0.016 SE, 0.016 × 0.022 SE, 0.018 × 0.025 SE, 0.019 × 0.025 SS.
Alternative treatment strategy: n/a.
Active treatment time: 10 months.
Retention: three-dimensional retention with Hawley retainers.

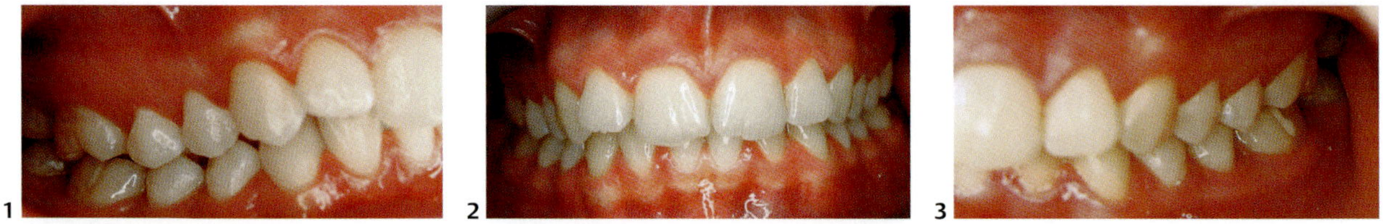

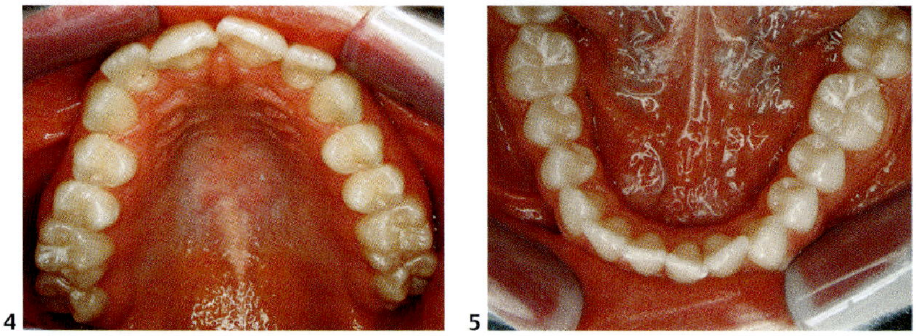

Fig. 9.5 1–23
1–5 The pretreatment situation shows a deep bite with an accentuated curve of Spee. The diagnostic work-up revealed a dentoalveolar cause, with adequate skeletal bases.

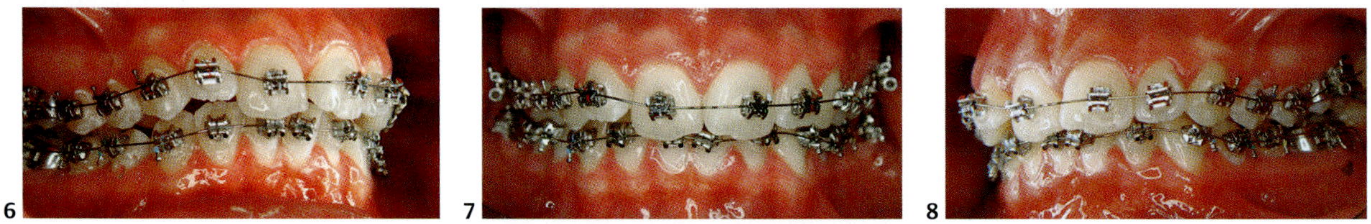

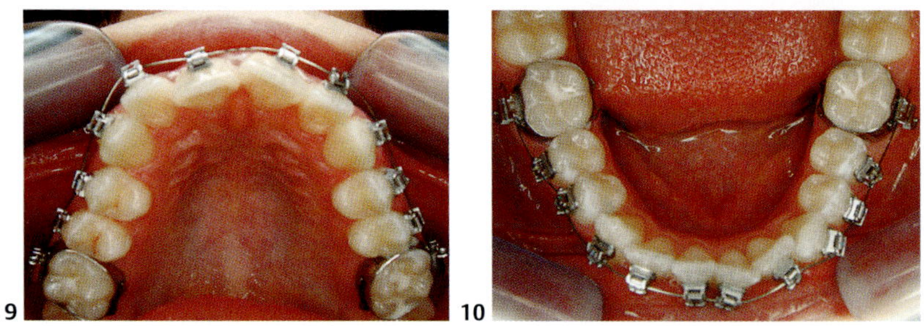

6–10 Self-ligating brackets with a ligated 0.012 SE archwire. The fixed-appliance therapy was supported by anterior bite planes, which allowed for extrusion of buccal segments, and intrusion of incisors. Anteroposterior correction with elastics. The treatment aims were achieved in 10 months.

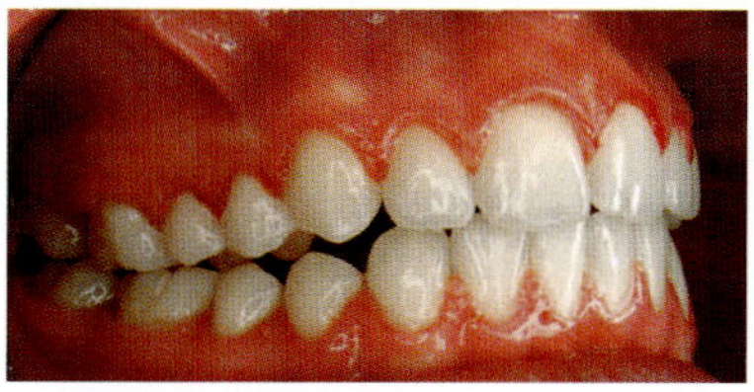
11
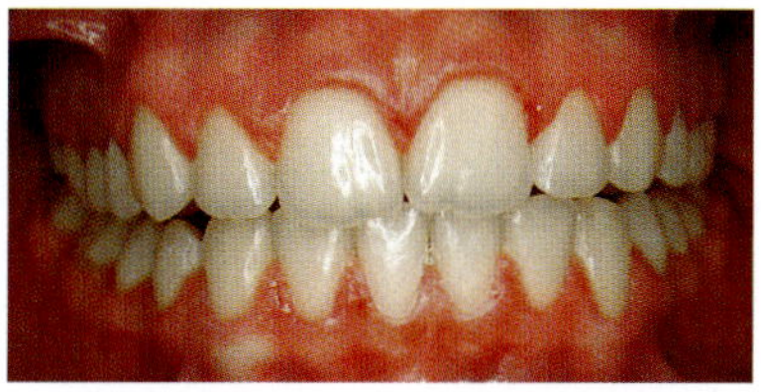
12
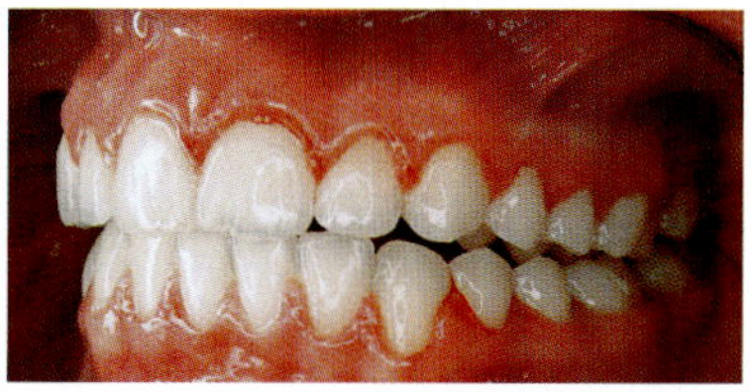
13

11–13 An inadequately settled posterior occlusion became apparent after debonding.

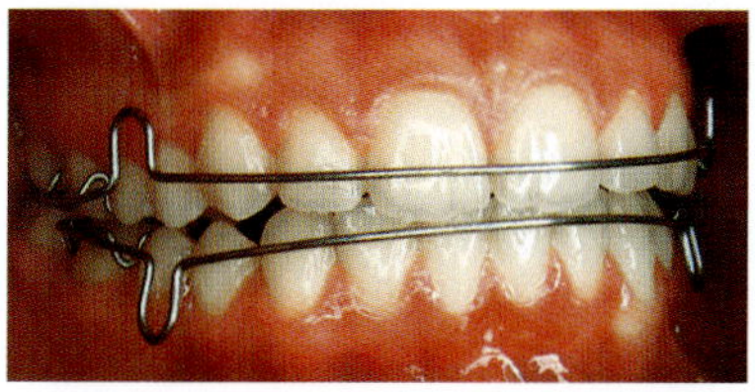
14
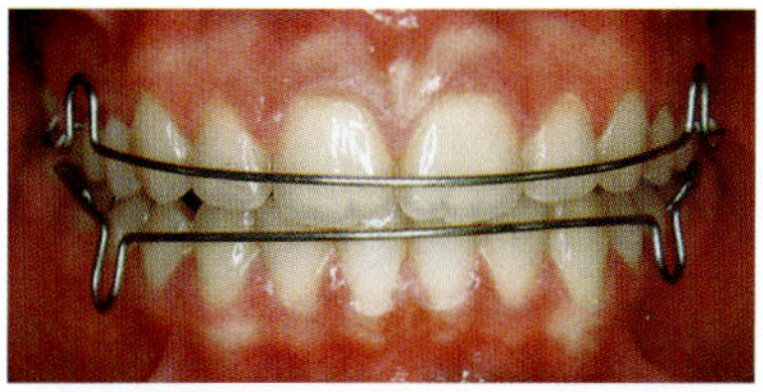
15
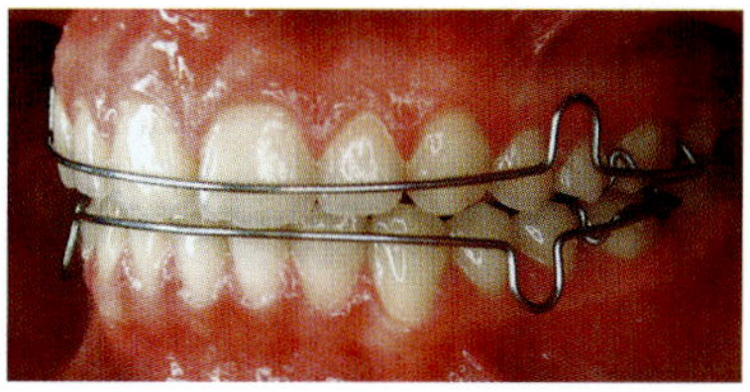
16
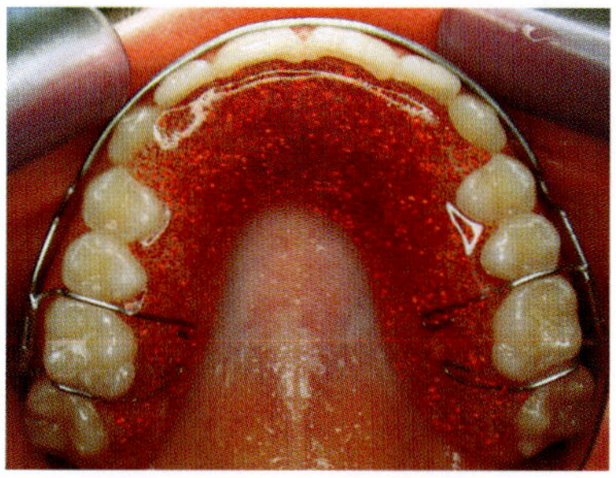
17
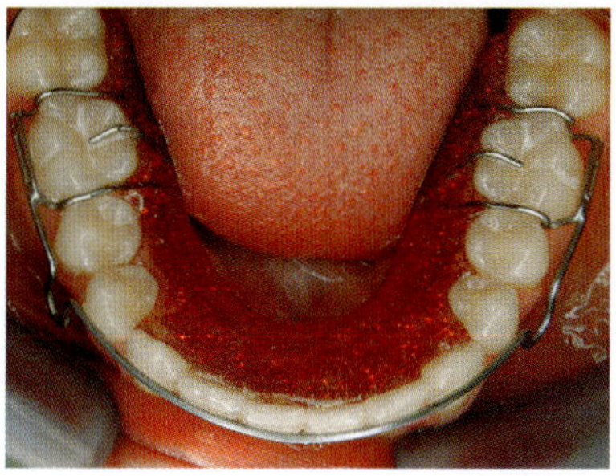
18

14–18 Maxillary and mandibular Hawley retainers were used for retention and to allow settling of the posterior occlusion.

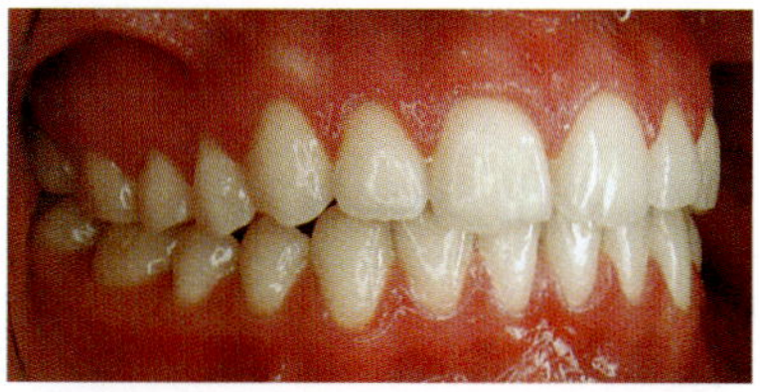
19
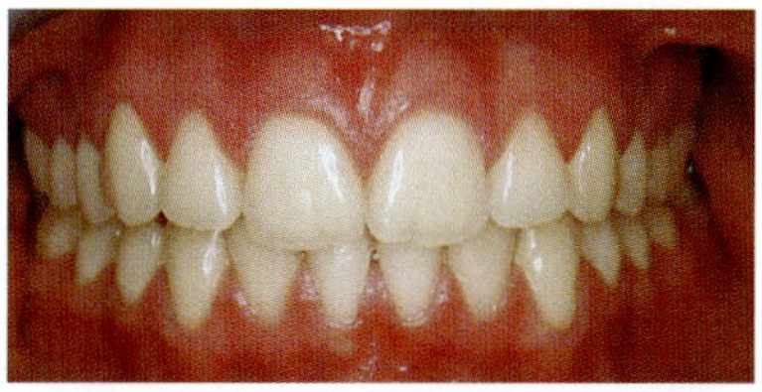
20
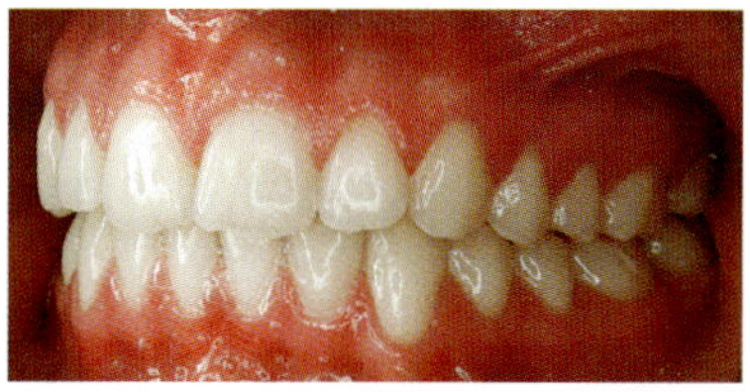
21
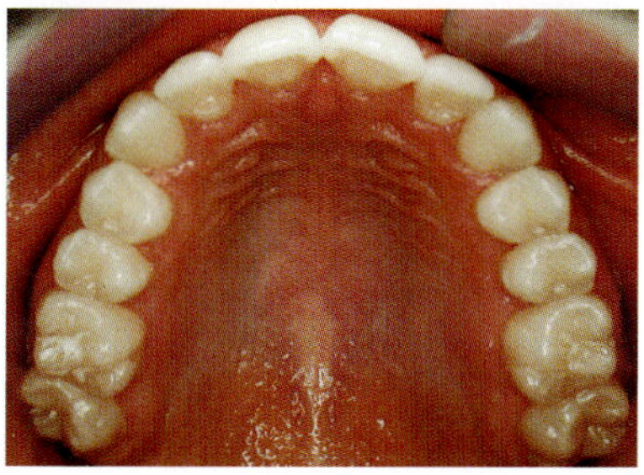
22
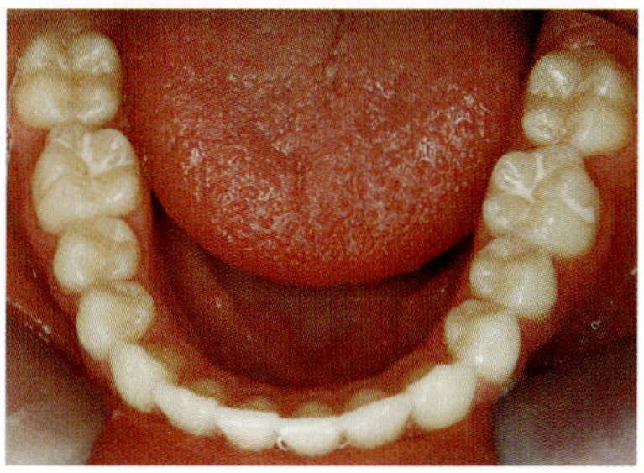
23

19–23 The result after 1 year of retention.

Retention of Transverse Corrections

After transverse corrections (particularly expansion of the upper jaw), a Hawley retainer or Schwartz plate is customarily used for retention. These can be fitted with a partially preexpanded midline screw. If the appliance is not worn for some time, the screw can be contracted, and the plate can be inserted again and then reexpanded to its original size.

Retention of Class II Cases

Orthodontically corrected skeletal discrepancies of the class II type often benefit from long-term retention of the sagittal correction. The present authors prefer to use vacuum-formed retainers fitted with the advancement components of Kinzinger's Functional Mandibular Advancer (FMA) (**Fig. 9.6**).[7,8] The vacuum-formed retainers provide good retention of the alignment of the labial segments while at the same time being rigid and retentive enough to allow forward positioning of the lower jaw. If required, minor tooth movement is possible with these retainers by means of an individual set-up (**Fig. 9.7**).

Retention in Class III Cases

Further developments in patients with a previously corrected class III malocclusion are difficult to anticipate, as the residual growth potential remains unknown. It therefore seems all the more important to achieve a final result with good cusp embrasure and anterior coupling, as a tight occlusal relationship is considered to be the best form of retention for class III patients. Tissue or tooth borne functional appliances (such as Fränkel III, 'Reverse Twin Block' and 'Reverse Double Plate' respectively) should also be considered for retention of treated class III malocclusions.

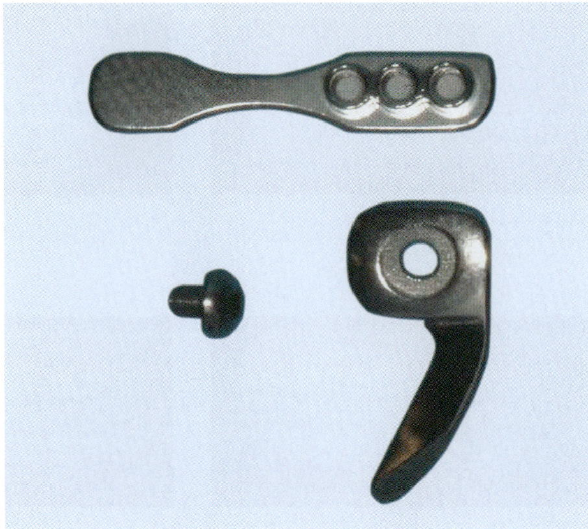

a

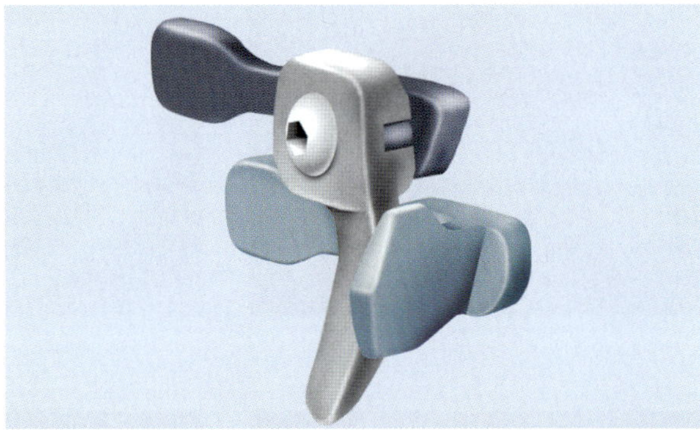

b

Fig. 9.6a, b Components of Kinzinger's Functional Mandibular Advancer (FMA). The guiding rods can be attached to the support bar with an Allen screw in three different positions. The appliance is fabricated to a protrusive wax bite with the guiding rods in the most distal position, allowing later activation by moving them mesially.

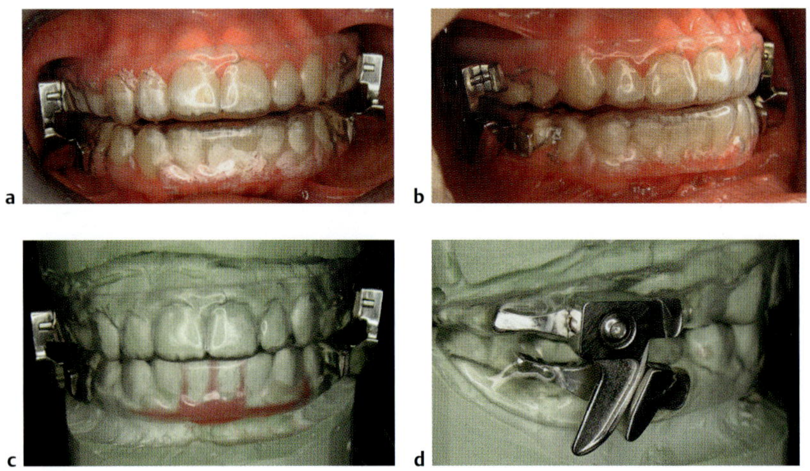

Fig. 9.7a–d Functional Mandibular Advancer splints in an overcorrected position. The working models shows the guiding mechanism of the appliance and an integrated set-up for the mandibular incisors. Simple removal of the guiding rods by unscrewing the fixtures allows for follow-up of the stability of the class II correction.

Retention after Treatment for Deep Bites

Patients who present with deep bites can benefit from long-term maintenance and retention of the corrected vertical components of their malocclusion. This can be done with a Hawley-type retainer with an anterior bite plane incorporated into it. This can be combined with fixed retention of the labial segments.

Retention after Treatment for Anterior Open Bites

Orthodontically treated anterior open bites are often challenging to maintain over the longer term. The ideal would be to have retention systems that do not depend on patient compliance. If the anterior open bite is associated with an anterior tongue thrust, we recommend fitting fixed spikes to the palatal surface of the upper incisors (**Fig. 9.8**). This strategy is associated with some patient discomfort, particularly initially. However, the spikes are usually tolerated well after the initial phase.

In addition, it is advisable to plan for myofunctional therapy in cases with lip incompetence due to hypotonic perioral muscles (**Fig. 9.9**).

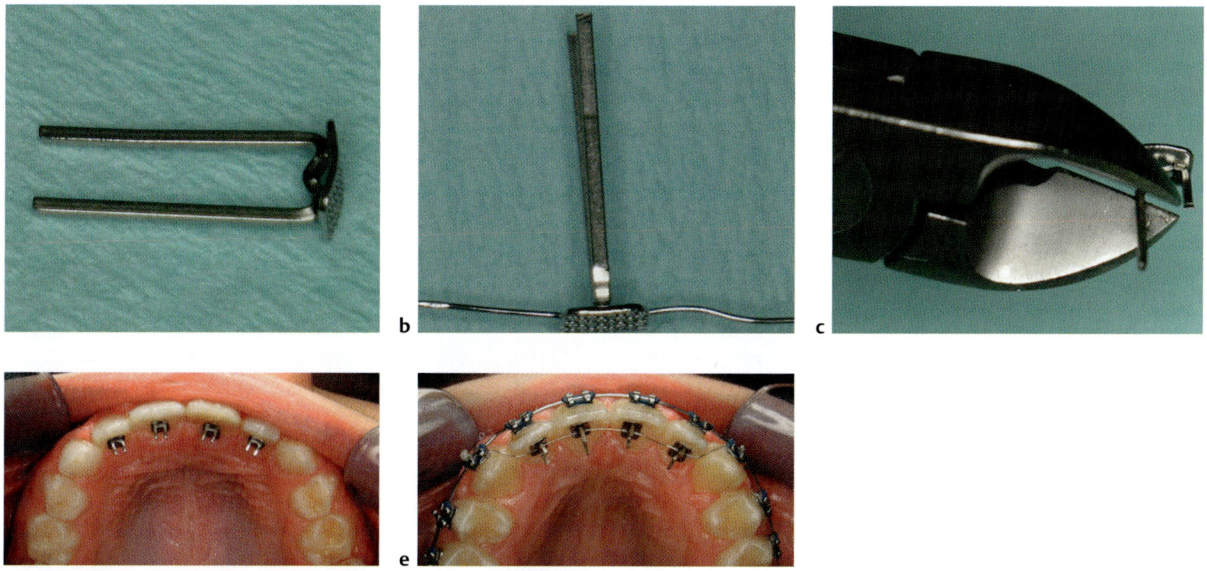

a b c d e

Fig. 9.8a–e Direct bonding of palatal spikes.
a–c Prefabricated spikes with an eyelet for attaching a ligature wire to prevent aspiration (PhD C. Sander). The length of the spikes is reduced as needed with a hard wire cutter.
d, e The spikes in place. The ligature wire is threaded through the eyelets and secured laterally to the brackets or bonded to the tooth surface.

CLINICAL PEARL

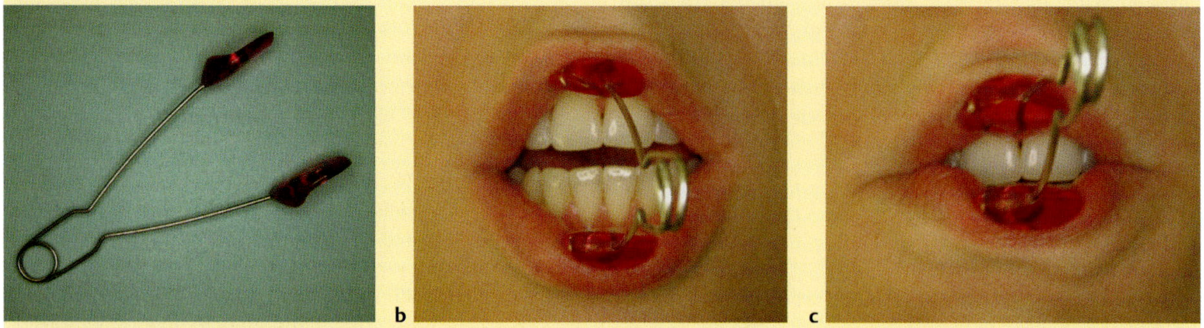

Fig. 9.9a–c Anterior open bites may be due to insufficient muscle activity of the lips.
a The lip position can be trained using the Dass lip activator.
b, c First application of the appliance in this patient. Compressing the spring requires considerable force (as the lip strain visible in **c** shows).

Retention after Correction of Significant Rotations and Severe Crowding

Retention, particularly in the lower anterior segment, is extremely important, especially in patients who present with severe crowding and rotations at the outset of treatment. Movement of the lower anterior teeth occurs naturally throughout life, independently of any previous orthodontic treatment, and is regarded as physiological. Minor changes in lower incisor alignment are therefore no longer regarded as relapse, but rather as normal occurrences.[6,23]

However, patients tend to expect and require stability for the lower front teeth following orthodontic treatment. Fixed retention may therefore best address the patient's wish to have a stable long-term result,[1] and it is the method of choice for most contemporary orthodontists. A variety of fixed retainers are available today. The main difference between retainers is whether only the canines are fixed to a rigid bar, or whether a wire or chain is attached to all six front teeth. Within these two major designs, there are a number of permutations.[19,22,26–28] No relevant side effects have been reported in the literature as long as adequate hygiene and regular recall intervals with the orthodontist are maintained. It is worth noting that poor oral hygiene of fixed retainers is associated with a higher incidence of recession of the front teeth. The claim that fixed retention as such may damage the periodontal ligament has been disproved.[21,25] The mobility of individual teeth is somewhat reduced, but it is still within the functional physiological limits for a healthy periodontium (**Fig. 9.11**).

CLINICAL PEARL

Retention of the labial segments using fixed retainers is a contemporary strategy for maintaining the alignment of the front teeth. It is important to remember that these retainers are likely to break at some stage, and this is often due to either abrasion of the adhesive (**Fig. 9.10**) or fracture of the wire.[2,19,22,24] Patients need to be advised accordingly before these retainers are fitted. In our practice, we generally combine fixed retention with removable retention; the latter provides some additional back-up if fixed retention fails.

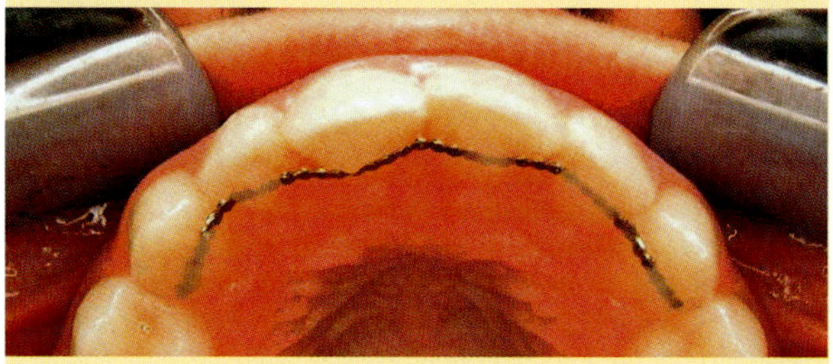

Fig. 9.10 A six-point bonded retainer, with a defect in the wire fixation on tooth 11.

Table 9.1 lists a selection of the various techniques and materials available for fixed retention.

Table 9.1 Procedures and materials for fixed retainers

Design	Manufacturer	Advantages	Disadvantages	Clinical application
Two-point retainers				
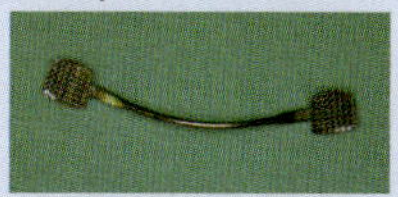 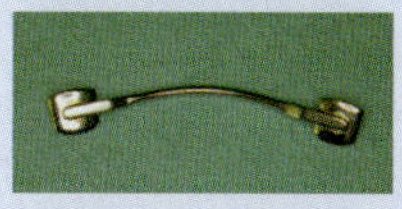	Available prefabricated in different sizes	• Quick installation • No laboratory procedure	• Size selection • Adaptation to the lingual arch shape required • Only limited application in the maxilla (due to thickness of the wire) • Plaster cast required for precise adaptation	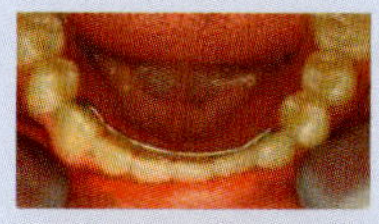 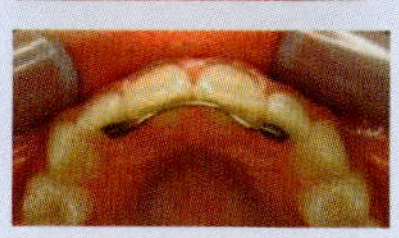
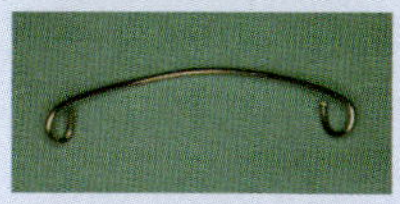	Custom-bent Blue Elgiloy wire (0.032"–0.036")	• Custom adaptation • No laboratory procedure	• Adaptation to the lingual arch shape required • Only limited application in the maxilla • Plaster cast required for precise adaptation	
Six-point retainers				
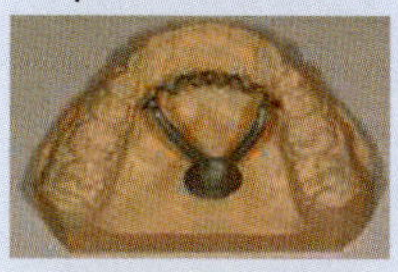	Laboratory-made retainer, cast from titanium[12]	• Exact fit through custom molding	• Complex laboratory procedure • Increases costs	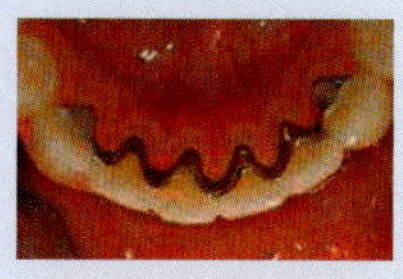
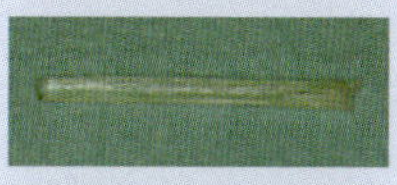 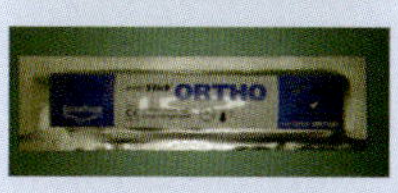	Glass fiber everStick Ortho[16]	• Translucent and esthetic • Direct bonding • Esthetic temporary splinting an option for spaced, periodontally compromised teeth	• Photosensitive during processing • Failure of the composite structure possible • Fiber fractures → semi-permanent retention • Difficult to clean	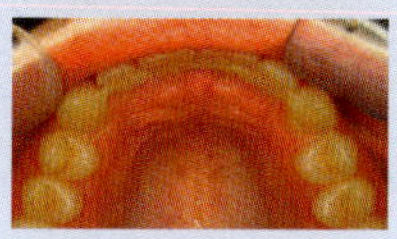
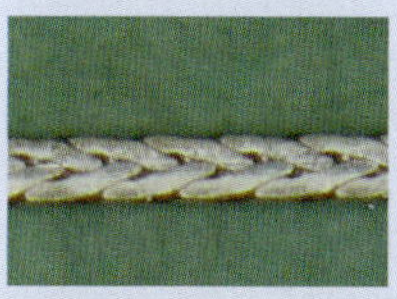	Bond-a-Braid (Reliance Orthodontic Products) eight-stranded braided band designed by Hilgers	• Simple adaptation due to moldable quality • No laboratory procedures • Rectangular shape for 3 D control	• Working model recommended	
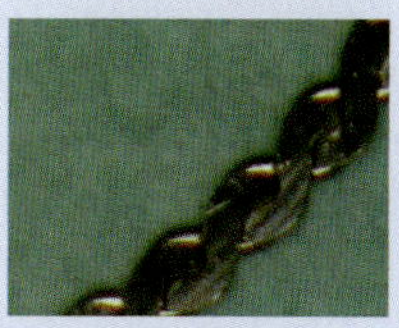	Ortho-FlexTech (Reliance Orthodontic Products), made of white gold alloy 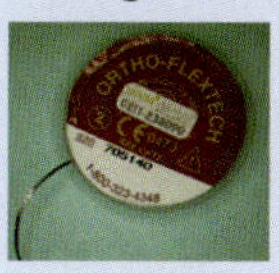	• Flexible braided chain • Direct intraoral bonding • No laboratory procedure • No models required	• Flexibility	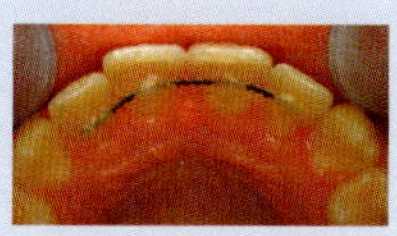
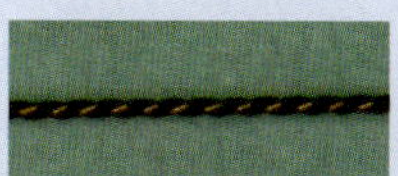 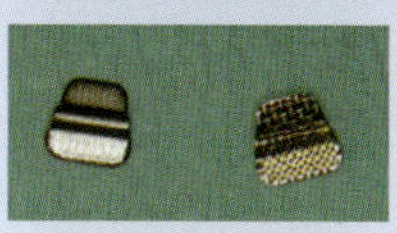 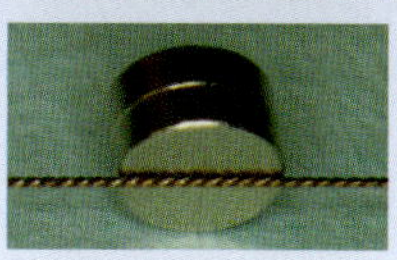	Six-stranded braided wire with pad fixation 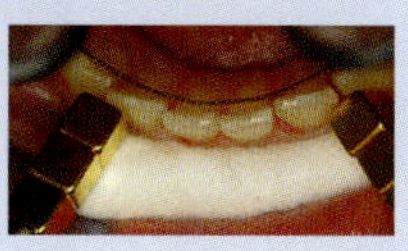	• Simple adaptation due to moldable quality • No laboratory procedures • Can be used with pads • Magnetic	• Coarse surface and structure	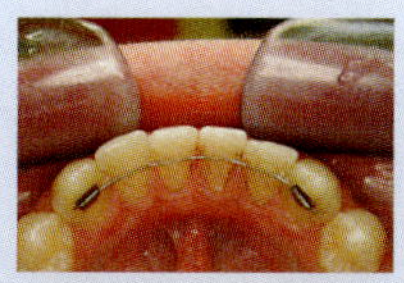 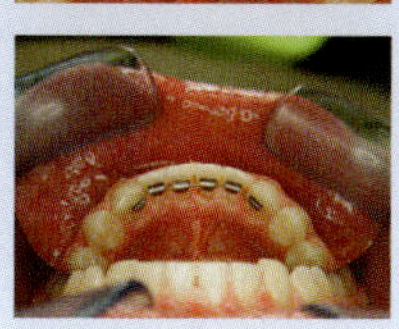

CLINICAL PEARL

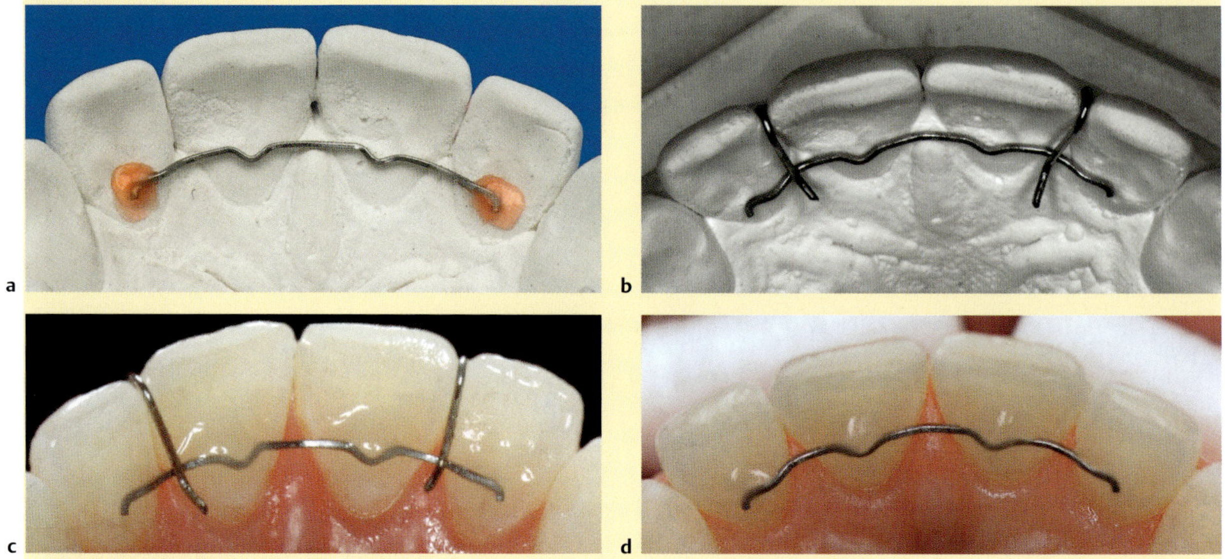

Fig. 9.11 a–d Fabrication of the retainer.
a The 0.016 × 0.016 inch stainless steel wire with optional v-bends. The areas to be bonded are sandblasted.
b Two s-shaped auxiliary hooks are welded interdentally to facilitate repositioning.
c Note the close-fitting devolution of the wire.
d This set-up facilitates bonding the stiff wire with the required passivity. (Method acc. to the protocol of the Univ. of Zurich, case report by Raphael Patcas)

The Spaced Dentition

In patients with missing teeth (congenitally or otherwise) orthodontic space management requires spaces of adequate size for dental restorations unless space closure is planned. Ample space at the root level and root parallelism are also required if the aim is to restore the edentulous sites with dental implants. Implants are generally not placed until skeletal growth has ceased, as these do not follow the growth of the facial skeleton. This means that the spaces have to be retained until implants can be inserted. Retention can be achieved in a variety of ways. Traditionally, removable appliances are used, but these require good compliance and tolerance. Particularly when anterior teeth are missing, removable retainers with pontics providing adequate esthetic results, but they cannot be worn during meal times and reveal the unrestored edentulous site. Recent developments and improvements in resin composites now make it possible to use techniques that no longer require wear of bulky appliances such as Hawley retainers that incorporate missing teeth. In our practice, we often use temporary adhesive bridges, which are made of composite (**Fig. 9.12**). The result is esthetically pleasing, but the application is costly and involves considerable chairside time. It is also important to remember that atrophy of the underlying bone will occur during the retention period.

Cortical anchorage for restoration of an edentulous site is another option in the anterior segment. This requires vertical insertion of an orthodontic mini-implant into the alveolar process, similar to a dental implant. The head of the implant is subsequently used as an abutment for the prosthetic replacement of the lateral incisor. It is important to remember that these teeth should not be in functional occlusion with the opposing arch, as mini-implants are not designed to withstand occlusal loads over prolonged periods of time (**Fig. 9.13**). This type of restoration provides very good esthetic results while at

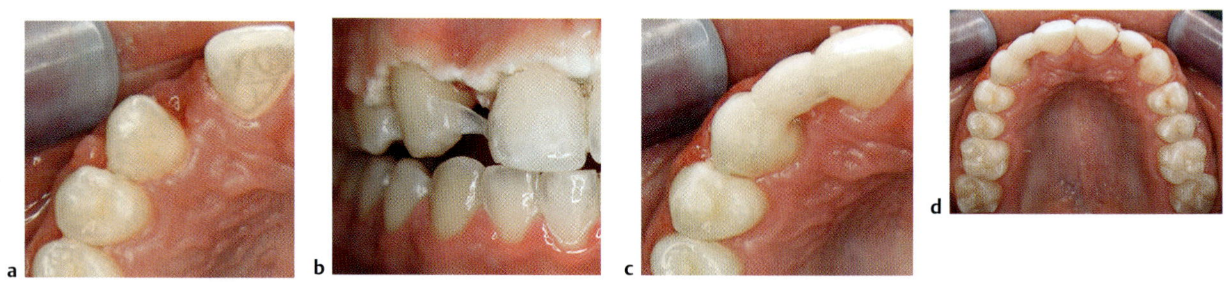

Fig. 9.12 a–d Chairside restoration of the edentulous site using a glass-fiber splint (everStick Ortho) and subsequent addition of composite.

Case Study 9.3 (Fig. 9.13)

Patient: S.S., male, age 15.
Diagnostic records: models, panoramic radiograph, lateral cephalometric radiograph, intraoral/extraoral photographs.
Main findings: hypoplastic maxilla, prognathic mandible, congenitally missing teeth 12 and 22, with maxillary and mandibular crowding.
Treatment aims: maxillary transverse development, archwire coordination, open spaces for restorations of missing teeth 12 and 22.
Appliances: Self-ligating brackets, hybrid rapid palatal expansion (RPE; see Chapter 8), temporary restoration of spaces 12 and 22.
Archwire sequence: 0.012 SE, 0.016 SE, 0.016 × 0.022 SE, 0.018 × 0.025 SE, 0.019 × 0.025 SS.
Alternative treatment strategy: traditional RPE or orthognathic surgery in adulthood.
Active treatment time: 14 months.
Retention: three-dimensional retention with a Hawley retainer, leaving temporary restorations in place until definitive implant replacement of teeth 12 and 22.

1 2 3
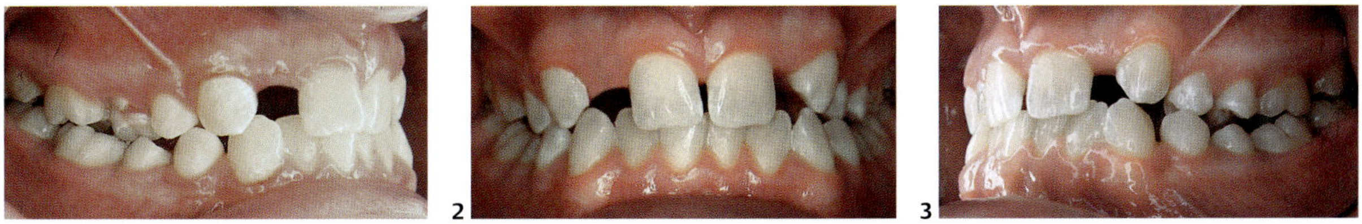

Fig. 9.13 1–18
1–3 The initial situation. Due to the underdeveloped maxilla and mandibular prognathism, canine substitution for the missing lateral incisors was not an option. The treatment plan consisted of maxillary transverse development and temporary restoration of the edentulous sites.

4 5 6 7 8 9
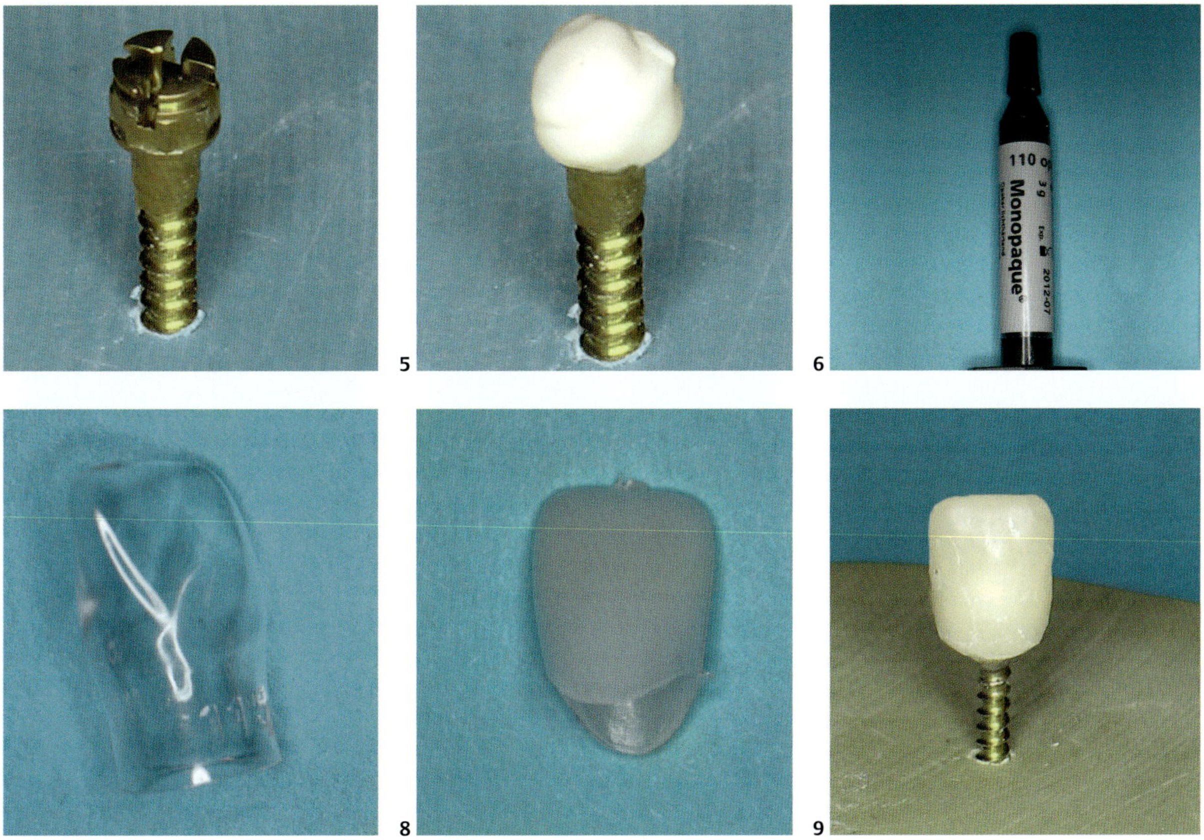

4–9 Miniscrew implants can retain temporary crowns and help to restore an edentulous site quickly and predictably. The crown length of a maxillary lateral incisor is on average 8.6 mm. To avoid unfavorable loads, screws at least 10 mm long are required. After insertion, the implant head is covered with opaque composite. Using templates (e.g., Frasaco crowns) allows quick fabrication of the crown by filling the template with composite, positioning it on the implant head, and light-curing it. Excess material needs to be removed, and the transition to the gingiva has to be contoured to allow for good oral hygiene and prevent soft-tissue irritation. The crown should be adjusted to have no static or functional occlusal contacts, to avoid loosening of the miniscrew implant.

10
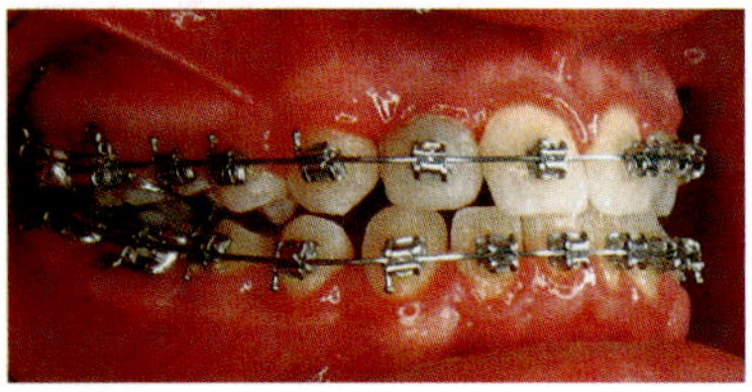
11
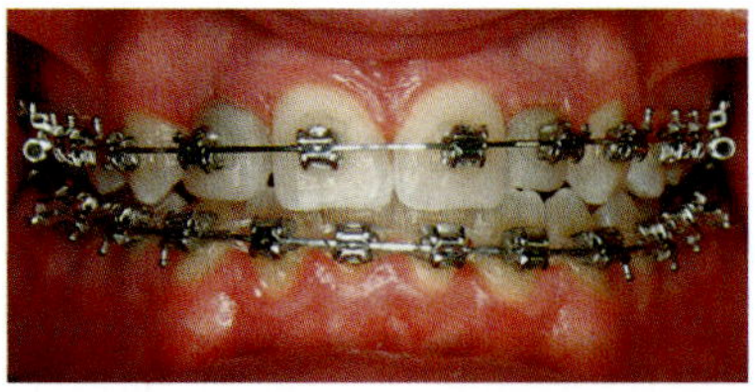
12
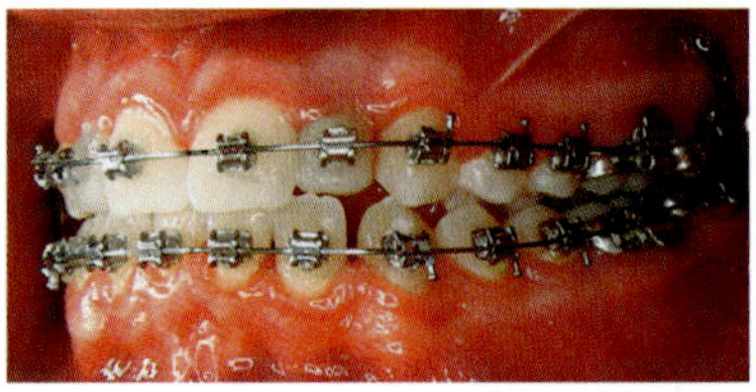

10–12 The miniscrew implants were already inserted during the active treatment phase and used as anchorage for space management. As the space grows larger, composite can be added to the crown to maintain contacts and the esthetic appearance.

NOTE

During the active phase of tooth movement, inserting a mini-implant requires at least 3.6 mm of interradicular space. The mini-implant diameter should be at least 1.6 mm, and the circumferential bone thickness should be no less than 1 mm.

13
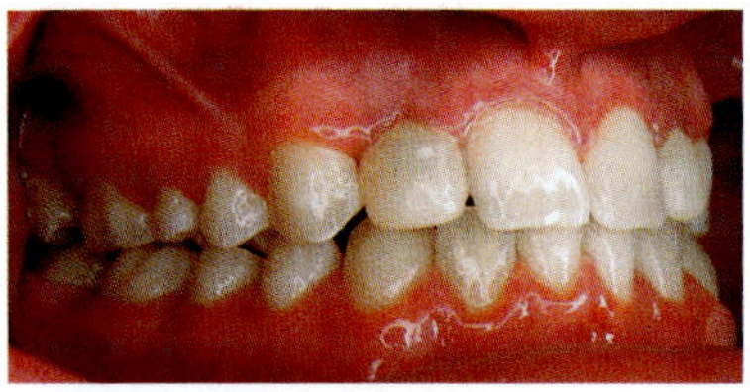
14
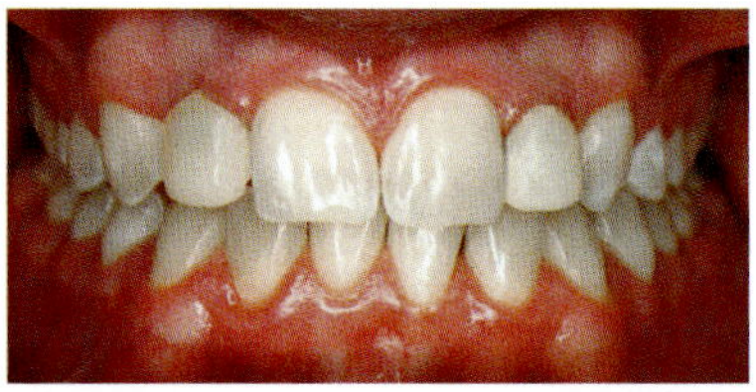
15
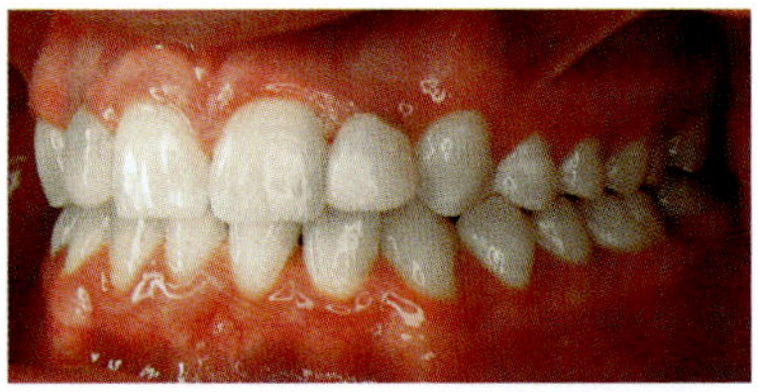
16
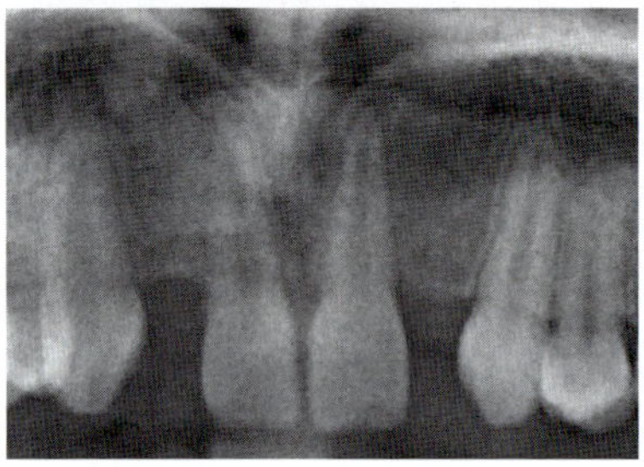
17
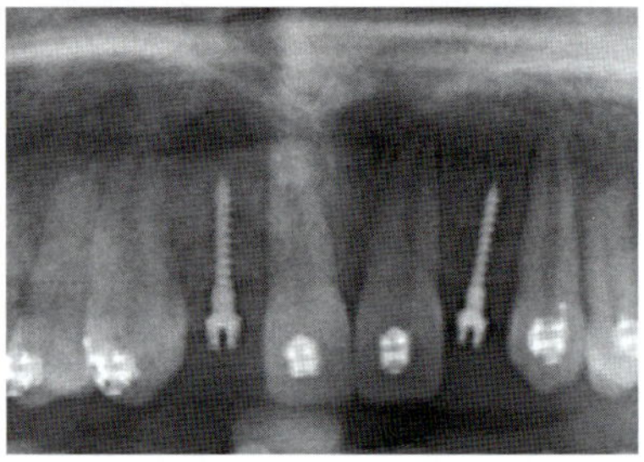
18
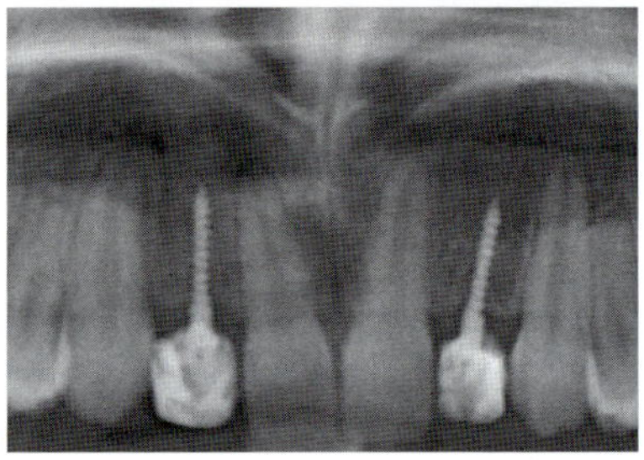

13–18 The situation after 1 year of retention. The miniscrew implants are stable and the crowns have been replaced for long-term esthetic retention of the edentulous sites. After cessation of growth, the implants will be removed and replaced with permanent dental implants and restorations.

CLINICAL PEARL

Mini-Implant versus Adhesive Bridge

Inserting mini-implants may be able to prevent atrophy of alveolar bone in the buccal–lingual direction, which is often associated with the use of adhesive bridges. This is most likely to be due to the physiological load that mini-implants transmit to the surrounding alveolar bone.

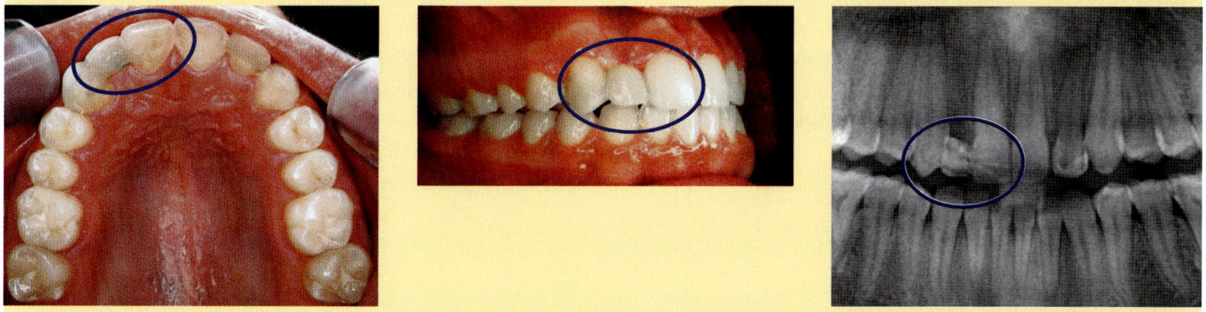

Fig. 9.14 A bonded temporary bridge. In this case, a bonded glass-fiber framework and an individually molded crown were used to restore the edentulous site. While a resin-bonded bridge meets both functional and esthetic requirements, it does not affect the bone of the alveolar process that will later retain the definitive implant.

ERRORS AND RISKS

The inclination of the adjacent teeth needs to be carefully considered before the mini-implant is inserted; the insertion direction should ideally be parallel to the adjacent teeth. Panoramic and lateral cephalometric views can be used as guides (**Fig. 9.15**).

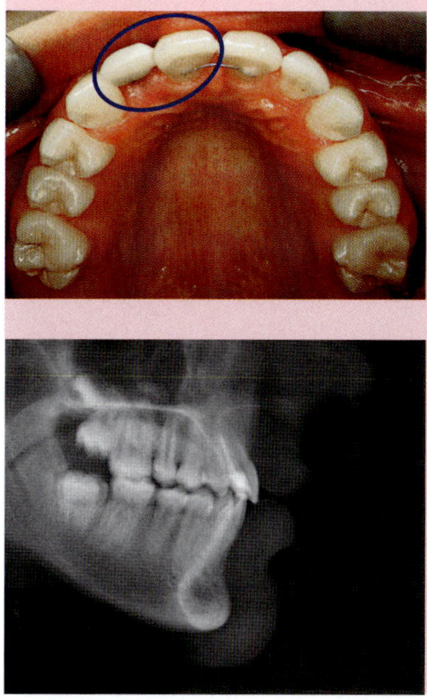

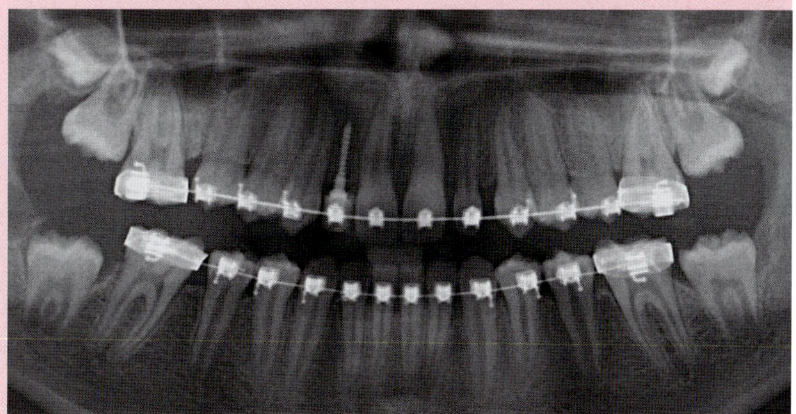

Fig. 9.15 Comparison of implant versus incisor angulation in the lateral cephalometric and panoramic projections.

the same time offering the advantage of potentially reducing or preventing buccal–lingual bone loss at the edentulous site.[5] There is some uncertainty regarding the effect of this mini-implant on the vertical development of the alveolar process in particular. The implant cannot “go along for the ride”—the alveolar process and the periodontal ligament of the teeth drive the vertical development of the alveolus, which is missing at the edentulous site. Whether this technique causes a significant vertical defect or whether it is comparable to having a normal edentulous site remains to be established. It is a relatively new technique and long-term results need to be evaluated yet. When skeletal growth has stopped, the mini-implants are removed and the patient is referred for permanent dental implant placement.

Management of Relapse

Interproximal Enamel Reduction (Stripping)

Irregularity or mild crowding of the lower incisors can be treated with interproximal reduction (IPR) of the enamel, also known as "stripping" (see Chapter 7). The underlying assumption is that the teeth can align once enough space has been created. This does not work reliably when the teeth to be aligned are rotated. The following technique should be considered as an adjunct.

Case Study 9.4 (Fig. 9.16)

Patient: J.Z., female, age 16.
Diagnostic records: models, panoramic radiograph, lateral cephalometric radiograph, intraoral/extraoral photographs.
Main findings: class I occlusion with anterior misalignment.
Treatment aims: alignment.
Appliances: set-up trays, IPR.
Alternative treatment strategy: multiple-bracket appliance.
Active treatment time: 9 months, with three set-up trays.
Retention: fixed retention.

1 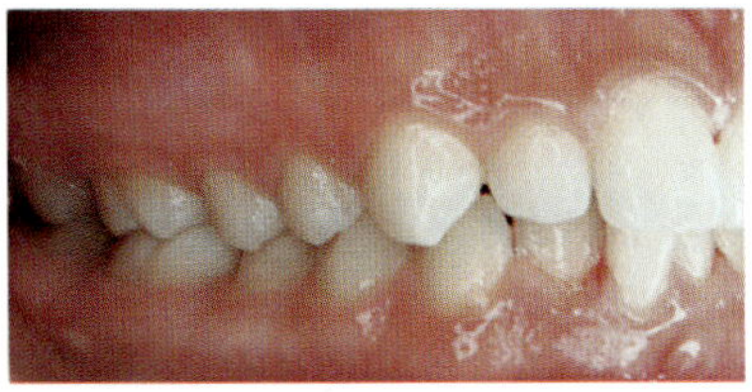
2 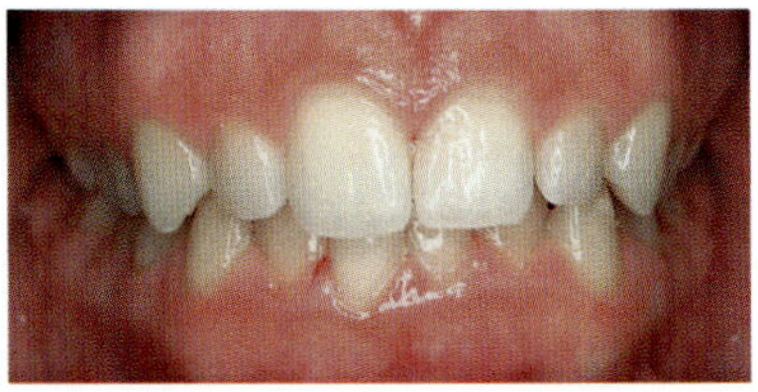
3 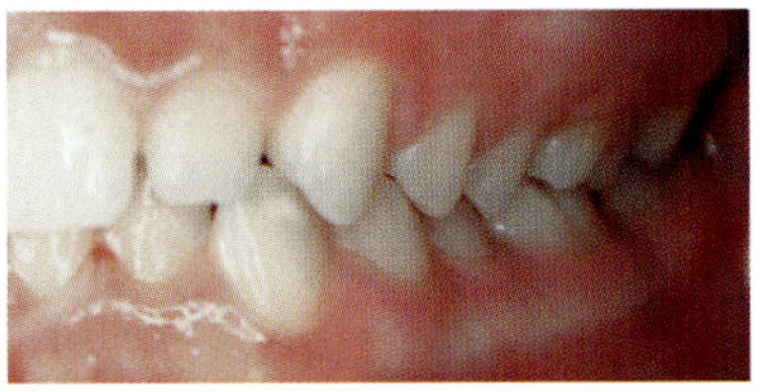
4 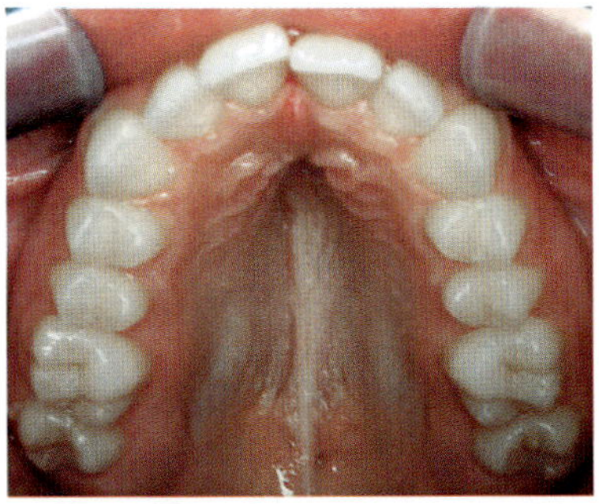
5 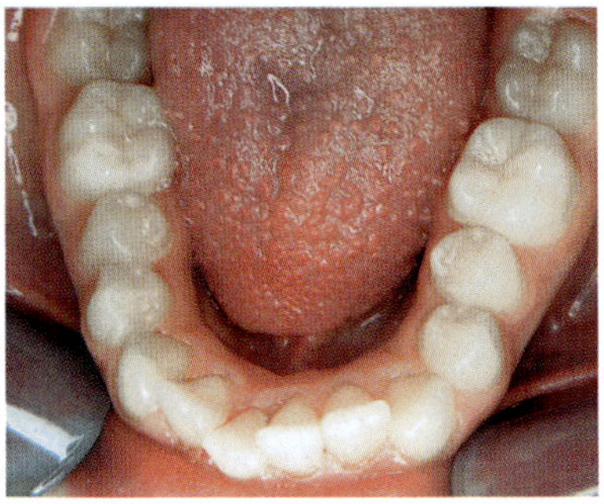

Fig. 9.16 1–15
1–5 The patient requested improved anterior alignment.

6 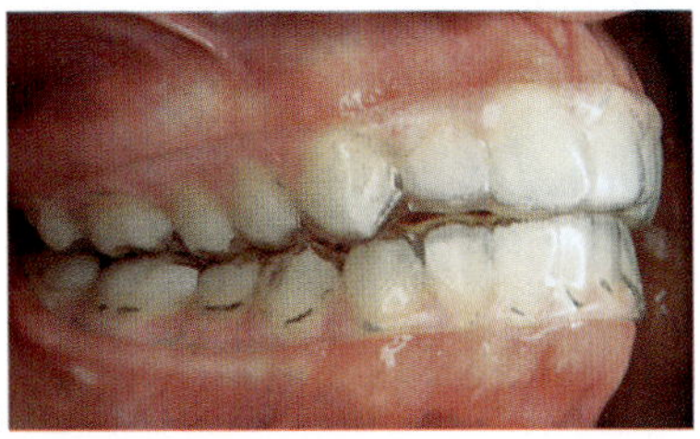
7 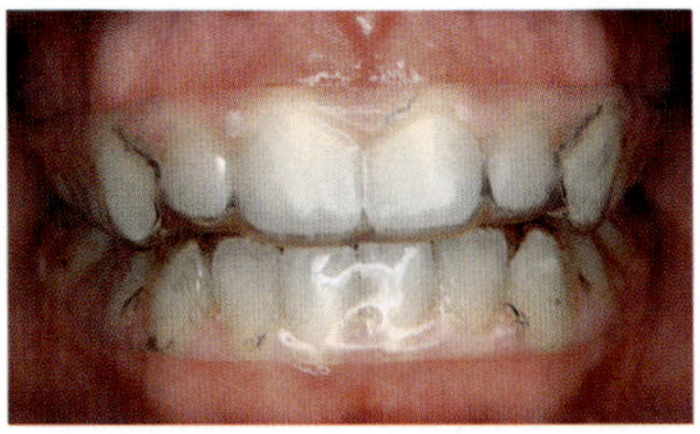
8 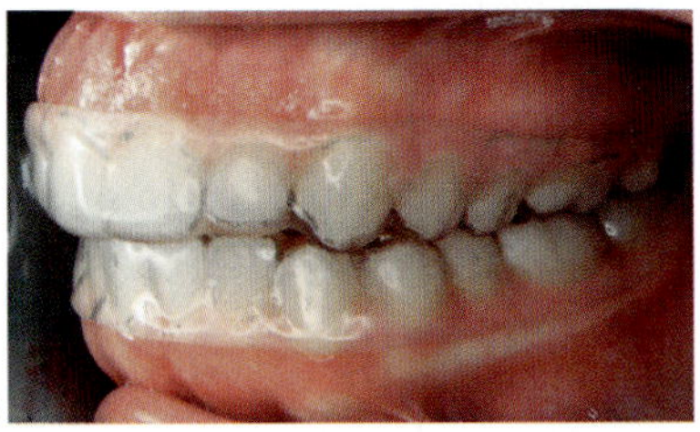
9 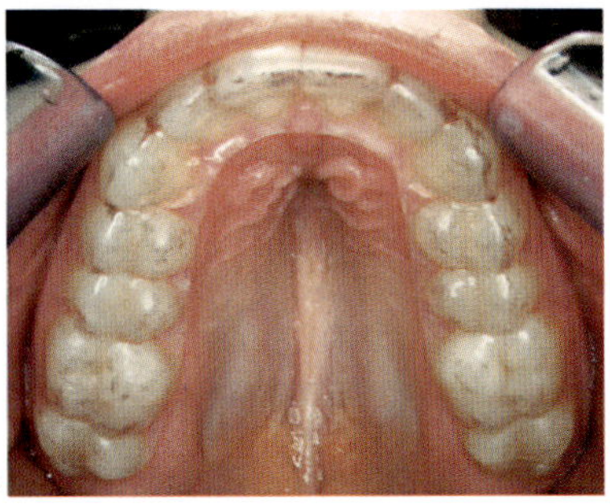
10 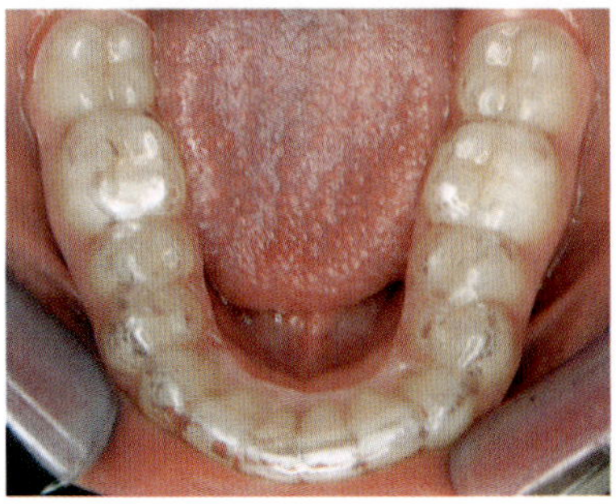

6–10 Stepwise IPR; the second set-up tray is in place.

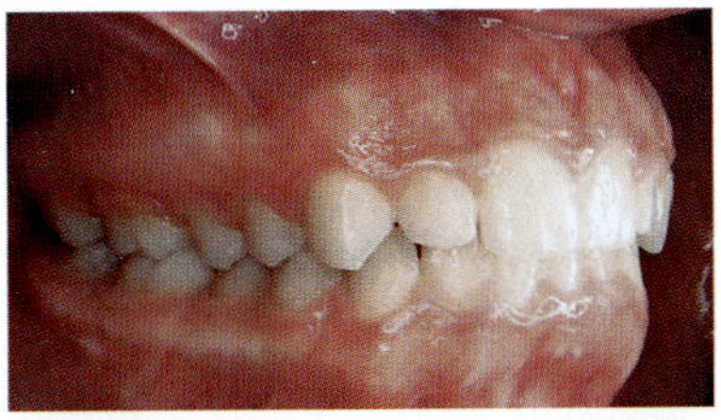
11

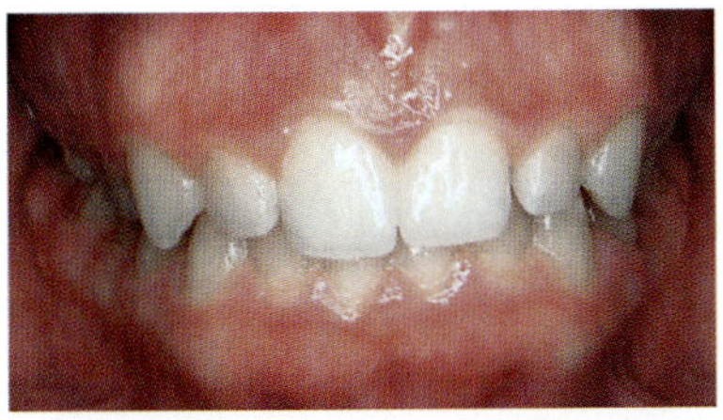
12

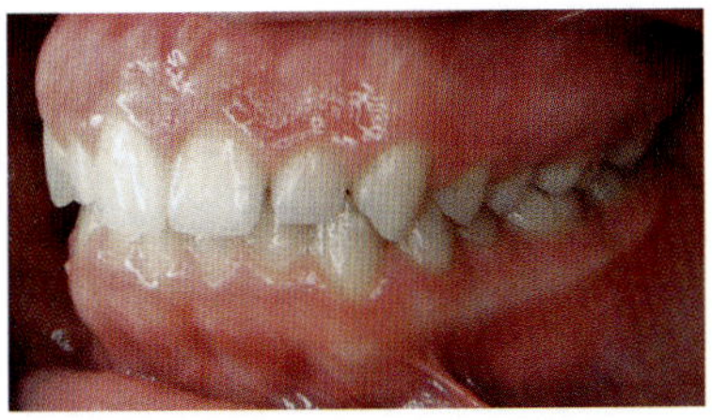
13

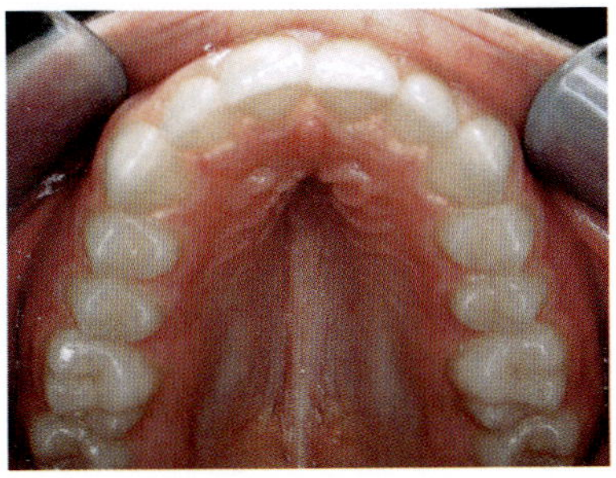
14

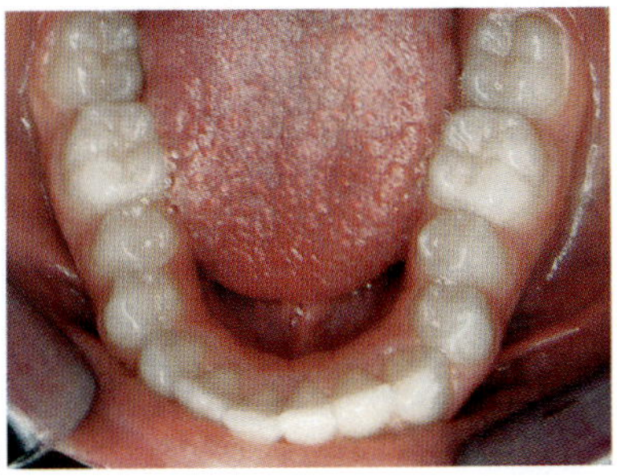
15

11–15 The situation before retention. The patient, who was satisfied with the results, was not disturbed by the minor rotation of tooth 33, which was therefore not corrected.

Individual Set-up for Vacuum-Formed Aligners

This well-known principle (developed by Sheridan) has been marketed as alignment with Essix aligners. A number of companies (e.g., Invisalign) offer a more comprehensive system in which all of the laboratory work is undertaken outside the dental practice. Here a plaster model-based set-up correcting the irregularity of the lower labial segment can be used for repeat treatment of postorthodontic relapse of the labial segment in particular. The last aligner can be used for long-term retention (**Fig. 9.16**).

CLINICAL PEARL

Mild lower incisor imbrication or crowding can be aligned using vacuum-formed retainers and individual set-ups. However, it is important to inform the patient that aligners need to be worn on a full-time basis, at least initially, in order to be successful.

SOX Retainers

SOX is an abbreviation for the 'social six' front teeth, and SOX retainers are designed to maintain the alignment of the upper and/or lower anterior teeth. The device was originally designed as a retainer, but it can also be used for tooth movement and correction of minor overlaps or irregularity of the anterior teeth. It was originally described by Philippe (**Fig. 9.17**).[13,17] The system is also known as a two-dimensional lingual bracket, and does not provide torque control. All of the archwires are round and will only provide derotation, intrusion, or extrusion, or changes in angulation. It is not possible to apply torque,

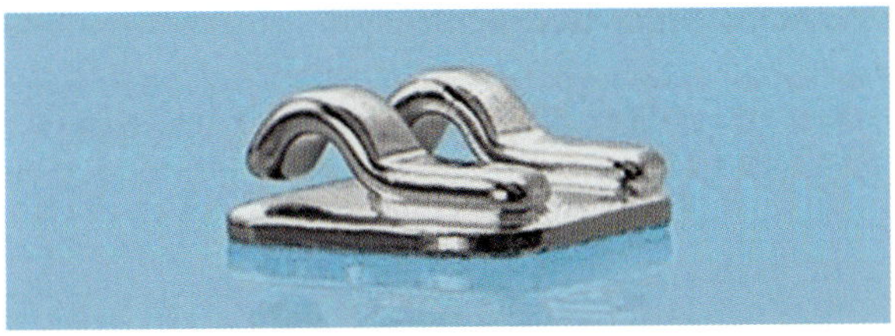

Fig. 9.17 The basic conformation of the bracket developed by Philippe. The ligation wings have a rounded inner surface and press the wire against the bracket base. The round slot is activated by pressing the wings against the bracket base.

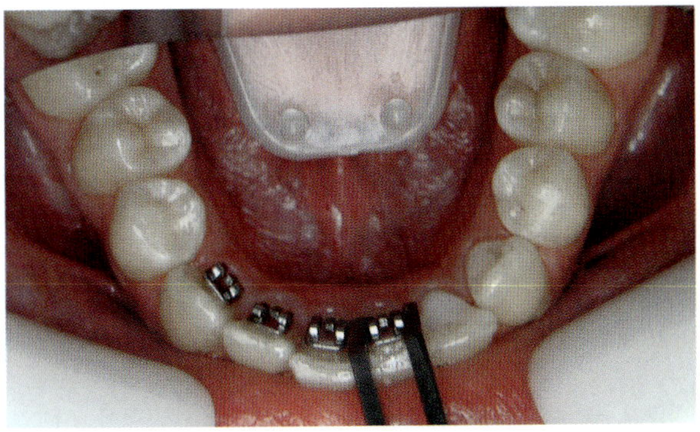

Fig. 9.18 The enamel surfaces are conditioned in the conventional way using phosphoric acid or a self-etching primer. Orthodontic light-cure composite is used to bond the brackets.

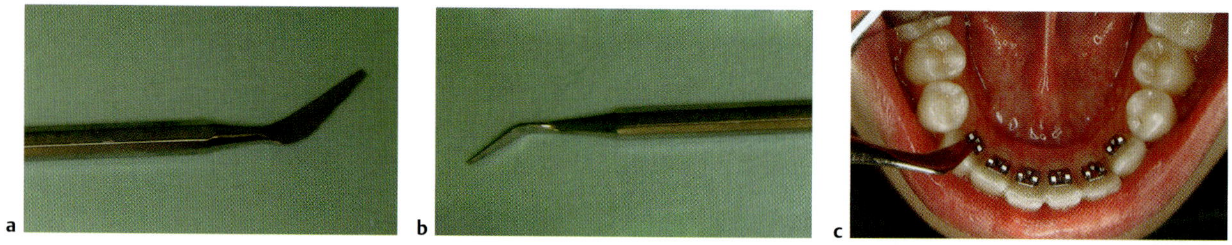

Fig. 9.19 a–c The bracket is self-ligating by means of two adjustable ligation wings that are open in the occlusal direction, allowing easy access for the wire. A special flat instrument is used to open the clip (**a, b**). The instrument is placed in the space between the bracket base and the retention clip and is used like a lever to open the bracket.

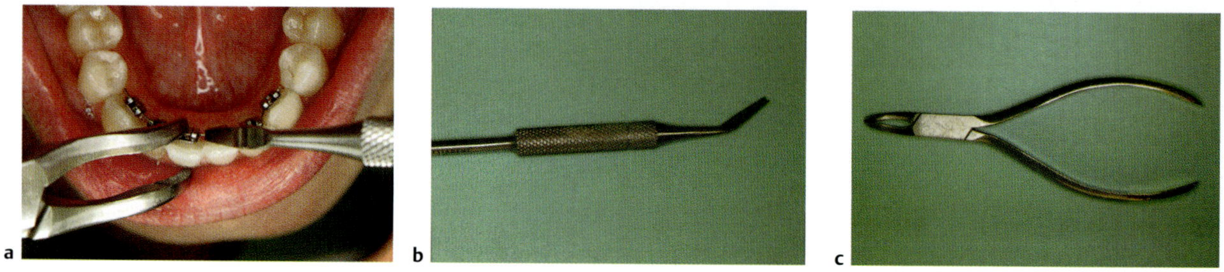

Fig. 9.20 a–c The lingual archwire (**a**) is held in place by a wire director (**b**) and locked into the bracket by pressing the ligation wings against the bracket base using small Weingart pliers (**c**). To protect the buccal tooth surface, one tip of the Weingart pliers can be covered with protective rubber tubing.

as there is no rectangular slot. In most cases, anterior alignment relapse is usually confined to small in–out discrepancies and rotations and this can be easily treated with this appliance. Due to its two-dimensionality, a universal bracket can be used on all teeth, which may lead to reduced inventory. The brackets are individualized by modifying their position on individual teeth. **Figs. 9.18–9.21** show clinical applications for bracket placement and ligation of an archwire.

The advantage of this concept is that it is possible to use the appliance as a retainer after successful alignment (see Case Study 9.5). To convert the appliance to a retention device, the last wire, usually 0.018 stainless steel, remains in the brackets and is then permanently locked into the individual brackets using a fluoride-containing, flowable composite.

The overall height of the bracket is only 1.4 mm, and patient comfort is improved in comparison with other lingual brackets, which are usually thicker and wider. The wearing comfort is similar to that of a fixed retainer, as the size is very similar.

It is widely known that even fixed retainers allow slight movement of contact points from their original position. With a SOX retainer, it is possible to reopen the retainer and adjust the archwire to correct very minor relapse or tooth movement; especially in adults, where long-term retention appears to be indicated. Many adult patients who have undergone orthodontic treatment experience postorthodontic changes in the alignment of the front teeth in particular. The range of retainers available today may offer these patients the reliable long-term retention they were hoping for after their original orthodontic treatment.

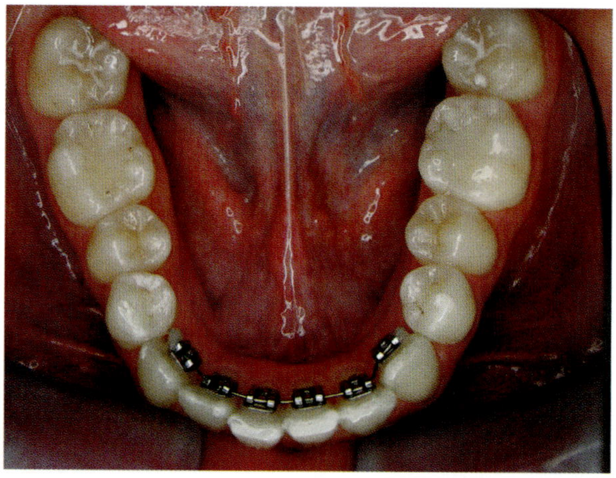

Fig. 9.21 Depending on the initial findings, either a regular buccal 0.010 or 0.012 superelastic NiTi wire can be used.

Case Study 9.5 (Fig. 9.22)

Patient: D.H., female, age 18.
Diagnostic records: models, panoramic radiograph, lateral cephalometric radiograph, intraoral/extraoral photographs.
Main findings: late anterior crowding.
Treatment aims: esthetic alignment of the maxillary and mandibular anterior teeth.
Appliances: two-dimensional lingual brackets, IPR.
Archwire sequence: buccal 0.010 SE, 0.012 SE and 0.016 SE preformed lingual archwires, custom-bent 0.016 SS lingual archwire.
Alternative treatment strategy: n/a.
Active treatment time: 6 months.
Retention: bonded retainer.

1 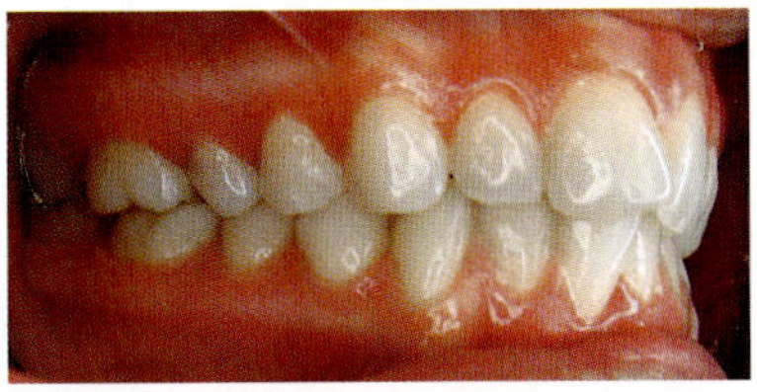
2 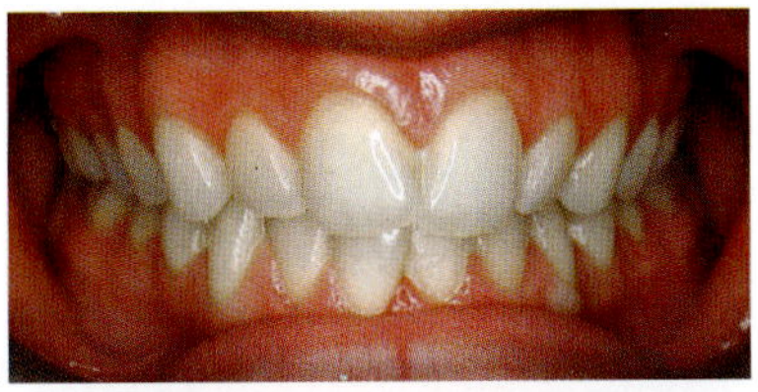
3 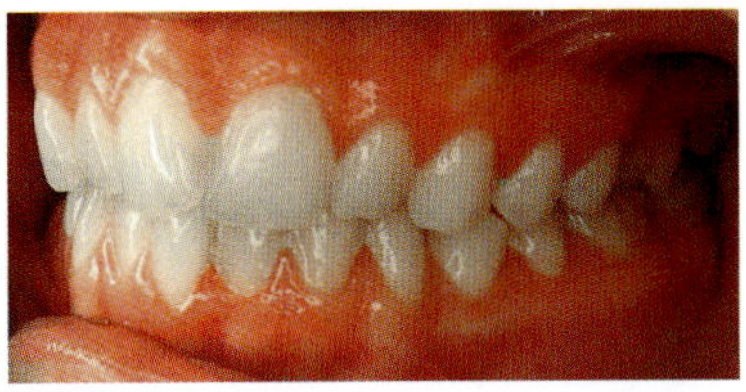
4 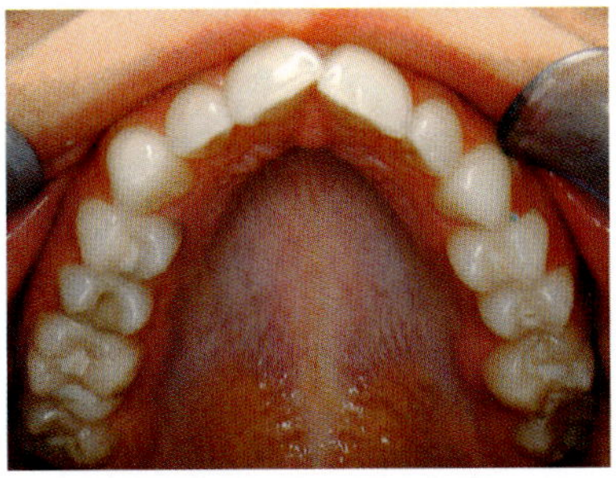
5 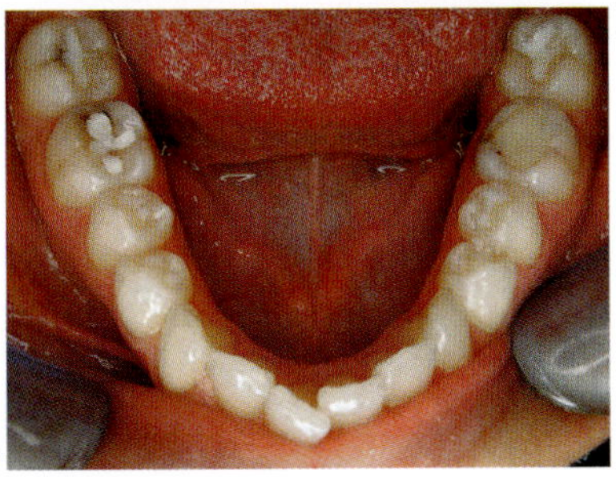

Fig. 9.22 1–20
1–5 Typical manifestation of late crowding and poor contact points on teeth 11 and 41.

6 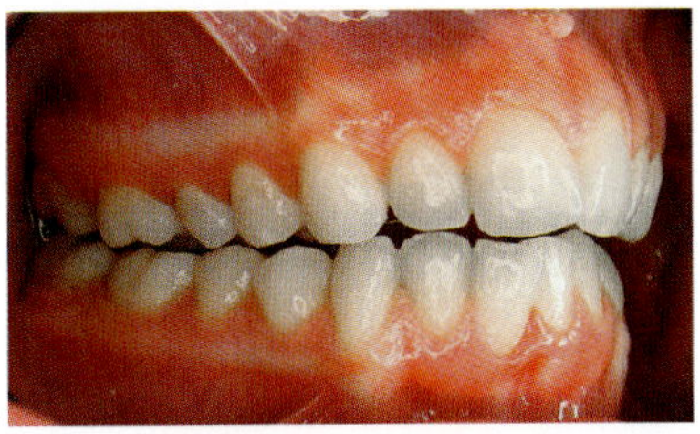
7 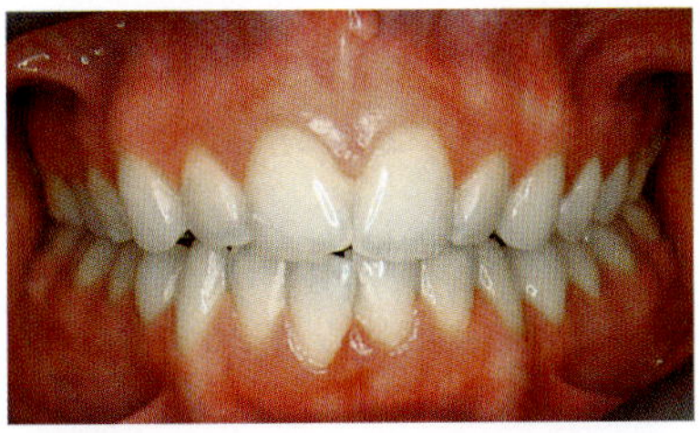
8 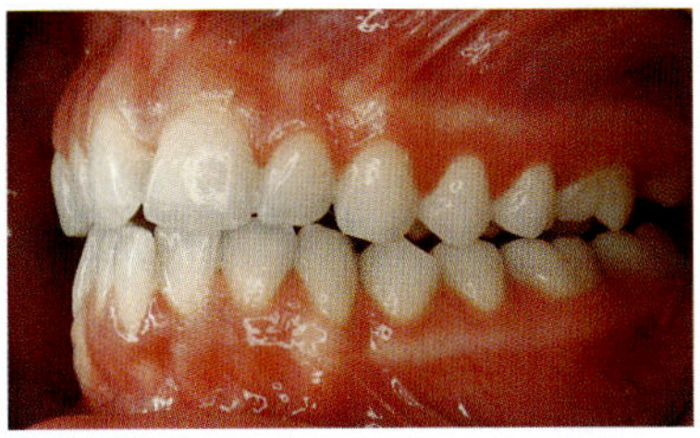
9 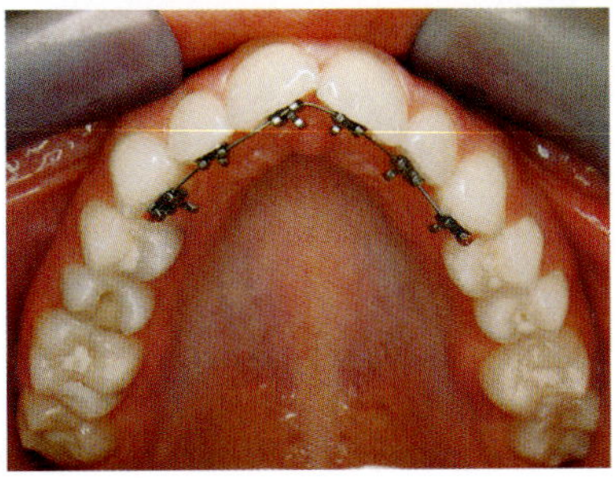
10 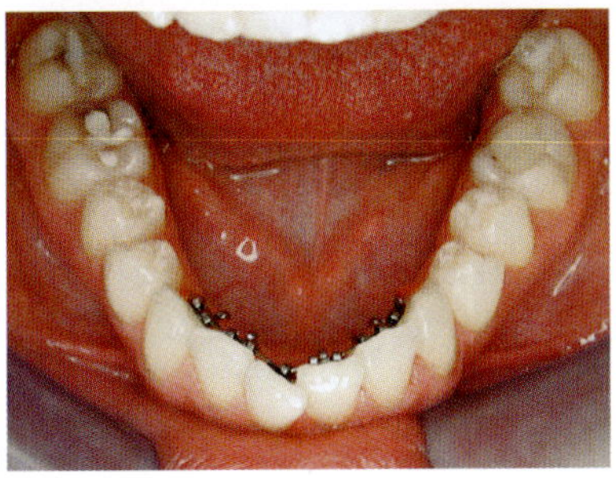

6–10 Two-dimensional lingual brackets in both arches bonded from canine to canine and 0.010 SE archwires in place. Due to the limited access on the lingual tooth surface, tooth 41 is bonded with a smaller, single-wing bracket.

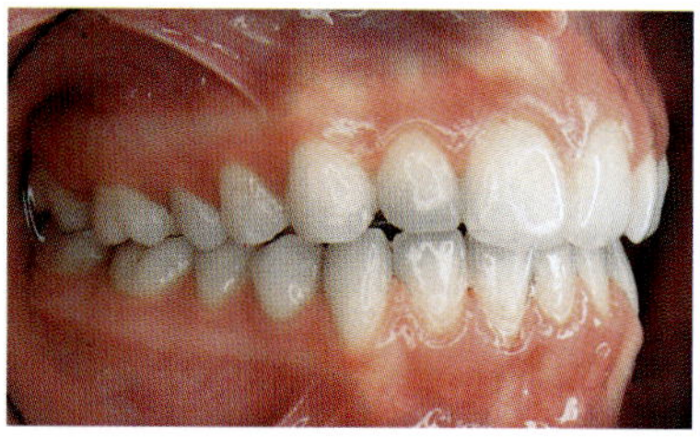
11

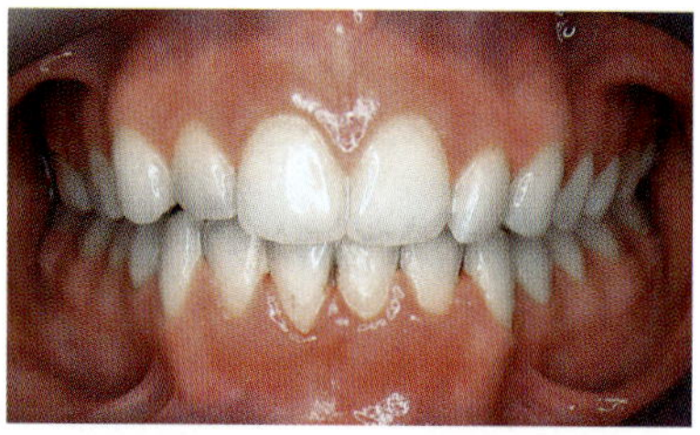
12

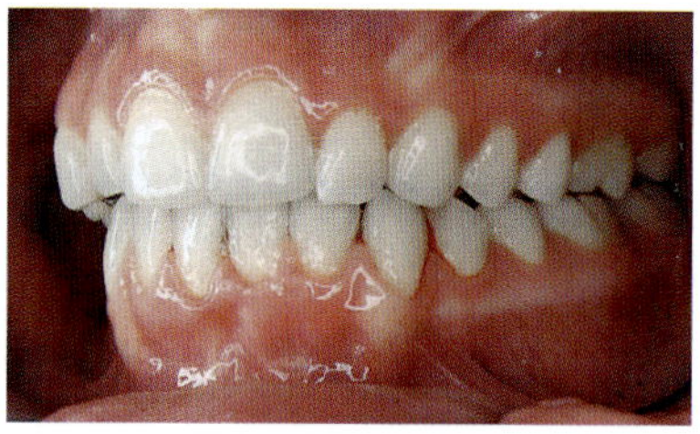
13

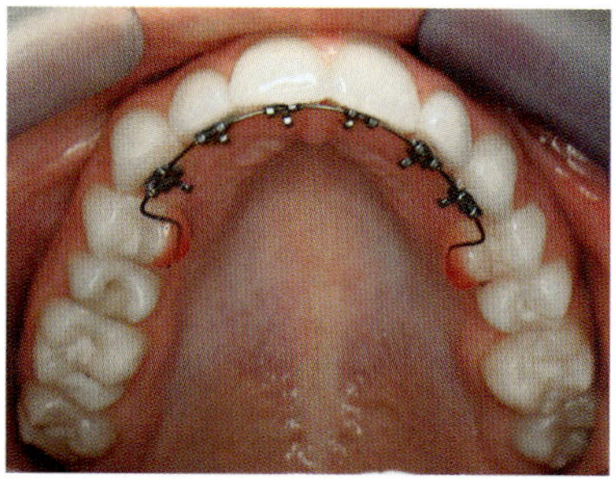
14

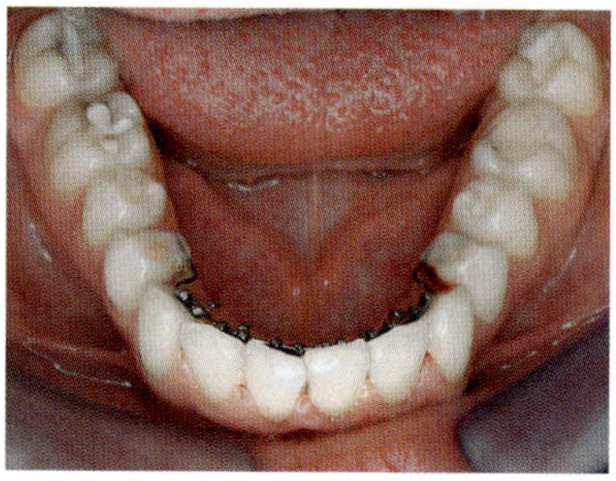
15

11–15 The situation after insertion of preformed 0.016 SS lingual archwires: the space for tooth alignment was created by IPR. In the meantime, tooth 41 was bonded with a regular two-dimensional lingual bracket. The wire was extended to the premolars to improve anterior arch shape.

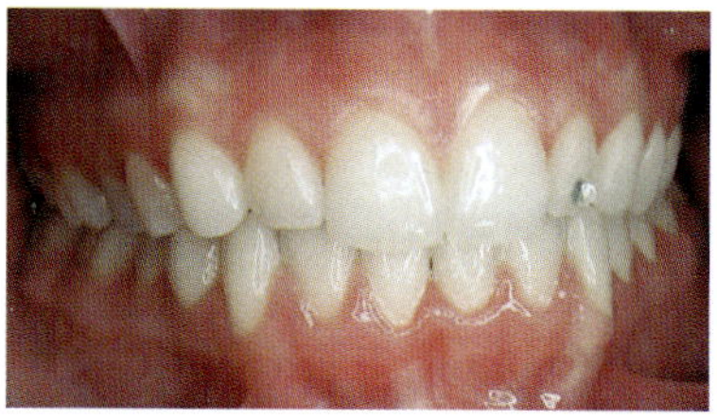
16

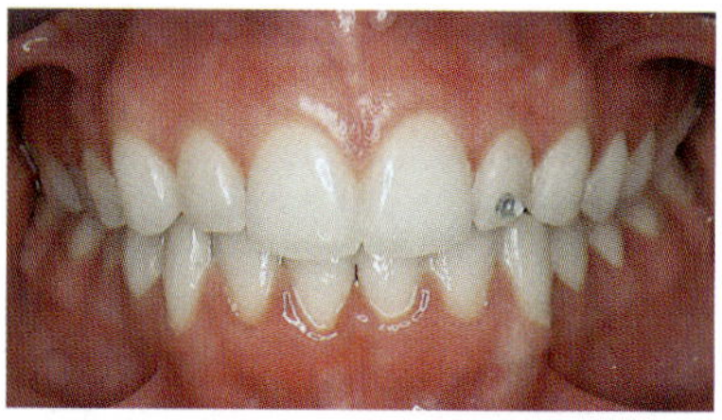
17

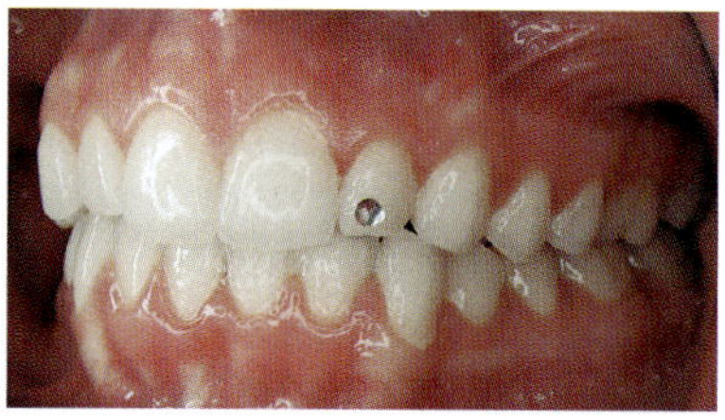
18

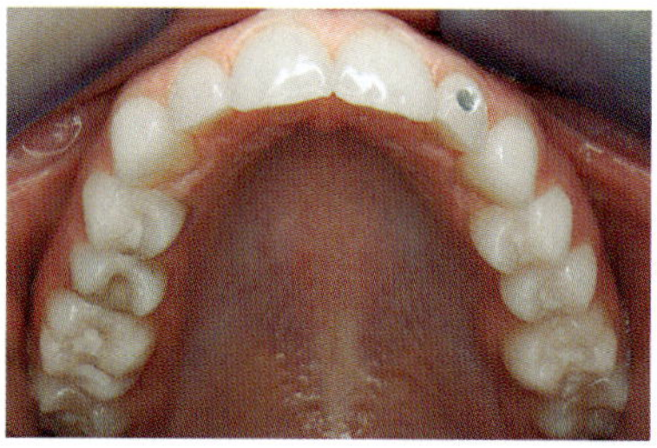
19

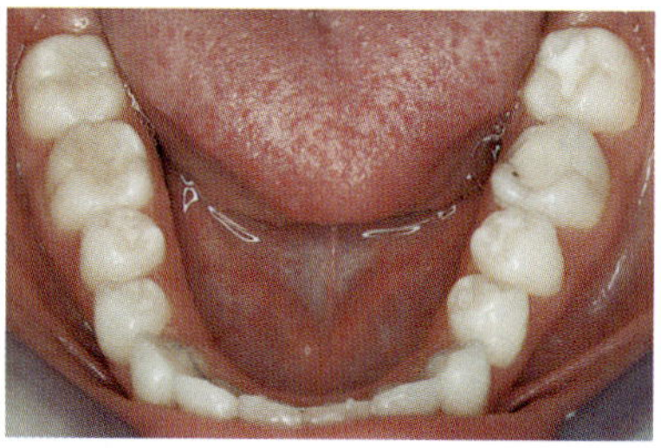
20

16–20 The final result in retention.

CLINICAL PEARL

- Lingual surfaces that are difficult to reach (due to crowding and/or rotation of teeth) can often be bonded with a reduced-width two-dimensional lingual bracket.
- It is recommended to initiate movement using 0.010 superelastic archwire, which we use for buccal alignment as well.
- It is often advisable to induce tooth movement by incorporating the first and second premolars in the fixed appliance. We tend to use a high-flow composite for adhesion of the wire, without the need for bracket placement on these teeth.

REFERENCES

1. Al Yami EA, Kuijpers-Jagtman AM, van't Hof MA. Stability of orthodontic treatment outcome: follow-up until 10 years post-retention. Am J Orthod Dentofacial Orthop 1999;115(3):300–304
2. Årtun J, Spadafora AT, Shapiro PA. A 3-year follow-up study of various types of orthodontic canine-to-canine retainers. Eur J Orthod 1997;19(5):501–509
3. Behrents RG, Harris EF, Vaden JL, Williams RA, Kemp DH. Relapse of orthodontic treatment results: growth as an etiologic factor. J Charles H Tweed Int Found 1989;17:65–80
4. Graber TM, Vanarsdall RL, Vig KWL. Orthodontics. 4th ed. Current principles and techniques. Chapter 27. Amsterdam: Elsevier; 2005
5. Graham JW. Temporary replacement of maxillary lateral incisors with miniscrews and bonded pontics. J Clin Orthod 2007;41(6): 321–325
6. Huck L, Kahl-Nieke B, Schwarze CW, et al. Postretention changes in canine position. Results of a long-term follow-up. J Orofac Orthop 2000;61(3):199–206
7. Kinzinger GS, Diedrich PR. Bite jumping with the Functional Mandibular Advancer. J Clin Orthod 2005;39(12):696–700, quiz 715
8. Kinzinger G, Diedrich P. Skeletal effects in class II treatment with the functional mandibular advancer (FMA)? J Orofac Orthop 2005;66(6):469–490
9. Lang G, Alfter G, Göz G, et al. Retention and stability – taking various treatment parameters into account. J Orofac Orthop 2002;63:26–41
10. Little RM, Riedel RA, Årtun J. An evaluation of changes in mandibular anterior alignment from 10 to 20 years postretention. Am J Orthod Dentofacial Orthop 1988;93(5):423–428
11. Little RM. Stability and relapse of dental arch alignment. In: Hösl E, Baldauf A, eds. Retention and long-term stability. 8th Int Conf for Orthodontists. Heidelberg: Hüthig; 1993:83–94
12. Ludwig B, Glasl B, Kappel F, et al. Vorstellung eines modellgegossenen Lingualretainers für die Frontzähne. Kieferorthopädie 2006;20:267–271
13. Macchia A, Tagliabue A, Levrini L, Trezzi G. Philippe self-ligating lingual brackets. J Clin Orthod 2002;36(1):42–45
14. Masella RS, Meister M. Current concepts in the biology of orthodontic tooth movement. Am J Orthod Dentofacial Orthop 2006; 129(4):458–468
15. McNamara JA, Brudon WL. Orthodontics and dentofacial orthopedics. Ann Arbor: Needham Press; 2004
16. Moser U, Moser L. Langzeitretention mit geklebten lingualen Glasfaserretainern. Kieferorthopädie 1996;10:85–94
17. Philippe J. L'orthodontie de l'adulte. Paris: Éditions SID; 1989
18. Proffit WR, Fields HW Jr, Sarver DM. Contemporary orthodontics. 4th ed. St. Louis: Mosby; 2007:Ch. 17.
19. Radlanski RJ, Zain ND. Stability of the bonded lingual wire retainer-a study of the initial bond strength. J Orofac Orthop 2004; 65(4):321–335
20. Reitan K. Principles of retention and avoidance of posttreatment relapse. Am J Orthod 1969;55(6):776–790
21. Schwarze J, Bourauel C, Drescher D. Frontzahnbeweglichkeit nach direkter Klebung von Lingualretainern. J Orofac Orthop 1995;56:25–33
22. Segner D, Heinrici B. Bonded retainers—clinical reliability. J Orofac Orthop 2000;61(5):352–358
23. Staufer K, Landmesser H. Effects of crowding in the lower anterior segment—a risk evaluation depending upon the degree of crowding. J Orofac Orthop 2004;65(1):13–25
24. Störmann I, Ehmer U. A prospective randomized study of different retainer types. J Orofac Orthop 2002;63(1):42–50
25. Watted N, Wieber M, Teuscher T, et al. Comparison of incisor mobility after insertion of canine-to-canine lingual retainers bonded to two or to six teeth. A clinical study. J Orofac Orthop 2001;62(5):387–396
26. Zachrisson BU. Long-term experience with direct-bonded retainers: update and clinical advice. J Clin Orthod 2007;41(12): 728–737, quiz 749
27. Zachrisson BU. Clinical experience with direct-bonded orthodontic retainers. Am J Orthod 1977;71(4):440–448
28. Zachrisson BU. Geklebter 3-3 Unterkieferlingualretainer der dritten Generation. Inf Orthod Kieferorthop 1995;27:369–379

Index

Page numbers in *italics* refer to illustrations or tables

M

N

O

P

Q

R

S